International Handbooks of Quality-of-Life

Aims and Scope

The International Handbooks of Quality-of-Life Research offer extensive bibliographic resources. They present literature reviews of the many sub-disciplines and areas of study within the growing field of quality of life research. Handbooks in the series focus on capturing and reviewing the quality of life research literature in specific life domains, on specific populations, or in relation to specific disciplines or sectors of industry. In addition, the Handbooks cover measures of quality of life and well-being, providing annotated bibliographies of well-established measures, methods, and scales.

More information about this series at http://www.springer.com/series/8365

Joar Vittersø
Editor

Handbook of Eudaimonic Well-Being

Springer

Editor
Joar Vittersø
UiT The Arctic University of Norway
Tromsø, Norway

ISSN 2468-7227 ISSN 2468-7235 (electronic)
International Handbooks of Quality-of-Life
ISBN 978-3-319-42443-9 ISBN 978-3-319-42445-3 (eBook)
DOI 10.1007/978-3-319-42445-3

Library of Congress Control Number: 2016951487

Printed on acid-free paper

This Springer imprint is published by Springer Nature
The registered company is Springer International Publishing AG Switzerland

I dedicate this volume to my wife, Astrid Musland, for her enduring love and support. Thank you.

Acknowledgments

The idea of this handbook originated in my office, some years ago, when Professor Joe Sirgy was visiting Tromsø, in conjunction with our Northern Insights work, funded by the Research Council of Norway. We had not seen each other for quite a while and had a lot to catch up on. During our conversation, the word eudaimonia kept popping up, and at some point, Joe proposed that the time might have come for a handbook on eudaimonic well-being. I am very grateful to Joe for this idea and for the everlasting enthusiasm he dedicates to the science of well-being. Without it, this book would not have been realized (at least not in its current form).

I am thankful to Esther Otten and Hendrikje Tuerlings at Springer for their helpful and patient guidance on the project—from beginning to end. I am also grateful to UiT The Arctic University of Norway for being such a wonderful place to work in.

My deepest gratitude goes to the authors for writing and reviewing chapters. Without your efforts, enthusiasm, talents, and insights, this book would not have existed.

Contents

Contributors

Jack J. Bauer University of Dayton, Dayton, OH, USA

Lorraine L. Besser Middlebury College, Middlebury, VT, USA

Andrew G. Christy Texas A&M University, College Station, TX, USA

Sara E. Dahill-Brown Department of Politics and International Affairs, Wake Forest University, Winston-Salem, NC, USA

Alexander F. Danvers Department of Psychology, Arizona State University, Temple, AZ, USA

Hartley Dean Department of Social Policy, London School of Economics, London, UK

Paul Dolan London School of Economics, London, UK

Olivia Efthimiou Murdoch University, Perth, Western Australia, Australia

Julie J. Exline Case Western Reserve University, Cleveland, OH, USA

Leah J. Ferguson College of Kinesiology, University of Saskatchewan, Saskatoon, SK, Canada

Blaine J. Fowers Department of Educational and Psychological Studies, University of Miami, Coral Gables, FL, USA

Zeno E. Franco Department of Family and Community Medicine, Clinical and Translational Science Institute, Medical College of Wisconsin, Milwaukee, WI, USA

Barbara L. Fredrickson Department of Psychology, University of North Carolina at Chapel Hill, Chapel Hill, NC, USA

Katie E. Gunnell The Healthy Active Living and Obesity Research Group, The Children's Hospital of Eastern Ontario, Research Institute, Ottawa, ON, Canada

Claudia Harzer Section on Psychological Assessment, Department of Psychology, University of Kassel, Kassel, Germany

Daniel M. Haybron Saint Louis University, St. Louis, MO, USA

Joshua A. Hicks Texas A&M University, College Station, TX, USA

Johannes Hirata Hochschule Osnabrück, University of Applied Sciences, Osnabrück, Germany

Veronika Huta University of Ottawa, Ottawa, Canada

Eranda Jayawickreme Department of Psychology, Wake Forest University, Winston-Salem, NC, USA

Jay Kimiecik Department of Kinesiology and Health, Miami University, Oxford, OH, USA

Laura A. King University of Missouri, Columbia, MO, USA

Hans Henrik Knoop Department of Education, University of Aarhus, Aarhus N, Denmark

Laura Kudrna London School of Economics, London, UK

Alan Law Bremen International Graduate School of Social Sciences, Bremen, Germany

Brian R. Little University of Cambridge, Cambridge, UK

Frank Martela University of Helsinki, Helsinki, Finland

Francis Mckay University of Chicago, Chicago, IL, USA

Ragnhild Bang Nes Department of Psychology, University of Oslo, Oslo, Norway

Norwegian Institute of Public Health, Oslo, Norway

Makenzie J. O'Neil Department of Psychology, Arizona State University, Tempe, AZ, USA

Anthony D. Ong Department of Human Development, Cornell University, Ithaca, NY, USA

Kenneth I. Pargament Bowling Green State University, Bowling Green, OH, USA

Alicia Patterson Department of Philosophy, Cornell University, Ithaca, NY, USA

Carmel Proctor PPRC, St. Peter Port, Guernsey, UK

Espen Røysamb Department of Psychology, University of Oslo, Oslo, Norway

Norwegian Institute of Public Health, Oslo, Norway

Richard M. Ryan Institute for Positive Psychology and Education, Australian Catholic University, Sydney, NSW, Australia

Carol D. Ryff Institute on Aging/Department of Psychology, University of Wisconsin-Madison, Madison, WI, USA

Rebecca J. Schlegel Texas A&M University, College Station, TX, USA

Barry Schwartz Psychology, Swarthmore College, Swarthmore, PA, USA

Kennon M. Sheldon University of Missouri, Columbia, MO, USA

International Laboratory of Positive Psychology of Personality and Motivation, National Research University Higher School of Economics, Moscow, Russia

Michelle N. Shiota Department of Psychology, Arizona State University, Tempe, AZ, USA

M. Joseph Sirgy Pamplin College of Business, Virginia Polytechnic Institute & State University, Blacksburg, VA, USA

Ursula M. Staudinger Columbia Aging Center, Columbia University, New York, NY, USA

Robert A. Stebbins University of Calgary, Calgary, Canada

Michael F. Steger Colorado State University, Fort Collins, CO, USA

North-West University, Vanderbijlpark, South Africa

Neil Thin University of Edinburgh, Edinburgh, Scotland

Valerie Tiberius University of Minnesota, Minneapolis, MN, USA

Roger Tweed Kwantlen Polytechnic University, Surrey, BC, Canada

Muzaffer Uysal Pamplin College of Business, Virginia Polytechnic Institute & State University, Blacksburg, VA, USA

Robert J. Vallerand Laboratoire de Recherche sur le Comportement Social, Département de Psychologie, Université du Québec à Montréal, Montreal, QC, USA

Australian Catholic University, Sydney, NSW, Australia

Dianne A. Vella-Brodrick Melbourne Graduate School of Education, Centre for Positive Psychology, University of Melbourne, Melbourne, Victoria, Australia

Joar Vittersø UiT The Arctic University of Norway, Tromsø, Norway

Sarah J. Ward University of Missouri, Columbia, MO, USA

Serena Wong Bowling Green State University, Bowling Green, OH, USA

Amy Wrzesniewski Yale School of Management, New Haven, CT, USA

Philip G. Zimbardo Stanford University, Stanford, CA, USA

The Most Important Idea in the World: An Introduction

1

Joar Vittersø

It has been said that Darwin's theory of evolution is "the best idea in the world" (Dennett, 1995). Such praise has hardly been offered to the concept of eudaimonic well-being, but the idea of eudaimonia has another advantage: it matters more to us than anything else. Eudaimonia asks not how life evolved, but at what our lives should be aimed. The idea boldly proposes that, given the right circumstances, humans can deliberately develop into beings that both act good and feel well. If this notion is true, what can possibly be more important?

We may speculate that Darwin had a hunch about these insights. At least, it turns out, he reminded himself to "Begin the discussion by saying what happiness is." It is not entirely clear what Darwin meant by this sentence, but he penned this plan to say something about happiness in one of his notebooks (McMahon, 2006, p. 410). Other thinkers and scientists have articulated the eudaimonic idea more explicitly than Darwin, partly by developing arguments about why a proper understanding of morality and the meaning of life is not only the most important, but also the most difficult of all intellectual problems (Flanagan, 2007). The Handbook of Eudaimonic Well-Being offers a collection of comprehensive and updated reviews on these imperative matters and its 38 chapters provide an overview of what we currently know—and don't yet know—about individual and societal goodness.

1.1 Everyone Wants to Be Happy

Happiness is the only thing in life worth having. That is what Voltaire told us (Tatarkiewicz, 1976, p. 327), echoing Aristotle and summarizing the essence of the eudaimonist axiom.[1] Socrates went even further. He said that merely asking the question is a silly thing to do "since it would be absurd to deny it" (Annas, 2002, p. 5). Any reasonable person must, therefore, ask himself or herself how to live. The answer to this question is "the person's conception of eudaimonia" (Nussbaum, 2001, pp. 31–32).

These perspectives bring forward very broad notions of a life that is going well. However, when it comes to concreteness such philosophical eudaimonism offers nothing more than "a thin specification" of what happiness or "the final end" is (Annas, 1993). Aristotle realized that this basic assumption of eudaimonia by itself was not very useful, as people disagree widely about what happiness is. For instance, in

J. Vittersø (✉)
UiT The Arctic University of Norway,
Tromsø, Norway
e-mail: Joar.vitterso@uit.no

[1] The eudaimonist axiom is defined by Jost (2002, p. xiv) as the doctrine that "Happiness is desired by all human beings as the ultimate end (telos) of all their rational acts."

J. Vittersø (ed.), *Handbook of Eudaimonic Well-Being*, International Handbooks of Quality-of-Life,
DOI 10.1007/978-3-319-42445-3_1

Table 1.1 Twelve conceptions of happiness in the ancient era

Source	Ideas about the good life
Homer's heroes	Wealth, physical health and attractiveness, strength of character, courage, justice, generosity, and piety
Hesiod	Flourishing and prosperous communities populated by honest people, living in peace, and enjoying the fruits of their labor, with an absence of worries and disease
Pythagoras	The unobservable harmony within an unobservable entity, which is the immortal soul
Heraclitus	Maximization of desire satisfaction is neither necessary nor sufficient for the good life
Empedocles	A transmigrating soul-like daimon within each individual that ultimately experiences a current good or bad life and accumulated credits
Protagoras	Features depend on individual preferences
Antiphon	Careful and accurate observations of nature, thinking "correctly" about what causes "distress" and "joy," and generally following nature's guides to a long and pleasant life
Democritus	Unobservable orderly and harmonious atomic activity
Plato	External goods like wealth and goods of the body like health are important, but goods of the mind like moral virtue are even more important
Iamblichus	Trust and law-abidingness for good human relations
Aristotle	Living well and doing well. It is achieved insofar as one deliberately engages in the unimpeded excellent exercise of one's capacities for the sake of doing what is fine, excellent, or noble, provided that the deliberation and activities are undertaken from a virtuous character and accompanied by an appropriate amount of external goods and pleasure
Epicurus	Pleasure, as consisting of a healthy body, peace of mind, and moral virtue

Note: Adapted from Michalos and Robinson (2012)

a review of the different conceptions of happiness in ancient times, Michalos and Robinson (2012) identified a dozen distinct conceptions of happiness in the period from the eighth to the third century BCE. A summary of this review is given in Table 1.1.

There is perhaps a vague communality across these ideas. Hudson was, for instance, able to identify three primary meanings of eudaimonia in the ancient texts written between the fifth and fourth centuries BCE: prosperity, pleasure, and moral attainment (Hudson, 1996, p. 62). To me, the most striking feature in Table 1.1 is rather the large variety of meanings even the ancients applied to the word happiness. Today the number of definitions and conceptualizations is much higher and quite overwhelming. The many meanings of "happiness" is so large that it is actually hard to understand what Tolstoy had in mind when he wrote the famous opening sentence in *Anna Karenina*, suggesting that "All happy families resemble one another" (Tolstoy, 1993, p. 1). No person knowledgeable about the scientific literature on happiness could have written these words. Hence, rather than finding a "Tolstoyian alikeness" as I battled my way through the literature on eudaimonia, I identified with George Eliot's character Edward Casaubon. In her classic novel Middlemarch, Eliot (1985) portrays the Reverend Casaubon as a pedantic clergyman who is obsessed with finding a common structure among the major religions in the world. His scholarly project is to write the definitive book in the tradition of syncretism, i.e., the idea that different and often contradictory beliefs from mythologies and religions can be combined into a consistent whole. Casaubon's book was never finished.

1.2 Jingles and Jangles

In 1890 the economist William Jevons complained that "Perhaps the most common cause of bad reasoning is the use of ambiguous terms, which mean one thing in one place and another thing elsewhere. A word with two distinct meanings is really two words" (Jevons, 1890, p. 114; cited in Cabanac, 2009, p. 234). The problem certainly applies to the study of happiness. As recognized by the authors of the handbook, a commonly accepted conceptual language remains to be established for eudaimonia. To some extent, this state of affairs may be a good thing, according to Tiberius (Chap. 38, this volume), who suggests that concluding prematurely about the nature and causes of human happiness is not what we want. We should aim, rather, toward a better articulation of the different positions must be an ideal toward which happiness research should aim. The goal for the Handbook of Eudaimonic Well-Being is therefore to nourish this striving toward a clearer conceptualization and better understanding of what good lives and good societies look like. The plan is to present chapters that articulate the varieties of human goodness, while carefully considering the many complexities that confront such an endeavor. This introduction starts with a warning against two common fallacies in the literature, followed by examples of how such misconceptions create unnecessary confusion in the study of eudaimonia.

Røysamb and Nes (Chap. 16, this volume) comment on the jingle and jangle fallacies, and how they hamper research on well-being. According to Thorndike (1913), the jingle fallacy was originally introduced by a "Professor Aikins," who described it as the mistake of interpreting different things to be the same because they have similar names, or as the "unthinking acceptance of verbal equality as a proof of real equality" (Thorndike, 1913, pp. 10–11). The jangle fallacy was introduced by Kelley somewhat later, and defined to be "the use of two separate words or expressions covering in fact the same basic situation, but sounding different, as though they were in truth different" (Kelley, 1927, p. 64). The literature on well-being is teeming with jingle/jangle fallacies and the most dramatic one comes from ignoring the distinction between happiness as "a state of mind" and happiness as "a complete life that goes well for the person leading it".

1.2.1 The Two Cultures About Happiness

Happiness researchers comprise a large community, and within it, more or less isolated tribes have arisen. Tribes everywhere foster their own language and classifications in order to organize a view of their world. As noted by the French anthropologist Levi-Strauss (1966), conceptual schemes often evolve as binary oppositions, and the communities of happiness researchers are no exception. Some of them speak of objective versus subjective qualities of life (Glatzer, 2015), others about cognitive versus affective well-being (Schimmack, 2008), including variants such as experiential well-being versus evaluative well-being (Stone & Mackie, 2013), or being happy IN your live versus being happy WITH your life (Kahneman & Riis, 2005). But the most vivid duality in the literature on happiness is the one between happiness as something "mental" versus happiness as something commonly agreed upon as "complete" (e.g., Haybron, 2011; Tiberius, 2013).

The philosopher Alasdair MacIntyre has expressed his view on this difference as "a fundamental contrast between man-as-he-happens-to-be and man-as he-could-be-if-he-realized-his-essential-nature" (MacIntyre, 1981, p. 52). Haybron argues (using different terms for these two kinds of happiness) that "psychological and prudential happiness[2] are not different theories, or conceptions, of happiness; they are different concepts altogether, and denote different things" (Haybron, 2000, p. 211).

As illustrated in the above quotes, the task of finding appropriate and commonly agreed upon names turns out in itself to be a challenging mission. For instance, the "state of mind" kind of happiness has been referred to as "psychological

[2]Prudential happiness is a term that seems to have been introduced by Griffin: "I am using 'prudence' here in the philosopher's especially broad sense, in which it has to do not just with a due concern for one's future, but with everything that bears on one's self-interest" (Griffin, 1986, p. 4).

happiness" (Haybron, 2011), "psychological well-being" (Bradburn, 1969; Vallerand, Chap. 13, this volume), "subjective well-being" (Diener, 1984), and "hedonic well-being" (Kahneman, Diener, & Schwarz, 1999), to mention only some of the most commonly applied terms. The words used to describe "complete happiness" vary just as much. Badhwar (2014) calls it "the highest prudential good," Foot (2001) prefers "deep happiness," Broadie (2007) speaks of "complete happiness," Nussbaum (2001) about a "complete human life," Tiberius (2013) makes use of the word "well-being," and Haybron draws on both "prudential happiness" and "well-being." In this chaotic situation it is tempting to adopt the strategy brought forward by Evans and Over (1996) for the study of thinking and decision making: The good old jangle fallacy had bewitched this domain with a conglomerate of words used for the same phenomenon, and to sort things out Evans and Over suggested simply employing the term "Type I rationality." A different plurality of words was used to refer to another phenomenon and Evans and Over suggested conversion to the term "Type II rationality." This strategy was later implemented with great success by Kahneman (2011), who relabeled Type I and Type II rationality into System 1 and System 2 thinking, respectively.

Comparably, it might be easier to communicate about the two major forms of happiness if they simply were referred to as Happiness 1 and Happiness 2. Sticking to the analogy from cognitive science, in which System 1 thinking is the quickest and least sophisticated form of reasoning, Happiness 1 should be the term used for the "subjective" or "state of mind" kind of happiness. On the other hand, Happiness 2 should refer to a kind of happiness that is more reflective or complex in the sense of being "complete," "deep," "prudential," or describing a life that in all respects "goes well for the person leading it."

A life that is good in the Happiness 2 sense has to be "complete" in some way or another, and a person's own judgments about how well his or her life is going will <u>never be a sufficient criterion</u> for this kind of goodness. If a person thinks she is happy, she is happy according to Happiness 1, but not necessarily according to Happiness 2. To illustrate the distinction between the first-person perspective of Happiness 1 and the third-person perspective of Happiness 2, Haybron uses the example of a man named George: "Imagine that George is living a cheerful life with his family and friends. George considers himself to be satisfied. However, George's family and friends can't really stand him, they are only pretending that they like him because of his money. If George was to discover these facts, he would have been devastated. But George never finds out. He remains ignorant his entire life" (Haybron, 2013, p. 304).

Michalos and Robinson (2012) have classified this distinction between objective[3] and subjective elements of a good life into four possible categories, or rather places, in which people can be happy.

1. Real paradise (people living in good conditions who evaluate their lives as good)
2. Real hell (people living in bad conditions who evaluate their lives as bad)
3. Fool's paradise (people living in bad conditions but evaluate their lives as good)
4. Fool's hell (people living in good conditions but evaluate their lives as bad)

From the perspective of Happiness 1 there is of course no fool's paradise or fool's hell, since a person's evaluation of his or her life is all there is to a happy life. Nevertheless, both Happiness 1 and Happiness 2 claim to conceptualize the goodness of a life as a whole. For instance, most Happiness 1 researchers seem to act as if the idea behind a complete life really can be measured by the use of questionnaires. Ever since Gurin, Veroff, and Feld (1960) started to investigate self-reported well-being in representative samples, the phrase "taking all things together" has been commonly used as an introduction for items about avowed happiness. And many well-being researchers reason that since they ask people to

[3]There are complexities related to the distinction between objective and subjective that I will not discuss here, but an interested reader will find a recent treatment in Badhwar (2014).

respond considering "all things," the data collected must consequently inform us about "all things." Good illustrations of this assumption are found in Stiglitz, Sen, and Fitoussi (2009), claiming that the "all things together items" provide information about everything important in people's lives, and in Oishi (2012) who, in his otherwise excellent book, suggests that survey questions about well-being capture virtues just as well as they capture pleasant experiences. Finally, Diener and Tov (2012, p. 139) argue that "subjective well-being is a concept that includes all the various ways that a person evaluates his or her life in a positive manner."

Julia Annas (1993, 2011) disagrees with the assumption that self-reports truly taps into the idea of a "complete life", and has taken great efforts to clarify just how different the concepts of Happiness 1 and Happiness 2 really are. If I should embark on the impossible task of reducing her extensive writings to a slogan, it might be that Happiness 2 is the overall end a person aims at by living well, something that applies to the person's life *as a whole* and not merely to what he or she thinks or feels about it.

The "as a whole" part is important to Annas. According to Michalos and Robinson (2012), it occurs about 90 times in her 455 page book on the Morality of Happiness (Annas, 1993). Another neo-Aristotelian, Martha Nussbaum, speaks of Happiness 2 as: "a kind of living that is active, inclusive of all that has intrinsic value, and complete, meaning lacking in nothing that would make it richer or better" (Nussbaum, 2008, p. S90). As articulated in another of her texts, the meaning of "the whole" when used about a good life can be explained as follows: "if one can show someone that [a person] has omitted something without which she would not think her life complete, then that is a sufficient argument for the addition of the item in question" (Nussbaum, 2001, p. 32).

It is important to note that subjective experiences are included in the notion of "the whole." A good life is simply not complete without positive feelings. Even if the good life cannot be just pleasure, Annas (2011) writes, pleasure must be woven into it. According to Annas, there is no separation between well-being as felt and well-being as motivation or behavior. Aristotelian pleasure is something that comes along with, or supervenes upon, the activity. Pleasures completes virtuous activity like "the bloom on the cheek of a healthy young person" (Nussbaum, 2008, p. S88). Hudson (1996) explains that "there is not a single version of classical eudaimonism that does not depict the happy person possessing some manner of desirable mental state" (p. 63).

The "completeness" of Happiness 1, on the other hand, is constrained by its first person perspective. It is therefore operating on a different scale than the completeness of Happiness 2, and if these differences are ignored, severe jingle fallacies easily emerge. For example, when Ryan and Martela (Chap. 7, this volume) argue that for Aristotle, happiness was not the primary aim of living, they must be referring to Happiness 1. Another reminder about the two cultures of happiness is provided by Sirgy and Uysal (Chap. 32, this volume). Their chapter categorizes prudential happiness as a Happiness 1 concept, whereas philosophers would typically locate it under the Happiness 2 umbrella (e.g., Griffin, 1986; Haybron, 2011; Qizilbash, 1997). Law and Staudinger (Chap. 9, this volume) enter the landscape of happiness duality with a discussion about morality. The authors point out that several psychological theories of eudaimonia seem to ignore the issue of moral goodness, which is a limitation that Law and Staudinger attempt to correct by including a sense of moral-practical in their own conceptualization of eudaimonia. This is a very delicate issue at the core of the Happiness 1 versus Happiness 2 debate. Philosophers such as Annas (e.g., 1993) maintain that eudaimonia under Happiness 2 does not allow for a separation between the moral good (i.e., acting without violating other people's moral rights) and the prudential good (i.e., concerning only the goodness of the person whose life it is). Within the domain of Happiness 1, such a merging of morality and well-being is not easily achieved.

Ryff's classic 1989 article also illustrates the different meanings of Happiness 1 and Happiness 2. The title of her article asks if "Happiness is everything," which, as we have heard from Socrates, is a silly question to ask. But as a critique of mainstream approaches to Happiness 1 research, Ryff's reflection is timely. It has helped give birth to a new branch of happiness studies. As one would expect with the rise of a new tribe, a set of novel binary terms appeared in their vocabulary as well, such as psychological eudaimonia versus philosophical eudaimonia (Tiberius, 2013), psychological eudaimonics versus philosophical eudaimonism (Haybron, Chap. 2, this volume), hedonic enjoyment versus personal expressiveness (Waterman, 1993), and hedonic well-being versus eudaimonic well-being (Ryan & Deci, 2001).

The complexities of Happiness 1 and Happiness 2 are not easily articulated, but a daring attempt to portray a simplified depiction of some of their characteristics is offered in Fig. 1.1. In the taxonomy, Happiness 1 is presented as comprising two sub-components, which roughly correspond to the distinction between bipolar concepts such as affective well-being and cognitive well-being (Schimmack, 2008), emotional well-being and life evaluations (Kahneman & Deaton, 2010), experiential well-being and evaluative well-being (Stone & Mackie, 2013), and between psychological happiness and prudential happiness (Sirgy & Uysal, Chap. 32, this volume), to name a few. Happiness 2 is considered one-dimensional in this taxonomy.

1.3 Conceptualizing Eudaimonia

The meaning of the term eudaimonia is woven into a complex fabric of etymological, historical, cultural, philosophical, and psychological conceptualizations. Hence, trying to define it once and for all is still a premature endeavor, although some clues exist as to how the term may be applied.

1.3.1 The Etymology

Contrary to popular belief, Aristotle didn't originate the concept of eudaimonia (εὐδαιμονία). It was included in the Greek vocabulary hundreds of years before he was born (Haybron, Chap. 2, this volume; McMahon, 2006). Actually, Aristotle never seemed particularly interested in the etymology of eudaimonia and the term had little influence on his thinking (Kraut, 2010). The reason is, Kraut suggests, that Aristotle regarded "eudaimon" as a mere substitute for the more important expression of eu zên ("living well").

Beyond debating Aristotle's use of the term, opinions diverge when it comes to the exact etymological meaning of eudaimonia. The Encyclopedia Britannica declares that the term literally means "the state of having a good indwelling spirit, a good genius." Kraut (2010) points out that the term is composed of two parts: 'eu' meaning well and 'daimon' meaning divinity or spirit. Other scholars, such as Dean (Chap. 34, this volume) translate 'eu' into good or wellness, but maintains that 'daimon' originally referred to what might be regarded as a person's soul or essence, or to what Kant would later describe as the 'noumenal self.' Accordingly, the translation of 'daimon' into demon, alluding to supernatural spirits, came later. Waterman (personal communication, October 2015) asserts the syllable 'ia' at the end of a Greek word refers to a feeling, like in

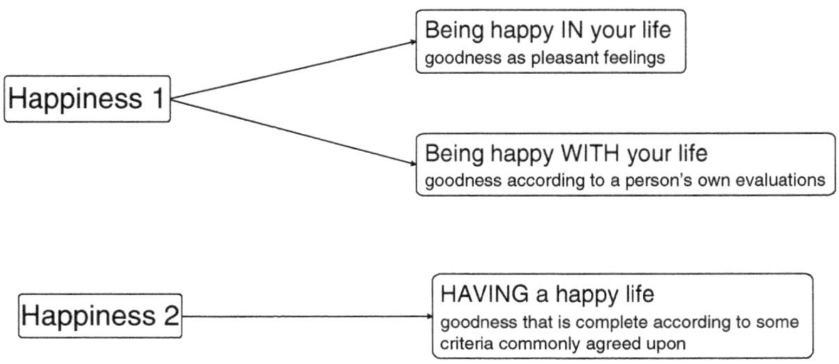

Fig. 1.1 A schematic difference between happiness 1 and happiness 2

euphoria, melancholia, and anhedonia. Expressed as eudaimonia then, an experiential element in the term is indicated. Hence, to Waterman eudaimonia translates into a subjective interpretation "centering on the feelings present when acting in a manner consistent with the daimon." The position that eudaimonia is a subjective experience that is lived and felt is also defended in the chapter by Kimiecik (Chap. 23, this volume).

As is the case with the term happiness, the noun eudaimonia can be used as an adjective (eudaimon) and as an adverb (eudaimonically). Eudaimonia can also be used in referring to an ideology (eudaimonism). Haybron (Chap. 2, this volume) further makes the distinction between a psychological version (eudaimonic), and a philosophical version (eudaimonistic).

Finally, eudaimon may be spelled 'eudeamon', which is an anglicization of the Greek word and not commonly used anymore. Eudaimon comes closer to the Greek origin, and the "eudaemon" spelling has, according to Nussbaum (2001, p. 31), acquired some hedonistic connotations by its associations of human goodness to a pleasant feeling state.

1.3.2 Translating Eudaimonia into English

Over the centuries, eudaimonia has almost universally been translated into English as happiness (Jost, 2002). One reason is that, historically, the English word happiness used to be associated with civic duties and social obligations, i.e., as Happiness 2 (Austin, 1968; Hudson, 1996; McMahon, 2006; Oishi, 2010). As discussed, however, Happiness 1 is now the concept more commonly used for "happiness," hence translating eudaimonia as happiness has become troublesome to many philosophers. Starting with Anscombe (1958), eudaimonia has therefore become rendered in English as flourishing, a tradition followed by other philosophers (e.g., Cooper, 1975; Flanagan, 2007; Kristjánsson, 2013; Nagel, 1972). Eudaimonia is also translated into well-being (e.g., Haybron, 2008) and proper functioning (e.g., Casebeer, 2003). Yet, some authorities still prefer to translate eudaimonia as happiness (e.g., Annas, 2011; Russell, 2013), while being very clear that happiness is more than just subjective feelings and/or life satisfaction. Russell writes: "By 'happiness' here we do not mean a mood or a feeling but a life that is rich and fulfilling for the one living it" (Russell, p. 7). It goes without saying that when Annas and Russell refer to eudaimonia as happiness, it is in the Happiness 2 sense of the word.

Another analysis is offered by Ross, in his 2009 introduction to The Nicomachean Ethics. Ross writes: "Defining happiness as outstanding rational activity may seem puzzling to those who assume happiness is a mental state, a state of subjective well-being. To ease the problem, some have suggested that eudaimonia should instead be translated 'flourishing' or 'fulfilment.' Clearly by 'happiness' Aristotle is not speaking of any kind of mental state, still less of one where subjects' self-reports are invited and treated as definitive" (Ross, 2009, p. vii). Sumner (2002, p. 37) argues along similar lines: "We understand eudaimonia as more or less equivalent to well-being." Sumner even suggests that the interpretation of eudaimonia as happiness is silly and absurd, whereas interpreting it as well-being may, given a lengthy philosophical argument, be sensible. Sumner must have had Happiness 1 in mind when writing his comment about happiness, because elsewhere in the book he holds that eudaimonia "corresponds much more closely to our notion of welfare (= well-being): a complete state of being and doing well" (Sumner, 1996, p. 69).

Jost (2002) reviews the translation debate in some detail and includes a juicy statement given by Gregory Vlastos, a philosopher. Vlastos ridiculed the attempt to translate eudaimonia into well-being. Eudaimonia would and should be translated as happiness, he insisted, as well-being "has no adjectival or adverbial forms. This may seem a small matter to armchair translators, philosophers dogmatizing on how others should do their jobs. Not so if one is struggling with its nitty-gritty, trying for clause-by-clause English counterparts that might be faithful to the sentence structure, no less than the sentence, of the Greek original. And 'well-being' suffers from a further liability: it is a stiff bookish phrase, bereft of the ease and grace with which the living words of a natural language perform in a wide diversity of contexts. Eudaimonia fits perfectly street-Greek and Aristophanic slapstick" (Jost, p. xxii). Referring to its "street-Greek" and "slapstick" jargon, we are encouraged by Vlastos to use the term happiness rather than well-being when translating eudaimonia into English.

Another disadvantage of translating eudaimonia into 'flourishing' is that "animals and even plants can flourish but eudaimonia is possibly only for rational beings" (Hursthouse, 2013, p. 9). A third argument against translating eudaimonia into a more "catchy" word is presented by Besser (Chap. 5, this volume). She reminds us that using the term well-being or flourishing or some other fancy word would not help us much unless the conceptual understanding of the new term is properly established. A survey that includes a few items about "flourishing" comes no closer to the idea of Happiness 2 than one using items such as "everything considered, how happy are you with your life?" A survey participant may still be completely wrong about his or her own Happiness 2, whether or not it is referred to as "flourishing." In the philosophical meaning of flourishing, a person simply can not decide for herself whether she is flourishing or not (Hursthouse).

A different problem with translation appears in the literature on subjective well-being. In "Dienerology," as Haybron (2008) half-jokingly calls it, happiness and well-being are typically used interchangeably (e.g., Hirata, Chap. 3, this volume). Hence, in these circles, the suggestion to change the translation of eudaimonia from happiness to well-being makes no sense. Neither do statements such as "Aristotle had no theory of happiness. He had a theory of well-being" (Haybron, p. 32). As pointed out by Thin (Chap. 37, this volume), the title of the present tome testifies to this confusion, since, according to some translations of eudaimonia, it is to be read "Handbook of Well-being Well-being" or "Handbook of Eudaimonistic Eudaimonia" (see Haybron, Chap. 2, this volume). Another confusion created from these different meanings and translations of eudaimonia is illustrated by Sheldon (Chap. 36, this volume). From a Happiness 1 perspective, which Sheldon subscribes to, well-being is a subjective experience. By contrast, eudaimonia as Happiness 2—and with reference to what G. E. Moore named the "naturalistic fallacy"—subjective experiences cannot be a defining characteristic of well-being. Consequently, Sheldon argues that eudaimonia cannot be defined as well-being.

In several authoritative interpretations of eudaimonia, however, positive feelings are presented as an integrated part of eudaimonia: "Happiness in eudaimonist thinking does not exclude pleasure, but it excludes the idea that happiness could just be pleasure. It answers to our thoughts that happiness must in some way have pleasures 'woven into it'" (Annas, 2011). Similarly, Broadie (1991, p. 313) advocates that "Aristotle maintains that the highest good is necessarily pleasant."

Finally, it is worth remembering that not every psychologist treats happiness and well-being synonymously. Seligman (2011), who now concludes that well-being and happiness are very different concepts, is an example in case. His new theory advocates that happiness cannot account for all the important elements of a good life, but well-being can. Note that Seligman speaks of well-being as a construct and not as a concept, a terminological twist with some unfortunate implications (Michell, 2013). Happiness, Seligman suggests, is neither a concept nor a construct, but a "thing"—a thing that is "so overused that it has become almost meaningless" (Seligman, loc. 256).

1.3.3 Psychological Theories of Eudaimonia

The literature on psychological eudaimonics is dominated by three "big" theories: Waterman's Eudaimonic identity theory (Waterman, 1984, 1993), Ryff's version of Psychological well-being

(Ryff, 1989)[4] and Deci and Ryan's Self-determination theory (SDT; Ryan & Deci, 2001). All three are rooted in a nature-fulfillment philosophy (Haybron, Chap. 2, this volume), in humanistic and existential psychology, and to some extent in clinical psychology. All three theories link the good life to the fulfillment of the ultimate purpose of being human, with the concept of ultimate purpose typically taken to mean an optimally functioning life. More concretely, Waterman, whose "Two concepts of well-being" article from 1993 is the most cited text on eudaimonia (according to Google Scholar), defines eudaimonia as both a feeling and a condition. Self-realization in the sense of identification and development of one's best potentials is the most important part of Waterman's theory. The concept of "feelings of personal expressiveness" is also essential, since such feelings signal that the present activity of the individual is in harmony with the daimon, that is, the true self. Ryff's theory of eudaimonic well-being comprises six dimensions, or "ultimate purposes in life," that include, but are not restricted to, Aristotle's version of eudaimonia (Ryff, Chap. 6, this volume). The dimensions—autonomy, environmental mastery, personal growth, positive relationships, purpose in life, and self-acceptance—are discussed by most authors in the Handbook, including Bauer, Proctor and Tweed, Ferguson and Gunnell, and Jayawickreme and Dahill-Brown. Self-determination theory is influenced by the literature on intrinsic motivation, by Rogers (e.g., 1963), and by the idea that needs are necessary in order to explain human motivation. Ryan and Deci's link between goodness and ultimate purpose is articulated as a stepwise process. It starts with activities aimed at regulating one's life in an intrinsic, autonomous, and reflective manner. Such activities will in turn produce feelings of autonomy, competence, and connectedness. Then, in a third step, the feelings of autonomy, competence, and connectedness will generate subjective experiences such as positive affect, fulfillment, life satisfaction, happiness, thriving, wellness, meaning, vitality, and depth. These experiences are, however, not included in the concept of eudaimonia, but are rather considered to be hedonic by-products of eudaimonia (Ryan & Martela, Chap. 7, this volume). The eudaimonics of SDT are widely used in the literature on well-being, and most chapters in the present handbook make reference to it. For instance, Sirgy and Uysal (Chap. 32, this volume) show how these principles are applicable to areas such as tourism research.

The big three of psychological eudaimonics differ in their ideas about what it takes to fulfill the ultimate purpose of being human. A critical distinction concerns the role of subjective experience and particularly the feeling of pleasure. Pleasure has been a central element in all philosophical theories of happiness since the dawn of western thinking (e.g., Haybron, 2008), but Ryff's theory of Psychological well-being is silent about it. In Self-determination theory (Ryan & Deci, 2001), pleasure is excluded from the concept of eudaimonic well-being, but not from hedonic well-being. In the scheme of goodness presented by Waterman (1993), pleasure is at the core of eudaimonia, in the form of "higher pleasure" or "feelings of personal expressiveness."

1.3.4 Other Understandings of Eudaimonia

The different conceptualizations offered by the big three reflect only a fraction of the variability that exists in understanding psychological eudaimonics. As underscored by several critics (e.g., Kashdan, Biswas-Diener, & King, 2008), the broad range of eudaimonia interpretations that have been proposed represents a problem for the possibility of developing a coherent science of eudaimonic well-being. To illustrate this problem, I have assembled a small "convenience sample" of definitions and descriptions of eudaimonia that have been proposed (Table 1.2). The table is not intended to be exhaustive and readers inter-

[4] Competing conceptualizations also referred to as Psychological well-being include those developed by Bradburn (1969), Su, Tay, and Diener (2014), and Vallerand (2012).

Table 1.2 Some descriptions of eudaimonia

	Description	Author(s)
1	The ancient Greeks saw the concept of eudaimonia as denoting a "broad idea of a life's going well"	Annas (1993)
2	The emotional state associated with full engagement or optimal performance in meaningful activity	Averill and More (2000)
3	Eudaimonic well-being deals with the appraisal that one feels good while explicitly considering one's sense of meaningfulness in life	Bauer, McAdams, and Pals (2008)
4	[To Aristotle happiness comes from] the pleasure that one takes in certain doings or activities – especially those that involve capacities that one has made an effort to develop	Benditt (1974)
5	A life experienced as valuably meaningful and as engaging	Berridge and Kringelbach (2013)
6	The fulfillment of one's true nature, including both self-actualization and commitment to socially shared goals. Today this approach to the study of well-being comprises a wide range of constructs, such as self-actualization and self-acceptance, perception of purpose and meaning, self-determination, cultivation of competences, trust in relationships, and cooperation	Delle Fave (2013)
7	The eudaimonic component, referred to as psychological well-being, is conceptualized as the search and attainment of meaning, self-actualization, and personal growth	Donaldson, Dollwet, and Rao (2015)
8	A self-realization theory that makes happiness or personal well-being the chief good for man (…) "What is eudaimonia?" is then the same question as "What are the best activities of which man is capable?"	Encyclopedia Britannica
9	Acting in an exemplary or extraordinary fashion	Fishman and McCarthy (2013)
10	The meaningful life	Gallagher, Lopez, and Preacher (2009)
11	In the sense of the classical Greeks is "having a good guardian spirit," that is "the state of having an objectively valuable life"	Griffin (2007)
12	The ultimate source of meaning in life	Halusic and King (2013)
13	A sense of purpose, meaning, and engagement with life	Heller et al. (2013)
14	Encompassing a wide range of possible content other than subjective satisfaction, although that is not excluded	Hudson (1996)
15	Being fully functional (i.e., realizing or developing one's potential)	Huppert (2005)
16	Seeking to use and develop the best in oneself, in congruence with one's values and true self	Huta (2013)
17	The well-being of individuals sought as their own good	Jost (2002)
18	Eudemonic measures refer to underlying psychological needs, encompassing various dimensions of wellness, such as autonomy, personal growth, or purpose in life, which contribute towards well-being independently of any positive affect they may convey	Kapteyn, Lee, Tassot, Vonkova, and Zamarro (2015)
19	Meaning and purpose; taking part in activities that allow for the actualization of one's skills, talents, and potential	Kashdan et al. (2008)
20	Embodying a value judgment about whether a person is leading a commendable life	Kesebir and Diener (2008)
21	"my activity" (not a state 'arising' in me) that is explicated in terms of living virtuously	Keyes and Annas (2009)

(continued)

Table 1.2 (continued)

	Description	Author(s)
22	An inner imperative, a feel of living in truth to oneself that is unique for each person. When an individual is living this feel, he or she flourishes in many ways	Kimiecik (2011, p. 782)
23	The fulfillment (including positive feelings) that comes from engagement in meaningful activity and the actualization of one's potential	King (2008)
24	A life is well-lived, embedded in meaningful values, together with a sense of engagement in that life. This is the cognitive or Aristotelian ingredient of happiness	Kringelbach and Berridge (2009)
25	Achieved through the development and fulfillment of one's potentials	Linley (2013)
26	Expresses the more general notion of human prosperity and sense of well-being. (…) It refers to quality of life as a whole, and especially to an individual's virtuous functioning in life	Naor, Ben-Ze'ev, and Okon-Singer (2014)
27	A lived experience whereby the "individual experiences the whole of his life in every act, and he experiences parts and whole together as necessary, such that he can will that nothing be changed"	Norton (1976)
28	A sense of meaning and purpose in life, or good psychological functioning	OECD (2013)
29	Eudaimonic well-being, measured with the satisfaction with life scale and a short version of the psychological well-being scale	Philippe, Koestner, Beaulieu-Pelletier, Lecours, and Lekes (2012)
30	Not pursued for the sake of pleasure, it is the end achieved by living a virtuous life in accordance with reason—pleasure is a byproduct of exercising good character	Proctor, Tweed, and Morris (2015)
31	Focuses on meaning and self-realization and defines well-being in terms of the degree to which a person is fully functioning	Ryan and Deci (2001)
32	The idea of striving toward excellence based on one's unique potential"	Ryff and Singer (2008)
33	Focus on becoming a better person by leading a virtuous life and achieving important goals	Schueller and Seligman (2010)
34	People's perceptions of the meaningfulness (or pointlessness), sense of purpose, and value of their life—a very broad set of considerations	Stone and Mackie (2013)
35	A complete state of being and doing good	Sumner (1996)
36	The life which is worth living or good in itself	Telfer (1980)
37	Ingredients of well-being that go beyond positive affect and life-satisfaction	Tiberius (2013)
38	Denotes that simply feeling good is not everything. The essence of a good life is seen in "living good" rather than in "enjoying life" and living good is seen as "psychological development"	Veenhoven (2013)
39	"feelings of personal expressiveness"	Waterman (2008)
40	A lifestyle characterised by the pursuit of virtue/excellence, meaning/purpose, doing good/making a difference, and the resulting sense of fulfillment or flourishing	Wong (2011)
41	The good composed of all goods; an ability which suffices for living well; perfection in respect of virtue; resources sufficient for a living creature	Wikipedia

ested in a more complete analysis may be better informed by reading the work of Huta (Chap. 15, this volume; Huta & Waterman, 2014). Rather, what the table offers is a non-pretentious attempt to illustrate how the task of defining eudaimonic well-being has turned into something of a conceptual cottage industry.

1.4 Conceptual Controversies

Already St. Augustine, in his book "The City of God," complained about the number of theories about happiness that the ancient philosophers had produced. He counted 288 competing theories, although it has been held against Augustine that his calculation was an exaggeration (Hudson, 1996, p. 63). As testified by Table 1.2, the tradition of proposing definitions and taxonomies about the good life is not restricted to the ancient era. Indeed, Benjamin, Kimball, Heffetz, and Szembrot (2014) recently published a list of 136 "aspects of well-being," which, according to the authors, represented "the most comprehensive effort to date to construct such a compilation." Work by the Australian Centre on Quality of Life may have escaped the attention of Benjamin and his co-authors, though, as the Australians ended up with a list of 173 domains of well-being and no less than 447 measures of quality of life (reported in Rapley, 2003). The chapter by Jayawickreme and Dahill-Brown (Chap. 31, this volume) also discusses lists of well-being taxonomies in some detail.

It is in this unfortunate situation that Nussbaum (2008) calls for a break, in order for happiness researchers to rethink their concepts and models. In her "Who Is the Happy Warrior?" paper, Nussbaum takes issue with the empirical literature on happiness, criticizing it for being "so riddled with conception confusion and normative naïveté that we had better pause and sort things out before going any further" (p. S108). The Handbook of Eudaimonic Well-Being aspires to offer such a pause, and its authors were invited to comment on Nussbaum's concerns. Several chapters in the book are partly written as a response to Nussbaum's critique.

But the Handbook is not only responding to Nussbaum's challenge by re-*thinking* the good life. The best way forward may not be by reflection alone—the study of happiness has certainly had its share of that, over the millennia. To the contrary, Thagard (2012) argues that philosophers' attempts to "analyze" concepts have not been very successful simply because we cannot trust reason to generate fruitful scientific taxonomies. The structure of the atom or vitamin C are not intuitively given to us, and neither is geometry—despite Kant's insistence of its a priori nature. Harris (2010) has even proposed that the scientific principle of confronting theoretical reasoning with empirical observations also applies to the science of goodness and morality. Relatedly, Thin (Chap. 37, this volume) asks if Nussbaum's own strategy towards conceptual clarity has been such a success. After all, how clarifying is her defense of the Aristotelian idea of the good life as a complete life in the sense of "lacking in nothing that would make it richer or better"? Not very, Thin suggests, characterizing such a conceptualization of eudaimonia as "obviously absurd."

Perhaps the problem in the science of happiness is not so much that researchers do not acknowledge the importance of conceptual clarity. Indeed, all the present chapters consider the current state of conceptual ambiguity as unfortunate. Rather, the crisis may be hidden in a general unwillingness to confront old ideas with new knowledge. Mill seized this phenomenon eloquently in his portrayal of Bentham as "[failing] in deriving light from other minds" (cited in Nussbaum, 2008, p. S83), and the problem is not limited to happiness research. The lack of conceptual progress in economics drove John Maynard Keynes to write that "The difficulty lies, not in the new ideas, but in escaping from the old ones, which ramify, for those brought up as most of us have been, into every corner of our minds" (Keynes, 1936, p. viii).

Few scholars have articulated this problem better than the biologist Ernst Mayr. His highly respected book on the growth of biological knowledge (Mayr, 1982) convincingly shows how science progresses more rapidly from conceptual improvements than from the discovery of new facts: "it seems to me that progress in the biological sciences is characterized not so much by individual discoveries, no matter how important, or by the proposal of new theories, but rather by the gradual but decisive development of new concepts and the abandonment of those that had previously been dominant. In most cases the development of major new concepts has not been due to individual discoveries but rather to novel integration of previously established facts" (Mayr, p. 856).

An excellent analysis of knowledge and its role in the development of taxonomies is provided by Thagard (1992), who also offers several paradigmatic examples of taxonomic and conceptual developments throughout the history of science. They all include the abandonment of the old conceptual schemes. One example is the celestial bodies and how the systems of their classification have changed. As commonly known, the planet Earth was given a privileged position as a unique "major" celestial body in the taxonomy describing the universe before the scientific revolution. With the introduction of the heliocentric worldview, its status was reduced to an ordinary planet on par with others in our solar system. The taxonomy changed dramatically. Another illuminating example comes from Nersessian (2008), who details how the taxonomy of birds started out according to some rather primitive schemas. One of the old classification systems was, for instance, based exclusively on the bird's beak and foot. As knowledge in biology grew, the taxonomies also became more sophisticated. Today ornithologists use a much broader range of properties to catalogue birds, drawing on aspects of the feather, plumage, and tarsus as well as the beak and feet.

Trivial as these examples may seem, their wisdom bears on how taxonomies develop as a consequence of improved knowledge. For example, some "boxologies" in our own field make a distinction between hedonic well-being and eudaimonic well-being, with the first category typically comprising both pleasant feelings and life satisfaction (e.g., Henderson & Knight, 2012). This move leaves the concept of life satisfaction in an ambiguous position, however. Thus, for the dichotomy to be fruitful, an agreement must be reached about the nature of life satisfaction. Is it a hedonic concept, as Vittersø (Chap. 17, this volume) suggests? Or is such an understanding deeply mistaken, as Haybron (Chap. 2, this volume) argues? According to Haybron, the term hedonic has to do with pleasure, and life satisfaction "is not hedonic in any plausible sense of the word." But Vittersø maintains that from a psychological point of view, both pleasant feelings and judgments about life satisfaction seem to be subcategories of the same overarching class of good-bad evaluations. In order for such disputes to be solved, better knowledge on the nature of pleasure and evaluations must be integrated in the theories of happiness. And once a unified concept has emerged, the old ideas must be retired.

According to Mayr (1982, p. 840), nothing strengthened the theory of natural selection as much as the refutation, one by one, of all the competing theories. This important part of scientific development was popularized in a recent book edited by Brockman (2015), and the Handbook of Eudaimonic Well-Being promotes these important insights as well. In what follows, highlights of some of the most pressing issues will be presented. The review starts with the concept of eudaimonia and asks if it is necessary for a theory of Happiness 1.

1.4.1 Do We Really Need the Concept of Eudaimonia?

The most fundamental dispute in the Handbook—and it is a big one in the general happiness literature as well—concerns the question of whether the concept of eudaimonic well-being is warranted at all. Three chapters, written by Ward and King (Chap. 35, this volume), Sheldon (Chap. 36, this volume), and Thin (Chap. 37, this volume), are particularly critical of this term. Rather than contributing to our knowledge of human goodness, these authors suggest, the concept of eudaimonia just makes things unnecessarily complicated.

There is no reason to propose complex models of well-being if we don't have to. After all, the appeal of hedonic well-being, in the narrow sense of proposing that an abundance of pleasure is the only good worth having, is precisely that it offers a one-dimensional view of happiness. As pointed out by Hirata (Chap. 3, this volume), such simplicity has the great advantage of reducing the multitudes of goodness and badness to something that can be maximized. And we can only maximize goodness if it can be represented along a single dimension. As both Hirata and Thin (Chaps. 3 and 37, this volume) explain, a taxonomy of happiness that comprises more than one dimension of goodness cannot be submitted to the principles of maximization, because intensifying one dimension may hamper another, thus reducing the individual's total well-being.

The importance of parsimony persuaded a scholar of Kahneman's stature to promote the idea of hedonic well-being for many years. However, Kahneman shifted his stance as he came to realize that humans also value things other than pleasant feelings. Goals and projects are important in our lives as well, whether or not they bring pleasure (see Little, Chap. 19, this volume). Thus, a one-component definition doesn't work for happiness, Kahneman argues, "because you cannot ignore life satisfaction as a measure of well-being" (Kahneman, 2012, p. 27). But adding the concept of life satisfaction to a one-dimensional taxonomy of human goodness makes the model quite complex, since a balance between two distinct forms of goodness must be established. This problem remains unexplained in the literature on subjective well-being.

Aristotle's version of eudaimonia purports to have solved the problem by its argument that happiness is "one single thing" (White, 2006, p. 18). Russell (2013) makes note of some passages in the Nicomachean Ethics that underline the unidimensionality of classic eudaimonia theory. According to Aristotle, "there is exactly one final end per person, and what's more, it is the same final end for each of us" (Nicomachean Ethics, I.2, cited in Russell, p. 9). Besser (Chap. 5, this volume) concludes that the classical notion of eudaimonia is a holistic one and that accordingly, a life cannot be well lived if it is divided into a set of "wellness dimensions" (see also Vella-Brodrick, Chap. 26, this volume).

Applying this one-facet model from philosophical eudaimonism to psychological eudaimonics will not take us very far, however. As Besser (Chap. 5, this volume) points out, carving up the concept of goodness into separate dimensions seems unavoidable in empirical research, and she thinks that this state of affairs segregates philosophical and psychological approaches to eudaimonia. Confronted with the history of science more generally, Besser's prediction is probably correct. The history of scientific advancement is ripe with examples of concepts that were first conceived of as homogenous, but could not be properly understood until they were partitioned into finer components. In physics, the concept of the atom is a well-known example; in biology, a longstanding debate about the concept of telos was not resolved until it was dissected into four subcomponents. Hence, from a scientific point of view, the Aristotelian idea of a telos cannot be considered a single thing. It must be divided into at least four different dimensions (Mayr, 1982).

Thus, as a scientific concept, psychological eudaimonics must be multi-dimensional. The only way to justify the notion of psychological eudaimonics against more parsimonious competitors is therefore to identify at least one psychological element of a life well lived that cannot be accounted for by pleasure or life satisfaction, even if it is a first-person perspective that defines its goodness. The most promising place to look for such a subjective goodness is within our human nature.

1.5 Fulfilling the Intrinsic Values of Human Nature

Aristotle's entry point for debating goodness was the identification of an intrinsic value, or ultimate purpose, of the human nature. This strategy led him to the notion of functioning, and from functioning to virtue, or arête, which he regarded as necessary but not sufficient for the good life (see the Chap. 4 by Fowers, Chap. 2 by Haybron, and Chap. 27 by Mckay in this volume). The Aristotelian concept of virtue means something like excellence of character, or excellence in the sense of fulfillment of human capacities. Badhwar, a philosopher, translates Aristotelian virtues as "an integrated intellectual-emotional disposition to think, feel, and act at the right time, about the right things, towards the right people, for the right end, and in the right way" (Badhwar, 2014, p. 143). From a scientific point of view, this formulation is quite a mouthful. Nevertheless, a few elements may, perhaps, be translated into something researchable without throwing the baby out with the bathwater.

Schwartz and Wrzesniewski (Chap. 8, this volume) give a brilliant example of how such an endeavor can be carried out. Their chapter strikes a balance between the scientific ideas of excellence and the classical thinking of Aristotle. The authors line up behind the eudaimonic view that well-being follows from certain forms of activity, and that there are certain features about activities that make them eudaimonic. The goal of the activity, or telos, is such a feature. The goodness of human life is associated with the development of excellence, and this development requires effort and a strenuous pursuit that cannot be categorized as pleasure or amusement. Schwartz and Wrzesniewski lean toward the neo-Aristotelian Alasdair MacIntyre, and his definition of "a practice" when clarifying what this means. MacIntyre (1981) pointed out four salient features of the concept of a practice, summarized as complexity, excellence, integration of means and ends, and continuous development of the practices and the goods toward which they are aimed. The latter element of a practice implies that as individuals continue to practice, their standards of excellence change. In his work on leisure, Stebbins (Chap. 33, this volume) has identified some parallels between different leisure practices and the features described by MacIntyre. In what Stebbins refers to as serious leisure, many of the characteristics of optimal functioning can be observed.

In his chapter on virtues and culture, Mckay (Chap. 27, this volume) probes further into MacIntyre's concept of practice and how it applies to anthropological accounts of the good life. The role of culture, Mckay advocates, is basically overlooked as a foundation for the realization of virtues, and to overcome this limitation, his chapter promotes an approach referred to as critical eudaimonics. As noted by Proctor and Tweed (Chap. 18, this volume), thorough perspectives on virtues like the one proposed by Mckay are hard to find in the psychological literature on eudaimonia. Due to their minimal representation of virtue, most measures of psychological eudaimonics are incomplete. A much-noted exception to this lack of interest in virtues is the project launched by Peterson and Seligman (2004) that has evolved into a massive, global research paradigm. Several chapters of the Handbook present results from this research program (e.g., Røysamb and Nes; Proctor and Tweed) and a comprehensive report is provided by Harzer (Chap. 20, this volume). Her chapter provides a review of the "Values in Action (VIA) Classification of Strengths and Virtues" and documents that some of these strengths and virtues, like zest and hope, correlate with the mainstream indicators of SWB. Other strengths and virtues, such as love of learning and judgment (a kind of openness to experience dimension) are not correlated with indicators of SWB. Rather, these strengths and virtues correlate with indicators of personal growth, illustrating again how measures of SWB fail to account for central elements of a good life.

Dean (Chap. 34, this volume) employs the terms virtue and practice from a societal perspective in his justification of eudaimonia. It is essential for individuals to flourish, Dean says, but we want them to do so as members of good societies. The contemporary priority of a 'work-first' policy is on par with hedonic and utilitarian principles, but not with solidaristic and eudaimonic principles. As an alternative to the 'work-first' policy, he has developed a set of principles referred to as a 'life-first' ethic, which is both consistent with and inspired by eudaimonic thinking. It may even be extended to encompass the idea that eudaimonic well-being is a social right. "Its simple meaning is that human life is about more than individual utility and that this provides a foundation for social policy making" (Dean, Chap. 34 this volume).

Investigating excellence and virtue from the perspective of wisdom, Law and Staudinger (Chap. 9, this volume) write with insight on what a scientific approach to the elusive issue of *virtue research* may look like. The chapter defends the view that wisdom (phronesis) is the perfect integration of mind and virtue. Law and Staudinger offer a series of important arguments for why pleasure and satisfaction cannot account for the concept of wisdom, and how it sometimes even hampers it. The contradiction between satisfaction on the one hand, and the development of an "excellent character" on the other was evident already in the work of Erik H. Erikson. In the last of Erikson's developmental stages, the one concerning the conflict between integrity and despair, satisfaction is achieved by individuals able to adapt to the losses experienced over the years. As Law and Staudinger point out, the reward for such integrity is high levels of hedonic well-being at the cost of reduced eudaimonic well-being. The abandoning of aspirations and life goals might well lead to satisfaction, but it will not lead to continued growth and goal attainment. In other words, personal growth and hedonic well-being are under some circumstances not only independent, they are in opposition to each other. A similar argument is put forward by Bauer (Chap. 10, this volume). From a narrative perspective on self-identity, it has been repeatedly documented that wisdom is not positively correlated with hedonic happiness. To the contrary, pleasure can sometimes reduce it.

Virtue can also be approached through studying another prototypical example: the hero (Franco, Efthimiou & Zimbardo, Chap. 22, this volume). In their chapter, heroism is considered as the pinnacle of human excellence and virtue in history, and the authors review a series of links between eudaimonia and the traits of a hero. Of particular interest is the elements they identify as being good without being perceived as pleasant.

Taken together, the above chapters show that some elements of a good life, things we value from a subjective point of view, are not necessarily associated with pleasure or life satisfaction. The principal indicators of subjective well-being simply do not reflect these ways of being well, and this important point is sometimes overlooked by critics of psychological eudaimonics.

For example, Ward and King (Chap. 35, this volume) are concerned with Mill's "dissatisfied Socrates," who illustrates a different kind of eudaimonic goodness than the one defined by subjective well-being. But the character portrayed as eudaimonically happy in the literature on psychological eudaimonics is typically a person who lives well in the SWB sense of leading a good life, with the possible exception that the eudaimonic person is even more happy. "Whenever eudaimonic goodness is articulated, good feelings and life satisfaction are never far away," Ward and King write, reminding us that when eudaimonic self-report instruments are examined more closely, they overlap substantially with measures of SWB—in the area of 0.80 or even above (see also Disabato, Goodman, Kashdan, Short, & Jarden, 2016; Røysamb & Nes, Chap. 16, this volime). The weakness of this argument, however, is a heavy reliance on a limited set of self-report measurements about eudaimonia. As elaborated by Proctor and Tweed (Chap. 18, this volume), the complexity of eudaimonic goodness does not lend itself easily to quantification and statistical treatment. The information extracted from the current measures of eudaimonic well-being may therefore not be a precise reflection of the eudaimonic idea. For example, Vittersø (Chap. 17, this volume) illustrates how eudaimonic self-report scales are contaminated with a bias toward hedonia.

The subjective well-being approach holds that the concept of life satisfaction is able to capture concepts like goal importance and goal achievement (e.g., Kahneman, 2011). In mainstream SWB research, therefore, a quick response obtained from self-reported survey items about life satisfaction is proposed to adequately capture everything important in a person's life, including the process of identifying and pursuing important life goals. This assumption is shown by several chapters of the Handbook to lack psychological credibility. The importance of having personal goals and striving to reach them, for example, is an argument in favor of expanding the notion of well-being beyond both pleasure and life satisfaction. The concept of life satisfaction cannot incorporate goal importance for several reasons, and Nussbaum (2008) articulates one of them. Although Nussbaum agrees with Kahneman that well-being must include the pursuit of goals, she disagrees with the assumption that satisfaction accounts for the development and striving that are inherent in the idea of goal importance. Rather to the contrary, Nussbaum claims that "if I ever notice myself feeling feelings of satisfaction, I blame myself and think that, insofar as I have those feelings, I am like Mill's 'pig satisfied' or Aristotle's 'dumb grazing animals,' and thus, reflectively, I report dissatisfaction with my life as a whole" (Nussbaum, p. S83).

Sheldon (Chap. 36, this volume) takes issue with Nussbaum and suggests that satisfaction is a mental state perfectly capable of sustaining personal struggles toward excellence. In Sheldon's view, satisfaction is just the kind of "go-signal" an individual needs in order to strive towards the goals and projects that Nussbaum is concerned about. He draws on an organismic perspective in the humanistic tradition of Carl Rogers in order to explain his position. According to these views, human beings have a natural growth instinct that pushes them to become more differentiated, integrated, and embedded within other people. The modus operandi for organismic growth is satisfaction, and self-determined growth will, given the right circumstances, be intrinsically motivated. If this assumption—further articulated in Sheldon's Self-concordance model (Sheldon, 2014)—is correct, feelings of pleasure and satisfaction are not antithetical to growth; "rather, they are essential for growth!"

A related perspective is developed in the Broaden-and-build theory (Fredrickson, 1998, 2013). Within this framework, Fredrickson (Chap. 12, this volume) considers eudaimonia to include kinds of engagement that "transcend immediate gratification and enable individuals to experience themselves as connected to the higher callings of purpose, meaning, contribution, and interconnectedness." This development towards growth and betterment is supported by hedonic feelings. The positive emotions stimulate the person experiencing them to broaden his or her awareness. In such an uplifted state, people will typically see their environment from a broader perspective, and this enables them to "to perceive the many ways in which they contribute to, and are interconnected with others, or are otherwise called to a higher purpose or meaning." From this perspective, Fredrickson says, eudaimonia becomes one of the many positive outcomes of hedonia, and we should thus stop thinking in terms of either eudaimonia or hedonia. She argues they are both valuable kinds of well-being and it is the interaction between them that creates good lives. The chapter written by Vallerand (Chap. 13, this volume) also subscribes to the logic that pleasure supports goal striving. His chapter proposes that passion triggers positive emotions, which in turn creates eudaimonic well-being, also referred to by Vallerand as "adaptive outcomes."

1.5.1 Purpose and Meaning

Meaning is essential to the notion of eudaimonia as the fulfillment of the intrinsic values of our human nature. Aristotle's functioning argument, for instance, places purpose at the center of eudaimonia in the sense that the ultimate end of life is to give one's life meaning (Russell, 2013; Haybron, Chap. 2, this volume). Aristotle's idea that we will get a better grasp of the concept of goodness once we have determined what the purpose (or function) of a human life is, suggests that a person will be in his or her best state when that purpose is achieved. Thus, there is an important connection between the essence of being human and the function of a human life. "The connection between the essence and function is that the essence explains the thing's characteristic behavior and explains it as the thing's purpose, what the thing is (metaphorically) meant to do" (Megone, 1994, p. 37).

In Aristotle's teaching, the purpose to be found in life is the same for all of us (e.g., Russell, 2013), but this idea is not easily confirmed by empirical studies. For instance, the chapter by Danvers, O'Neil and Shiota (Chap. 21, this volume) defines meaning as something that connects things that would be otherwise unconnected. The making of these connections is not inherent, Danvers et al. explain, but must be identified by each individual. Positive emotions, and perhaps awe in particular, play a distinct role in such meaning-making. Connecting the unconnected often requires schematic accommodation, which in itself is typically experienced as aversive. Because awe opens up our minds to the unknown, however, this emotion prompts an effort to understand the "bigger picture" and to expand one's self into something greater. In the chapter by Schlegel, Hicks and Christy (Chap. 14, this volume), the personal uniqueness of meaning is exemplified through the notion of one's "true" self. People perceive their "true" selves as a hub of meaning in their lives, and the research presented by Schlegel et al. illustrates how individuals are concerned about something deeper than pleasures in their lives, and that those who feel "in touch" with their true self also perceive more meaning in their lives. The chapter by Pargament, Wong and Exline (Chap. 25, this volume) reviews how individual meaning systems can be organized individually, even within a framework of wholeness.

Ferguson and Gunnell (Chap. 28, this volume) address another Achilles heal in Aristotle's teaching—the issue of gender. Classic eudaimonism is criticized for being snobbish, partly because it excluded large groups of people, like women and children, from the list of those who could potentially lead good lives (e.g., Thin, Chap. 37, this volume). Defenders of Aristotle's view claim that this limitation must be understood in the context of his life, including his role as a teacher of elite male Athenian citizens in the fourth century BCE (e.g., Annas, 2011), and they maintain that the ancient theories are open for "considerable revisions of content, as long as its role and formal structure remain the same (Annas, 2002, p. 11). As new evidence and knowledge accumulate, however, the question becomes how long we can keep trusting "Aristotle's embarrassingly smug effort in Nicomachean ethics to persuade us that the only good life is that of the philosopher" (Thin, 2012, p. 41).

Ong and Patterson (Chap. 24, this volume) illustrate how the purpose of an activity may depend on the human life cycle and lifespan developments, whereas the chapter by Vella-Brodrick (Chap. 26, this volume) documents that not all of us respond to well-being interventions in similar ways. Individual experience and interpretation of a positive intervention can influence intervention outcomes, Vella-Brodrick writes, pointing out how so-called "fit" factors are important determinants of intervention effectiveness. Røysamb and Nes (Chap. 16, this volume) discuss how individual variation in eudaimonia makes sense from a heritability perspective. Building on their concept of gene-environment matchmaking, the unique interplay between genes and environmental factors explains how activities that provide opportunities to express (partly) genetic talents and potentials for some people are not necessarily the same activities that will provide such opportunities for others.

A life may be experienced as meaningful if it is "felt to have significance beyond the trivial or momentary, to have purpose, or to have a coherence that transcends chaos" (King, Hicks, Krull, & Gasio, 2006, p. 180). Following up on this experiential understanding of meaning, with roots going back at least to Osgood, Suci, and Tannenbaum (1957), Dolan and Kudrna (Chap. 29, this volume) suggest that the experience of meaning, or *purpose* in their vocabulary, is different from the experience of pleasure. The chapter suggests that purpose and pleasure are two types of well-being that can be further divided into levels of evaluation and experience. Types (i.e., pleasure and purpose) and levels (i.e., evaluations and experience) can be combined into nine different forms of well-being, with "satisfaction with yesterday" as the most comprehensive.

Dolan and Kudrna consider both pleasure and purpose to be hedonic (*sentimental hedonism* in their vocabulary). By contrast, many well-being researchers think of meaning as something non-

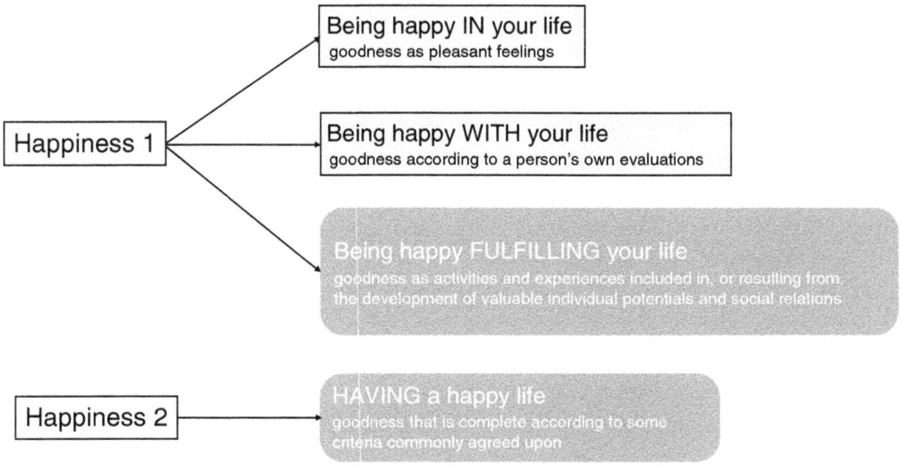

Fig. 1.2 A schematic difference between happiness 1 and happiness 2, including a categorization into hedonic well-being (*gray boxes*) and eudaimonic well-being (*dark boxes* with *rounded corners*)

hedonic (cf. Table 1.2), including Steger (Chap. 11, this volume) who regards the search for meaning as eudaimonic. The search for meaning is known from existential philosophy and psychology, such as through the work of Victor Frankl and books entitled "Man's Search for Meaning" and "The Will to Meaning" (Frankl, 1945, 1970). According to Steger, the search for meaning dimension is uncorrelated, or negatively correlated, with measures of subjective well-being (King & Hicks, 2009; Steger, Frazier, Oishi, & Kaler, 2006; Steger & Kashdan, 2006; Ward & King, Chap. 35, this volume). There is, however, another form of meaning in life, and Steger describes it as a kind of meaning that is already present in a person's life. This kind of meaning is typically correlated with indicators of pleasure and life satisfaction, but despite this overlap, pleasure and the presence of meaning seem to reflect at least partly independent elements of well-being (e.g., Baumeister, Vohs, Aaker, & Garbinsky, 2013; Jayawickreme & Dahill-Brown, Chap. 31, this volume).

The Handbook of Eudaimonic Well-Being presents a variety of ideas about the good life. In the current section, attempts were made to articulate some of their common elements. The existence of a subjective goodness left unexplained by pleasure and life satisfaction was tentatively suggested as one such commonality, backed by an argument about how psychological eudaimonics may account for the gap. At the core of this reasoning is Aristotle's idea of how elements of human nature help us to understand how to identify goodness. Translated into a modern language, the essence of psychological eudaimonics may be articulated as something like **activities and experiences included in, or resulting from, the development of valuable individual potentials and social relations**.

The tension between psychological eudaimonics and philosophical eudaimonism remains. The former appears as a subcomponent in the Happiness 1 taxonomy, whereas philosophical eudaimonism is complete and unidimensional. According to the Happiness 1 approach, pleasure and life satisfaction are elements of a good life, but they are not elements of psychological eudaimonics. In contrast, the Happiness 2 approach considers pleasure and satisfaction to be inseparable from the notion of eudaimonia, and from this perspective it makes no sense to speak of a hedonic component and a eudaimonic component of well-being. Figure 1.2 tries to sketch the gist of the above reasoning in schematic form.

1.6 Conclusion

Karl Popper, discussing progress in science, once used Hegel's definition of electricity to illustrate how a lack of conceptual clarity may lead us astray. Electricity, Hegel claimed, "is the purpose of the form from which it emancipates itself, it is the form that is just about to overcome its own indifference; for electricity is the immediate emergence, or the actuality just emerging, from the proximity of the form, and still determined by it—not yet the dissolution, however, of the form itself, but rather the more superficial process by which the differences desert the form which, however, they still retain as their condition, having not yet grown into independence of and through them" (Popper, 1963, p. 332). Needless to say, there would have been no street lamps or computers around if Hegel's conception was the common understanding of electricity. It is also easy to see how Hegel's analytical approach falls short of the scientific practice of constraining theoretical assumptions to empirical observations. But quantification in science makes no sense until we have a proper understanding of what we would like to measure. Empirical tests offer no replacement for the tedious task of gradually improving our knowledge by continuously refining our concepts—and by retiring the old and confusing ones.

The aim of the Handbook of Eudaimonic Well-Being is to let leading scholars of happiness present both cutting-edge research and elaborated analytical thinking. The impressive result of this effort is now gathered between two covers. But the most remarkable outcome of the book is arguably its large-scale relevance; a most crucial message to us as human beings. Ryan and Martela (Chap. 7, this volume) correctly remind us that the more we know about the good way of living, the more we are in a position to build a society that can be supportive and offer opportunities for such a way of living for all of its citizens. The notion of eudaimonia is unique in this respect, with its promise of a knowledge that explains how doing good and being well can come together. If we believe in science, we should also trust "its promise for accumulating knowledge about human behavior that can advance the quality of the human condition" (Open Science Collaboration, 2015). Understanding goodness and what our lives ought to be aimed at is just the kind of knowledge needed to move humankind in this direction. The notion of eudaimonia offers such insights, by specifying why our world cannot be called a good place until it provides all of us with opportunities to fulfill the intrinsic values of our human nature.

References

Annas, J. (1993). *The morality of happiness [kindle version]*. New York: Oxford University Press.

Annas, J. (2002). Should virtue make you happy? In L. J. Jost & R. A. Shiner (Eds.), *Eudaimonia and well-being* (pp. 1–19). Kelowna, Canada: Academic Printing & Publishing.

Annas, J. (2011). *Intelligent virtue [kindle version]*. Oxford, UK: Oxford University Press.

Anscombe, G. E. M. (1958). Modern moral philosophy. *Philosophy, 33*, 1–19.

Austin, J. (1968). Pleasure and happiness. *Philosophy, 43*, 51–62.

Averill, J. R., & More, T. A. (2000). Happiness. In M. Lewis & J. Haviland-Jones (Eds.), *Handbook of emotions* (2nd ed., pp. 663–676). New York: Guilford.

Badhwar, N. K. (2014). *Well-being: Happiness in a worthwhile life [kindle]*. New York: Oxford University Press.

Bauer, J. J., McAdams, D. P., & Pals, J. L. (2008). Narrative identity and eudaimonic well-being. *Journal of Happiness Studies, 9*, 81–104.

Baumeister, R. F., Vohs, K. D., Aaker, J. L., & Garbinsky, E. N. (2013). Some key differences between a happy life and a meaningful life. *The Journal of Positive Psychology, 8*, 505–516. doi:10.1080/17439760.2013.830764.

Benditt, T. (1974). Happiness. *Philosophical Studies: An International Journal for Philosophy in the Analytic Tradition, 25*, 1–20. doi:10.2307/4318819.

Benjamin, D. J., Kimball, M. S., Heffetz, O., & Szembrot, N. (2014). Beyond happiness and satisfaction: Toward well-being indices based on stated preference. *The American Economic Review, 104*, 2698–2735.

Berridge, K. C., & Kringelbach, M. L. (2013). Towards a neuroscience of well-being: Implications of insights from pleasure research. In H. Brockmann & J. Delhey (Eds.), *Human happiness and the pursuit of maximization* (pp. 81–100). Dordrecht, The Netherlands: Springer.

Bradburn, N. M. (1969). *The structure of psychological well-being*. Chicago: Aldine.

Broadie, S. (1991). *Ethics with Aristotle*. New York: Oxford University Press.
Broadie, S. (2007). *Aristotle and beyond: Essays on metaphysics and ethics*. Cambridge, UK: Cambridge University Press.
Brockman, J. (Ed.). (2015). *This idea must die: Scientific theories that are blocking progress [kindle]*. New York: Harper Collins.
Cabanac, M. (2009). *The fifth influence. The dialectics of pleasure*. Bloomington, IN: iUniverse.
Casebeer, W. D. (2003). *Natural ethical facts: Evolution, connectionism, and moral cognition*. New York: Cambridge University Press.
Cooper, J. (1975). *Reason and human good in Aristotle*. Cambridge, MA: Harvard University Press.
Delle Fave, A. (2013). The exploration of happiness: Present and future perspectives. In A. Delle Fave (Ed.), *The exploration of happiness* (pp. 3–14). Dordrecht, The Netherlands: Springer.
Dennett, D. C. (1995). *Darwin's dangerous idea: Evolution and the meanings of life*. New York: Simon & Schuster.
Diener, E. (1984). Subjective well-being. *Psychological Bulletin, 95*, 542–575.
Diener, E., & Tov, W. (2012). National accounts of well-being. In K. C. Land, A. C. Michalos, & M. J. Sirgy (Eds.), *Handbook of social indicators and quality of life research* (pp. 137–157). Dordrecht, The Netherlands: Springer.
Disabato, D. J., Goodman, F. R., Kashdan, T. B., Short, J. L., & Jarden, A. (2016). Different types of well-being? A cross-cultural examination of hedonic and eudaimonic well-being. *Psychological Assessment, 28*, 471-482. doi:10.1037/pas0000209.
Donaldson, S. I., Dollwet, M., Rao, M. A. (2015). Happiness, excellence, and optimal human functioning revisited: Examining the peer-reviewed literature linked to positive psychology. *Journal of Positive Psychology 10*, 185–195.
Eliot, G. (1985). *Middlemarch*. New York: Bantham Books. Original work published 1871–1872.
Evans, J. S. B. T., & Over, S. E. (1996). *Rationality and reasoning*. Sussex, UK: Psychology Press.
Fishman, S. M., & McCarthy, L. (2013). Conflicting uses of 'happiness' and the human condition. *Educational Philosophy and Theory, 45*, 509–515. doi:10.1111/j.1469-5812.2012.00856.x.
Flanagan, O. (2007). *The really hard problem. Meaning in a material world*. London: The MIT Press.
Foot, P. (2001). *Natural goodness*. Oxford, UK: Oxford University Press.
Frankl, V. (1945). *Man's search for meaning. An introduction to logotheraphy*. New York: Washington Square Press.
Frankl, V. (1970). *The will to meaning*. New York: Plume.
Fredrickson, B. L. (1998). What good are positive emotions? *Review of General Psychology, 2*, 300–319.
Fredrickson, B. L. (2013). Positive emotions broaden and build. In D. Patricia & P. Ashby (Eds.), *Advances in experimental social psychology* (Vol. 47, pp. 1–53). Burlington, MA: Academic Press.
Gallagher, M. W., Lopez, S. J., & Preacher, K. J. (2009). The hierarchical structure of well-being. *Journal of Personality, 77*, 1025–1049.
Glatzer, W. (2015). Monitoring and analyzing quality of life – an introduction. In W. Glatzer, L. Camfield, V. Møller, & M. Rojas (Eds.), *Global handbook of quality of life: Exploration of well-being of nations and continents* (pp. 1–11). Dordrecht, The Netherlands: Springer.
Griffin, J. (1986). *Well-being. Its meaning, measurement, and moral importance*. Oxford, UK: Clarendon.
Griffin, J. (2007). What do happiness studies study? *Journal of Happiness Studies, 8*, 139–148.
Gurin, G., Veroff, J., & Feld, S. (1960). *Americans view their mental health*. New York: Basic Books.
Halusic, M., & King, L. A. (2013). What makes life meaningful: Positive mood works in a pinch. In K. D. Markman, T. Proulx, & M. J. Lindberg (Eds.), *The psychology of meaning* (pp. 445–464). Washington, DC: American Psychological Association.
Harris, S. (2010). *The moral landscape: How science can determine human value*. London: Bantam Press.
Haybron, D. M. (2000). Two philosophical problems in the study of happiness. *Journal of Happiness Studies, 1*, 207–225.
Haybron, D. M. (2008). *The pursuit of unhappiness. The elusive psychology of well-being*. Oxford, UK: Oxford University Press.
Haybron, D. M. (2011). Happiness. In E. N. Zalta (Ed.), *The Stanford encyclopedia of philosophy*. Stanford, USA: Stanford University Press. Available from: http://plato.stanford.edu/archives/fall2011/entries/happiness.
Haybron, D. M. (2013). The nature and significance of happiness. In S. David, I. Boniwell, & A. C. Ayers (Eds.), *The Oxford handbook of happiness* (pp. 303–314). Oxford, UK: Oxford University Press.
Heller, A. S., van Reekum, C. M., Schaefer, S. M., Lapate, R. C., Radler, B. T., Ryff, C. D., et al. (2013). Sustained striatal activity predicts eudaimonic well-being and cortisol output. *Psychological Science, 24*, 2191–2200. doi:10.1177/0956797613490744.
Henderson, L. W., & Knight, T. (2012). Integrating the hedonic and eudaimonic perspectives to more comprehensively understand wellbeing and pathways to well-being. *International Journal of Wellbeing, 2*, 196–221. doi:10.5502/ijw.v2i3.3.
Hudson, D. W. (1996). *Happiness and the limits of satisfaction*. London: Rowman & Littlefield Publishers.
Huppert, F. (2005). Positive mental health in individuals and populaitions. In F. Huppert, N. Baylis, & B. Keverne (Eds.), *The science of well-being* (pp. 307–340). Oxford, UK: Oxford University Press.
Hursthouse, R. (2013). Virtue ethics. In E. N. Zalta (Ed.), *The Stanford encyclopedia of philosophy* (Spring 2014 ed.). Available from: https://leibniz.stanford.edu/friends/members/preview/ethics-virtue/

Huta, V. (2013). Pursuing eudaimonia versus hedonia: Distinctions, similarities, and relationships. In A. Waterman (Ed.), *The best within us. Positive psychology perspectives on eudaimonia* (pp. 19–38). Washington, DC: American Psychological Association.
Huta, V., & Waterman, A. S. (2014). Eudaimonia and its distinction from hedonia: Developing a classification and terminology for understanding conceptual and operational definitions. *Journal of Happiness Studies, 15*, 1425–1456. doi:10.1007/s10902-013-9485-0.
Jevons, W. S. (1890). *Pure logic and other minor works*. London: Macmillan.
Jost, L. J. (2002). Introduction. In L. J. Jost & R. A. Shiner (Eds.), *Eudaimonia and well-being* (pp. ix–xxxiii). Kelowna, Canada: Academic Printing & Publishing.
Kahneman, D. (2011). *Thinking, fast and slow*. New York: Penguin Books.
Kahneman, D. (2012). A machine for jumping to conclusions. *APA Monitor, 43*(2), 24-27. Retrieved from http://www.apa.org/monitor/2012/02/conclusions.aspx
Kahneman, D., & Deaton, A. (2010). High income improves evaluation of life but not emotional well-being. *Proceedings of the National Academy of Sciences, 107*, 16489–16493.
Kahneman, D., Diener, E., & Schwarz, N. (Eds.). (1999). *Well-being: The foundations of hedonic psychology*. New York: Russel-Sage.
Kahneman, D., & Riis, J. (2005). Living, and thinking about it: Two perspectives on life. In F. Huppert, N. Baylis, & B. Keverne (Eds.), *The science of well-being* (pp. 285–304). Oxford, UK: Oxford University Press.
Kapteyn, A., Lee, J., Tassot, C., Vonkova, H., & Zamarro, G. (2015). Dimensions of subjective well-being. *Social Indicators Research, 123*, 625–660. doi:10.1007/s11205-014-0753-0.
Kashdan, T. B., Biswas-Diener, R., & King, L. A. (2008). Reconsidering happiness: The costs of distinguishing between hedonics and eudaimonia. *The Journal of Positive Psychology, 3*, 219–233.
Kelley, T. L. (1927). *Interpretation of educational measurements*. Oxford, UK: World Book.
Kesebir, P., & Diener, E. (2008). In pursuit of happiness: Empirical answers to philosophical questions. *Perspectives on Psychological Science, 3*, 117–125. doi:10.1111/j.1745-6916.2008.00069.x.
Keyes, C. L. M., & Annas, J. (2009). Feeling good and functioning well: Distinctive concepts in ancient philosophy and contemporary science. *Journal of Positive Psychology, 4*, 197–201.
Keynes, J. M. (1936). *The general theory of employment, interest and money*. London: Macmillan.
Kimiecik, J. (2011). Exploring the promise of eudaimonic well-being within the practice of health promotion: The "how" is as important as the "what". *Journal of Happiness Studies, 12*, 769–792. doi:10.1007/s10902-010-9226-6.
King, L. A. (2008). Interventions for enhancing subjective well-being. Can we make people happier, and should we? In M. Eid & R. J. Larsen (Eds.), *The science of subjective well-being* (pp. 431–448). New York: Guilford Press.
King, L. A., & Hicks, J. A. (2009). Detecting and constructing meaning in life events. *The Journal of Positive Psychology, 4*, 317–330.
King, L. A., Hicks, J. A., Krull, J. L., & Gasio, A. K. (2006). Positive affect and the experience of meaning in life. *Journal of Personality and Social Psychology, 90*, 179–196.
Kraut, R. (2010). Aristotle's ethics. In E.N. Zalta (Ed.), *The Stanford encyclopedia of philosophy* (Summer 2010 ed.). Available from: http://plato.stanford.edu/archives/sum2010/entries/aristotle-ethics/
Kringelbach, M. L., & Berridge, K. C. (2009). Towards a functional neuroanatomy of pleasure and happiness. *Trends in Cognitive Sciences, 13*, 479–487. doi:10.1016/j.tics.2009.08.006.
Kristjánsson, K. (2013). *Virtues and vices in positive psychology*. New York: Cambridge University Press.
Levi-Strauss, C. (1966). *The savage mind*. Chicago: University of Chicago Press.
Linley, P. A. (2013). Human strengths and well-being: Finding the best within us at the intersection of eudaimonic philosophy, humanistic psychology, and positive psychology. In A. Waterman (Ed.), *The best witin us: Positive psychology perspectives on eudaimonia* (pp. 269–285). Washington, DC: American Psychological Association.
MacIntyre, A. (1981). *After virtue* (Vol. 99). Notre Dame, IN: University of Notre Dame Press.
Mayr, E. (1982). *The growth of biological thought. Diversity, evolution, and inheritance*. Cambridge, MA: Harvard University Press.
McMahon, D. (2006). *The pursuit of happiness. A history from the Greeks to the present*. London: Allen Lane.
Megone, C. (1994). Quality of life: Starting from Aristotle. In S. Baldwin, C. Godfrey, & C. Propper (Eds.), *Quality of life: Perspectives and policies* (pp. 28–41). London: Routledge.
Michalos, A. C., & Robinson, S. R. (2012). The good life: Eighth century to third century BCE. In K. C. Land, A. C. Michalos, & M. J. Sirgy (Eds.), *Handbook of social indicators and quality of life research* (pp. 23–61). Dordrecht, The Netherlands: Springer.
Michell, J. (2013). Constructs, inferences, and mental measurement. *New Ideas in Psychology, 31*, 13–21. doi:http://dx.doi.org/10.1016/j.newideapsych.2011.02.004.
Nagel, T. (1972). Aristotle on eudaimonia. *Phronesis, 17*, 252–259.
Naor, N., Ben-Ze'ev, A., & Okon-Singer, H. (2014). The modern search for the Holy Grail: Is neuroscience a solution? *Frontiers in Human Neuroscience, 8*, 388. doi:10.3389/fnhum.2014.00388.
Nersessian, N. J. (2008). *Creating scientific concepts*. Cambridge, MA: MIT Press.

Norton, D. L. (1976). *Personal destinies: A philosophy of ethical individualism*. Princeton, NJ: Princeton University Press.
Nussbaum, M. C. (2001). *Upheavals of thought. The intelligence of emotions*. New York: Cambridge University Press.
Nussbaum, M. C. (2008). Who is the happy warrior? Philosophy poses questions to psychology. *The Journal of Legal Studies, 37*, s81–s113.
OECD. (2013). *OECD Guidelines on measuring subjective well-being*. Retrieved from http://dx.doi.org/10.1787/9789264191655-en
Oishi, S. (2010). Culture and well-being: Conceptual and methodological issues. In E. Diener, J. F. Helliwell, & D. Kahneman (Eds.), *International differences in well-being* (pp. 34–69). Oxford, UK: Oxford University Press.
Oishi, S. (2012). *The psychological wealth of nations. Do happy people make a happy society?* Sussex, UK: Wiley-Blackwell.
Open Science Collaboration. (2015). Estimating the reproducibility of psychological science. *Science, 349*, aac4716-4711–aac4716-4718. doi:10.1126/science.aac4716.
Osgood, C. E., Suci, G. J., & Tannenbaum, P. H. (1957). *The measurement of meaning*. Urbana, IL: University of Illinois Press.
Peterson, C., & Seligman, M. E. P. (2004). *Strengths and virtues: A handbook and classification*. Washington, DC: American Psychological Association.
Philippe, F. L., Koestner, R., Beaulieu-Pelletier, G., Lecours, S., & Lekes, N. (2012). The role of episodic memories in current and future well-being. *Personality and Social Psychology Bulletin, 38*, 505–519. doi:10.1177/0146167211429805.
Popper, K. R. (1963). *Conjectures and refutations. The growth of scientific knowledge*. London: Routledge and Kegan Paul.
Proctor, C., Tweed, R., & Morris, D. (2015). The naturally emerging structure of well-being among young adults: "Big Two" or other framework? *Journal of Happiness Studies, 16*, 257–275. doi:10.1007/s10902-014-9507-6.
Qizilbash, M. (1997). Needs, incommensurability and well-being. *Review of Political Economy, 9*, 261–276. doi:10.1080/751245295.
Rapley, M. (2003). *Quality of life research: A critical introduction*. London: Sage.
Rogers, C. R. (1963). The concept of the fully functioning person. *Psychotherapy: Theory, Research & Practice, 1*, 17–26. doi:10.1037/h0088567.
Ross, W. D. (2009). *Aristotle: The nicomachean ethics*. Oxford, UK: Oxford University Press.
Russell, D. C. (2013). Virtue ethics, happiness, and the good life. In D. C. Russell (Ed.), *The Cambridge companion to virtue ethics [kindle version]* (pp. 7–28). Cambridge, UK: Cambridge University Press.
Ryan, R. M., & Deci, E. D. (2001). On happiness and human potentials: A review of research on hedonic and eudaimonic well-being. *Annual Review of Psychology, 52*, 141–166.
Ryff, C. D. (1989). Happiness is everything, or is it? Explorations on the meaning of psychological well-being. *Journal of Personality and Social Psychology, 57*, 1069–1081. doi:10.1037/0022-3514.57.6.1069.
Ryff, C. D., & Singer, B. H. (2008). Know thyself and become what you are: A eudaimonic approach to psychological well-being. *Journal of Happiness Studies, 9*, 13–39.
Schimmack, U. (2008). The structure of subjective well-being. In M. Eid & R. J. Larsen (Eds.), *The science of subjective well-being* (pp. 97–123). New York: Guilford Press.
Schueller, S. P., & Seligman, M. E. P. (2010). Pursuit of pleasure, engagement, and meaning: Relationships to subjective and objective measures of well-being. *Journal of Positive Psychology, 5*, 253–263.
Seligman, M. E. P. (2011). *Flourish. A visionary new understanding of happiness and well-being [kindle version]*. New York: Free Press.
Sheldon, K. M. (2014). Becoming oneself: The central role of self-concordant goal selection. *Personality and Social Psychology Review, 18*, 349–365. doi:10.1177/1088868314538549.
Steger, M. F., Frazier, P., Oishi, S., & Kaler, M. (2006). The meaning in life questionnaire: Assessing the presence of and search for meaning in life. *Journal of Counseling Psychology, 53*, 80–93. doi:10.1037/0022-0167.53.1.80.
Steger, M. F., & Kashdan, T. B. (2006). Stability and specificity of meaning in life and life satisfaction over one year. *Journal of Happiness Studies, 8*, 161–179. doi:10.1007/s10902-006-9011-8.
Stiglitz, J. E., Sen, A., & Fitoussi, J.-P. (2009). *Report by the commission on the measurement of economic performance and social progress*. Paris: Commission on the Measurement of Economic Performance and Social Progress. Retrieved from, http://www.stiglitz-sen-fitoussi.fr/en/index.htm.
Stone, A. A., & Mackie, C. (2013). *Subjective well-being: Measuring happiness, suffering, and other dimensions of experience*. Washington, DC: National Academies Press.
Su, R., Tay, L., & Diener, E. (2014). The development and validation of the Comprehensive Inventory of Thriving (CIT) and the Brief Inventory of Thriving (BIT). *Applied Psychology: Health and Well-Being, 6*, 251–279. doi:10.1111/aphw.12027.
Sumner, L. W. (1996). *Welfare, happiness, and ethics*. Oxford, UK: Clarendon Press.
Sumner, L. W. (2002). Happiness then and now. In L. J. Jost & R. A. Shiner (Eds.), *Eudaimonia and well-being* (pp. 21–39). Kelowna, Canada: Academic Printing & Publishing.
Tatarkiewicz, W. (1976). *Analysis of happiness*. The Hague, Netherlands: Nijhoff.
Telfer, E. (1980). *Happiness*. New York: St. Martin's Press.
Thagard, P. (1992). *Conceptual revolutions*. Princeton, NJ: Princeton University Press.
Thagard, P. (2012). *The cognitive science of science*. Cambridge, MA: The MIT Press.

Thin, N. (2012). *Social happiness. Theory into policy and practice*. Bristol, UK: The Policy Press.

Thorndike, E. L. (1913). *An introduction to the theory of mental and social measurements* (2nd ed.). New York: Teachers College Press (Original work published 1904).

Tiberius, V. (2013). Recipes for a good life: Eudaimonism and the contribution of philosophy. In A. Waterman (Ed.), *The best within us. Positive psychology perspectives on eudaimonia* (pp. 19–38). Washington, DC: American Psychological Association.

Tolstoy, L. (1993). *Anna Karenina*. New York: Random House (Original work published 1878).

Vallerand, R. J. (2012). The role of passion in sustainable psychological well-being. *Psychology of Well-Being: Theory, Research and Practice, 2*, 1–21. doi:10.1186/2211-1522-2-1.

Veenhoven, R. (2013). Notions of the good life. In S. David, I. Boniwell, & A. C. Ayers (Eds.), *The Oxford handbook of happiness* (pp. 161–173). Oxford, UK: Oxford University Press.

Waterman, A. S. (1984). *The psychology of individualism*. New York: Praeger.

Waterman, A. S. (1993). Two conceptions of happiness: Contrasts of personal expressiveness (eudaimonia) and hedonic enjoyment. *Journal of Personality and Social Psychology, 64*, 678–691. doi:10.1037/0022-3514.64.4.678.

Waterman, A. S. (2008). Reconsidering happiness: A eudaimonist's perspective. *Journal of Positive Psychology, 3*, 234–252.

White, N. (2006). *A brief history of happiness*. Oxford, UK: Blackwell.

Wong, P. T. P. (2011). Positive psychology 2.0: Towards a balanced interactive model of the good life. *Canadian Psychology/Psychologie Canadienne, 52*, 69–81. doi:10.1037/a0022511.

Part I

Philosophical Eudaimonism

The Philosophical Basis of Eudaimonic Psychology

2

Daniel M. Haybron

2.1 Introduction[1]

A recent collection of papers on eudaimonic psychology sports a pair of photographs on its cover: one of an acorn, and the other of a grove of healthy-looking old oaks (Waterman, 2013). Many observers have noted, and lamented, the lack of consensus among eudaimonic researchers about what their measures of well-being should look like. There is, as well, a decided lack of philosophical clarity about the motivation behind these metrics, despite the admirable efforts of psychologists in this area to engage seriously with the philosophical literature. Yet for all that, there is a cluster of recurrent themes in this field that resonate far beyond academic circles, and there is arguably a coherent philosophical core behind it. And that book cover aptly depicts the ideal in question: of well-being as the realization of one's potential. *Flourishing*, in the fullest sense of the term.

That, at any rate, is what I will propose in this chapter. The proposal is hardly radical: most if not all authors in this area have made similar claims. But the philosophical justification for such contentions remains unclear, and the connection between this root ideal and the particular measures employed by eudaimonic researchers is often somewhat mysterious. As well, there are important, and often underappreciated, theoretical choices to be made within the eudaimonic approach. Finally, the need for eudaimonic metrics, and their relation to measures of subjective well-being, could also be a good deal clearer.

In what follows I will first discuss the philosophical tradition from which eudaimonic psychology draws inspiration, "welfare eudaimonism."[2] Eudaimonistic accounts of well-being center on ideals of nature-fulfillment, which have distinctive attractions and draw similar objections, but also can vary widely. Aristotle's account is just one member of a diverse family of theories, which divide notably on several key questions, such as the role of virtue or species membership in well-being. The second half of this chapter discusses eudaimonic measures of well-being: what the

[1]I am grateful to Joar Vittersø and an anonymous referee for helpful feedback on an earlier version of this chapter.

[2]That is, eudaimonism about well-being. As noted below, this is simply a view of well-being and is distinct from, e.g., ethical eudaimonism, which takes all of ethics to be grounded in eudaimonia. Ancient eudaimonists tended to hold both views, but one could be a eudaimonist about well-being while rejecting the ancients' effort to ground morality in the individual's own well-being. Mill is arguably a good example of a welfare eudaimonist, though he was certainly not an ethical eudaimonist.

D.M. Haybron (✉)
Saint Louis University, St. Louis, MO, USA
e-mail: haybrond@slu.edu

J. Vittersø (ed.), *Handbook of Eudaimonic Well-Being*, International Handbooks of Quality-of-Life,
DOI 10.1007/978-3-319-42445-3_2

rationale for such measures might be, and what form they should take. I sketch a core schema for eudaimonic scales that outlines what seem to be the most important sorts of indicators for eudaimonic instruments to include, nearly all of which are already highly prominent in the empirical literature. The actual task of scale design is of course best done by empirical researchers, who will also want to vary the schema according to their theoretical inclinations and operational needs. But I hope to make it clear that eudaimonic psychology is a more coherent and principled enterprise, than has often been supposed.

Before proceeding, some terminological clarity would be helpful. 'Well-being', 'welfare', 'flourishing' and 'eudaimonia' will be the terms used for the kind of value in question here, namely prudential value, which concerns matters of benefit and harm. While 'happiness' is frequently employed, particularly in discussions of eudaimonistic theories and translations of historical work, as a further term for this value, I will usually restrict the term to its purely descriptive contemporary meaning, where it refers simply to a psychological condition. Whereas Aristotelians take it to be obvious that "happiness" in the well-being sense is all that matters for human welfare—indeed it seems to be a tautology—they are less enthusiastic about the importance of "happiness" in the psychological sense: one might be happy in an experience machine, say, yet have a pathetic life—happy, yet failing to lead a happy *life*, in the well-being sense of the term.

I will follow the usual practice of using 'eudaimonic' to denote, among other things, the empirical research paradigm that interests us in this volume. The related philosophical accounts of well-being such as Aristotle's, however, I will term 'eudaimonist' or 'eudaimonistic', as this usage is more standard in the philosophical literature and helps us keep the distinction between the empirical and philosophical schools in view. Similarly, 'hedonic' is normally used when referring to an approach in psychology as well as a kind of mental state or value, whereas the associated philosophical doctrines are usually characterized as 'hedonistic'.

2.2 The Approach

Eudaimonic psychologists claim inspiration from Aristotle and other philosophers in the eudaimonist tradition of ancient Greece. In this tradition, ethical theories were founded on the notion of *eudaimonia*—that is, well-being or flourishing.[3] Specifically, *ethical eudaimonism* grounds morality and other values in the agent's own well-being: the ultimate reason to be virtuous, for instance, is that you need to be virtuous to flourish. Epicurus, for instance, thought injustice would render life unpleasant, so we should be just for that reason. This does not mean that we should be focused on our own well-being in everyday practice, only that morality and other values ultimately matter because they are good for us. Eudaimonistic ethics, then, offers a general framework for living founded on the notion of well-being.

For our purposes, the more important question is: *what is well-being*? In principle, eudaimonists could endorse any theory of well-being, since 'eudaimonia' just was the ancient Greek term for well-being, and commonsense Greek views of eudaimonia were varied and sometimes low-minded, just as people today have many different views about the happy life. Eudaimonist philosophers too held diverse opinions: Aristotle and the Stoics, for example, identified well-being roughly with virtue, while Epicurean hedonists equated it

[3]Perhaps the best survey of ancient eudaimonism is (Annas, 1993). Since 'eudaimonia' just was the ancient Greek term for well-being, rather than a term for a certain view of well-being, it is slightly odd to talk about "eudaimonistic" or "eudaimonic" theories of well-being, since one might just as well call them eudaimonistic theories of eudaimonia! I use it here to denote theories of well-being that exhibit characteristic features from the ancient tradition.

with pleasure. In their basic content, these views could hardly be more different.[4]

If even a hedonist can be a eudaimonist, then what makes a theory of well-being eudaimonistic—an instance of what I'll call *welfare eudaimonism*? Philosophers are divided on this question, with many using the term to denote theories that identify well-being with virtue; this usage has the awkward result that many ancient eudaimonists, like Epicureans, did not have eudaimonistic accounts of well-being. A second option is to deem theories eudaimonistic if they figure in a eudaimonistic ethical theory, in which moral and other norms are all grounded in the individual's well-being. But this makes the characterization of a theory of well-being entirely dependent on how it is used in a broader ethical theory, and independent of what the theory itself is like. If you just want to know what well-being is, and haven't committed to any particular moral theory, this sort of classification isn't going to be helpful. Maybe you favor a kind of Aristotelian theory of well-being, but want to use it in a deontological moral theory. In that case, the theory ceases to be eudaimonistic.

A third option seems preferable: focus on the main feature that seemed to be shared by all accounts of well-being in the eudaimonist tradition: the teleological idea that well-being consists in *nature-fulfillment*: the fulfillment of one's nature (Annas, 1993). Nature-fulfillment theories ground well-being in facts about how we are constituted, and so tie their ideals of well-being to views about human nature, or the self. To flourish, on this sort of approach, is to live in accordance with the sort of being one is. Where theorists disagree is on what the relevant nature is, what we are actually like, and what it means to fulfill those natures. Epicureans regard human beings as fundamentally pleasure-seekers whose nature is accordingly fulfilled in the pleasant life. Whereas Aristotelians view us as essentially rational and active, so that our well-being centers on rational activity done well: a life of virtuous activity. Identifying welfare eudaimonism with nature-fulfillment views has the further benefit of fitting with eudaimonic psychology, which also seems to center on such ideals.

Thus understood, eudaimonistic accounts of well-being can be found in many traditions and historical periods into the contemporary period, including not just ancient Greeks and Romans and their contemporary followers but also—at least arguably—Thomists, Marxists, Hegelians, Mill, Green, Nietzsche, existentialists, Maslow, and today's eudaimonic psychologists, among many others. Welfare eudaimonism also appears at least in other quite different cultural settings, including Hindu ideals of self-realization, the writings of Mencius in China, and doubtless many other places.[5]

2.3 Objections

So diverse are eudaimonistic theories that one might ask what the alternatives could be. In fact, most modern theorizing about well-being has done without any clear reliance on teleological notions of nature-fulfillment. The main alternatives are (most modern forms of) *hedonism*, *desire* theories, and *list* theories of well-being (Crisp, 2005). Typically, these views are defended on grounds having no apparent connection with nature-fulfillment. Most modern hedonists, for instance, might just point to the intuitive appearance that pleasure and suffering matter for what they are like, as experiences. They need not stake any claims about human nature, or about what people ultimately seek, as Epicureans did.[6] (Mill

[4]Epicureans indeed went to great lengths to argue for a strong link between well-being and virtue, but this was an (extremely bold and likely false) empirical claim. Today's Benthamite hedonists can make it as well, if they wish, but it is no part of their philosophical theory about the nature of well-being, as it is for Aristotelians and the like.

[5]For some recent philosophical discussions, see (Annas, 1993; Besser-Jones, 2014, 2015; Brink, 2003, 2013; Feinberg, 1992; Gewirth, 1998; Haybron, 2007, 2008a, 2008b; Hurka, 1993; Keyes & Annas, 2009; Kim, 2015; LeBar, 2013; Russell, 2013; Tiberius, 2013).

[6]This is not to say that they don't tacitly rely on substantial views of human nature or even eudaimonistic ideals. The point is just that they can and typically do defend their position without harnessing it to claims about what is essential to, characteristic of…human beings. For

seems to be a notable exception here, as his discussion of individuality in *On Liberty* is a paradigm defense of an ideal of nature-fulfillment, with a distinctly modern, individualistic spin on it.) Desire theorists, for their part, might focus on grounds like agent sovereignty: what's ultimately good for us has to be for us to decide. The rationale has to do with a commitment to subjectivist principles, not eudaimonist ones. Finally, list theorists simply identify well-being with some list of ultimate goods, such as friendship, accomplishment, knowledge, pleasure, and so forth. Other than intuitive plausibility, there may be no further rationale for the theory: these things just matter, period, and not as fulfillments of our nature.

Eudaimonistic approaches to well-being, then, appear to be in the minority among contemporary scholars. Opposition to welfare eudaimonism takes at least three major forms, one being that it somehow implicates us in a "naturalistic fallacy," deriving normative conclusions from descriptive facts about human nature. From the fact that something is part of our nature, for instance, it doesn't follow that fulfilling it is good. Maybe human nature is something we are supposed to rise above, as Katharine Hepburn proclaimed in *The African Queen*. But nature-fulfillment theories need not involve such mistakes, and few contemporary eudaimonists seem to make them: theorists standardly recognize the need to develop a substantive account of which aspects of our natures are ethically significant and which are not. They do not assume that human nature, or the self, is a biological given from which we can mechanically derive norms. It is also important to recognize that from the fact that something is good *for* a person, it does not follow that it is good, period, or that there is good reason to do it. One might think a happy Comanche warrior a paradigm of human flourishing, yet deem his ruthless treatment of outsiders deeply immoral, and hence disapprove of his way of life. (This would not of course be a move Aristotle could sanction, but again, welfare eudaimonists can depart from his views in many ways.)

A second objection has to do with the *teleological* character of eudaimonistic theories: teleology is widely thought to be a relic of pre-modern metaphysics, discredited by modern science. Nature does not have purposes built into it. This sort of objection may indeed have force against many pre-modern eudaimonists like Aristotle, whose ethical views were embedded in a teleological metaphysics that most contemporaries reject. But again, most eudaimonists today take their teleology to be part and parcel of their broader ethical theories, not a freestanding fact gifted us by biology, physics or whatever. *Self-fulfillment* theories, for instance, take nature-fulfillment to focus on the fulfillment of those features of us that define the self: who one is.[7] But philosophical accounts of the self tend not to posit a distinct entity, a "self," in their ontologies, akin to an immaterial soul. They might simply be identifying certain aspects of our psychologies that seem particularly important to us, playing a certain role in the way we think about each other.

Another way to look at it is to note that every theory of well-being faces deep metaphysical problems: desire theories might seem unmysterious, because one might think they need posit only desires, along with states of desire-fulfillment. Yet they must also posit something further: that

---

instance, you can simply point to the pleasantness of pleasant experience and say, *that* is what matters; and the reason it matters is simply because of its phenomenal quality. The claim that prudential value is grounded in the quality of experience is completely independent of any views about human nature, since it isn't a claim about human beings at all. It certainly doesn't rest on any interesting claims about human nature, the way Aristotelian theories do.

[7] The notion of self-fulfillment seems to figure at least tacitly in many if not most modern nature-fulfillment views, for instance those of the existentialists, humanistic psychologists, and Mill. The use of this notion is made explicit in, e.g., (Haybron, 2008a, 2008b; Yelle, 2014). Complicating matters is that many authors use 'self-fulfillment' and similar terms loosely, as roughly equivalent to nature-fulfillment, without clearly linking them to the notion of the self. As I use the terms here, it is quite possible to hold a nature-fulfillment theory that, say, bases well-being on species norms without coupling this view in some way to an account of the self, or even thinking that there need be any such coupling. This would not be a self-fulfillment view, as understood here.

desire-fulfillment is *valuable*, is *worth* pursuing for one's own sake, or the sake of one's child, that we have *reason* to care about it (instead of, say, Aristotelian excellence), etc. Making sense of such claims is one of the deepest metaphysical problems in philosophy, and desire theories have the problem no less than Stoic accounts, or any other theory of well-being. All of us need to solve it, and once we've dealt with that problem, it is not obvious that the needed teleology couldn't come along for the ride. For example, many theorists of a naturalistic bent loosely follow Hume in taking value to be somehow a product of human sensibilities—something we project on the world, for example. If that's right, then why couldn't value take a teleological form? Perhaps human beings tend to project value according to a teleological paradigm. We see wolves, for instance, as having a certain nature, and wolf flourishing as involving the fulfillment of that nature: living in packs, and hunting. A wolf locked alone in a cage, even if drugged to be happy, might seem to be languishing, a sad waste of potential—not because of any weird physical or supernatural reality that is being contravened, but simply because that's how we are wired to think about the living world. Note, in this connection, that teleological language is common in biology: hearts and other organs have functions, for instance. Indeed, a plausible conjecture is that biologists, at least in certain fields like ecology, tend tacitly to assume a eudaimonistic approach to well-being—the happily drugged caged wolf, for instance, seems unlikely to inspire joy in many biologist's hearts. Similarly, suggestions by animal welfare advocates that it might be desirable to end predation tend to elicit howls of outrage from biologists, and probably not just because they betray a stupendous ignorance of biology. They may also take offense at the notion that a world of lupine Lotus Eaters, cheerfully lazing about munching on drug-laced wolf chow, is something to be welcomed.

The third objection to eudaimonistic approaches is that ideas like nature-fulfillment or self-fulfillment are simply too *obscure*. Even if one can live with the idea of teleology, one might doubt that it has enough, or clear enough, content to be a useful guide to theorizing. The notion of the self, for instance, is notoriously unclear and difficult to adjudicate. To found a theory of well-being on the idea of the self-fulfillment, then, may seem to involve a leap from frying pan to fire. This is a sensible concern, but the proof is in the pudding: what do eudaimonistic theories actually look like? If you can give a reasonably clear, principled and persuasive defense of a nature-fulfillment theory of well-being, then who cares if the project sounded unpromising in the abstract? Note as well that philosophical theorizing often appeals to some fundamental rationale that, at the start of inquiry, lacks a very clear or determinate content. Many opponents of eudaimonism, for instance, begin from a *subjectivist* ideal: well-being must be fundamentally grounded in the person's subjectivity. But what this means is also obscure and up for grabs: for some, it has to do with what the person's experience is like—thus perhaps favoring hedonism—while for others it concerns what the individual cares about—thus perhaps favoring a desire theory. But there are other interpretations, and even these readings need further specification—a fiendishly difficult task to pull off while still getting a believable theory of well-being. (How, for instance, do you respect both the idea that people are sovereign about their welfare and the obvious fact that people make mistakes?)

2.4 Attractions

2.4.1 Four Theoretical Virtues

The basic idea of grounding well-being in some ideal of nature-fulfillment has several major attractions. First, it seems to fit well with common ways of thinking about the living world, which are rife with teleological notions. Biologists and laypeople alike freely attribute functions to hearts and other biological entities, and as the wolf example illustrates, very many of us seem at least tacitly committed to eudaimonistic ideals in the way we think about well-being in living things. (Recall also the acorn analogy with which we started, variants of which might prove to be near-universal across cultures.) Second, eudaimonism offers an appealingly unified approach to thinking about flourishing across different life forms. The same basic theory applies to oaks, wolves and human beings, differing in each case because of differences in the organisms' natures. Hedonists and desire theorists, by contrast, have a harder time extending their views beyond a limited class of cases, and seem committed to denying that anything can be good or bad for nonsentient organisms. (And if your account of well-being is grounded in an ideal of agent sovereignty, what do you say even about children and dogs?) Even among sentient creatures, one might doubt that such accounts are sensitive enough to the *differences* between organisms: whereas hedonists notoriously have difficulty distinguishing human well-being very strongly from cat well-being—both are just a matter of pleasant experience—eudaimonists can point to sharp differences in their natures, so that the same theoretical structure supports a strongly differentiated view of well-being for different kinds of living things.

A third point favoring eudaimonism also relates to its unifying power, allowing us to posit a plurality of ultimate goods while framing it in an elegant theoretical structure that offers a principled basis for including each item. Among objectivist theories, the main alternatives are list theories, which tend to be unsatisfying from a theoretical point of view, whatever their other virtues: they just posit some list of ultimate goods, such as knowledge, achievement, and love, typically with no further rationale than that, on reflection, they all seem to belong on the list. The result can seem like an unprincipled, ad hoc fabrication that also does little to explain why any of these things are good for us: what do knowledge and love, for instance, have in common such that they both belong on the list? Why these items, and not others? Eudaimonistic accounts can offer a principled answer: each, for instance, speaks to a different aspect of human nature.

Fourth, eudaimonistic theories can diminish worries about *alienation* that commonly attend objectivist approaches to well-being: such views allow that something could be part of our good even if we do not want or like it. This gives rise to objections that our good could be alien to us on such views, too divorced from our own concerns or perspectives to plausibly count as our good. Eudaimonistic forms of objectivism, however, at least ground well-being in the individual's nature: it is because of the kind of being I am that, say, accomplishment is good for me. It isn't just a brute fact that holds independently of what I am like. Aristotelians, for instance, might deem knowledge a good for us because of our status as human beings, whose nature is partly realized through it.

Whether one finds such claims persuasive or not, it is important to understand that objectivists need not be vulnerable to one common sort of alienation complaint: they need not, and generally do not, claim that you could be flourishing even if you hated your life. Virtually all major schools of thought maintain that ideally, our lives will be satisfying and pleasant. Aristotle deemed a life of virtuous activity to be the most pleasant life we could lead, and it essentially involves a wholehearted engagement with one's activities. What makes these views objective is perhaps better understood in terms of a negative claim: crudely, *certain things are such that their absence in one's life is something to be regretted, making one worse off, regardless of one's likes or wants.* To say that accomplishment is objectively good for us need not require saying that a life of accomplishment would be a happy life for you, even if you despised it. Perhaps it is also essential that you value it. It may only be to say that it is lamentable—bad for you—for your life to be devoid of accomplishment.

2.4.2 Two Substantive Virtues: Authenticity and Impoverishment

So far we've discussed the theoretical attractions of eudaimonism. It also has some substantive features that make it appealing to many. One has to do with common intuitions about the importance of *authenticity* for well-being—generally relating to what we might call the "be yourself" intuition.[8] Take, for instance, the Repressed Artist: a dutiful Victorian woman who subordinates her love of painting to lead a quiet, respectable life as a "good daughter and wife." Or, similarly, a gay man straitjacketed into a heterosexual lifestyle. Many find such cases problematic: these individuals are failing to express their true nature, living in conflict with who they are. The problem seems naturally expressed in terms of authenticity: their way of life frustrates the authentic expression of their personalities. The same sort of concern arises in cases of drug-based happiness (*soma*) or other manipulated forms of happiness, such as a happy lobotomy patient, or the subjects of certain future human enhancement technologies. Psychiatric contexts provide especially revealing examples of the role of authenticity ideals in everyday thinking. How people feel about antidepressant use, for instance, depends partly on whether they think their depressed mood reflects who they really are, or is rather a disorder suppressing their personalities, so that medication might either seem to undermine authenticity ("it's not really me") or enhance it ("I'm finally myself again").

The value of authenticity is quite at home in a eudaimonistic framework: we do not fulfill our natures, it seems, when living inauthentically. Standard varieties of hedonism and the desire theory, by contrast, seem unable to make sense of this intuition.[9] It is easy to underestimate the broad appeal of the notion of authenticity because the term itself tends to be associated with modern Western, individualistic cultural norms (as does the term 'self-fulfillment'). Yet authenticity has no essential link with individualism—in more collectivist cultures authenticity might take a highly relational, communal form such that "being yourself" requires a high degree of conformity to certain social roles, deference to elders, and attentiveness to the needs of the family or community rather than oneself. That's who you are, and you could no more authentically lead the freewheeling life of Venice Beach-style eccentricity than you could authentically be a Vulcan. But it needn't be all there is to you, and even non-individualistic cultures do not, as far as I am aware, regard family members and friends as indistinguishable and replaceable. Nor does it seem likely that people anywhere would be happy to have beloved Granny's brain scrambled, yielding a radically different personality, even if the result might otherwise have seemed an improvement. In New Delhi just as in New York, people probably want the people they care about, including themselves, to be themselves.

Concerns about authenticity are an important motivation for eudaimonistic approaches, but they have gotten far less attention in the literature than a different sort of worry, having to do with *impoverishment*, which we might crudely summarize as the "be all you can be" intuition. In a nutshell, the concern is that it seems possible to be happy in a stunted, impoverished life. Moreover, you might have no desire for anything more, and perhaps you'd be no happier in a richer, more well-rounded life. Impoverishment worries have taken many forms since at least Plato, who has Socrates inquire whether it would really be good to have the life of someone who is content to do nothing but scratch an itch all day, day in and day out (*Gorgias*), and elsewhere suggested that a life of nothing but pleasure would be the life of an oyster (*Philebus*). In Rawls, we encounter the specter of a man who finds happiness doing nothing but counting blades of grass, and in Foot, a lobotomy patient content just picking up leaves (Foot, 2001; Rawls, 1971). From a practical perspective, impoverishment worries take their best-known form in concerns that have been raised especially regarding adaptive preferences and related phenomena: happy slaves, oppressed housewives, and others who content themselves with "small mercies," as Sen put it (Elster, 1983; Nussbaum, 2000; Sen, 1987).

Contemporary interest in eudaimonic psychology, however, may be rooted more in worries

[8]This paragraph is adapted from "Eudaimonism, Ancient, and Modern" (ms).

[9](Haybron, 2008a, 2008b). A seminal account of authenticity in the context of well-being is (Sumner, 1996), whose "authentic happiness" theory centers on life satisfaction and rests on a subjectivist, rather than eudaimonist, foundation.

about life in the consumer society, where—at least according to popular stereotypes—one might pass a comfortable, contented yet pointless existence as a passive couch potato whose most challenging activity is a day at the shopping mall. Caricatures of this sort abound in popular culture, for instance in films like *Wall-E* or *Idiocracy*. Such thoughts tend to be associated with affluent intellectuals, but they are hardly confined to those circles: you might well spot a bow-hunting t-shirt proclaiming "live life at full draw" on a West Virginian who also enjoys monster truck rallies. For that matter, the U.S. Army probably was not aiming for the Harvard demographic in its "be all you can be" recruiting campaign. Such slogans illustrate the broad appeal of impoverishment's positive counterpart: a rich, fully realized life in which we exercise our capacities in worthwhile activities. I am unaware of data on this question, but it would not be surprising if the great majority of people valued such a life for themselves, across a wide range of cultures (and indeed ideals of self-realization are prominent in many traditions, such as Hindu thought). It may indeed be that eudaimonistic accounts of well-being accurately express the way most people think about well-being *in their own lives*—the minority status of such views owing substantially to a reluctance to "impose" such ideals on others. Who really watches *Idiocracy* and thinks, "right, that's the life for me"? (A reluctance to extend such reasoning to others may be confused, since one might hold an objective account of well-being, believing that people can be fundamentally mistaken about their own good, while insisting on others' right to pursue mistaken conceptions of the good, and even refusing in practice to pass judgment on others' views. Objectivists about well-being can be as committed to antipaternalistic principles as any subjectivist.)

2.5 Variants

2.5.1 Nature-Fulfillment: The Basic Idea, and Open Questions

The bare idea of well-being as nature-fulfillment gives us only this: that *certain facts about the sort of creature one is—one's nature—"point" to certain ideals, the fulfillment of which in turn constitutes one's well-being*. That is, certain ideals of well-being are implicit in the way one is constituted. To do well or flourish is to achieve those ideals: to fulfill one's nature. As noted above, the teleological "pointing" metaphor need not commit us to a teleological metaphysics where nature has supplied with the norms by which we are to live. The relevant conception of the facts about how we are constituted may itself already be informed by our values; or perhaps it is something we project onto the world.

Most varieties of welfare eudaimonism offer resources for addressing concerns about authenticity and impoverishment. But the approach can take a wide range of forms, and the next section discusses three of the most important theoretical choices facing eudaimonists:

1. Is virtue a fundamental constituent of well-being?
2. What is the basic structure of nature-fulfillment: capacity-fulfillment or goal-fulfillment?
3. Are the standards for well-being grounded entirely in the particular makeup of the subject, or in species norms or other subject-transcendent features?

2.5.2 The Role of Virtue: Perfectionism vs. Non-perfectionism

It is sometimes assumed that nature-fulfillment invariably takes the form of perfection: somehow becoming a better, more perfect version of the kind of being one is. Accordingly, some authors use 'perfectionism' as equivalent to 'welfare eudaimonism'. Yet this is a mistake: perfection is normally taken to refer to a kind of excellence or virtue. But the idea of nature-fulfillment need not take this form at all, as we see in the Epicurean case. Nature-fulfillment might simply involve the satisfaction of those desires or values that define who you are, or achieving the fulfillment of your emotional nature (say, being happy). Such views do not seem to involve any kind of perfection at all, yet they have the characteristic structure of eudaimonistic theories: they ground well-being in some prior account of the individual's nature, for instance the self. At any rate, this chapter will use 'perfectionism' to denote views that identify well-being somehow with excellence or virtue. To get a bead on what is meant by perfection, let's understand perfection—which in turn I'll treat as equivalent to excellence or virtue—broadly and roughly in terms of *that to which attitudes of admiration typically are* pro tanto *a fitting response*.[10] Aristotelian, Stoic and Platonic theories would be paradigm perfectionist theories, but again any theory that takes virtue or excellence to be a fundamental constituent of well-being will count.

Perfectionists normally understand virtue broadly, to include many kinds of non-moral excellence. But in the ancient eudaimonist tradition, perfectionists like Aristotle invariably placed a premium on moral virtue, since they could only defend the moral life on the grounds that it is somehow necessary to flourish. And it is on this question that the debate between perfectionist and non-perfectionist views takes its most familiar form: *can the wicked flourish, at least in principle*? Most moderns seem to think so, following Kant and the Utilitarians (Haybron, 2007, 2008b, 2013a). But intuitions divide on this question, and many people find it implausible that someone could profit from a life of immorality.

2.5.3 Two Ideals of Nature-Fulfillment: Actualization vs. Success

We know that nature-fulfillment views take many forms. But can we say more about their general structure? There seem to be two basic "sub-ideals" that theories can embody to one degree or another:[11]

1. Goal-fulfillment: success
2. Capacity-fulfillment: actualization

The ideal of capacity-fulfillment has to do with what we intuitively regard as realizing one's potential, or developing and exercising one's capacities—what I'll call *actualization* for short-hand (though "realization" would serve just as well). The acorn metaphor is one of the most familiar metaphors for this ideal, which in turn gives 'flourishing' much of its evocative power. And it is the notion of actualization that most plainly speaks to one of the chief attractions of eudaimonism, its apparent ability to address concerns about impoverished lives. Is capacity-fulfillment just the same thing as perfection? Or at least a genus, of which perfection is one species? Perhaps, but some of our interest in capacity-fulfillment is not obviously linked to issues of perfection or virtue, and vice-versa.

One way to see this is to consider the crude slogan associated with each ideal: "be all you can be," on the one hand, and "be the best you can be," on the other. These slogans can play out in different ways. Compare, for instance, the life of a brilliant and saintly medical researcher, who works long hours developing new medicines and has little time for other pursuits, with someone who leads a rich, active life involving sports, playing music, writing poetry, cooking, travel, socializing regularly with close friends, but nothing at any substantial degree of excellence or accomplishment. Someone might sensibly regard the latter person as leading a more fully actualized life, while the researcher exhibits greater excellence, both moral and nonmoral.[12] A third

[10]Resourcefulness, for instance, is a virtue to which admiration would typically be a fitting response, other things equal. When put in the service of immoral aims, however, admiration might not be called for.

[11]I am partly following Alan Gewirth here, but substituting 'goal-fulfillment' for 'aspiration-fulfillment', which has an overly narrow meaning (Gewirth, 1998), and further distinguishing perfection from the other two ideals.

[12]There's no consensus on exactly how to characterize the distinction between moral and nonmoral virtues. Roughly, when talking about character assessment (as opposed say to intellectual virtues), moral virtues concern at least our other-regarding obligations of, e.g., beneficence and

individual spends many years toiling in sweatshops and then, when her children are grown, incites a successful labor reform movement, for which she spends the rest of her life in a dank prison cell. She might have had little chance to develop, let alone exercise, her capacities, yet in crucial respects her life exhibits a high degree of perfection: it may indeed be morally exemplary. Readers may have varying responses to these three cases, but it should be clear enough that capacity-fulfillment and perfection or excellence are not *obviously* equivalent, and are profitably recognized as distinguishable ideals. Arguably, humanistic and eudaimonic psychologists have placed greater emphasis on capacity-fulfillment, while ancient and medieval eudaimonists focused more on perfection. The more admirable life—either morally, non-morally, or both—is not necessarily the more fully realized life. The eudaimonistic theorist needs to decide on an interpretation of nature-fulfillment that, if it employs these ideals at all, does so in a consistent and plausible manner.

This is not always easy. Aristotelians, in particular, seem to waver between "actualization" and "admirability" readings of their views, making for an elusive target. Much of the recent literature, for instance, emphasizes the importance of fulfilling our capacities, leading a full, rich, and richly human life.[13] Indeed, moral virtue seems nearly invisible in some writings. Yet it is essential to the orthodox Aristotelian approach that their account of flourishing gives an appropriate place in human life to *moral* virtue, because flourishing is the only place they can fit morality. And for most of us, morality is absolutely central to how we ought to live, in deciding which lives are choiceworthy and which are not. It is not obvious how to understand "virtuous activity" in an Aristotelian account of well-being so that it both gives morality its rightful place and makes good on the appealing idea that flourishing centers on richly exercising our capacities. For instance, a man who trades a very rich, highly actualized life for a much more cramped existence by taking in an orphaned child with severe disabilities (Haybron, 2008b, pp. 163–164). If Aristotelians put enough weight on the value of actualization, they can honor the appearance that he has sacrificed his interests in doing so; but how, then, can they still give sufficient weight to admirability, or moral virtue, which seems then to take a back seat to actualization? Would it then be ok to lie about one's merits, or even to murder, in order to beat a rival out for a scholarship that would enable escape from dire poverty into a life of many and varied accomplishments? Perhaps it is possible to answer these concerns; the point here is simply to note the tension and highlight the ways in which capacity-fulfillment and virtue might seem to diverge.

Nature-fulfillment can take a second form, which I'll call *goal-fulfillment*. Part of our constitution is not just that we have certain capacities, but that we have certain goals: we desire certain things, for instance. We can understand goals quite broadly, as something we may not always recognize in prospect but may rather discover only in retrospect: one way to have something as a goal is to be prone to meet it with joy, even if it never occurred to you to want it. Put another way, if you wanted to instill certain goals, such as companionship, into an organism, you might give it desires for those things; but you could also give it the propensity to be made happy by them, or unhappy by their absence. In fact, given that desires are often formed in ignorance of what their fulfillment would be like, the organism's evaluative response tendencies—what makes it happy or unhappy, brings it pleasure or pain—might be the most reliable metric of what its most important goals are. (People get all sorts of weird ideas about what's worth pursuing, but the things that make them happy tend to be less subject to whimsy.) Whereas merely giving an organism the *capacity* to do something seems not to be a way of giving it a goal at all. This might indeed be

justice, and arguably relate to how good or bad a person one is. Nonmoral virtues include, e.g. wit, resourcefulness, persistence, fortitude, grit, and concern norms that we don't ordinarily regard as moral norms (and might indeed be expressed in immoral projects). Aristotelians are keen to emphasize that well-being for them is not simply a matter of moral virtue, but centers also on nonmoral virtues.

[13] See especially Martha Nussbaum's work (Nussbaum, 2000).

taken as a point against capacity-fulfillment views of well-being, but here I mean only to circumscribe a distinctive approach to nature-fulfillment, on which flourishing has to do with *success*, as opposed to actualization or admirability. (Though again, a theory might combine these ideas; for instance, actualization might be embodied in a fuller, richer kind of success.) We might thus distinguish three types of norms that eudaimonistic views of well-being might embody, either alone or in combination, namely norms of:

1. Admirability (perfection)
2. Actualization (capacity-fulfillment)
3. Success (goal-fulfillment)

One might question whether goal-fulfillment is a variety of eudaimonism at all: aren't we just talking about good old-fashioned desire theories or hedonism? In general, no, because the present ideal has a characteristically eudaimonistic structure: the view of well-being is coupled to some account of the individual's nature, such as a theory of the self.[14] In one variant of the approach, for instance, well-being is identified with self-fulfillment and hence linked to the character of the self (Haybron, 2008a, 2008b). The self in turn is claimed to consist partly in the person's emotional nature: what ways of living tend to be emotionally fulfilling, making her *authentically happy*. Because it is plausible that the self is also partly constituted by the individual's commitments, desires or values, a further development of the account would likely incorporate a second component such as value-fulfillment: success regarding the values that help define who you are.[15] Indeed, the popularity both of desire theories of well-being and desire-based views of the self in the philosophical literature may be no coincidence: perhaps desire theorists tend tacitly to be relying on an appeal to the value of self-fulfillment. Be that as it may, most desire theorists make no explicit commitment to eudaimonistic foundations, defending their views on other grounds, and hence do not fall within the eudaimonist camp.

2.5.4 Does Your Well-Being Depend Entirely on Your Particular Makeup?

Another theoretical choice has not gotten much attention in the literature, but is quite important. The easiest way to see the issue is to note a well-known feature of Aristotelian theories: well-being is grounded in *species* or kind norms: what is distinctively or characteristically human. What's good for you, then, depends partly on what human beings are characteristically like. This is by no means to say that all people should live the same way. The theory allows lots of room for individual difference, and might even deem individuality among our characteristically human qualities (Badhwar, 2014; Russell, 2013). Human excellence has many faces. At the same time, certain things do seem important for well-being, no matter who you are: we are a social species, for instance, so that a psychopath with no capacity for normal human relationships is worse off for it: he is missing out on an important element of a full life for a human being. This might be the case even if he is happy and getting everything he cares about: to some extent the standards of well-being depend on factors that may be external to, or transcend, the particular features of the subject. Similarly, many find it intuitively plausible that deafness involves a kind of *deprivation*: while hearing-impaired persons might perfectly

[14]As noted above regarding hedonism, the question here isn't whether a theory of human well-being could be truly independent of any view of human nature; perhaps it cannot, and indeed I suspect that hedonists and desire theorists profit from a covert reliance on eudaimonistic ideals. But we are talking about the theories as they are, not as they should be; and as they are, subjectivist accounts are typically not grounded in any appeal to selves or human nature, and so are not eudaimonistic in their structure. They lack the teleological structure of eudaimonism.

[15]Recent defenses of value-fulfillment ideals of well-being—though not explicitly employing a eudaimonistic framework—include (Hall & Tiberius, 2015; Raibley, 2010, 2013; Tiberius, 2008, 2014). Benjamin Yelle defends an explicitly eudaimonistic value-fulfillment theory (Yelle, 2014). Accounts of the self centering on values include, e.g., (Doris, 2015; Frankfurt, 1971; Sripada, 2015; Watson, 1975; Wolf, 1993).

well thrive, and do better than many hearing people, perhaps there is still something missing in a life where one never hears music, songbirds, a loved one's voice (Haybron, 2013a). A deprivation need not be cause for sympathy or pity, but there is still something to regret. It strikes many as important to lead a truly full life, replete with the goods that human beings typically get to enjoy. We might call this the "no child left behind" intuition.

The example of deafness is instructive: many others have the opposite intuition. The only downside to being deaf, on this view, is whatever frustration it may bring, especially in a world built to favor the hearing. Indeed deafness brings its own distinctive satisfactions, different ways of perceiving and relating. In itself there is nothing worse about being deaf; it is just a different way of being. More generally, we might say that what's good for you must depend entirely on the particularities of what *you* are like, however idiosyncratic or atypical: it must depend wholly on what your wants, likes, values, hedonic or emotional propensities, or physical makeup are like. Call this idea *subject-dependence*: what's ultimately good for a welfare subject depends entirely on the arbitrarily idiosyncratic particulars of that individual's makeup. Call the contrary claim *subject-transcendence*. (I originally referred to this notion as "welfare internalism" and called the opposing view "welfare externalism," but given the proliferation of internalisms and externalisms in the literature I will follow Hall and Tiberius in the present terminology (Hall & Tiberius, 2015; Haybron, 2007, 2008b).) According to subject-dependence, that sociality or hearing are characteristic features of human life has nothing to do with what's good for you. Likewise, that beauty, knowledge or whatever have intrinsic value is irrelevant to whether they are good for you, except to the extent that they somehow fit with your personal makeup.

Subject-dependence is easily confused with subjectivism, which is the best-known form of the view. But objectivists could make well-being subject-dependent, for instance by grounding it in features of the subject other than her attitudes. Physical health might be one example, and indeed hedonism might be one on some understandings of objectivism (given that hedonists claim pleasure is all that's good for you regardless of whether you care about other things). And any view that takes well-being to consist partly in unconscious states, as one account incorporating happiness as emotional well-being does, could be subject-dependent without being subjectivist: unconscious mental states are not comfortably regarded as subjective states (Haybron, 2008b).

Within the welfare eudaimonist tradition, subject-dependence is closely associated with, and may indeed be coextensive with, a certain family of nature-fulfillment theories, *self-fulfillment* views.[16] The term 'self-fulfillment' is sometimes used interchangeably with 'nature-fulfillment', but here I understand it in a strict sense: as referring to the fulfillment of the self and not, say the fulfillment of one's nature *qua* human being. This move makes the theory of well-being parasitic on our theory of the self. If the self is defined by one's desires, then self-fulfillment involves desire-fulfillment; if by one's values, then value-fulfillment; if by a narrative, then perhaps narrative-role-fulfillment; if by one's emotional makeup—what makes one happy—then happiness; etc. The ideal of self-fulfillment is especially characteristic of modern forms of eudaimonism, as befits moderns' greater focus on the self. Mill's paean to individuality in *On Liberty* is perhaps the best expression of self-fulfillment as an ideal of human flourishing. Unfortunately, the term 'self-fulfillment' has acquired connotations of extreme individualism if not a kind of New Age narcissism. Such views need not of course have these features, and indeed could be quite non-individualistic if the self is conceived in relational or communal terms: in parallel with the earlier remarks about authenticity, if who you are is defined by your relationships and social roles, then self-fulfillment will likely depend strongly on how your relationships and loved ones fare, and how well you fulfill those social roles.

[16] For discussion of the notion of self-fulfillment, see (Haybron, 2008a, 2008b).

I hope it is clear that both subject-dependent and subject-transcendent approaches to well-being have significant attractions. Both are popular approaches because they answer to strong and widely shared intuitions about human well-being.

2.6 Justifying Eudaimonic Measures

2.6.1 Why Employ Eudaimonic Measures?

It is time to descend from the airy heights of eudaimonistic philosophy and consider how one might operationalize its insights—no trivial matter given both the variety of philosophical options and the prominence of hard-to-measure notions like virtue in that tradition. Fortunately, the utility of eudaimonic measures does not require researchers to assume, tendentiously, that a eudaimonistic account of well-being such as Aristotle's is *true*. As should be clear by now, such theories of well-being have endured in philosophy because they answer to widely shared and deeply felt intuitions about human welfare. Whatever the correct theory of well-being may be, the fact remains that very many people consider things like the realization of one's potential, or authenticity, to be important elements of our good.

The mere fact that so many people value eudaimonic goods, and are not obviously mistaken in doing so, is itself reason to want eudaimonic measures. Subjective well-being researchers sometimes resist such measures on the grounds that doing so involves adopting the mantle of philosopher-king and foisting alien standards of well-being on people: "we know what's best for you, and that's how we're going to judge your quality of life." The risk of paternalistic practices is indeed reason for caution, but it is reason for caution in using *any* measures of well-being: for example, if you employ certain metrics on the grounds that a subjectivist or any other theory of well-being is true, then you will invariably be contravening the best judgment of many of those you study. Many ordinary citizens are not subjectivists about well-being; if you assume subjectivism, then, you are effectively saying they have the wrong view about their own welfare. Even if you grant that it's good for them to get whatever they happen to want, you may still be saying effectively that, for example, Aristotelians' desires for their lives are founded on a superstition. When those employing the measures wield power over the individuals in question, the result may be what Nussbaum has called "expressive subordination."[17] Where no significant power relation holds, the practice might be harmless; the point is just that the "philosopher king" worry can arise no matter what theory of well-being one employs.

At any rate, just from a practical standpoint it seems wise for researchers to avoid shackling their studies to tendentious value commitments any more than they have to: they'll not likely persuade many colleagues to change philosophical convictions, and risk needlessly limiting the audience for their work. Not to mention that most empirical researchers lack the expertise in philosophical theories of well-being to adjudicate the deep disagreements within the field; even the experts should admit, when talking to outsiders, that they cannot claim the backing of most of their colleagues in their views. Humility seems to counsel an expansive approach to well-being metrics, taking seriously the range of people's cherished values and aspirations—including, arguably, their eudaimonic aspirations.

At this point the subjective well-being researcher might object that their metrics *already* do that: as is too-infrequently appreciated, measures like life satisfaction are meant to allow for almost limitless variation in people's values. If you value an active life of achievement, your life satisfaction reports should reflect that; if you value a pig's life, then that too should register in your life satisfaction. If you belong to a strongly collectivist culture and don't much value personal satisfaction, *that too should turn up in your life satisfaction judgments*: you'll evaluate your

[17](Nussbaum, 2011). For further discussion of these issues, see (Haybron & Tiberius, n.d.).

life more by the social and collective values you care about, and put less weight on your own enjoyment, success, etc. In fact it is not clear that life satisfaction or other life evaluation measures need privilege any cultural orientation, except perhaps the very idea of evaluating your life and reporting the judgment to others, which may indeed be alien to certain cultures. So: if eudaimonic values are widespread, then they will pervasively influence life satisfaction reports, and we don't need eudaimonic metrics. The only reason to use them, the argument goes, would be a conviction that those are the *right* metrics: subjectivists are wrong, and life satisfaction measures defer too much to mistaken views about well-being.

But this isn't quite right: even setting aside the plausible idea that some people have mistaken views about their ultimate interests—as they might themselves discover during a deathbed reckoning—there are at least two reasons for thinking we need eudaimonic measures, and not just life evaluation measures. First, all measures involve error, and no one should deny that life evaluation reports will often omit important information or otherwise fail to give a perfectly faithful picture of how people's lives are going relative to their values. Indeed it is plausible that a major impetus for eudaimonic psychology is a worry that the modern consumer society tends to distract us from some of our deepest concerns, directing our attention away from the relationships and meaningful activities that, on reflection, we most care about, and instead toward trivial matters like owning the latest iPhone. Even if everyone had eudaimonic values, their life evaluations might give a spotty indication of how things are going regarding those values, because our lifestyles make less important matters more salient on a day-to-day basis (Haybron, n.d.-b).

Second, all parties should likewise agree that whole life evaluation metrics are too coarse-grained for many purposes. We don't just want to know how people are doing *on the whole*; we want to know what's going right and what's going wrong. We need a variety of well-being measures to help us build a richer portrait of people's quality of life than just a single number. The single number is useful in its own right, to be sure. But no one should think that's all we need. In this connection, it is worth mentioning that different metrics may be suited to different purposes. For instance, policymakers face one set of demands, including the risks that attend power, while therapists and other practitioners face another, including the need sharply to discount many patients' global self-reports and delve more deeply into the specifics of their lives; when the patient with badly mutilated forearms says "I'm fine doc," it would probably be wise not to stop there.

In short, we have good reason to seek eudaimonic measures regardless of what the right theory of well-being is: they assess values with broad and enduring appeal, which many experts have long deemed to be essential elements of human welfare. There is no reason to discount these views; on the contrary, we ought to take them seriously, if only out of respect for the viewpoints of the individuals whose quality of life we wish to understand. And for all we know, they might be right.

I have not really addressed empirical questions about whether subjective well-being measures might after all track eudaimonic goods; partly for reasons already noted, I doubt they do so well enough to make eudaimonic measures otiose. In any case, there are reasons of face validity to employ eudaimonic measures: if well-being research is going to serve the needs of non-researchers, its measures need to *look* like valid well-being measures. As well, policymakers and the public will be more accepting of the research if it at least appears to address the values they care about.

2.6.2 A Note in Defense of Subjective Well-Being Metrics

Before we get into the substance of eudaimonic indicators, we should pause to note a crucial feature of subjective well-being metrics that researchers sometimes get wrong: subjective well-being research is often characterized as "hedonic," and indeed that's a fairly standard contrast to make with eudaimonic psychology. Subjective well-being researchers themselves have sometimes encouraged this practice, but it is misguided: *the most popular subjective well-being measures, for instance life satisfaction measures, are not hedonic in any plausible sense of the word.* Subjective well-being might be most usefully understood as a blanket category encompassing the various mental states to which the term 'happiness' tends to refer in contemporary English: judgment-like states such as life satisfaction, on the one hand, and affective states like pleasure and emotional well-being, on the other. Strictly speaking, the "hedonic" has to do with pleasure, pain, suffering: the pleasantness of our experience. It is dubious even to call emotional well-being a hedonic matter, since our emotional conditions run much deeper than the hedonic quality of our experience; depression is not merely an unpleasant experience but a complex emotional syndrome with both hedonic and non-experiential aspects (Haybron, 2001, 2008b).

But as we saw above, life satisfaction has far more to do with people's judgments about their lives than pleasant experiences, and in fact life satisfaction metrics are properly seen as *alternatives* to hedonic indicators: most people care about things other than simply leading pleasant lives—love, accomplishment, contributing to the community, etc.—and can accordingly be satisfied even when their lives aren't enjoyable. That's the attraction: maybe New Yorkers prefer lives of accomplishment to lives of pleasure, and so are satisfied with their lives even if they don't feel good. Life satisfaction is useful in such cases precisely because it conveys *non-hedonic* information. In terms of life satisfaction Wittgenstein, by appearances having led one of the more unpleasant lives in recent philosophical history, might have done quite well, if he really did regard his life as "wonderful." If we wish to call a life of suffering a hedonic success, then we seem to have lost all sight of what 'hedonic' is supposed to mean. Hedonists have varied a good deal in their understandings of the pleasant life; but I don't believe they have ever allowed that the pleasant life could be realized through an unpleasant life.[18] It is a serious mistake to assimilate all subjective well-being research to "hedonic" psychology.

The significance of this point is not merely verbal: one of the putative attractions of eudaimonic metrics is that subjective well-being supposedly does not track important values like meaning, relationships, autonomy, personal growth, and so forth. However, life satisfaction measures, as we noted above, can (in principle) register how people are doing in relation to all these values, so long as people care about them, and know how they are doing in those areas. Indeed, there is a particularly close link between life satisfaction and subjective perceptions of meaning in life, a classic eudaimonic metric: to see your life as meaningful presumably has something to do with what you value; are you engaged in worthwhile activities, for instance, that seem to you valuable? But so too is life satisfaction concerned with what you value, and it would be odd to judge your life meaningless while also thinking it going well relative to the things you care about. Indeed it seems incoherent. This is not to deny that there are differences in the metrics; but they are not so different as many have thought (Haybron, n.d.-b).

---

[18]My other discussions of life satisfaction cited here explore these issues in much greater depth, but as some readers will likely want to push back on these claims, let me note, first, that some hedonists understand pleasure as something more like a judgment and hence akin to life satisfaction in that respect (Feldman, 2004). A standard complaint about such views is precisely that they miss their target: what they call "pleasure" is about something other than the pleasantness of one's experience, and is not what hedonists have traditionally cared about. But even these views would have the result that Wittgenstein's life was hedonically bad. A second objection is that suffering might preclude life satisfaction insofar as one has to feel good to truly be satisfied. The short answer is, that's a possible view, but it isn't what current measures, which assess judgments, are tracking; and at any rate it seems poorly motivated: feeling good is one thing, judging that you've achieved the things you care about, even if you don't feel good, is quite another. Life satisfaction loses its distinctive attractions as a metric if we build very much in the way of pleasant feelings into it.

Why do so many well-being researchers get this fact about subjective well-being measures wrong? Perhaps because, prior to reflection about the point of life evaluation metrics, we might think of life satisfaction as a *feeling*: that pleasant feeling of satisfaction you get when thinking about how well your life is going. But, first, such feelings are not what life satisfaction instruments actually seem to be measuring; the questionnaires usually focus on asking people to evaluate their lives, not describe their feelings, and even people who report feeling depressed not-uncommonly claim to be satisfied with their lives (Glatzer, 1991).[19] Second, if all we cared about was a good feeling, why bother? Why not just use straightforwardly hedonic or emotional metrics? Whatever the role of good feelings in life satisfaction might be, the central motivation for employing life satisfaction instruments in subjective well-being is plainly non-hedonic: we want to know how people think their lives are going, by their own standards. We're mainly after a judgment, not a feeling.

I suspect that the animus of many researchers toward life satisfaction measures has a further source: the remarkably positive results that tend to emanate from life satisfaction studies, and the ease with which we can imagine people proclaiming satisfaction even when doing badly by any reasonable standard. It just may not seem very important that people be satisfied with their lives, or at least that they are prone to make that judgment. There is indeed excellent reason to doubt that people's lives are going as well, even by their standards, as self-reports might suggest, due to a mix of positivity bias, poorly designed measures in some cases, and a misunderstanding of what life satisfaction means—namely, that one sees one's life as good *enough*, which is not to say good (Haybron, 2008b, 2011). You might be satisfied when you think life is going badly, say because even a hard life is something to be grateful for. We cannot conclude from positive reports of life satisfaction that people see their lives as going well for them (though perhaps the story is different with life evaluation measures that don't focus on satisfaction, like the Cantril ladder scale). More generally, current subjective well-being measures offer little grounds for drawing conclusions about absolute levels of well-being—whether people are happy, or doing well. *But they might still, and do, provide useful information about relative levels of well-being: who is doing better or worse* (Diener, Inglehart, & Tay, 2012; Haybron, n.d.-b). And that is the more important question, as well as the question on which validation protocols focus. Indeed, in mainstream welfare economics it is the only question: we can speak intelligibly of one state being preferable to another, but not of someone's doing *well*, in absolute terms.

2.7 What to Measure: A Core Schema for Flourishing Scales

2.7.1 Deciding What to Measure

One of the difficulties facing eudaimonic researchers is the lack of consensus on theoretical approaches and measures, which can often look quite different. Diversity is good to a point, but questions arise about whether there is any principled way of deciding between different approaches. Many worry, not unreasonably, that the composition of eudaimonic measures depends too much on the investigator's whimsy: what seems important to her. Can philosophers offer any guidance? I would suggest that we can, and in this section will discuss some of the most plausible candidates for inclusion in eudaimonic measures, based on those values that turn up most consistently in eudaimonistic philosophy, as well as among eudaimonic psychologists themselves. These will likely be the easiest measures to justify to a broad audience. This of course is not the

[19] See also (Ponocny, Weismayer, Stross, & Dressler, 2015). It may be that life satisfaction reports are heavily driven by affective processes, but that is different from the question of what's being asked of participants, and what they are doing when answering: they are being asked for a judgment about their life, and that's what they seem to be giving. Whether the judgment is caused by rational deliberation, induced by mood, or whatever, is a different question.

place to design questionnaires, and most of the work of scale development will best be done by empirical researchers themselves. Here I will focus simply on sketching, in general terms, what the most broadly acceptable eudaimonic measures will likely want to assess, at least as primary indicators of eudaimonic well-being (some values, like authenticity, might be highly important but not so important to measure in most contexts). I will focus on self-report-based scales, but sometimes other measures will be preferred, for instance objective measures of educational attainment.

The eudaimonic literature is large and diverse, but I will focus on the following five approaches as representative examples:

- Self-Determination Theory (Ryan & Deci, 2001; Ryan, Huta, & Deci, 2008)
- Psychological Well-Being (Keyes, 2007; Ryff, 1989; Ryff & Singer, 2008)
- Personal Expressiveness (Waterman, 1993; Waterman, Schwartz, & Conti, 2008)
- PERMA (Seligman, 2011)
- The Flourishing Scale (Diener et al., 2009)

Diener and colleagues of course are not normally associated with eudaimonic psychology. But for the same reason their scale of flourishing, which is meant to assess just the sorts of variables that typically concern eudaimonic theorists, is instructive, since they are not particularly invested in any specific approach.

To help motivate the discussion, a few examples are in order. These are meant to be stylized cases that either illustrate the appeal of eudaimonic approaches or caution against the risk of cultural chauvinism—concerns about which animate much of the opposition to such measures:

1. <u>The sweatshop worker</u>: illiterate and lacking in skills, having little choice but to labor for long hours under the thumb of controlling supervisors in a mindless, meaningless job that leaves little time for other pursuits in life
2. <u>The couch potato</u>: content to while away his life in an existence of passive consumption, with few skills or interests, and little concern for anything outside his own amusement and comfort
3. <u>The architect</u>: a loving mother with many interests and talents who works a fulfilling job as an architect. Well read, well versed in history, the arts, math and science, and also active in the community, she plays piano and participates in team sports on a weekly basis. Though leading an exceptionally rich and active life, she manages it without being stressed and her exuberant, high-spirited nature is infectious
4. <u>The hunter</u>: a member of a hunter-gather tribe blessed with a largely agreeable forest environment, he is extremely capable and knowledgeable about the natural world, the making of tools, shelter, and other useful artifacts. Visiting biologists are, by comparison, oafish, and ignorant of the world around them. Child mortality and other hazards are not-infrequent causes for sorrow or pain, but life on a typical day is relaxed, good-humored and richly social, and he enjoys deep ties of affection with most members of his band. Coercion is all but taboo, and while he has few career options he spends his days as he alone chooses, with no one telling him what to do. "Work," such as it is, consists mainly of doing the things he loves best, especially hunting, at which he is highly skilled.

I make no claim that these are common scenarios. The point is just to illustrate eudaimonic ideals of flourishing, in the last two cases, and eudaimonic views of languishing, in the first two. The last case hopefully makes clear that eudaimonic approaches need not commit to parochial notions of "happiness for yuppie New Yorkers." Some eudaimonists might be so committed—the philosophical literature often carries more than a whiff of it—but then so much the worse for their views. Arguably, the hunter might strongly realize his human capacities and thrive, perhaps no less than the architect (Haybron, 2008b). However challenging the ancestral environment might have been, it would be surprising if flourishing for human beings were impossible under any conditions remotely approximating those in which we evolved. Human flourishing should not just be accessible to individualistic moderns with elite frequent flier status.

With this background in place, we can lay out some core eudaimonic metrics—a *core schema for flourishing scales*: not a scale, but merely a schema for thinking about the kinds of eudaimonic measures we might seek. Researchers will doubtless want to vary or depart from the schema to fit their own theoretical inclinations and practical purposes; I have no expectation that anyone will want follow it exactly. Rather, the aim is chiefly to help clarify the justification for commonly used eudaimonic measures. I use the term 'flourishing' rather than 'eudaimonic' purely for strategic reasons: measures are more likely to get traction in policy circles and elsewhere to the extent that we use ordinary language to frame them. I suspect it will be hard to get many politicians to stump for the "eudaimonic" well-being of their citizens. But this is a practical question on which others may reasonably differ.

As it happens, the most popular eudaimonic scale items seem to correspond fairly neatly to familiar ways of thinking about the different aspects of human nature. Accordingly, our schema will center on four types of good relating to the facts that:

1. We are *agents* who express our natures through activity: agency
2. We are *social* beings: relationships
3. We are *rational* agents with values, not just desires: meaning or worth
4. We are *emotional* beings: emotional well-being

2.7.2 Agency

This is a broad category corresponding roughly to competence and autonomy in the self-determination theory framework, and it centers on two goods:

- Personal development: developing one's capacities or competence (e.g., education)
- Exercising one's capacities or competence (e.g., skilled activity)

Some theorists, including Aristotle on a standard reading, regard personal development as important purely for the activity it makes possible. But one might value such development for its own sake, and at any rate well-being researchers will sometimes want to measure both items. Policymakers, for example, might want to assess both educational attainment (say, literacy) and the extent to which people exercise the abilities they have acquired (say, reading). Economic calamity, for instance, often results in people doing work that makes little use of their abilities, for instance surgeons displaced by the collapse of the Soviet Union who ended up working as dishwashers.

A closely related good of agency is *accomplishment* or achievement (e.g., Bradford, 2015; Hurka, 2010; Seligman, 2011). However, these terms tend to emphasize the product of the activity, and connote activities that are both difficult and have especially valuable products: landing on the moon, inventing the light bulb, curing cancer. Whereas the skillful playing of a sonata, or a deftly executed yet failed football play, are not the first things that come to mind when we think of accomplishments or achievements, though they plainly involve the exercise of competence. You can exercise your capacities to a very high degree yet still fail to accomplish very much, as we ordinarily think about it. This is not to say that accomplishment is the wrong place to focus: perhaps accomplishment matters more than the mere exercise of competence, or perhaps both matter. It is just to note that they are different goods, and hence may require different measures. For conventional Aristotelian forms of eudaimonism, at least, it seems that the exercise of competence is what primarily matters: virtuous activity.

A further good of agency is quite common in eudaimonic measures: *autonomy*. Autonomy can be understood in many ways, but the root idea has to do with self-determination or self-governance. This may have various conditions, for instance acting freely rather than from weakness of will, acting according to values that are truly one's own, or being in control of one's choices rather than being subject to the will of others. As noted earlier, the ideal of autonomy is controversial, as it is associated with Western individualism, but it should be clear by this point that autonomy need not be understood in individualistic terms. There is good reason to think that people in a wide range of cultures, if not all cultures, prefer not to be under another's thumb, and fare best when their actions accord with their internal motivations (Chirkov et al., 2010; Chirkov, Ryan, Kim, & Kaplan, 2003). Arguably, healthy human agency crucially involves making one's own decisions and not acting under compulsion, though of course this could involve a high degree of deference to social roles and the wishes of others. It is also worth distinguishing autonomy in one's daily activities from "macro" autonomy in major life choices, such as whom to marry or what to do for a living. While it is unlikely that constant browbeating and micromanaging contribute to flourishing in any society, it is less obvious that people need autonomy at the macro level to do well.

In short, agency metrics plausibly merit a central place in eudaimonic psychology, as they speak most directly to the ideal of being "all you can be." Indeed, one or more of the other metrics discussed below, like relationships, might reasonably be deemed to matter as further aspects of agency; I treat them separately because this connection is not obvious, and it is useful for many purposes to separate them out. For instance, promoting agency goals, as we ordinarily think of them, may often conflict with sociality: a population that is better able to pursue rewarding careers, say, may have weaker social connections as a result.

Agency metrics as understood here, then, will likely center on goods such as (with some tinkertoy survey items to illustrate):

- Personal development: the development of competence (e.g., "can you play a musical instrument?")
- Skilled activity: the exercise of competence (e.g., "how many times have you engaged in that activity this week?")
- Accomplishment or achievement (e.g., "I have recently accomplished something I am proud of")
- Autonomy (e.g., "I often have to do things against my will")

2.7.3 Relationships

It is difficult to imagine a credible notion of human nature that doesn't take our sociality seriously: if nature-fulfillment for human beings involves anything, it surely involves, for the great majority of us at least, lives in relationship with others. Eudaimonic measures accordingly tend to involve some assessment of sociality (see especially Keyes, 2007). This in turn can take multiple forms, and researchers need to consider which are most important to measure. For example:

- Close personal relationships, for instance confidants. Feeling understood, respected and supported
- Social enjoyments: socializing, or time spent enjoying the company of others
- Community: living among people you like and trust, with whom you feel a sense of belonging

The first two items are readily confused but quite distinct: you might have an active social life yet no one you can really trust or rely on for anything sensitive, or you may have close friends or family you hardly see.

2.7.4 Meaning

A sense of meaning, or that one's activities are worthwhile, is one of the most common targets of eudaimonic instruments, yet the connection with ideals of nature-fulfillment is less than clear. Agitation about the question of "leading a meaningful life" seems more characteristic of the modern than the ancient era (and I suspect would be utterly incomprehensible in many small-scale societies). I would suggest that it relates to the fact of our practical rationality—we are not just agents, but rational agents who (at least sometimes) deliberate and act for reasons, on the basis of things we don't merely want but *value*: that we see as worth wanting, as meriting our pursuit. (Human rationality might also be the basis for another common eudaimonic good discussed below, virtue, and indeed Aristotle took virtue to be the proper expression of our rational natures. Not coincidentally, Aristotelian views of well-being sometimes closely resemble popular theories of meaning—cf. (Darwall, 2002; Wolf, 2014).) We are valuers, and fulfill our natures partly by living in ways that are, or at least seem to us, valuable and worthwhile. And to say that you lead a life that is and seems to you worthwhile at least resembles the thought that your life is meaningful (Wolf, 2010). Perhaps it is just the same thing. The life of passive consumption, in service of one's appetites seems empty, the opposite of fulfilling. And it can seem a waste of one's potential—a waste of one's life.

It may be more useful to speak of worthwhileness rather than meaning, as the former arguably has a plainer meaning. Be that as it may, we need to distinguish several types or dimensions of meaning or worth. For starters:

- Subjective meaning: the sense that one's activities or life are meaningful
- Objective meaning: one's activities or life actually being worthwhile or meaningful

A genocidal dictator may subjectively regard his life as meaningful, but his pursuit may objectively be meaningless or worthless (putting it mildly). And a depressed saint's good deeds may make for a highly worthwhile life, though she fails to recognize its merits and sees herself and her efforts as worthless. Philosophers differ on whether a meaningful life depends on subjective meaning, objective, or both, though perhaps the leading contemporary account of meaning requires both, holding that meaning arises when "subjective attraction meets objective attractiveness" (Wolf, 2010). One difficulty for measurement is that we aren't sure how to measure objective worthwhileness, if there is such a thing, and attitudes about which lives are most worthwhile vary sharply. There seem at least to be *moral* standards that don't depend on the subject's attitudes, and some of those are widely agreed on (theft, betrayal), but offhand it is hard to tell what a metric of "objective worthwhileness" would look like, let alone how we would devise reliable instruments for measuring it.

We can also distinguish what we might call:

- Global meaning: a general sense that one's life has a purpose or is worthwhile. (E.g., "I feel that on the whole, my life is focused on worthwhile goals")
- Local meaning: experiencing one's activities as meaningful or worthwhile, as they happen (White & Dolan, 2009); Dolan & Kudrna, Chap. 29, this volume). (E.g., "My activities at that time felt worthwhile and fulfilling")

This distinction is quite important for empirical research: global meaning is much easier to assess and hence more commonly assessed, through general questions like "do you feel you have a purpose in life?" or "do you feel that your life is meaningful?" But the harried sweatshop worker might sincerely offer affirmative answers to such questions though her daily toils are experienced as utterly meaningless and unfulfilling, like Sisyphus pushing his stone. Perhaps her religious beliefs underwrite a global belief that it all serves some worthy purpose in a larger scheme, even as the local evidence of her daily experience offers only emptiness and futility. From an operational standpoint, the difficulty here is that the experience of meaning is very difficult to grasp even for the individual having it, and indeed many people may not have any explicit recognition of it all. And if they do, they may not cognize it under the mantle of 'meaning'. (Hunting can be a richly meaningful experience for the hunter, but he may be too focused on the matter at hand to be reflectively aware of the fact, and may at any rate lack the concept of a meaningful experience—what use would hunter-gatherers have for such a concept?) The difficulty of measuring this experience is a major challenge, arguably, for well-being research.

Our natures as valuers may warrant positing a further aspect of nature-fulfillment: success in relation to our values, or value-fulfillment (Haybron, 2008a b; Raibley, 2010; Tiberius, 2014; Yelle, 2014). This is a variant of desire-fulfillment that focuses more narrowly on a person's values: what she cares about and sees as grounding reasons for her, as worth pursuing, and as justifying her choices. You might want a new iPhone but not value it; rather, what justifies the purchase is the pleasure you expect to get from it, and you value pleasure. From a practical standpoint, the focus on values should be attractive to eudaimonic researchers: it is one thing for people to satisfy their everyday consumer preferences, as perhaps the couch potato does, and some might register satisfaction with their lives on that basis if they are sufficiently unreflective. But it is another thing to lead a life rich in the things one actually *cares* about: time with friends and family, meaningful work, engaging leisure activities, happiness... And it is cliché that we can too-easily pass through life generally getting what we want, only to discover in our final survey that we failed badly in the areas of life that we most valued. Perhaps we fulfill our natures partly by succeeding in those areas: by leading lives we see as actually valuable. It would be hard, at least, to lead a fulfilling life otherwise.

As noted above, life evaluation measures can offer a way of getting at value-fulfillment, and there is good evidence that they do track value-fulfillment to some extent (Diener et al., 2012; Schimmack & Oishi, 2005). But to sort out success regarding values from success regarding mere wants—where, e.g., the distracted consumer has lost sight of the big picture—we may want more reflective instruments, for instance inviting participants to undertake a "life review" and identify the things that ultimately matter to them before assessing their lives. Perhaps assessments of value-fulfillment could be derived from life narratives themselves.

2.7.5 Emotional Well-Being

Emotional well-being is normally associated with subjective well-being metrics and, depending on what exactly we want from eudaimonic measures, might reasonably be dropped from this schema. But there are also good reasons to include it, starting with the fact that our emotionality is central to our natures, and it is difficult to imagine human beings fulfilling their natures without also leading emotionally fulfilling lives. Consider how utterly pervasive and profound the effects of depression are on a person's psyche; virtually everything about the mind that makes us human is impacted. Not coincidentally, eudaimonic researchers sometimes look to mental health instruments for inspiration, and in some cases have been modeled explicitly on depression and other mental health measures (Huppert & So, 2011; Keyes, 2002; Ryff & Singer, 1998). Flourishing is often contrasted with languishing, a term closely associated with depression. If it could make sense to build a eudaimonic scale by inverting depression and anxiety instruments, then it probably makes sense to include emotional well-being in our eudaimonic measures generally: very crudely speaking, emotional well-being just *is* the opposite of anxiety and depression.[20] I have argued elsewhere that emotional well-being measures should in fact be modeled on anxiety and depression scales, which better reflect the psychological complexity and depth of our emotional conditions than popular affect scales such as PANAS (Haybron, n.d.-b, 2008b, 2013b).

Crucially, emotional well-being differs from hedonic balance, which focuses entirely on the pleasantness of the flow of experience. Pleasure is an important well-being concern in its own right, but seems not to be a matter of nature-fulfillment: what makes pleasure good, and suffering bad, is

[20] For further discussion of emotional well-being, or the emotional state theory of happiness, see (Haybron, 2005, 2008b, 2013a, 2013c).

just what the experience is like and not, it seems, that it involves the fulfillment of one's nature. Unfulfilling sexual activity usefully illustrates the difference: it involves highly pleasant sensations—"pleasure" in the colloquial sense—but emotionally leaves you flat, empty. Hedonic balance concerns the flow of experience, while emotional well-being concerns, essentially, the condition of the psyche; we might call it *psychic flourishing* (Haybron, 2005, 2008b).

Emotional well-being also makes sense as a eudaimonic concern when we consider its various aspects. I have conjectured that it has three dimensions, two of which correspond to two of the five items in Seligman's PERMA framework (Seligman, 2011). "Positive emotion" is the most obvious, or what I have called the *endorsement* dimension: emotional states that function to respond to successes or failures, gains or losses, such as joy and sadness. The second aspect of emotional well-being, *engagement*, also appears (more or less) in PERMA: states that function to respond to conditions of opportunity, or lack thereof. Is one's life worth investing in and engaging with? One aspect of this is the condition of flow, where one is so caught up in an activity that one isn't aware of feeling anything, yet which also clearly involves a desirable emotional condition. Another kind of engagement is exuberance or vitality: feeling alive, being full of energy, as opposed to being bored, or withdrawn and listless, as in depression. This too is a common eudaimonic concern (Waterman, 1993). The third aspect of emotional well-being is perhaps the least familiar in eudaimonic research: *attunement*, which concerns one's emotional response to conditions of security or threat. Tranquility or peace of mind is the classic state here, but also important are a sense of confidence and an expansive orientation that, taken together, represent one's being psychically at home in one's life: you are in your element, a safe place where you can relax and fully be yourself. Anxiety and stress are the most salient negative counterparts to attunement; stress in particular is probably the most important item to measure in this regard, as chronic stress—not the good kind that keeps us engaged but the bad kind that gives us heart attacks—is so pervasively corrosive in its effects on human life. It is surprising, in fact, that eudaimonic psychologists don't focus more on stress, since it is difficult to imagine any attractive notion of nature-fulfillment in which we fulfill our natures very well whilst being stressed out. From a biological perspective, avoiding serious stress is generally deemed a top priority—"above all, don't stress the animal"—yet for some reason contemporary research tends to exempt human beings from this generalization. Arguably, the attunement dimension of emotional well-being is one of the cornerstones of eudaimonic well-being: truly to fulfill one's nature, one needs first to be able to function without substantial impediment, inhibition, or fear. It is hard to be yourself, much less be all you can be, if you're constantly looking for the hammer to drop.

2.7.6 Other Possibilities: Authenticity, Knowledge, Virtue

Clearly, this is a selective list, and eudaimonic researchers will likely want to measure items not discussed above. One significant omission is *authenticity*, which I noted as a major ideal animating eudaimonistic views of well-being. Beyond the ways in which agency or emotional well-being metrics already get at matters of authenticity, it is not clear how important it is to measure authenticity in the general case, or for that matter what plausible measures would look like (but see Waterman, 1993). The question is whether there are relatively untendentious standards of authenticity that we can measure, and that vary enough in the general population to merit inclusion in our primary well-being instruments. For psychologists to tell people that their happiness isn't really authentic, for instance, is a dicey business, and it isn't clear how often that obtains in any event. From a practical standpoint, human enhancement technologies may raise weighty concerns about authenticity in coming decades—if such technology bothers you, there's a good chance it has something to do with authenticity—but it is not obvious how that should affect measures, especially given that those using such technologies are unlikely to accept a measure that deems their authenticity to be compromised.

From a philosophical standpoint, our schema has at least two significant omissions: first, *knowledge* or understanding. For we are not just practically rational creatures; we are rational creatures period, capable also of theoretical reasoning. We are thinkers and inquirers with a profound need to understand the world around us, and so we fulfill our natures partly by acquiring knowledge (Hurka, 1993, 2010). I did not include knowledge in the schema for two reasons: it does not generally figure in eudaimonic psychology, and agency metrics might already cover the relevant ground sufficiently for practical purposes. It is not clear, for instance, that we generally need further measures beyond personal development instruments tracking, for instance, education levels and the kind of knowledge needed for skilled activity. Purely theoretical knowledge, such as a well-read attorney's understanding of obscure mathematics or physics, may confer some intrinsic benefit to the individual—which is highly controversial, note—but it seems unlikely that general metrics of well-being of the sorts we have been discussing would be far off the mark if they simply didn't bother assessing it.

Perhaps the most awkward omission from the schema—indeed, perhaps the most awkward topic for eudaimonic psychology period—is *virtue*. Aristotle, the paradigm eudaimonist, literally defined well-being as virtuous activity. So it is odd that neither 'virtue' nor 'excellence' makes its way into most eudaimonic scales; nor do they include obvious stand-ins for virtue. To be sure, Aristotelians and other perfectionist eudaimonists understand virtue very broadly so that potentially any kind of worthwhile activity could count as virtuous; consequently, metrics of skilled activity, sociality, meaning and the like are at least relevant to the assessment of virtue. But it is not hard to think of all manner of examples of people who lead mediocre or vicious lives yet do well on standard eudaimonic measures. Someone might take pride in a rich array of hobbies like singing, yet be clueless about his ineptitude in most of them, like an inability to sing on key. Another person might deem it meaningful to devote many hours to amassing the world's largest collection of string, yet if this is an accomplishment at all, it may not in fact be meaningful, or a worthwhile way to spend one's life. Compare a brilliant novelist who holds a more modest view of her own achievements: is her life really less worthwhile or meaningful, or accomplished, than that of the proud string-hoarder? And of course, it is essential on most perfectionist views, certainly Aristotle's, that we also be *morally* virtuous. Yet most eudaimonic instruments do not even attempt to assess moral virtue (but see Keyes, 2007). And when they do, they leave the verdict to the subject: a self-righteous but morally grotesque zealot might hold his moral qualities in high esteem, yet in fact be a cruel, dishonest, manipulative hypocrite.

This is not the place to resolve such difficulties, but they may not be entirely insuperable. First, it is highly controversial even within the eudaimonist tradition that well-being essentially involves virtue, as we saw earlier. One reason not to include it in the core eudaimonic schema, then, is simply that so many people don't conceive of well-being in terms of virtue. For many of us, it is perfectly possible that a vicious person could thrive—for instance, a happy warrior in a tribe that sanctions ruthless treatment of outsiders, like perhaps the Comanche or Iroquois. Of course, it is plausible that virtue tends generally to promote one's own well-being; but that is not the perfectionist claim, which is that flourishing just *is* virtue, at least in part. There is no question that people should be morally and otherwise virtuous; it is better to be good. But that it is necessarily good *for* you is a much more controversial proposition, particularly in an age where subjectivist sensibilities tend to dominate (Haybron, 2007, 2008b). That alone is a good reason not to build virtue into core well-being metrics.

But suppose we do want to include measures of virtue. (We should probably want someone to study virtue in the population at any rate, since it obviously matters whether we live in a society of finks.) There may be ways of doing so. Note, first, that most researchers just need measures that are close enough to make broad discriminations across large populations; we don't need to handle all the weird cases, and we can hope that most people aren't that delusional about their merits. Second, some errors might be corrected through informant reports; do acquaintances corroborate people's self-assessments? (The singer's family probably knows if he's tone-deaf.) Third, the lack of consensus on which lives are most virtuous or admirable does not mean people's opinions are all over the map. Hollywood wouldn't know how to make money if they were; no one could agree on whom to root for. Measures might center on those areas where we have broad agreement: in the moral case, for instance, that it is better to be loath to tell lies, to betray friends, to break promises, to steal, to visit harm on others; as well, that it is better to be kind, compassionate, and generous. It is not implausible that instruments could help make rough discriminations along these lines; it should be possible, for instance, to distinguish relatively Hobbesian societies characterized by ruthless selfishness from highly prosocial societies where cooperation and caring predominate.

Before concluding, let's return to the idea that virtue tends to be a good bet for well-being, no matter what theory of well-being we have (Kesebir & Diener, 2014; Ricard, 2015). Perhaps the best evidence we have for this relates to *prosociality*, or "altruism." Caring and doing for others is well-known to be a potent source of subjective well-being, and there is little doubt that people who care a great deal for others tend to fare better than the selfish. This is part of our sociality, and indeed it is hard to see how we could reliably pull off successful relationships if it were not the case. If this association is strong enough, and if assessing prosocial orientation and activity allowed us sufficiently to make discriminations in well-being beyond those afforded by other measures like relationships, then we may want to include prosociality items in eudaimonic scales *even if we reject welfare perfectionism*—that is, even if we think Aristotle and others are wrong to identify well-being at all with virtue. It may be that, at least for the great majority of us, we cannot fulfill our natures without a high degree of genuine other-concern. Moreover, we might flourish, even on our own terms, only when possessed of a substantial degree of virtue.

Here a word of caution is in order: certain settings, like therapeutic contexts, require far more than just making crude generalizations about large populations. We need to get *a specific individual's* well-being right. It is one thing to infer that people in Hobbesylvania are generally lower in well-being given their odious personalities. It is quite another to make that attribution of one's patient, who might simply have an unusual makeup; maybe she manages just fine without much caring about others, and might reasonably be indignant at the suggestion that she's a sad case. "Who are you to say?" In this instance, at least, the charge might be just. What counts as a satisfactory measure for large groups may be unacceptable for use in individual contexts.

2.8 Conclusion

I have argued that eudaimonic psychology is rooted in a long and diverse philosophical tradition, welfare eudaimonism, that in turn is motivated by deeply and widely felt concerns about the character of human well-being. While not a majority approach among philosophers of well-being—likely no approach is—eudaimonism's focus on nature-fulfillment has much to recommend it, and is less problematic than many have imagined. Moreover, the values most commonly studied by eudaimonic psychologists tend to be widely shared; even if we reject the theories of well-being that inspire them, we should take those values seriously and study them. Very many people, perhaps most, deem it important to lead a full, rich life in which one realizes something of one's potential; no one grows up aspiring to be a couch potato. Well-being research needs at least to acknowledge such convictions.

Those drawn to a eudaimonistic philosophical theory of well-being have some choices to make: Aristotle did not own the word 'eudaimonia'. It belonged no less to Stoics, hedonists, and basically anyone else fluent in ancient Greek.

Among the key questions dividing eudaimonistic philosophers are these:

1. Perfectionism or non-perfectionism?
2. Capacity-fulfillment or goal-fulfillment?
3. Subject-transcendence or subject-dependence?

Aristotle took the first position on each of these questions, whereas the Mill who valorized individuality in *On Liberty* is arguably an example of a philosopher who takes the second, in keeping with the more individualized, liberal spirit of modernity (a clear example in the contemporary literature is Haybron, 2008a, 2008b). Indeed we might profitably divide eudaimonists crudely along "Aristotelian" and "Millian" lines.[21] Eudaimonic psychologists and their humanistic predecessors are not always clear on these counts, but some seem closer to the Millian model than the Aristotelian (e.g., Waterman, 1993), and Aristotle's emphasis on virtue is not especially prominent in their work.

Fortunately, we do not need to resolve the philosophical debate to identify some of the key goods that eudaimonic measures should likely target. Drawing on several lines of evidence, including existing eudaimonic measures and common views about the important dimensions of human nature, I sketched a core schema for flourishing measures. Each item corresponds to a different aspect of human nature that has often been deemed to be ethically significant: our status as agents; our sociality; our status as rational agents or valuers; and our emotionality. To wit:

1. Agency
   (a) Personal development (the development of competence)
   (b) Skilled activity (the exercise of competence)
   (c) Autonomy
2. Relationships
3. Meaning
4. Emotional well-being

We could roughly sum up the resulting picture of well-being as follows: *happiness in a meaningful life that is rich in relationships and the free exercise of one's capacities* (cf. (Badhwar, 2014)). Not all eudaimonists would accept this as even part of their view, but most would probably deem it a plausible summary of what, to a large extent, human flourishing tends to look like in practice. A key ambiguity in this formula is the reference to "meaningful," which in some cases will involve a more or less subjective standard of meaning. But for Aristotle and many others, it would entail an objectively worthwhile life.

This, again, is not meant to be a definitive list, just a starting point for thinking about the sorts of eudaimonic goods we have reason to measure. As I noted earlier, investigators could well draw on these reflections and employ measures of such goods without committing to any "eudaimonic" school of thought, or taking a significant stand on the right theory of well-being. They might simply regard eudaimonic psychology as offering a useful toolbox of items that might be worth studying, in addition to the usual subjective well-being metrics. It may indeed be that empirical researchers will want largely to sidestep philosophical debates over whether well-being is subjective, eudaimonistic, or whatever, that even professional philosophers have trouble coping with. It might be plausible enough that your studies of meaning or accomplishment convey significant information about well-being, even if you leave it open just which philosophical framework best explains their importance.

It bears remarking, in this regard, that when (for example) researchers equate subjective well-being with well-being *simpliciter*, they are trading in some weighty and tendentious value judgments: for instance, that laid-back Louisianans high in subjective well-being are *better off* than high-achieving New Yorkers with lower subjective well-being. In terms of self-interest, at least, they have better lives. And any-

[21] I explore this suggestion in (Haybron, n.d.-a). A difficulty with the "Millian" label is that Mill's better-known discussion of well-being in *Utilitarianism* distinguishes pleasures by a metric of "quality," and it is not clear that this view is really subject-dependent. But his discussion of individuality in *On Liberty* is arguably one of the finest articulations of a subject-dependent ideal of well-being.

one who thinks otherwise, like those New Yorkers, is simply wrong. Likewise, *mutatis mutandis*, for eudaimonic psychologists whose views entail that the New Yorkers are better off. The science of well-being cannot hope to be value-free, but I suspect many investigators will not wish to wade quite so deeply into these waters. This is not to say that empirical researchers can safely ignore the philosophical debates about well-being; some may want to be more theoretically committed than others, and all well-being researchers should understand the philosophical reasoning that motivates concern for various goods, and favors some metrics and methods over others.

I hope it is apparent that eudaimonic metrics are theoretically and practically well-motivated. We shall hardly want to abandon subjective well-being measures, which concern goods virtually everyone deems centrally important for well-being, and hence might still offer the best candidates for headline measures in policy contexts among others. But eudaimonic measures also have an important role to play.

References

Annas, J. (1993). *The morality of happiness*. New York: Oxford.

Badhwar, N. K. (2014). *Well-being: Happiness in a worthwhile life*. Oxford, UK: Oxford University Press.

Besser-Jones, L. (2014). *Eudaimonic ethics: The philosophy and psychology of living well*. New York: Routledge.

Besser-Jones, L. (2015). Eudaimonism. In G. Fletcher (Ed.), *The Routledge handbook of philosophy of well-being* (pp. 187–196). New York: Routledge.

Bradford, G. (2015). *Achievement*. Oxford, UK: Oxford University Press.

Brink, D. O. (2003). *Perfectionism and the common good: Themes in the philosophy of T.H. green*. New York: Oxford.

Brink, D. O. (2013). *Mill's progressive principles*. Oxford, UK: Oxford University Press.

Chirkov, V. I., Ryan, R. M., Kim, Y., Kaplan, U. (2003). Differentiating autonomy from individualism and independence: A self-determination theory perspective on internalization of cultural orientations and well-being., *84*(1), 97–110. http://doi.org/10.1037/0022-3514.84.1.97

Chirkov, V. I., Sheldon, K. M., Ryan, R. M., Chirkov, V. I., Ryan, R. M., & Sheldon, K. M. (2010). *Cross-cultural advancements in positive psychology* (Vol. 1). Dordrecht, The Netherlands: Springer.

Crisp, R. (2005). Well-being. In E. N. Zalta (Ed.), *The stanford encyclopedia of philosophy*. URL = http://plato.stanford.edu/entries/well-being/

Darwall, S. (2002). *Welfare and rational care*. Princeton, NJ: Princeton University Press.

Diener, E., Inglehart, R., & Tay, L. (2012). Theory and validity of life satisfaction scales. *Social Indicators Research, 112*, 497–527. doi:10.1007/s11205-012-0076-y.

Diener, E., Wirtz, D., Tov, W., Kim-Prieto, C., Oishi, S., & Biswas-Diener, R. (2009). New well-being measures: Short scales to assess flourishing and positive and negative feelings. *Social Indicators Research, 97*(2), 143–156. http://doi.org/10.1007/s11205-009-9493-y.

Doris, J. M. (2015). Talking to our selves, 1–262.

Elster, J. (1983). *Sour grapes*. New York: Cambridge University Press.

Feinberg, J. (1992). Absurd self-fulfillment. In J. Feinberg (Ed.), *Freedom and fulfillment* (pp. 297–330). Princeton, NJ: Princeton University Press.

Feldman, F. (2004). *Pleasure and the good life*. New York: Oxford.

Foot, P. (2001). *Natural goodness*. New York: Oxford University Press.

Frankfurt, H. (1971). Freedom of the will and the concept of a person. *Journal of Philosophy, 68*(1), 5–20.

Gewirth, A. (1998). *Self-fulfillment*. Princeton, NJ: Princeton University Press.

Glatzer, W. (1991). Quality of life in advanced industrialized countries: The case of West Germany. In F. Strack, M. Argyle, & N. Schwarz (Eds.), *Subjective well-being* (pp. 261–279). Elmsford, NY: Pergamon Press.

Hall, A., & Tiberius, V. (2015). Well-being and subject dependence. In G. Fletcher (Ed.), *The Routledge handbook of philosophy of well-being* (pp. 175–186). New York: Routledge.

Haybron, D. M. (2001). Happiness and pleasure. *Philosophy and Phenomenological Research, 62*(3), 501–528.

Haybron, D. M. (2005). On being happy or unhappy. *Philosophy and Phenomenological Research, 71*(2), 287–317.

Haybron, D. M. (2007). Well-being and virtue. *Journal of Ethics & Social Philosophy, II*(2), i.

Haybron, D. M. (2008a). *The pursuit of unhappiness: The elusive psychology of well-being*. New York: Oxford University Press.

Haybron, D. M. (2008b). Happiness, the self and human flourishing. *Utilitas, 20*(01). http://doi.org/10.1017/S0953820807002889

Haybron, D. M. (2011). Taking the satisfaction (and the life) out of life satisfaction. *Philosophical Explorations, 14*(3), 249–262. http://doi.org/10.1080/13869795.2011.594959.

Haybron, D. M. (2013a). *Happiness: A very short introduction*. New York: Oxford University Press.

Haybron, D. M. (2013b). The nature and significance of happiness. In I. Boniwell & S. David (Eds.), *The Oxford handbook of happiness*. New York: Oxford

Haybron, D. M. (2013c). The value of positive emotion: Philosophical doubts and reassurances, 1–20.

Haybron, D. M. (n.d.-a). *Eudaimonism, ancient and modern*.

Haybron, D. M. (n.d.-b). Mental state approaches to well-being. In M. D. Adler & M. Fleurbaey (Eds.), *The Oxford handbook of well-being and public policy*. New York: Oxford.

Haybron, D. M., & Tiberius, V. (n.d.). Well-being policy: What standard of well-being? *Journal of the American Philosophical Association.*

Huppert, F. A., & So, T. T. C. (2011). Flourishing across Europe: Application of a new conceptual framework for defining well-being. *Social Indicators Research.* doi:10.1007/s11205-011-9966-7.

Hurka, T. (1993). *Perfectionism.* New York: Oxford.

Hurka, T. (2010). *The best things in life: A guide to what really matters.* New York: Oxford University Press.

Kesebir, P., & Diener, E. (2014). In N. E. Snow & F. V. Trivigno (Eds.), *A virtuous cycle: The relationship between happiness and virtue* (pp. 287–306). New York: Routledge.

Keyes, C. L. M. (2002). The mental health continuum: From languishing to flourishing in life. *Journal of Health and Social Behavior*, 207–222.

Keyes, C. L. M. (2007). Promoting and protecting mental health as flourishing: A complementary strategy for improving national mental health. *American Psychologist, 62*(2), 95–108. http://doi.org/10.1037/0003-066X.62.2.95.

Keyes, C. L. M., & Annas, J. (2009). Feeling good and functioning well: Distinctive concepts in ancient philosophy and contemporary science. *The Journal of Positive Psychology, 4*(3), 197–201.

Kim, R. (2015). Well-being and confucianism. In G. Fletcher (Ed.), *The Routledge handbook of philosophy of well-being* (pp. 40–55). New York: Routledge.

LeBar, M. (2013). *The value of living well.* New York: Oxford University Press.

Nussbaum, M. C. (2000). *Women and human development: The capabilities approach.* New York: Cambridge University Press.

Nussbaum, M. C. (2011). Perfectionist liberalism and political liberalism. *Philosophy & Public Affairs, 39*(1), 3–45.

Ponocny, I., Weismayer, C., Stross, B., & Dressler, S. G. (2015). Are most people happy? Exploring the meaning of subjective well-being ratings. *Journal of Happiness Studies*, 1–19. http://doi.org/10.1007/s10902-015-9710-0

Raibley, J. (2010). Well-being and the priority of values. *Social Theory & Practice, 36*(4), 593–620.

Raibley, J. R. (2013). Values, agency, and welfare. *Philosophical Topics, 41*(1), 187–214. http://doi.org/10.5840/philtopics20134119.

Rawls, J. (1971). *A theory of justice.* Cambridge, MA: Harvard University Press.

Ricard, M. (2015). *Altruism: The power of compassion to change yourself and the world.* New York: Little, Brown and Company.

Russell, D. (2013). *Happiness for humans.* New York: Oxford University Press.

Ryan, R. M., & Deci, E. L. (2001). On happiness and human potentials: A review of research on hedonic and eudaimonic well-being. *Annual Review of Psychology, 52*(1), 141–166.

Ryan, R. M., Huta, V., & Deci, E. L. (2008). Living well: A self-determination theory perspective on eudaimonia. *Journal of Happiness Studies, 9*(1), 139–170. http://doi.org/10.1007/s10902-006-9023-4.

Ryff, C. D. (1989). Happiness is everything, or is it? Explorations on the meaning of psychological well-being *57*(6), 1069.

Ryff, C. D., & Singer, B. (1998). The contours of positive human health, *9*(1), 1–28.

Ryff, C. D., & Singer, B. H. (2008). Know thyself and become what you are: A Eudaimonic approach to psychological well-being. *Journal of Happiness Studies, 9*(1), 13–39. http://doi.org/10.1007/s10902-006-9019-0.

Schimmack, U., & Oishi, S. (2005). The influence of chronically and temporarily accessible information on life satisfaction judgments *89*(3), 395–406. http://doi.org/10.1037/0022-3514.89.3.395

Seligman, M. (2011). *Flourish: A visionary new understanding of happiness and well-being.* New York: Simon & Schuster.

Sen, A. (1987). *On ethics and economics.* Oxford, UK: Basil Blackwell.

Sripada, C. (2015). *Self-expression: A deep self theory of moral responsibility.*

Sumner, L. W. W. (1996). *Welfare, happiness, and ethics.* New York: Oxford.

Tiberius, V. (2008). *The reflective life: Living wisely with our limits.* New York: Oxford.

Tiberius, V. (2013). Recipes for a good life: Eudaimonism and the contribution of philosophy. In A. S. Waterman (Ed.), *The best within us: Positive psychology perspectives on Eudaimonia* (pp. 19–38). Washington, DC: American Psychological Association.

Tiberius, V. (2014). How theories of well-being can help us help. *Journal of Practical Ethics, 2*(2), 1–19.

Waterman, A. S. (1993). Two conceptions of happiness: Contrasts of personal expressiveness (eudaimonia) and hedonic enjoyment., *64*(4), 678.

Waterman, A. S. (2013). *The best within us: Positive psychology perspectives on eudaimonia.*

Waterman, A. S., Schwartz, S. J., & Conti, R. (2008). The implications of two conceptions of happiness (hedonic enjoyment and eudaimonia) for the understanding of intrinsic motivation. *Journal of Happiness Studies, 9*(1), 41–79. http://doi.org/10.1007/s10902-006-9020-7.

Watson, G. (1975). Free agency. *Journal of Philosophy, 72*(8), 205–220.

White, M. P., & Dolan, P. (2009). Accounting for the richness of daily activities. *Psychological Science, 20*(8), 1000–1008. http://doi.org/10.1111/j.1467-9280.2009.02392.x.

Wolf, S. (1993). *Freedom within reason.* Oxford University Press, Incorporated.

Wolf, S. (2010). *Meaning in life and why it matters.* Princeton, NJ: Princeton University Press.

Wolf, S. (2014). *The variety of values: Essays on morality, meaning, and love* (1st ed.). Oxford, UK: Oxford University Press.

Yelle, B. (2014). Alienation, deprivation, and the well-being of persons. *Utilitas, 26*(04), 367–384. http://doi.org/10.1017/S095382081400017X.

3 Ethics and Eudaimonic Well-Being

Johannes Hirata

3.1 What Is the Normative Core of EWB?

For Aristotle, eudaimonia was primarily a matter of virtue, much more than of positive feelings (Aristotle, 1934, 1177a, 1179a).[1] When modern positive psychologists claimed to stand in that same tradition and translated 'eudaimonia' with 'happiness', however, philosophers (Hossenfelder, 1998, pp. 176–177) and linguists (Wierzbicka, 1999, pp. 51–54) pointed out that the meaning of the word 'happiness' in today's English lexicon is much more a matter of positive emotion than was the case with the word 'eudaimonia'.

In fact, positive psychologists (and empirical sociologists, economists and others who study such data) do not use the word 'happiness' all that much, with the notable exception of article titles. They prefer other terms to make it clear that they refer to self-report data that do not equal the respondents' actual happiness but rather their possibly inaccurate answer to a survey question about their happiness, satisfaction or about a related state of mind. This construct is typically called 'subjective well-being' (SWB).

This practice of relying on self-reports can be interpreted as a distancing by the researcher from the underlying construct such as happiness. Rather than claiming to learn something about actual happiness, the claim is much more moderate and defensible, namely to learn something about what people say about how happy or satisfied they are. This practice also liberates the researcher from having to specify actual well-being or happiness because that is now a matter of the shared understanding of the survey question by the language community.

The fact remains, however, that the question respondents have to answer aims at actual happiness or satisfaction, and of course we must have reason to believe that there is a reasonable degree of correspondence between actual and reported happiness for these studies to be meaningful at all. To give credence to this view, researchers have verified that survey answers do actually correlate reasonably well with other more objective variables that are commonly taken to be associated with happiness, such as smiling frequency (Diener, 1984, p. 551), brain wave patterns

[1] While eudaimonia is now almost always understood in the Aristotelian tradition, there are several classical accounts of eudaimonia that differ in important respects from Aristotle's view (cf. Haybron, 2008, pp. 35–36).

J. Hirata (✉)
Hochschule Osnabrück, University of Applied Sciences, Caprivistr. 30a, 49076 Osnabrück, Germany
e-mail: j.hirata@hs-osnabrueck.de

J. Vittersø (ed.), *Handbook of Eudaimonic Well-Being*, International Handbooks of Quality-of-Life,
DOI 10.1007/978-3-319-42445-3_3

(Davidson, 1992) or assessments by close friends (Diener, Sandvik, Pavot, & Gallagher, 1991, p. 47).

In this context, it should be noted that the underlying concepts which respondents are asked to assess carry undeniable normative undertones. Saying that a person is very happy or rather happy with her life is generally understood to also express a value judgment in the sense that being happy is better, *ceteris paribus*, than being unhappy (cf. Tiberius, 2013b, p. 25). This is simply a matter of the semantic substance of the question asked and can be verified by noting that a statement like "She is unhappy but overall her life is good." strikes us as paradoxical. While this suggests that happiness is a necessary aspect of a good life, saying that happiness is a normative concept does not imply nor require that it is a sufficient aspect.

The methodological distancing from the underlying normative concepts may seem to bring the researcher back to the safe territory of purely positive (i.e., descriptive and value-free) research. After all, she merely observes and analyzes answers to survey questions without judging herself how well the respondents' lives are going. This position, however, is difficult, if not impossible, to defend, and it is so for a number of reasons.

First, the idea that there can be such a thing as value-free research at all is heavily disputed on methodological grounds: the very act of rational arguing, the choice of one's research question and of one's variables in empirical research and the identification of a theoretical framework and of admitted methods all rest on normative convictions of good scientific practice and of legitimate and valuable research interests (cf. Weber, 1985).

Second and more specifically, trying (successfully or not) to abstain from any kind of value judgment would make psychological research much less intelligible and less relevant to real-world questions. A researcher could no longer say that, e.g., the negative effect of unemployment on SWB is worrying or even that it is large, or that people with certain personality traits "cope better" with adversity than others. Moreover, research into well-being is confronted with normative expectations by the general public which takes it for granted that well-being research provides answers to normative questions about what constitutes a life worth living, and these expectations cannot simply be ignored (Tiberius & Hall, 2010, see also Tiberius, Chap. 38, this volume).

Third, explicitly normative concepts or objectives ("optimal functioning", "maturity"; cf. Ryff, 1989, p. 1071) abound in positive psychology, and someone trying to remain value free would have to avoid these concepts and try to find alternative ways of describing related ideas without any valuational content or undertones.

While purely positive research on SWB may be impossible even if one tried, it would not even be desirable in the first place. Without a normative interest in learning something about actual well-being and the good life, one would risk using meaningless concepts and pursuing irrelevant questions. In order to make sense of SWB research, we need to understand how the construct of SWB relates to actual well-being, and this requires a normative conception of the good life. In any case, there is nothing wrong with being normative in science as long as the reasons one has for one's normative choices are transparent (Weber, 1985, pp. 510–511). Being value free as such is no quality criterion for scientific inquiry.

It is precisely because subjective well-being corresponds very imperfectly with a normative idea of the good life that the concept of eudaimonic well-being (EWB) has been put forward by psychologists (cf. Ryan & Deci, 2001, pp. 145–146; Ryan & Martela, Chap. 7, this volume). In other words, the *raison d'être* of the concept of eudaimonic well-being is that it is supposed to better describe how well, evaluatively speaking, a person's life is going, even if its empirical measurement remains imperfect. That this is the role of EWB can be verified by observing that it is typically framed as a response to the shortcomings of measures of hedonic well-being (HWB) when this is assessed against a standard of a good life, e.g. the discrepancy between SWB measures and measure of healthy living (cf. Ryan & Deci, p. 146) or the discrepancy between how one experiences life and how life is actually going when one is deluded, as in Robert Nozick's (1989) famous thought experiment of a happiness machine (Tiberius, 2013b, p. 22). In other words, eudaimonic well-being is a more comprehensive good than subjective well-being or hedonic well-being because it avoids their occasional incongruence with what is taken to be a good life, and EWB is therefore more relevant to most of the questions asked.

Being an intentionally normative concept, EWB must get it roughly right about what makes a life go well. Whatever the precise role EWB is supposed to play—a comprehensive and exhaustive conception of well-being or an essential but non-exclusive component of the good life—the concept of EWB needs to be responsive to the ethical complexity of what people think of as a good life. This does not mean, however, that the only way to conceptualize EWB can or should be as a comprehensive and exhaustive conception of well-being itself. A normative conception of EWB can also be more modest and occupy a subordinate position as a non-exclusive but perhaps still constitutive aspect, or content, of the good life.

In the following, I will try to characterize some formal aspects of a normatively adequate conception of eudaimonic well-being. In particular, I will try to shed light on the role of prudence for well-being (Sect. 2) and on the relationship between eudaimonic well-being and morality (Sect. 3). The fourth section will then bring together the moral aspects of eudaimonic well-being and show how they relate to one another.

3.2 Prudence and Eudaimonic Well-being[2]

Arbitration between competing ends is an integral part of life and consequentially of a conception of well-being. All types of well-being theories—objective or subjective—must come up with an answer to the question of how to arbitrate between different goods that are in conflict with one another. Some theories, such as desire-based theories, relegate the issue to the individual, trusting that she will be the best judge of how to prioritize different goods in the interest of her own well-being, but this merely passes the responsibility for the judgment along rather than eliminating it. In any case, even for an objectivist account of well-being, there must be some room for subjective valuation when it comes to the comparative valuation of different goods.

Whatever one's preferred theory of well-being, one of the central and inescapable normative challenges is judging how far to go in pursuing each specific good when this compromises some other good. Another central normative question, even prior to the previous one, is what qualifies as a good for you in the first place (and here objectivist theories clearly differ from subjectivist accounts). These two questions are at the core of what philosophers call prudence, but I will focus on the former question of prudential judgments wherever we have to arbitrate between goods.[3]

Certain tradeoffs are clearly inferior to others. Let us take the case of the two goods 'sleeping' and 'being active'. Sleeping for only 2 h a day and being active for 22 h is clearly a poor tradeoff for a person's well-being, absent extraordinary circumstances. Turning the choice around, sleeping or resting 22 h and being active for 2 h, does not make things much better: there clearly is a better way (i.e., better for one's well-being) to use the 24 h of the day. But what choice exactly is in the best interest of my well-being?

At this point, it is tempting to think of well-being as something to be maximized by playing with the various goods. Going from 2 h of sleep to 3 and to 4, at the expense of a corresponding amount of active time, certainly improves one's well-being. This is a value judgment that can be justified in different ways, for example by

[2]Some of the following arguments were first published in Hirata (2011), chapter 4.

[3]Similar questions can be asked with regard to choice behavior, but my interest here is on valuation rather than choice, and I do not subscribe to the view (prevalent in economics) that choice behavior and valuation ("preferences") coincide perfectly (for a critique of this view, cf. Sen, 1977).

showing how sleep deprivation increases a person's risk of suffering an accident (in an objective theory of well-being) or by invoking the stated preferences of people for more than 2 h of sleep (in a subjective theory of well-being). But where should we stop? Are 8 h of sleep better for a given person's well-being than 7, taking into account the sacrifice in active time? Even without a way of determining the exact optimal amount of sleep to the minute (due to unsurmountable practical limitations), one criterion might seem obvious: the optimum amount of sleep is whatever amount maximizes that person's well-being (including the possibility that there be many equally optimal tradeoffs within a certain "optimum range").

As obvious as this may sound, however, saying that well-being—or the good in general—can be maximized at all is an audacious statement. It involves the claim that well-being is a very specific kind of phenomenon with a systematic, stable and determinate structure. It also implies a deterministic view of the good, and I will try to demonstrate that these views are fundamentally inconsistent with the way we are used to think and speak of well-being and of the good.

Before tackling the question of maximization as such, one should note that maximization can refer to two distinct types of goods, namely either to subordinate goods or to the final good ("summum bonum"). Subordinate goods are rather specific goods like wealth, autonomy or health, i.e. goods that may be valued for very good (intrinsic or extrinsic) reasons but that do not individually suffice for a good life. "The more the better" will generally, though not always, be true for these goods in a relative, *ceteris paribus* sense (cf. Tiberius, 2013a, p. 66), but not in an absolute sense because the pursuit of any one of these goods competes with the pursuit of other goods. For example, more health is better than less *ceteris paribus*, but since actually pursuing better and better health will eventually come at the expense of other goods, certain pro-health choices may not be prudent for a given person because the concomitant sacrifice in terms of other goods is out of proportion with—i.e. would not be justified by—the health benefits gained.

It is easy to see, therefore, that prudence demands something different than maximizing a subordinate good. In fact, caring about maximizing only a single subordinate good would rather seem deeply irrational. As far as the maximization of financial wealth is concerned, e.g., John Maynard Keynes diagnosed "[t]he love of money … [as] a somewhat disgusting morbidity, one of those semi-criminal, semi-pathological propensities which one hands over with a shudder to the specialists in mental disease." (Keynes, 1972/1928, p. 329) Maximizing a subordinate good is clearly not the same as optimizing one's well-being. This also implies that those who criticize the idea of maximization or optimization of well-being for being imprudent (e.g., because well-being requires moderation of desire fulfillment rather than maximization) are criticizing a half-baked conception of well-being.[4] They are simply barking up the wrong tree.

The final good, or "*summum bonum*" ("highest good") to use the formula coined by Cicero, is different. (I am still talking about well-being here, so my use of *summum bonum* in this context does not include moral concerns, at least not any that are independent from well-being). Since the *summum bonum* does not, by definition, have any rival goods, there is no obvious reason for which to limit oneself in its pursuit. Any argument brought forward against furthering the *summum bonum* to the utmost will therefore appear to be self-contradictory.[5] In this terminology, therefore, maximizing the *summum bonum* would be the same as optimizing one's well-being.

To say that well-being is a matter of maximization therefore requires as a necessary condition that one's conception of well-being be a final good in this sense, rather than a subordinate good. But this is only a necessary condition, not a sufficient one. In addition, for well-being to be a matter of maximization, it would have to be possible—in principle, not in practice—to deter-

[4] For an example of such a critique, see Bayertz (2013).

[5] For example, saying that it is better to balance the pursuit of the *summum bonum* against, say, following one's irrational passions would imply the paradoxical conclusion that one can do better than pursue what is best.

mine the well-being effects of any given kind of choice or circumstance. There may be many reasons for which to doubt this possibility, for example because of complex interactions between different variables, because of the non-linearity of the effects of certain influences, or because of the interdependence of desires or preferences. All of these objections, however, are merely a matter of the practical challenges of complexity that do not cut to the bone of the issue and which are easily refuted or accommodated by the defendants of maximization-of-well-being conceptions. The only objection that shatters the foundation of the maximization view of well-being is directed against the determinacy of the good that any maximization theory of well-being must presume.

Maximization of well-being requires determinacy of the good because without determinacy it is logically impossible to rank all alternatives. For certain (but not for all) comparisons between two scenarios A and B one simply would not be able to say whether A is better for a given person's well-being than B not because of the complexity of the effects to be considered but because a sufficiently precise specification of that person's well-being does not exist in the first place.

As an example, consider the question whether ordering a coffee after dinner will enhance your well-being or not. Let us assume that you very much like coffee and would distinctly enjoy drinking a coffee in this situation, but that having a coffee at this time of the day will mean you will fall to sleep about 1 h later than you would otherwise and that you are well aware of this effect (let us also assume there is no third alternative). In the eyes of a well-being-maximization theorist, you then face a tradeoff between the current enjoyment and the price you have to pay later on, and the right tradeoff will be a matter of how the advantages of having the coffee (enjoyment, socializing etc.) relate to the disadvantages (later sleep with all its consequences) as you see them (I suppose that this would be a clear example for a situation in which even objective-list theorists would see a role for subjective weighting). Finding the answer to this apparently simple question may involve complex considerations, but—to the maximization theorist—there will ultimately be a single clear answer out of three possible ones: (1) drinking the coffee is good for (i.e. will maximize) your well-being; (2) drinking the coffee will be bad for (i.e. will fall short off maximizing) your well-being; or (3) drinking the coffee and not drinking the coffee are equivalent as far as your well-being is concerned.

Let us suppose you decide against drinking the coffee mainly because you remember how intensely you disliked not being able to sleep right away last time you had coffee after dinner. This looks like a decision that maximizes your well-being. Now imagine a scenario in which you decide to drink the coffee and take a resolution not to feel irritated about not being able to sleep at the usual time. You plan to read a book for an extra hour in bed and to take it lightly if you feel sleepy the next day, so the disadvantages of having the coffee will be rather insignificant. In this scenario, drinking the coffee actually looks like it maximizes your well-being. Which decision, coffee or not, will maximize your well-being therefore depends on how you will feel about the lost hour of sleep.

The point is that as long as you think of yourself as a person with a free will, it is you who determines how exactly you will feel about the lost hour of sleep. By extension, your resulting well-being will depend as much on your free valuation as it depends on the coffee. If you have a free will, the way you feel about losing an hour of sleep is not pre-determined: you are not doomed to feel irritated about losing an hour of sleep—you may as well make up your mind to make the best of it and consciously downplay the negative consequences of drinking the coffee. This is not to say that we can freely choose our values and our affective responses without any limits; we clearly cannot. If the coffee did not cost you 1 h of sleep but the entire night's sleep, you would probably not be able to sufficiently downplay the irritation at having to stay awake all night and the drowsiness the following day. The important insight is that if there is some range of values over which you can decide freely, then the idea of maximizing well-being breaks down because of the fundamental indeterminacy of the process giving rise to well-being.

Of course the well-being-maximization theorist can reply that this is just one more reason to reject the idea of a free will, and that this argument is merely speculative. In some formal sense he might indeed be consistent if he maintained the well-being-maximization hypothesis and rejected the existence of a free will. The problem is that one cannot reject the free will without at the same time rejecting a whole system of beliefs and convictions about human nature and social relations that are very close to most people's hearts and minds. In a world without a free will, one cannot make sense of concepts like guilt, desert, willpower or even choice because these ideas and many others depend on a person's freedom to choose and to value. The very idea of the person as an agent who takes decisions would lose its meaning and be replaced by the idea of a self-aware robot that reacts to external stimuli by executing decision algorithms it received from an equally external environment.

All of this is not a proof for the existence of a free will. It just means that a lot depends on the free will and that the way we think and talk about ourselves and the world is inconsistent with a rejection of the free will. This has very far-reaching implications for the well-being-maximization theorists and others who reject the free will: to be consistent, they will have to stop using all those words and making all those arguments and statements that presuppose the existence of a free will. What is more, they will no longer be able to engage in any rational discourse in the common sense of the word because that requires the recognition of the discourse participants' ability to freely evaluate the validity of arguments (Apel, 1973, p. 413). Someone who rejects the free will and tries to convince (rather than manipulate) his interlocutors of this view by rational arguments is committing a performative contradiction because he implicitly presupposes that his interlocutors can freely accept arguments they recognize as the better ones.

In this light, sticking with the free will and rejecting the well-being-maximization hypothesis does not look like such an undesirable option. In fact, the main objection against a conception of well-being that embraces the free will is rather weak: it is about the uncomfortable indeterminacy of such a conception. If there is freedom of choice in my valuations, there is no firm yardstick for well-being and there is often no way of ranking different alternatives in terms of well-being. This is a weak objection, however, because the fact that a determinate conception of well-being better suits our desire for a powerful theory is just not the right kind of argument. Adopting a determinate theory despite believing that it is wrong would mean committing the fallacy of misplaced concreteness that Aristotle already warned against when he said that "it is the mark of an educated mind to expect that amount of exactness in each kind which the nature of the particular subject admits" (Aristotle, 1934, 1094b).

In order to think of well-being as something indeterminate, the distinction between two different kinds of ultimate end is helpful: a dominant end and an inclusive end (Hardie, 1965, p. 279). A dominant end is determinate and subject to maximization. Substantive goods (such as sleep and active time) contribute to the dominant end, and they are valuable exactly to the degree that they contribute to the dominant end. This implies that substantive goods can in principle be substituted for each other because what matters ultimately is the resulting degree of well-being and nothing else. To put it differently, only the dominant end has intrinsic value while substantive ends are only of instrumental value.

If well-being is thought of as an inclusive end, by contrast, it is used merely as an umbrella term for a multidimensional construct that is ultimately indeterminate. In this perspective, the various substantive goods (perhaps not all of them, but quite a few) have intrinsic value and cannot be substituted. They cannot be thought of as contributing to or causing well-being, but rather as the irreducible content of well-being. A good night's sleep does not *cause* well-being to increase, it *is* well-being (or an integral part of it), just as the clarinets in a Mozart symphony do not merely *contribute to* the music, they *are* the music (Spaemann, 2000/1989, p. 23).

When well-being is thought of as an indeterminate, inclusive end, prioritizing and finding a balance between competing goods is not a matter of optimization, but more of an art that draws on our distinctly human faculty of actively taking a stance towards the world around us and towards ourselves (Spaemann, 2000/1989, p. vii; Tiberius, 2013a, p. 62). That is what we mean when we speak of human beings as having agency. This resonates with the concept of eudaimonic well-being in its various specifications in which concepts like agency, autonomy and self-determination (Tiberius, 2013b, p. 30) take center stage. In this view, we do not simply have preferences, we rather can—within limits—affirm and reject them, and we *care* (Frankfurt, 1999, p. 157; Tiberius, p. 63) about certain preferences because we have reasons to do so, especially when we regard these as meaningful. This is a qualitatively different perspective than the hedonic one of maximization, in which hedonic well-being is ultimately only about myself because it is my own well-being that is to be maximized. Others are only of instrumental value to my hedonic well-being (though perhaps not to my conscience), giving rise to a self-referential conception of hedonic well-being that can best be described as solipsistic. This is in contrast to eudaimonic well-being in which other persons or even abstract ideals (such as beauty or truth) may be part of my well-being in the sense that I care about them intrinsically, leading to a conception of well-being that goes beyond the ego and which is perhaps best described as self-transcendent well-being (Hirata, 2011, p. 96).

Saying that well-being is self-transcendent in this sense is meant to specify prudence. Self-transcendent well-being should not be understood as a matter of morality or righteousness in the sense that it is primarily a matter of caring about the moral dimension of how we relate to others. It merely extends the domain of prudence by including the consideration of others in their own right, i.e. by recognizing that there are intrinsic reasons for taking an interest in other people. It means *that* I care about others in their own right, but not that I do so for moral reasons or in a morally unobjectionable way. When two persons love one another, for example, their love will be a paramount prudential aspect of their respective (self-transcendent) well-being that is not dominated by the moral aspects involved. Similarly, a person may experience self-transcendent well-being through meaningful relations to friends but at the same time violate moral principles in his relation to strangers without necessarily compromising his well-being thus defined.

These two dimensions, prudence and morality, can probably not be neatly separated from one another in many cases. Both have a role to play in eudaimonic well-being, and it is not possible to think of one entirely separated from the other. Self-transcendent well-being probably does not go well together with outright malice, and the demands of morality would have no object without a conception of prudential well-being. The next section will therefore discuss the relation between EWB and morality.

3.3 Eudaimonic Well-being and Morality

Aristotle saw a very strong link between eudaimonia and morality: only a truly virtuous person was considered to have eudaimonia (cf. Hossenfelder, 1998, p. 176). Most contemporary authors on eudaimonic well-being do not maintain this strong link. But, as I will argue, morality still has some role to play in our understanding of eudaimonic well-being, and even of subjective well-being. For one thing, well-being seems to be compromised by a bad conscience. For another thing, moral considerations inform the distinction between justified and unjustified perceptions of deprivation that is important to EWB. I will discuss these two roles of morality in turn.

3.3.1 Well-being and Approval

Imagine a person who is enjoying a meal that she thinks is delicious. Half way through the meal she learns that what she thought was beef is in fact horse meat, and she happens to be a passionate horse rider and strongly disapproves of eating horse meat. She will no longer be able to enjoy the food, and even though the food tastes the same as before, eating it will no longer enhance her well-being.

This example illustrates that a person's moral convictions may set constraints on well-being contents. More specifically, for a person to experience (subjective or eudaimonic) well-being, she must not strongly disapprove of whatever good she enjoys, including the circumstances that lead to her enjoying the good. Other examples might be the case of a person who learns that the kidney transplant she received had an illicit origin; or a manager who learns that her job promotion was the result of racial discrimination of a better qualified colleague.

This moral aspect of well-being is different from Aristotle's requirement of perfect virtuousness.[6] First, the standard is the respective person's own ethos, rather than an external, impartial standard of virtue or morality. Well-being is impaired only if that particular person strongly disapproves of the benefit she enjoys, no matter whether her moral judgment is defensible from an impartial point of view. This is of course a purely subjective criterion, and it applies, I believe, to the idea of well-being in general, not only to eudaimonic well-being.

Second, only *strong* disapproval is incompatible with well-being, whereas minor violations of a person's own moral standards need not create problems for her well-being. For example, when a person is desperate to watch a newly released movie and buys an illegal copy against his conviction that it is wrong to do so, he may nevertheless enjoy the movie and benefit from it in terms of well-being. This is not to say that he comes to the conclusion that his desperation justifies his buying the illegal copy in the sense of constituting extenuating circumstances—if he did, he would not disapprove of his conduct in the first place. Rather, he bought the illegal DVD in spite of believing it to be unjustifiable, but as long as he categorizes this as a minor moral transgression it need not significantly tarnish his enjoyment of the movie. In short, well-being does not require a perfectly pure conscience, but it also does not go well together with a strong sense of guilt (cf. Hirata, 2011, p. 94).

Saying that EWB is a matter of subjective rather than objective moral standards does probably not imply that EWB is consistent with outright malice. This is because it appears questionable whether a person deriving satisfaction from malicious acts is capable of a self-transcendent perspective as a feature of prudent well-being in the first place. In addition, one might doubt whether a person committing acts of malice does not actually feel a strong sense of guilt or whether she is simply trying to keep such feelings under the surface.

Approval matters to well-being in yet another way. The previous argument was about the absence of strong disapproval as a sort of side constraint for enjoying a benefit, where the benefit in question may be purely self-regarding. By contrast, living up to, or even exceeding, one's own moral standards may actually be a source of well-being in its own right. For example, if I help a lost child find her parents in a crowded mall and as a consequence miss my train home, the inconvenience of having to wait for the next train will be mitigated or even made up by the thought that this is a result of a good deed, i.e. that I lived up to or exceeded my moral standards. Rather than experience my moral standards as a burden and grudgingly do what I believe is my moral duty, which would subtract from my well-being, I can embrace my moral standards and feel good about what I did. (Note that this does not imply in any way that my feeling good was the *motive* for me

[6]Dan Haybron (2008, p. 156) calls this view "welfare perfectionism". Chapter 8 of his book contains an elaborate critical analysis of the role of virtue for well-being, even though he is not specifically concerned with eudaimonic well-being.

helping the child; it may just be an incidental consequence). Positively affirming one's moral principles may align well-being and morality to a good degree.

3.3.2 Justified and Unjustified Perceptions of Deprivation

An important aspect of well-being is deprivation, or rather its absence. A person who is seriously deprived of elementary rights and freedoms is well-being-deficient on virtually every account of well-being, such as that by Amartya Sen (2009). Sen also highlights the difference between perceived deprivation and actual deprivation and makes it clear that the latter is normatively more important (in his framework, important for assessing a person's capabilities; cf. Sen, p. 283). In particular, he warns of taking self-reported well-being at face value when people declare being happy despite miserable living conditions because they "adjust their desires and expectations to what little they see as feasible" (Sen 2009, p. 283).

As far as eudaimonic well-being is concerned, however, perception still plays an important role and should not be left out of the equation. This is particularly relevant for the reverse case where someone with highly favorable living conditions feels deprived and unhappy out of sheer envy for his neighbors who are even better off. As long as that person feels unhappy, he lacks an essential ingredient of EWB, whether or not his unhappiness is self-inflicted.

With respect to deprivation, EWB therefore seems to impose two necessary conditions: first, the person must not *feel* deprived, and, second, he must not *be* seriously deprived as judged from an impartial point of view. The latter is of course an evaluative judgment that may often be highly contentious. It is indispensable nevertheless in order to address the problem rightly raised by Sen. Without an external standard of deprivation, the happy slave who has come to accept his oppression as an unobjectionable state of the world might have to be declared as high on EWB as anybody else, even though he would strongly object to his predicament if he were conscious of the impossibility to justify that state of affairs, and this would seem to compromise his degree of EWB.[7] Therefore, both the ignorant happy slave and the envious millionaire would not attain a high degree of EWB: the slave because he is unaware that others are actually depriving him of his rights, the envious millionaire because of self-inflicted feelings of deprivation.

Is it impossible, then, for a severely deprived person to have EWB? Such an absolute requirement would probably go too far. It would imply that a paraplegic person or entire generations of, say, South Africans under Apartheid had no chance of attaining EWB. A less rigorous requirement might demand that a person can attain a reasonably high level of EWB in spite of being and feeling deprived as long as she is aware of her deprivation (and deprivation can then still be reflected by the *degree* of EWB). In other words, (high) EWB would be out of reach for a person who is unaware of her deprivation as a result of a strong distortion of her standards of what constitutes a good life and of what she is morally entitled to. The slave who feels happy out of ignorance would not have EWB, but one who does so in full awareness of the injustice inflicted upon him might actually be regarded as having a high level of EWB.

3.4 Synthesis

Whereas for the ancients eudaimonia was a matter of leading a virtuous life, the modern notion of eudaimonic well-being is much less strictly tied to virtue or morality. As I argued above, however, there still seems to be a limited moral core to it, and I will try to connect the various arguments by way of a synthesis.

First of all, the way we think and talk about choices and values reveals a deep-seated conviction that we are autonomous agents endowed

[7]This is similar to Nozick's (1989) famous happiness machine objection, but here I am concerned with judgments that have culpably been distorted by others and therefore have a distinctly moral dimension.

with a free will. As a matter of consistency, we cannot at the same time portray well-being as a determinate, dominant end to be maximized. Instead, whether and by how much a given situation, choice or experience (such as a coffee after dinner) affects my well-being will depend crucially, though not exclusively, on my ultimately free decisions and valuations. We therefore need to think of well-being, eudaimonic or not, as an inclusive end the composition of which is (also) subject to our free judgment. Well-being is not a thing out there, but an idea that stands for a rational, indeterminate and revocable judgment.

Morality comes in as soon as the existence of a free will is acknowledged simply because it is the flipside of our freedom to choose: if and only if we have a choice, we have a moral responsibility to not make immoral choices. But this does not mean that well-being and morality are neatly aligned; they are not. Rather, eudaimonic well-being is constrained by moral aspects in two ways, of which one is subjective and one is objective. Subjectively, eudaimonic well-being requires that a person can approve of the experiences that give rise to her well-being, or at least that she does not strongly disapprove of these experiences and that she does not feel a strong sense of guilt. Objectively, eudaimonic well-being requires that, in the case of serious deprivation, the person is not ignorant of major violations of her moral rights.

An important question that remains to be answered is that of the precise moral status of EWB. Is EWB unconditionally good and is EWB all that matters for a comprehensively good life? The answer to both questions is no, and this follows from the previous considerations. Regarding the first question, it has been argued that EWB requires at least the absence of a strong sense of guilt, but this is merely a subjective criterion of morality. As long as an experience is justifiable by the moral convictions of the person in question, there is no basis for disqualifying it in terms of EWB. This may seem to lead to undesirable conclusions, but the alternative would be to impose external moral standards on the content of EWB, and this would be in conflict with the subjective nature of EWB. In particular, such an external moral standard would mean that a person's EWB will depend on what experiences exactly are justifiable in a world inhabited by seven billion people and threatened by climate change. If you believe that, say, air travel beyond a certain carbon budget is not justifiable, you might have to conclude that flying to a remote ski resort does not actually contribute to EWB, despite the eudaimonic merits of such an experience. Such an understanding of EWB conflates well-being and morality and is therefore not helpful.

EWB should therefore be understood as an amoral concept in the sense of not requiring justifiability of the reasons for someone's EWB from an impartial perspective. There is no logical contradiction in saying that, on the one hand, EWB has intrinsic worth and is desirable *ceteris paribus* but that, on the other hand, not all decisions and experiences that enhance a person's EWB are justifiable. In other words, saying that spending a week at a remote ski resort contributes to my EWB does not imply that this is justifiable and that it is good in a comprehensive sense.

We now also have an answer to the second question, namely whether EWB is all that matters for a good life. A good life in a comprehensive sense must be good for the person whose life is at stake, but it must also not be (excessively) bad for all others (cf. Haybron, 2008, p. 36; see also Haybron, Chap. 2, this volume). When these two conditions do not perfectly coincide, which I have just tried to demonstrate will not always be the case, then trying to lead a good life means realizing EWB only under the condition of legitimacy. This tension can be suspended to the degree that a person critically examines her values and desires in the light of moral considerations and adjusts her values accordingly, but it would be naïve to assume that this will do away with all conflicts between EWB and ethics. EWB is of paramount importance for the good life, but it is not everything.

Acknowledgements I am grateful for very helpful reviews of an earlier manuscript by Paul McNamara and by Lorraine Besser-Jones.

References

Apel, K.-O. (1973). Das Apriori der Kommunikationsgemeinschaft und die Grundlagen der Ethik: Zum Problem einer rationalen Begründung der Ethik im Zeitalter der Wissenschaft. In K.-O. Apel (Ed.), *Transformation der Philosophie, Vol. 2: Das Apriori der Kommunikationsgemeinschaft (engl.: Towards a Transformation of Philosophy, London: Routledge, 1980)* (pp. 358–435). Frankfurt a. M, Germany: Suhrkamp.

Aristotle. (1934). *Nicomachean ethics*. Cambridge, MA: Harvard University Press.

Bayertz, K. (2013). Happiness by maximization? In H. Brockmann & J. Delhey (Eds.), *Human happiness and the pursuit of maximization* (pp. 41–54). Dordrecht, The Netherlands: Springer.

Davidson, R. J. (1992). Anterior cerebral asymmetry and the nature of emotion. *Brain and Cognition, 20*(1), 125–151.

Diener, E. (1984). Subjective well-being. *Psychological Bulletin, 95*(3), 542–575.

Diener, E., Sandvik, E., Pavot, W., & Gallagher, D. (1991). Response artifacts in the measurement of subjective well-being. *Social Indicators Research, 24*, 35–56.

Frankfurt, H. G. (1999). *Necessity, volition, and love*. Cambridge, UK: Cambridge University Press.

Hardie, W. F. R. (1965). The final good in Aristotle's ethics. *Philosophy, 40*(154), 277–295.

Haybron, D. M. (2008). *The pursuit of unhappiness: The elusive psychology of well-being*. Oxford, NY: Oxford University Press.

Hirata, J. (2011). *Happiness, ethics, and economics*. London: Routledge.

Hossenfelder, M. (1998). Die Rolle des Glücksbegriffs in der Moralphilosophie. In J. Schummer (Ed.), *Glück und Ethik* (pp. 169–187). Würzburg, Germany: Königshausen und Neumann.

Keynes, J. M. (1972/1928). Economic possibilities for our grandchildren. In J. M. Keynes (Ed.), *Collected writings*, vol. IX (pp. 321–332). London: Royal Economic Society/Macmillan Press.

Nozick, R. (1989). Happiness. In R. Nozick (Ed.), *The examined life: Philosophical meditations* (pp. 99–117). New York: Simon and Schuster.

Ryan, R. M., & Deci, E. L. (2001). On happiness and human potentials: A review of research on hedonic and eudaimonic well-being. *Annual Review of Psychology, 52*, 141–166.

Ryff, C. D. (1989). Happiness is everything, or is it? Explorations on the meaning of psychological well-being. *Journal of Personality and Social Psychology, 57*, 1069–1081.

Sen, A. K. (1977). Rational fools: A critique of the behavioural foundations of economic theory. *Philosophy & Public Affairs, 6*(4), 317–344.

Sen, A. K. (2009). *The idea of justice*. London: Penguin.

Spaemann, R. (2000/1989). *Happiness and benevolence*. Notre Dame: University of Notre Dame Press.

Tiberius, V. (2013a). Maximization and the good. In H. Brockmann & J. Delhey (Eds.), *Human happiness and the pursuit of maximization* (pp. 55–67). Dordrecht, The Netherlands: Springer.

Tiberius, V. (2013b). Recipes for a good life: Eudaimonism and the contribution of philosophy. In A. S. Waterman (Ed.), *The best within us: Positive psychology perspectives on eudaimonia* (pp. 19–38). Washington, DC: American Psychological Association.

Tiberius, V., & Hall, A. (2010). Normative theory and psychological research: Hedonism, eudaimonism, and why it matters. *The Journal of Positive Psychology, 5*(3), 212–225.

Weber, M. (1985). Der Sinn der „Wertfreiheit" der soziologischen und ökonomischen Wissenschaften. In J. Winckelmann (Ed.), *Gesammelte Aufsätze zur Wissenschaftslehre* (6th ed., pp. 489–540). Tübingen, Germany: Mohr.

Wierzbicka, A. (1999). *Emotions across languages and cultures: Diversity and universals*. Cambridge, UK: Cambridge University Press.

Aristotle on Eudaimonia: On the Virtue of Returning to the Source

4

Blaine J. Fowers

4.1 Eudaimonia in Ancient and Modern Thought

The concept of eudaimonia has generated great interest among psychologists, with perspectives being offered from eudaimonic identity theory (Waterman, Schwartz, & Conti, 2008), the theory of psychological well-being (Ryff & Singer, 2008; Ryff, Chap. 6, this volume), psychological and social flourishing (Keyes, Shmotkin, & Ryff, 2002), Self-Determination Theory (Ryan, Huta, & Deci, 2008; Ryan & Martela, Chap. 7, this volume), and eudaimonic theory (Fowers, 2005, 2012; Fowers, Mollica, & Procacci, 2010). These and other authors have made a compelling case that eudaimonia is a fruitful focus of theoretical and empirical interest. The term *eudaimonia* has been adopted from ancient Greek philosophers. Most appropriations of this concept are attributed to Aristotle, although these appropriations are often inconsistent with his views. Aristotle's (1999) primary ethical text, the Nicomachean *Ethics* (NE)[1], contains a rich description of eudaimonia as the highest good for human beings. Because Aristotle is the most widely discussed philosopher of eudaimonia, I will focus this chapter on his views. Of course, other ancient eudaimonic theories can also be profitably explored and appropriated by contemporary scholars.

Eudaimonia is often translated as happiness, but this translation can be misleading as happiness generally connotes an affective state, particularly in psychology. Aristotle saw eudaimonia as living a fully realized human life. For these reasons, I will use the term flourishing as a translation. For the most part, I will use the term eudaimonia, occasionally employing flourishing as a synonym.

The revival of virtue ethics and eudaimonic theory began with Anscombe (1958) and a lively and sizable scholarly community has emerged. Psychologists first showed sustained interest in virtue and eudaimonia in the 1990s. Psychological researchers have primarily studied the concept of eudaimonia under the rubric of eudaimonic well-being (EWB), which is also the focus of this book. EWB has been studied primarily using self-report measures that include constructs such as meaning, purpose, personal growth, flow, and personal expression. Using the term "EWB" is helpful because it maintains a very clear distinction between a philosophically-based interest in a flourishing life and psychological research on the subjective experience of well-being. I will dis-

[1]To avoid repetitive date referencing, all citations of Aristotle (1999) will be to the NE (Nicomachean Ethics).

B.J. Fowers (✉)
Department of Educational and Psychological Studies, University of Miami, Coral Gables, FL, USA
e-mail: bfowers@miami.edu

J. Vittersø (ed.), *Handbook of Eudaimonic Well-Being*, International Handbooks of Quality-of-Life, DOI 10.1007/978-3-319-42445-3_4

cuss both eudaimonia and EWB, but my focus will be on the former as the more foundational and historically relevant concept.

In a lively exchange, a number of scholars (Biswas-Diener, Kashdan, & King, 2009; Kashdan, Biswas-Diener, & King, 2008; Keyes & Annas, 2009; Waterman, 2008) debated the value of the concept of eudaimonia. (See also Part III of this volume for critical viewpoints). Kashdan et al. (2008) highlighted important conceptual confusions and raised a number of methods-related concerns. Waterman (2008) countered that psychological scholarship on eudaimonia has only begun and is therefore an immature area of study requiring significant work to iron out these difficulties. Keyes and Annas (2009) pointed out the availability of many useful conceptual resources that can help to work toward a consensual view.

One of the chief shortcomings of the growing eudaimonia literature is that many psychologists have appropriated the term from Aristotle with rather tenuous reference to his philosophy. I suggest that the first step in refining the psychological study of eudaimonia and EWB is a return to the ancient Greek thinkers as the original sources. Aristotle has been the primary source for modern eudaimonia scholars, so I focus principally on his thought, but I recognize that the Stoics, Epicureans, and others also had important things to say about eudaimonia. High quality scholarship requires careful attention to the sources of our concepts. We must give these sources their due credit and provide cogent rationales for how we appropriate them rather than simply hijacking a venerable term for our idiosyncratic purposes.

To make Aristotle relevant to our time, we will inevitably reinterpret his formulations, but we must still acknowledge his original thought.[2] Some psychologists have done this by giving eudaimonia a humanistic gloss (e.g., Ryan & Deci, 2001; Waterman, 2008). This humanistic interpretation consists of strong emphases on personal self-realization, autonomous individuals, and a subjectively focused version of eudaimonia. The preoccupation with self-realization, autonomy, and subjectively defined values are thoroughly modern and diverge strongly from Aristotle's views. As Tiberius (2013) put it, "No one in the ancient world thought that what things are good for you could be determined by your own subjective attitudes…Subjectivism is so much the default now that we don't even see it as a view in need of any justification; it's like water to us fishes" (p. 29).

Contemporary appropriations of Aristotle can, of course, be made legitimately from humanistic or other standpoints, but the difficulty is that scholars have not clarified where and how much they have diverged from Aristotle's views, creating conceptual confusion and interpretive difficulties. One of the purposes of this chapter is to provide a close interpretation of Aristotle's and other ancients' views to allow us to more clearly compare and contrast contemporary psychological accounts with his. I hope that this chapter will be useful in clarifying Aristotle's views. It is perfectly reasonable to seek guidance about eudaimonia from other sources or to reinterpret Aristotle to enhance the relevance of his thought. Of course, this chapter is one such reinterpretation. I do quote Aristotle liberally to provide a baseline for my interpretations, but mine is far from the final word. What is not reasonable is to claim an Aristotelian heritage without clarifying how one's views are built on and/or diverge significantly from his work.

4.2 An Overview of Eudaimonia

Let me begin by highlighting nine facets of Aristotle's complex concept of eudaimonia. He defined eudaimonia as the best, most complete form of human life with the following features:

[2]It is important to note and disassociate myself from Aristotle's notoriously inegalitarian views. In accordance with his time, he viewed propertied male citizens as superior humans, with outsiders, women and slaves having a lesser status. In every modern appropriation of his ethics, including this one, these inegalitarian views are repudiated. His ethics can be relatively easily universalized to all human beings to square with contemporary views.

1. **Ethical Concept:** Aristotle introduced eudaimonia in the *NE*, making eudaimonia an inextricably ethical concept because it is about living the *best* kind of life. References to one's life as good, better, and best are ineluctably ethical characterizations.
2. **Nature-Fulfillment:** Aristotle defined eudaimonia as realizing one's full human potential as a particular kind of *natural* being. This formulation shows that he saw science and ethics as inseparable, suggesting exciting ways for science and ethics to inform one another.
3. **Activity:** Eudaimonia is a form of activity. That is, eudaimonia is a way of living and cannot be limited to a subjective state or process.
4. **Constitutive Activity:** Central human goods (e.g., friendship and justice) are constitutive goods because the actions necessary to enact them constitute them as goods. These activities cannot be separated from the good, which makes these activities themselves choiceworthy, not simply means to an end.
5. **Multiple Constituents:** Aristotle viewed humans as reasoning, social beings who flourish through enacting friendship, justice, the best form of politics, and many other choiceworthy goods, meaning that eudaimonia has multiple constituents.
6. **Pleasure:** Eudaimonia is inherently pleasant. Eudaimonic pleasure accompanies noble pursuits (e.g., learning), whereas a pleasure-focused life does not differentiate noble and base pursuits (e.g., gluttony). Thus, eudaimonia is pleasant, but excludes ignoble forms of pleasure.
7. **Virtue:** Eudaimonia is constituted by excellent activity or virtue. Eudaimonia is only possible when an individual acts with excellence.
8. **Complete Life:** Eudaimonia is comprised by a complete life, meaning that it is a matter of how one's life comes together as a whole rather than being comprised of a series of transitory psychological states.
9. **Final End:** Aristotle argued that eudaimonia is fully self-sufficient. He saw eudaimonia as living the best form of human life, which is the ultimate or final end.

Beginning with the ethical nature of eudaimonia, I expand on each aspect of this fascinating concept.

4.2.1 Eudaimonia as an Ethical Concept

Eudaimonia is the central concept of Aristotle's primary text on ethics, the NE, because he, like other ancient Greeks, understood ethics in terms of living a good life. Eudaimonia refers to the most desirable form of human life. Two contrasts to more familiar, contemporary approaches to ethics help to clarify Aristotle's approach. First, the two dominant contemporary approaches to ethics focus on acting rightly according to some general principle or duty (deontology) or in order to foster positive outcomes (consequentialism). In contrast, the core of Aristotle's ethics is the good life and actions are chosen because they help to constitute a good life. Second, familiar forms of contemporary ethics centers on how one should treat others, but have relatively little to say about how best to live one's own life where another person's welfare is not directly at stake. Although individual welfare is central to eudaimonia, Aristotle saw individual well-being as deeply dependent on good relations with others (Fowers, 2005).

Recognizing eudaimonia as an ethical concept at its core presents a dilemma for psychologists who want to maintain a strict separation between science and ethics, facts and values (Fowers, 2008). This is part of Kashdan et al.'s (2008) discomfort with eudaimonia research as they worry that there "is the implicit (and sometimes explicit) argument that there is a moral hierarchy to be found in happiness, with eudaimonic happiness being viewed as more objective, comprehensive, and morally valid than hedonic well-being" (p. 219). In particular, they urge scholars not to ascribe "moral judgment in our definition of happiness" (p. 220). Instead, we should "examine how the presence of values and goals…influence the experience of positive affect, feelings of belongingness, meaning in life, and other elements of the Good Life" (p. 220). In this way, they believe that we can minimize "the biases, interests, and values of any particular researcher" (p. 220). Ironically, they value a value-neutral science of well-being. Additional irony ensues because they do not recognize that "positive affect, feelings of belonging, meaning in life, and other elements in the Good Life" are themselves interests and values and express a modern individualistic bias. These values just happen to be so thoroughly internalized by twenty-first century American authors and that the values escape notice. Relegating values to the subjective sphere is itself a major pillar in the dominant value perspective known as individualism (Richardson, Fowers, & Guignon, 1999). Separating facts and values is very problematic, frequently leading researchers to smuggle in culturally syntonic values under the guise of objective science, as Kashdan et al. did.

Kashdan et al. (2008) are not unusual in struggling with the fact-value dichotomy and failing to recognize that many key psychological constructs entail strong value commitments and ethical claims. They follow a well-worn psychological path in attempting to avoid values in their work by focusing on subjective outcome variables. The breadth of this tendency is exemplified by the promotion of self-efficacy, an internal locus of control, and satisfaction with life, as well as attempts to reduce aggression, bullying, and depression, all emblematic of modern Western moral preoccupations with affirming ordinary life and reducing suffering (Taylor, 1989). The problematic nature of this fact-value distinction in psychology has been extensively argued elsewhere (Fowers, 2005; Cushman, 1995; Danziger, 1990; Richardson et al., 1999; Taylor, 1989). The key point for now is that eudaimonia is no more value laden than many other psychological constructs. Psychologists do not contest the idea that a reasonable degree of self-efficacy, internal locus of control, and life satisfaction is better than powerlessness and depression. A life with a positive hedonic valence seems obviously more desirable than an anhedonic life, all other things being equal. Similarly, I argue that a eudaimonic life is more desirable than a non-eudaimonic life. I recommend that we frankly admit these commitments rather than hiding behind putatively subjective preferences.

The question of whether science and ethics can be integrated is a large one with which psychology has been struggling since its inception. Investigators of eudaimonia have to come to terms with this question because eudaimonia is a frankly and historically ethical term. The standard response is to render the variable subjective so that researchers appear to avoid claims about objective well-being. Kashdan et al.'s (2008) imputation that eudaimonia is an "objective" concept of well-being seems to signal their disapproval of seeing well-being as anything other than a subjective concern. The question of whether eudaimonia is subjective or objective is very anachronistic because Aristotle did not divide the world that way. Many contemporary thinkers (cf., Richardson et al., 1999) reject the subjective-objective dichotomy because it obscures more than it reveals. Eudaimonia has both objective or consensually observable elements (physical health, tangibly meaningful activities, observably enacted purposes, and demonstrable aspects of a good life) and subjective or psychological elements (experiencing meaning, purpose, and belonging). Both subjective and objective aspects of eudaimonia are indispensible. Keyes and Annas (2009) discussed this in terms of one's feelings (subjective) and functioning (objective) both being essential to flourishing. Eudaimonia is best characterized by the seamless integration and harmony of personal experience and observable actions and outcomes.

Ultimately, decisions regarding the ethical character of eudaimonia and the wisdom of dividing the world into subjective and objective realms or value-laden and factual domains rest with the discipline as a whole. I am suggesting, however, that the attempt to maintain a fact-value dichotomy in inquiry on eudaimonia is at least as problematic as adopting a frankly ethical concept of human well-being.

4.2.2 Eudaimonia as Nature-Fulfillment

Aristotle clarified that eudaimonia is a natural phenomenon in the first book of the NE. He introduced the function argument, which suggests that the good for any being is defined in terms of its nature. In the function argument, eudaimonia is defined as the most complete expression of the natural characteristics of human beings. Aristotle emphasized particularly that humans are reasoning, social creatures, and that living well involves the full realization of those natural features. Interest in the function argument has been renewed recently in naturalized approaches to ethics (Arnhart, 1998; Fowers, 2015; Okrent, 2007). Thus, Aristotle saw no separation between an "objective" realm of human nature and what psychologists often see as the "subjective" human good.

The term function is a translation for *ergon*, which in various contexts could also be translated as work, product, result, or achievement (Ostwald, 1999). Using the translation of work is helpful because it connotes the work or function of human beings in much the way we refer to the works of a poet, artist, or craftsperson. Thus, ergon refers to characteristic human functions, and these functions are manifold and open-ended rather than unitary and pre-determined. The function argument also suggests that the good for humans is evaluated in terms of being members of the human species, and the characteristics, capacities, and interests of our species define what living well is for us.

If eudaimonia is a matter of living fully as a member of the *human species*, our natural characteristics make certain goods central for us. Of course, establishing what is natural for human beings is a very large question that is beyond the scope of this chapter, but I can suggest some broad outlines (See Fowers, 2015 for a more thorough treatment). If humans are social beings, then belonging and social harmony are likely central goods. If humans are reasoning beings, then gaining knowledge, planning our futures, and living meaningfully are likely central goods. Aristotle saw success in attaining characteristic human goods as essential for eudaimonia. Agency is indispensable because individuals pursue these (and other) characteristic human goods in their own particular ways.

Aristotle's approach is what philosophers term a nature-fulfillment theory (Tiberius, Chap. 38, this volume). He describes natural characteristics of humans as a species and ties them to what is good for human beings. For example, humans are a highly social species, and there is abundant evidence that social relationships are critical to individual well-being (e.g., Fowers, 2015). Aristotle suggested that social relationships are necessary for living the best kind of life whether an individual realizes it or not. That is, the importance of relational living is not a matter of subjective preference, but is an aspect of human nature. His point is not simply that individual well-being and social connections are correlated, but that participating in social relationships partly constitutes flourishing. That is, relationships are logically necessary for eudaimonia, not just simply correlative or even causal.

In contrast to Aristotle's focus on expressing *human* nature, some prevalent psychological approaches to eudaimonia emphasize *personal* self-expression. Striving to become an excellent human being and aiming to fully express my inner self may coincide, of course. Those two goals will only coincide in two conditions. First, Romantic philosophy suggests that humans are inherently good and expressing one's "true" inner nature will automatically allow one to become an excellent human being. In contrast, Aristotle stated that goodness and excellence are "implanted in us neither by nature nor contrary to nature" (NE, p. 33). Second, human excellence and self-expression coincide when one learns what is good and shapes one's habits to be conducive to the good. In Aristotle's view, excellence is a matter of cultivating good character and habits, not expressing the "truth" of an inner self.

For example, Waterman's (2008) definition of eudaimonia has been influential in psychology (cf. Ryan et al., 2008; Ryff & Singer, 2008). He followed a formulation by Norton (1976) that lacks any currency among Aristotle scholars in defining eudaimonia as being true to one's self, taking the prefix "eu" to mean true and "daimon" to mean self. The prefix "eu" means good, not true, as its usage in euphoria (good feelings) and eupraxia (good practices) exemplify. Scholars of ancient history and linguistics (Liddell & Scott, 1996; Martin, 2007) suggest that, for the ancient Greeks, eudaimonia included having a kind of guardian spirit or demigod (a daimon), with "eu" meaning good. Aristotle's usage suggests a life that is being guided toward worthwhile activities. He did not emphasize the daimon per se, only seeing eudaimonia as a blessed or flourishing condition. Moreover, ancient Greeks did not have a concept of an inner self to which one should or even could be "true" (Taylor, 1989). In contrast, Waterman (2008) defined eudaimonia in terms of "personal expressiveness" and "self-realization," both of which focus on bringing out the "true, inner self," adhering to modern views that "a self" is a natural human endowment. Waterman (2008) recognized this as a distinctly modern interpretation, and he adopted it as a way to "render eudaimonic concepts and principles in a form more congenial to psychological theorizing and empirical research" (p. 241). Nevertheless, his definition diverges strongly (and, from my viewpoint, unnecessarily) from Aristotle in relying on questionable modern assumptions of a real inner self to which one should be true.

Self-determination theorists have attempted to integrate eudaimonia into their theory and they also emphasize the concept of an inner self. Ryan et al. (2008) explicitly made "a broad claim that there are intrinsic values built into human nature and that these values are universal" (p. 148). They theorize that those values are the natural needs of the inner self: autonomy, competence, and social relatedness (Ryan & Deci, 2001). Thus, Self-Determination Theory (SDT) theorists agree with Aristotle that core human goods are components of human nature. The concept of eudaimonia has been only recently and partially incorporated into SDT (Ryan & Deci, 2001; Ryan et al., 2008), leaving three significant tensions between SDT and eudaimonic thought. First, the central theme in SDT is personal autonomy, which relates to an individual's ownership of goals and action (Ryan & Deci, 2001; Ryan et al., 2008). The SDT emphasis on individual ownership of goals and actions is partially consistent with Aristotle's view that the best kind of activities must be chosen wholeheartedly by the individual. Autonomy does not go far enough, from an Aristotelian perspective, because *choosing well* is at least as important as the autonomy of the choice. In other words, owning one's choices is independent of whether one has chosen well or not. One can fully own poor choices because having the autonomy to choose well presupposes the autonomy to choose poorly.

SDT researchers could counter that their attention to the content of goals (intrinsic vs. extrinsic) addresses the question of pursuing *worthwhile* autonomous goals. Ryan et al. (2008) define intrinsic goals as personal growth, affiliation and intimacy, community contribution, and physical health. This definition of goal content appropriately leaves significant latitude to individual choice, but it raises a second difficulty from an Aristotelian perspective. These goals represent formal characteristics rather than actual contents. The goals are contentless because individuals can attain them through virtually any self-chosen activity. Therefore, becoming an orchestral musician is no more intrinsic than devoting oneself to racial supremacy. Nothing in the list of intrinsic goals provides criteria for the worthiness of goals and activities. At least in theory, one could experience personal growth, affiliation and intimacy, and physical health while contributing to a supremacist community. In contrast, Aristotle would say that supremacists cannot have the best human life because they promote injustice. SDT and other psychological theories may have adopted contentless views on goals and flourishing to avoid taking an ethical stand. This avoidance backfires in failing to prevent clearly unacceptable aims from being described as intrinsic goals.

Third, the focus in SDT is on the satisfaction of *personal needs*, whereas Aristotle's emphasis is on fostering the best in ourselves *as human beings*. SDT proposes that the satisfaction of basic human needs will lead naturally to the expression of the best in human beings, but this is an article of humanistic faith. Aristotle explicitly denied natural individual goodness. In contrast, he believed that good habits, rather than need satisfaction, do the work of fashioning a eudaimonic life.

As noted above, Aristotle discussed the content of goals as an outgrowth of humanity's social and reasoning nature. In the domain of sociality, he famously said that "man is by nature a social and political being" (NE, p. 15). Therefore, he emphasized friendship, justice, and good governance. Aristotle made the good and virtue of friendship central in the NE, devoting two of the ten books to it. He suggested that "in order to be eudaimon, a man [sic] needs morally good friends" (NE, p. 267). In the domain of reasoning, he asserted that "what is by nature proper to each thing will be at once the best and the most pleasant for it. In other words, a life guided by intelligence is the best and most pleasant for man, inasmuch as intelligence, above all else, is man" (NE, p. 291). Therefore, he saw practical wisdom (good judgment), scientific knowledge, and contemplative wisdom as necessary components of eudaimonia.[3] Systematic contemporary arguments that link natural characteristics and eudaimonia have been advanced (Arnhart, 1998; Fowers, 2015; Okrent, 2007).

In pointing out these discrepancies between contemporary psychological writings and Aristotle, I am not insisting that scholars must accept Aristotle or my reading of him as authoritative. Waterman and his colleagues have presented an interesting model of well-being with some supportive evidence (see Waterman et al., 2008). Similarly, SDT scholars have developed an interesting model with corroborative evidence (Ryan & Deci, 2001; Ryan et al., 2008). Nevertheless, I believe that good scholarship requires us to accurately recognize the sources of our terms and concepts. The widespread adoption of the term eudaimonia could amount to an opportunistic capitalization on a venerable and impressively Greek term or it could open the way to careful examination of how we can fruitfully appropriate ancient wisdom to inform approaches to human flourishing in our time. The question is how adequately we document the manner and rationale for appropriating the term and clearly delineate how this might or might not be consistent with the original use of the term. The lack of such delineation is a primary reason why the psychological literature on eudaimonia is so conceptually confused. Theorists just do what they want with the term, seldom clearly explaining their choices. (See Huta (2013) for a good example of delineating similarities and differences from Aristotle).

[3] In part of Book X of the NE, Aristotle discusses contemplation as the highest human activity. There is a good deal of controversy regarding how this concept is to be integrated into the rest of Aristotle's account of eudaimonia. I have downplayed this concept and the controversy in this chapter because it does not seem pertinent enough to psychological scholarship to merit recounting it. For more on this question, see Broadie (1991).

4.2.3 Eudaimonia as Activity

Aristotle's insistence that eudaimonia is not a subjective state is also seen in his central claim that "eudaimonia is some kind of activity" (NE, p. 264), which he affirms throughout the NE. He clarifies that "the good of man (eudaimonia) is an activity of the soul (*psyche*) in conformity with excellence or virtue" (NE, p. 17). Aristotle specifies further that

> it does doubtless make a considerable difference whether we think of the highest good as…being a characteristic or an activity. For a characteristic may exist without producing any good result, as for example, in a man who is asleep or incapacitated in some other respect. An activity, on the other hand, must produce a result… (NE, p. 20)

He concludes that "obviously, eudaimonia must be classed as an activity" (NE, p. 286).

Some psychological aspects of eudaimonia are quite consistent with this view. Waterman's (2008) approach to assessing eudaimonia has focused on activities from the beginning. In particular, he emphasized the quality of an individual's activities as the marker of eudaimonia. Steger, Kashdan and Oishi (2008) found that eudaimonic activities were related to experiencing meaning and life satisfaction in a daily diary study (see also Steger, Chap. 11, this volume). Huta and Ryan (2010) conducted an experience sampling study of participants' activities and motives for those activities. They found clearly eudaimonic and hedonic motives. Hedonically motivated behavior was accompanied by positive affect and carefreeness whereas eudaimonically motivated behavior was accompanied by the experience of meaning. My colleagues and I (Fowers et al., 2010) reported that different modes of goal activity were associated independently with hedonic and eudaimonic well-being.

In contrast to Aristotle's emphasis on eudaimonia as activity, most psychologists rely on self-report measures of EWB that focus on subjective experiences such as engagement or meaning and on personal traits rather than concrete activities (e.g., Waterman et al., 2010). Other measures are not termed EWB scales, but researchers frequently use them for this purpose, such as the Scales of Psychological Well-being (Ryff, 1989) and the Orientation to Happiness Scale (Peterson, Park, & Seligman, 2005) that similarly emphasize subjective assessments. These measures can be very useful as indicators of the subjective elements of eudaimonia, but they are insufficient as assessments of an Aristotelian concept of eudaimonia, which requires incorporating both worthwhile activities and subjective experience. Thus, the important challenge here is to resist the temptation to fully psychologize eudaimonia.

4.2.4 Eudaimonia as Constitutive Activity

From the first paragraph of the NE, Aristotle stressed that eudaimonia is a specific form of activity: "Every art or applied science and every systematic investigation, and similarly every action and choice, seem to aim at some good… there is a difference in the ends at which they aim: in some cases the activity is the end, in others the end is some product beyond the activity" (NE, p. 3). I have called the latter orientation to goals instrumental, in which one seeks an end through means or actions that are separable from the outcome (Fowers, 2010). Obtaining wealth is a paradigm example because it can be obtained in many ways, including working very hard, marrying someone wealthy, or fraud. If the aim is strictly wealth possession, any of these means will do, and success is all that counts. This is because "where the end lies beyond the action the product is naturally superior to the activity" (NE, p. 3). That is, when one's actions are separable from the end product, the product is what is important and the actions are only instruments to that end. It is not just the strategies for obtaining wealth that are instrumental. Wealth itself is also an instrument to be used for other purposes. It is not choiceworthy in itself in a good life; wealth is only valuable in itself to the greedy and miserly.

When the "activity is the end," the actions and ends are inseparable. This inseparability means that the actions constitute the end, and such activities are called constitutive (Fowers, 2010). Examples of constitutive goal pursuit include artistic endeavors, friendship, and democracy. In each of these cases, the only way to attain the end is to enact it through creating art, acting as a friend, or participation in democratic activities. All of these ends are also choiceworthy in themselves. Whether or not art, friendship or democracy helps us to obtain other goals, we in the modern West tend to see them as worthy of choice. Aristotle emphasized the value and constitutive nature of these activities: "Activities desirable in themselves are those from which we seek to derive nothing beyond the actual exercise of the activity" (NE, p. 286). Constitutive activity has meaning and dignity because it is inseparable from the valued end.

Instrumental ends are clearly essential to a good life "for it is impossible or at least not easy to perform noble actions if one lacks the wherewithal. Many actions can only be performed with the help of instruments, as it were: friends, wealth, and political power" (NE, p. 21). Instrumental goals such as wealth are not choiceworthy in themselves, but they do facilitate the pursuit of constitutive goals. Although great wealth, power, and friendship networks are not necessary to live well, these resources are required to some degree.[4]

Eudaimonia is a constitutive good because the way to attain it is by realizing one's potential as a human being. There are no short-cuts or strategies; one can flourish only through the full expression of one's human capacities. For Aristotle, eudaimonia is the overarching constitutive goal for a human life because "we always choose eudaimonia as an end in itself and never for the sake of something else" (NE, p. 15). My colleagues and I have documented that constitutive goal pursuit is uniquely related to EWB, consistent with Aristotle's perspective (Fowers et al., 2010). In summary, constitutive activities aimed at choiceworthy goals comprise eudaimonia. Instrumental activity is important in providing the infrastructure for constitutive goal pursuit.

4.2.5 The Multiple Constituents of Eudaimonia

Although Aristotle saw eudaimonia as the highest good and as a cohesive way of life, it is constituted by the presence of multiple human goods or ends. That is, eudaimonia is unidimensional in that it a single, overarching way of life, but it has many constitutive elements (e.g. friendship, justice, intellectual activity). He clarified that "since there are many activities, arts, and sciences, the number of ends is correspondingly large" (NE, p. 3). Thus, there are many different ends one can seek. He discussed many instrumental ends, including wealth, fame, and power, as well as a number of constitutive ends, such as friendship, justice, and knowledge. None of these ends are sufficient by themselves for eudaimonia. Rather, a eudaimonic life is one that encompasses many choiceworthy ends and ties them together in a coherent whole (Broadie, 1991). There is no definitive form for a eudaimonic life, for differing talents, opportunities, and social relations shape eudaimonia for a given individual. Aristotle clarified that diverse worthwhile ends contribute to eudaimonia: "all the other goods are either necessary prerequisites for eudaimonia, or are by nature co-workers with it and useful instruments for attaining it" (NE, pp. 22–23).

Seeing eudaimonia as constituted by a variety of choiceworthy ends helps to address Kashdan et al.'s (2008) worry about its prescriptive moral content. It is reasonable to be concerned about a theory arrogating the role of prescribing choices and values. Because there are multiple constituents of flourishing, there is wide latitude in how one cultivates a good life, rendering prescription impossible.

Huta and Waterman (2014) identified four core content elements in most psychological accounts of eudaimonia: authenticity, meaning, excellence, and growth. They also highlighted four types of analyses: orientations (values, motives, and goals); behaviors; experiences; and functioning (mental health and flourishing). They organized various researchers' work in terms of these content elements and types of analysis. An Aristotelian perspective must include a large plurality of goods for eudaimonia. An adequate account of eudaimonia also requires that we employ all four forms of analysis (see also Huta, Chap. 15, this volume).

Measurement of EWB has generally incorporated multiple components. Ryff (1989), a pioneer in extending well-being research beyond positive and negative affect, designed the Scales of Psychological Well-being to assess six dimensions of well-being. The dimensions are: Self-acceptance, Purpose in Life, Environmental Mastery, Positive Relationships, Personal Growth, and Autonomy.

Peterson et al. (2005) created the Orientations to Happiness scale to assess the Life of Pleasure, the Life of Meaning, and the Life of Engagement as three independent and complementary orientations to happiness. The Life of Pleasure scale assesses how important pleasure is in one's life (a hedonic scale). The Life of Meaning scale assesses how meaningful a person views his or her life (a measure of EWB). The Life of

[4] Aristotle described three types of friendship: utility, pleasure, and character. A utility friendship, in which a friend is an instrument to one's end. He saw character friendship as a central human good because character friends seek ends that are good in themselves together and want one another to flourish (Fowers, 2005).

Engagement measures the degree to which an individual experiences "flow," the tendency to become absorbed in one's activities.

Waterman et al. (2010) developed the Questionnaire for Eudaimonic Well-being as a scale that is "closely grounded in contemporary philosophical understandings of eudaimonic functioning" that has "incremental value…to account for behavior beyond the contributions made by other conceptions of well-being" (p. 42). The scale development was "strongly theory driven" with items from "six inter-related categories with strong philosophical-psychological linkages: (1) self-discovery, (2) perceived development of one's best potentials, (3) a sense of purpose and meaning in life, (4) investment of significant effort in pursuit of excellence, (5) intense involvement in activities, and (6) enjoyment of activities as personally expressive" (p. 44).[5]

These prominent measures show that EWB is clearly conceptualized with multiple components. Recent structural equation modeling and confirmatory factor analytic studies also support this multicomponent approach to EWB (Fowers et al., 2010; Linley, Maltby, Wood, Osborne, & Hurling, 2009).

Psychologists have also assessed individuals' goals and activities as they relate to eudaimonia. Investigators generally study ideographic goals and activities rather than specifying a priori which goals and activities are eudaimonic (Fowers et al., 2010; Sheldon & Kasser, 1995; Sheldon, Chap. 36, this volume). Experience sampling techniques similarly study naturally occurring behavior (Huta & Ryan, 2010; Steger et al., 2008). These approaches are based on a multicomponent conceptualization of eudaimonia rather than a monolithic and prescriptive viewpoint.

4.2.6 Eudaimonia and Pleasure

Pleasure is an important aspect of well-being, and the relationship between eudaimonia and pleasure is complex in the NE. Aristotle examined whether pleasure is the highest good for humans. Pleasure could be the ultimate good because we choose it for its own sake. He also cited the strong relationship between pleasure and activity: "there is no pleasure without activity, and every activity is completed by pleasure" (NE, p. 282). By completion, he meant that pleasure emerges in activities that are carried out well. That is, pleasure is not distinct from the activity; rather it arises through the activity. "Pleasures differ in kind…each pleasure is intimately connected with the activity which it completes" (NE, pp. 282–283). For example, pleasures of taste (delicious food) differ from pleasant sights (beautiful vistas), and these differ from intellectual pleasures (solving theoretical problems).

The intimate connection between activity and pleasure helped Aristotle explain why pleasure cannot be the highest good for humans because "activities differ from one another in goodness and badness. Some are desirable, others should be avoided, and others again are indifferent. The same also is true of pleasures…the pleasure proper to a morally good activity is good, the pleasure proper to a bad activity evil" (NE, p. 284). Individuals find pleasure in very different activities. Some find pleasure in acting kindly toward others, while some find it in exploiting or dominating others. Aristotle suggested that "the sensation of pleasure belongs to the soul, and each man derives pleasure from what he is said to love" (NE, p. 20), whether in mutually supportive relations with others or in wielding unilateral power over others.

This discussion of pleasure brings us back to Aristotle's basic point that eudaimonia is an inherently moral concept. This is a difficult pill for many psychologists to swallow because we tend to relegate the experience and sources of pleasure to subjective preference. Aristotle's reminder that some people experience pleasure through activities that are deplorable reminds us that the sources of pleasure are not merely matters of subjective preference. As an illustration, the American Psychological Association has adopted and advocated specific public policy statements that repudiate activities that may

[5]Waterman et al. (2010) presented some evidence that these six categories can be summarized in a single dimension, but this evidence is based on an inappropriate use of confirmatory factor analytic methods.

provide pleasure by exploiting or dominating others (e.g., APA, 2003, 2010). Surely, we can recognize that finding pleasure in deplorable actions is morally problematic, not just a subjective preference. This amounts to recognizing a crucial distinction: "the good is the sort of thing which we wish for *because we think it good*, not something we think good because it is what we wish for" (Wiggins, 1980, p. 231).

Eudaimonic theory sees pleasure as completing activity, particularly when conducting the activity well. When an individual's activities are clear expressions of human excellence, these activities will be very pleasant. Because eudaimonia is the fullest expression of human excellence, Aristotle believed that eudaimonia provides the greatest human pleasure: "Eudaimonia is at once the best, noblest, and most pleasant thing, and these qualities are not separate" (NE, p. 21). Although eudaimonia is itself pleasant, there are some pleasures that are distinct from eudaimonia. Recognition of both the relatedness and distinctness of pleasure and eudaimonia is the mainstream position among eudaimonia researchers. In contrast, Kashdan et al. (2008) presented a belabored and unsubstantiated imputation of a dichotomy between pleasure and eudaimonia among eudaimonia investigators. Kashdan et al. implausibly recommended collapsing eudaimonia and hedonia rather than continuing to carefully and persistently examine the distinctions and relationship between these concepts.

Contra Kashdan et al. (2008), the predicted distinction between and relatedness of pleasure and eudaimonia have been regularly empirically documented. The vast majority of the literature on well-being has focused on what has been called subjective well-being (SWB). SWB is generally assessed in terms of positive and negative affect and life satisfaction (see Diener, 2012 for a review). These indicators of SWB are much more consistent with the concept of pleasure (hedonia) than with eudaimonia. This narrow focus on positive affect led a number of scholars to argue for a broadening of the study of well-being beyond SWB (e.g., Ryff, 1989; Waterman, 2008), ultimately resulting in the EWB literature. Subsequently, investigators have studied the relationship between SWB and EWB. Numerous investigations have produced results that are consistent with the distinctiveness of these forms of well-being (Fowers et al., 2010, Compton, Smith, Cornish, & Qualls, 1996; Huta & Ryan, 2010; Keyes et al., 2002).

This "related but distinct" result is not fully satisfying from an Aristotelian perspective. The reason for this is that Aristotle's views differentiated pleasures, but the current conceptualization and measurement of SWB remain undifferentiated. Thus, there is no way to tell how much of self-reported SWB is based on noble or base pleasure, or on well-earned or fatuous satisfaction. This discrimination may prove difficult due to the social desirability likely to be evoked by the concepts of nobility, baseness, dessert, or fatuousness. Therefore, a current challenge is to find a way to make this discrimination for a more thorough and interesting empirical exploration of Aristotle's concept of eudaimonia. The concepts of nobility and baseness are closely related to virtue, the next element of eudaimonia.

4.2.7 Eudaimonia and Virtue

No discussion of eudaimonia is complete without addressing the topic of virtue. For Aristotle, "eudaimonia is one of the most divine things, even if it is not god-sent but attained through virtue and some kind of learning or training. For the prize and end of excellence or virtue is the best thing of all" (NE, p. 22). Broadie (1991) explained that "…an excellence or virtue, as Plato and Aristotle understand that concept, is nothing but a characteristic which makes the difference between functioning and functioning well" (p. 37). The virtues just are the character strengths that make it possible to pursue worthwhile ends (Fowers, 2005). Recall that Aristotle's definition of the good life included living according to our natural characteristics (e.g., sociality and rationality). He adds that "this kind of life is an activity of the soul (*psyche*)…and if a man of high standards is he who performs these actions well and properly, and if a function is well performed when it is performed in accordance with the excellence appropriate to it; we reach the conclusion that the good of man is an activity of the soul in conformity with excellence or virtue" (NE, p. 17). To live a eudaimonic life therefore requires the virtues.

Aristotle discussed an array of virtues, ranging from courage and generosity to wit. He outlined a structure of virtue such that particular circumstances call for each virtue, and the virtue is defined in contrast to deficiency and excess. For example, situations involving significant risk call for the virtue of courage. The deficient response to risk is cowardice and the excessive response is recklessness. Courage occurs in the face of fear, not in its absence, as the courageous person "endures and fears the right things, for the right motive, in the right manner, and at the right time" (NE, p. 70). Because everyone has to face situations of risk, a flourishing life will include the ability to face those risks with courage. Of course, it makes sense to take risks only when something quite valuable is at stake. Courageous risk-taking is essential when protecting a loved one, struggling to maintain one's community, or preserving democracy. It is the value of the end that makes courage worthwhile. When nothing important is at stake, risk-taking devolves to recklessness or thrill-seeking (Fowers, 2008).

Practical wisdom (*phronesis*) is the ability to make good decisions about what is at stake in a situation, about which virtues are called for, and in what virtuous action consists, given the actor's aims and the relevant context. Aristotle saw practical wisdom as necessary for virtue and eudaimonia: "it is impossible to be good in the full sense of the word without practical wisdom or to be a man of practical wisdom without moral excellence or virtue" (NE, p. 172). Practical wisdom is a complex topic that has been treated extensively elsewhere (e.g., Fowers, 2005; Schwartz & Sharpe, 2010; Schwartz & Wrzesniewski, Chap. 8, this volume; Wiggins, 1980).

The virtues have cognitive, affective, and behavioral components. For Aristotle, an act is virtuous only if "the agent has certain characteristics as he performs it: first of all, he must know what he is doing; secondly, he must choose to act the way he does, and he must choose it for its own sake; and in the third place, the act must spring from a firm and unchangeable character" (NE, p. 39). In order to act virtuously, a person has to choose to act virtuously knowingly and be disposed to act well willingly.

Crucially, virtue must always show up in behavior, and virtue is characterized by consistently acting rightly in a particular domain (e.g., generosity). That is, virtue is a habitual form of action. For Aristotle, "the question of moral philosophy is not simply how I am to conduct myself in my life, but how I am to become the kind of person for whom proper conduct emanates characteristically from a fixed disposition" (Kosman, 1980, p. 103). The goal is to develop a "character that somehow has an affinity for excellence or virtue, a character that loves what is noble and feels disgust at what is base" (p. 296). The key to virtue, then, is to cultivate love for what is good. When this is accomplished, acting virtuously becomes second nature because one is drawn naturally to what is worthwhile because "each man derives pleasure from what he is said to love" (NE, p. 20).

Although eudaimonia and virtue mutually entail one another, most psychological discussions do not link them directly (e.g., Ryan & Deci, 2001; Ryff & Singer, 2008). Most discussions of eudaimonia do not even mention virtue and most discussions of virtue barely mention eudaimonia as the raison d'être of virtue (e.g., Baumeister & Exline, 1999; Peterson & Seligman, 2004). At times, this is simply due to limiting the domain of a particular study or argument to make it more manageable. If so, it seems appropriate to at least acknowledge that one is setting this important relationship aside in order to more fully address a narrower question. In other cases, virtues have been replaced by something like needs, as in most discussions of eudaimonia in SDT, where eudaimonia is seen as the result of fulfilling the three theorized human needs of autonomy, competence, and belonging rather than being constituted by virtuous action (cf. Ryan & Deci, 2001). Virtues are included in their most recent writings (e.g., Ryan and

Martela, Chap. 7, this volume), but they do not make the connection clear, suggesting only that autonomy and mindfulness are somehow related to virtue and indicating that universal human good will is related to the virtue of friendliness. Much greater specification of the role of virtue in the SDT understanding of eudaimonia is needed. When scholars do not make clear connections between the core concepts of eudaimonia and virtue, it leaves one to wonder just why they even chose to use the term eudaimonia.

4.2.8 Eudaimonia as a Complete Life

Aristotle made it very clear that eudaimonia is comprised by how one's life is coming together as a whole (consistent with eudaimonia being based on good character). He clarified that "the good of man is an activity of the soul (*psyche*)… But we must add 'in a complete life.' For one swallow does not make a spring, nor does one sunny day; similarly, one day or a short time does not make a man blessed and eudaimon" (NE, pp. 17–18). Once stated, this seems obvious because an individual who lived well for only a portion of his or her life would hardly be considered to have experienced the best kind of life. The best kind of life would clearly encompass its entirety. Aristotle referred to a complete life as one composed of the ongoing, reasonably successful pursuit of worthwhile, characteristically human ends. These pursuits are characterized by excellence and experienced as pleasant. In addition, the activities in a eudaimonic life should have a significant degree of coherence, so that the individual does not have to continually struggle with contradictory motives and ends. This will convey a degree of stability in that individuals "who are supremely eudaimon spend their lives in these activities most intensely and most continuously…The eudaimon will have the attribute of permanence" (NE, p. 25).

The concept of the complete life is daunting for psychological researchers because it implies investigating the entire length of individuals' lives. There are a few impressively extended longitudinal studies that tell us something about living well over an extended period of time (e.g., Terman, 1954). Such extended studies are rare, given the extraordinary devotion and stability of purpose required to conduct them. Scholars can examine the coherence and completeness of individuals' lives in shorter time frames by asking their respondents to assess the breadth and coherence of their aims and activities. For example, Sheldon and Kasser (1995) found that when individuals have goals that mutually facilitate one another, they had a greater degree of psychological well-being. Such investigations can also include retrospection on the longevity and progress in the individuals' aims and activities, as well as projections of their maintenance in the future. No doubt, many studies will involve short-term research on eudaimonic activity and experience as a matter of practicality. Nevertheless, incorporating the concept of a complete life into our conceptual frameworks would enrich eudaimonia research because the relative longevity of eudaimonic activity and experience is an important way they differ from hedonic experience.

The concept of a complete life is most easily understood in trait terms because a eudaimonic life is comprised by consistent virtuous action aimed at enduring human goods. In contrast, Huta (2013) summarized research on momentary eudaimonic experience or eudaimonic states through intensive longitudinal research (e.g., Huta & Ryan, 2010; Straume & Vittersø, 2012; Vittersø, Chap. 17, this volume). These investigators have found interesting differences in relationships between trait and state eudaimonic measures and many related constructs. Although it may seem that assessing states is inconsistent with the concept of a complete life, this is a superficial difference. A life is made up of innumerable moments, and the emotions, motives, goals, and behaviors in each of those moments contribute to the overall quality of one's life. A eudaimonic life will be comprised of a significant preponderance of momentary experiences, behaviors, and interactions that are eudaimonic in nature.

4.2.9 Eudaimonia as the Final End

The first book of the NE is an argument that if there is an overall or final end in human life, it must be eudaimonia. For Aristotle, the final end is the end that is chosen for its own sake and not for the sake of anything else, and is complete in itself, lacking nothing. He suggested that eudaimonia is that ultimate end "for we always choose eudaimonia as an end in itself and never for the sake of anything else." (NE, p. 15). Other ends, such as pleasure and knowledge, are good in themselves but they can be means to further ends as well. Aristotle suggested that whereas one might pursue pleasure as part of a flourishing life, one would not seek to flourish so that one could feel pleasure. He also concluded that "eudaimonia lacks nothing and is self-sufficient" (p. 286) because he believed that a eudaimonic life is everything humans can hope for in this world. Nothing can be added to a flourishing life it to make it better.

Using terms like "highest," "best," and "final" raises the question of whether eudaimonia and virtue are elitist concepts, a worry expressed by Kashdan et al. (2008). Is eudaimonia available only to a few people or is it accessible to all, or at least to most? Aristotle's answer is that because "eudaimonia depends on excellence, it will be shared by many people; for study and effort will make it accessible to anyone whose capacity for virtue is unimpaired" (NE, p. 22). Clearly, he saw it as widely available. In addition, eudaimonia is something one pursues within one's own life rather than in competition with others. It is not a commodity with a limited quantity. Available research indicates that growth stories associated with eudaimonic indicators "cut across gender, ethnicity, and socioeconomic status" (Bauer, McAdams, & Pals, 2008, p. 92; Bauer, Chap. 10, this volume). Yet the caveat about eudaimonia not being accessible to some is important because some people experience great misfortunes, such as severe child abuse or living under horrific conditions that can make virtue and eudaimonia extremely difficult to attain. Yet the path to eudaimonia is the pursuit of characteristically human ends through excellent activity, which is widely accessible rather than being limited to a small elite.

4.3 Conclusion

I have presented this discussion of eudaimonia and EWB as a dialogue between Aristotle and contemporary EWB researchers. No doubt my standpoint and commitments have colored this interpretation of Aristotle's views on eudaimonia, but I have tried to stay as close to the NE as possible. Moreover, I have critiqued EWB theory and research in some unorthodox ways. Nevertheless, this discussion highlights many features of eudaimonia and raises several important challenges for scholars of eudaimonia and EWB. Aristotle defines eudaimonia as an inherently ethical conception of a complete life that has multiple constituents and is inherently pleasant. His concept is ethical because it is comprised of constitutive activity that expresses human nature in its *best, most complete, and self-sufficient manner.* It has multiple constituents because humans are complex beings with many choiceworthy ends. It is pleasant because nature fulfillment is enjoyable.

The most pointed challenge raised by this discussion regards the quality of eudaimonia scholarship in psychology. Good scholarship is comprised of respect for the evidence and for the integrity of other scholars' work. It is essential that we avoid the temptation to pick and choose the words we want to appropriate from another scholar without respect to that scholar's overall conceptual scheme. If we want to appropriate Aristotle's terms, we need to be very familiar with what he meant by them. If one does not wish to follow his lead, there are two reasonable choices. One is to use different terms. The second is to redefine his terms through carefully reasoned arguments that make it as clear as possible what one has appropriated and how one has reinterpreted it. Simply appropriating a term and giving it an idiosyncratic, convenient, or anachronistic redefinition will not do. Respect is a scholarly virtue that is essential to advancing the good of knowledge, which is, in turn, a key part of eudaimonia. In contrast, the ongoing use of idiosyncratic and weakly justified definitions of eudaimonia dims our chances of progress.

Divergent views about the concept of eudaimonia, reasoned argument and debate are also constitutive of good scholarship. Aristotle himself did not believe that he had the last word on the good life. He noted that "the capacity of deliberating well about what is good…is regarded as typical of a man of practical wisdom," and he was not referring to limited aspects of life, but to "what sort of thing contributes to the good life in general" (NE, p. 152). This suggests that we will never have a final or complete concept of what is good because the human good itself is characterized by ongoing deliberation. As MacIntyre (1981) puts it, "the good life for man is the life spent in seeking for the good life for man, and the virtues necessary for the seeking are those which will enable us to understand what more and what else the good life for man is" (p. 204). That is, eudaimonia is an open-ended question rather than something that can be specified once and for all.

The second challenge for eudaimonia and EWB scholars is that eudaimonia is a frankly ethical concept, and psychologists generally have not come to terms with the ethical nature of living well. As difficult as it may be, we must accept the fact that terms like "virtue," "good," and "best" are unavoidably ethical terms. Using these terms without acknowledging the moral commitments involved is trying to talk out of both sides of one's mouth. The traditional solution has been to relegate questions about living well to subjective preference, which appears to free psychologists from making claims about what a good life is. As I have argued, the placement of values in the subjective realm is a core tenet of the ideology of individualism in which the individual and the individual's desires and goals are the goods with the highest priority. Individualism is now well known as an ethical viewpoint, but most psychologists have not recognized how thoroughly it permeates our discipline. Eudaimonia scholarship offers us the possibility to transcend that ideology if we approach the social and ethical core of this concept with appropriate seriousness.

The question of eudaimonia and ethics is just one more instance of the much broader issue of whether psychological science is inextricably bound up with ethical commitments. Psychologists tend to be uncomfortable with this possibility, but the issue has been raised over and over in the history of the discipline (e.g., Cushman, 1995; Danziger, 1990; Richardson et al., 1999), and there is no compelling explanation for how psychology can operate in a value-neutral manner, only assertions that it must do so. Clearly, this is not an issue that can be resolved in a single chapter, or, for that matter, just among eudaimonia scholars. Nevertheless, this thorny question is at the heart of eudaimonia scholarship and must be addressed directly rather than skirted. Scholars can take various positions and attempt to defend them in the intellectual marketplace or they can ignore the question and rely on the weight of tradition and popular opinion in the discipline, but these unscientific tactics do not make the question go away.

The third challenge is that the concept of eudaimonia calls upon us to overcome the modern dichotomy of subjectivity and objectivity. The standard resort of assigning well-being of all forms to the subjective realm has been an unsuccessful attempt to avoid owning our discipline's moral commitments. This is clearly inconsistent with Aristotle's concept of eudaimonia. Moreover, in my view, it is an awkward and unsustainable recourse for two reasons. Well-being obviously has a subjective dimension, but it also clearly transcends subjectivity (physical health, purposeful activity, observable joy, etc.). Although we can differentiate the subjective and extrasubjective dimensions, they cannot be cleanly and fully separated. Aristotle clearly and repeatedly emphasized that eudaimonia is activity. For him, activity cannot be conceived as either a subjective state or a purely objective event because he viewed activity as including intentions and observable actions in one inextricable whole. Philosophers also argue over whether living well is best seen in subjective or objective terms, but the attempt to relegate eudaimonia to either pole of this *modern* dichotomy is anachronistic and obscures more than it reveals.

Another reason against limiting eudaimonia to a purely subjective dimension is that a very promising area of eudaimonia scholarship its relationship to human evolution (e.g., Arnhart, 1998; Fowers, 2015; Okrent, 2007). Aristotle's function argument suggests that living well is a matter of living in accordance with our evolved nature. This gives us some grounds for identifying aspects of our nature that are demonstrably essential to living well. This is controversial, to say the least, but there are commonly studied features of human nature that appear to be essential to living well. One obvious example is that we are social creatures who flourish or languish depending on the quality of our social connections (cf., Fowers, 2015). Given our evolution as social creatures, we need social connections, take pleasure in them, and frequently find them to be a vital source of meaning. Therefore, artificially dichotomizing subjective and objective domains is both questionable and likely to obstruct scholarly progress.

In this chapter, I have returned to a primary source of the concept of eudaimonia and endeavored to set out what I think Aristotle meant by it. It is my hope that identifying some key definitional points and questions will help to give shape to our ongoing, shared deliberation about what we mean by eudaimonia. I also hope to encourage psychologists interested in eudaimonia to study the NE carefully and to read some of the excellent and accessible philosophical commentary on Aristotle and eudaimonia to enrich and deepen our discourse. There are few psychological topics that carry the intrinsic interest and import of human flourishing, which makes excellent scholarship highly desirable.

References

American Psychological Association. (2003). Guidelines on multicultural education, training, research, practice, and organizational change for psychologists. *American Psychologist, 58*, 377–402.

American Psychological Association. (2010). *Psychological issues related to child abuse and neglect*. http://www.apa.org/pi/families/resources/policy/neglect.aspx

Anscombe, G. E. M. (1958). Modern moral philosophy. *Philosophy, 33*, 1–19.

Aristotle. (1999). *Nicomachean Ethics* (trans: Ostwald, M.) Upper Saddle River, NJ: Prentice Hall.

Arnhart, L. (1998). *Darwinian natural right: The biological ethics of human nature*. Albany, NY: SUNY Press.

Bauer, J. J., McAdams, D. P., & Pals, J. L. (2008). Narrative identity and eudaimonic well-being. *Journal of Happiness Studies, 9*, 81–104.

Baumeister, R. F., & Exline, J. J. (1999). Virtue, personality, and social relations: Self-control as the moral muscle. *Journal of Personality, 67*, 1165–1194.

Biswas-Diener, R., Kashdan, T. B., & King, L. A. (2009). Two traditions of happiness research, not two distinct types of happiness. *Journal of Positive Psychology, 4*, 208–211.

Broadie, S. (1991). *Ethics with Aristotle*. Oxford, UK: Oxford University Press.

Compton, W. C., Smith, M. L., Cornish, K. A., & Qualls, D. L. (1996). Factor structure of mental health measures. *Journal of Personality and Social Psychology, 71*, 406–413.

Cushman, P. (1995). *Constructing the self, constructing America: A cultural history of psychotherapy*. Reading, MA: Addison-Wesley.

Danziger, K. (1990). *Constructing the subject: Historical origins of psychological research*. Cambridge, UK: Cambridge University Press.

Diener, E. (2012). New findings and future directions for subjective well-being research. *American Psychologist, 67*, 590–597.

Fowers, B. J. (2005). *Virtue and psychology: Pursuing excellence in ordinary practices*. Washington, DC: APA Press.

Fowers, B. J. (2008). From continence to virtue: Recovering goodness, character unity, and character types for positive psychology. *Theory & Psychology, 18*, 629–653.

Fowers, B. J. (2010). Instrumentalism and psychology: Beyond using and being used. *Theory & Psychology, 20*, 1–23.

Fowers, B. J. (2012). An Aristotelian framework for the human good. *Journal of Theoretical and Philosophical Psychology, 32*, 10–23.

Fowers, B. J. (2015). *The evolution of ethics: Human sociality and the emergence of ethical mindedness*. London: Palgrave/McMillan.

Fowers, B. J., Mollica, C. O., & Procacci, E. N. (2010). Constitutive and instrumental goal orientations and their relations with eudaimonic and hedonic well-being. *Journal of Positive Psychology, 5*, 139–153.

Huta, V. (2013). Pursuing eudaimonia versus hedonia: Distinctions, similarities, and relationships. In A. Waterman (Ed.), *The best within us: Positive psychology perspectives on eudaimonic functioning* (pp. 139–158). Washington, DC: American Psychological Association.

Huta, V., & Ryan, R. M. (2010). Pursuing pleasure versus virtue: The differential and overlapping well-being benefits of hedonic and eudaimonic motives. *Journal of Happiness Studies, 11*, 735–762.

Huta, V., & Waterman, A. S. (2014). Eudaimonia and its distinction from hedonia: Developing a classification and terminology for understanding conceptual and operational definitions. *Journal of Happiness Studies, 15*, 1425–1456.

Kashdan, T. B., Biswas-Diener, R., & King, L. A. (2008). Reconsidering happiness: The costs of distinguishing between hedonics and eudaimonia. *Journal of Positive Psychology, 3*, 219–233.

Keyes, C. L. M., & Annas, J. (2009). Feeling good and functioning well: Distinctive concepts in ancient philosophy and contemporary science. *Journal of Positive Psychology, 4*, 197–201.

Keyes, C. L. M., Shmotkin, D., & Ryff, C. D. (2002). Optimizing well-being: The empirical encounter of two traditions. *Journal of Personality and Social Psychology, 82*, 1007–1022.

Kosman, L. A. (1980). Being properly affected: Virtues and feelings in Aristotle's ethics. In A. O. Rorty (Ed.), *Essays on Aristotle's ethics* (pp. 103–116). Berkeley, CA: University of California Press.

Liddell, H. G., & Scott, R. (1996). *A Greek-English lexicon*. Oxford, UK: Clarendon.

Linley, P. A., Maltby, J., Wood, A. M., Osborne, G., & Hurling, R. (2009). Measuring happiness: The higher order factor structure of subjective and psychological well-being measures. *Personality and Individual Differences, 47*, 878–884.

MacIntyre, A. (1981). *After virtue: A study in moral theory*. Notre Dame, IN: University of Notre Dame Press.

Martin, D. B. (2007). *Inventing superstition: From the Hippocratics to the Christians*. Cambridge, MA: Harvard University Press.

Norton, D. L. (1976). *Personal destinies*. Princeton, NJ: Princeton University Press.

Okrent, M. (2007). *Rational animals: The teleological roots of intentionality*. Athens, OH: Ohio University Press.

Ostwald, M. (1999). Translator's notes in Aristotle's *The Nicomachean Ethics*. Upper Saddle River, NJ: Prentice Hall.

Peterson, C., & Seligman, M. E. P. (2004). *Character strengths and virtues: A handbook and classification*. Washington, DC: American Psychological Association.

Peterson, C., Park, N., & Seligman, M. E. P. (2005). Orientation to happiness and life satisfaction: The full life versus the empty life. *Journal of Happiness Studies, 6*, 25–41.

Richardson, F. C., Fowers, B. J., & Guignon, C. (1999). *Re-envisioning psychology: Moral dimensions of theory and practice*. San Francisco: Jossey-Bass.

Ryan, R. M., & Deci, E. L. (2001). On happiness and human potentials: A review of research on hedonic and eudaimonic well-being. *Annual Review of Psychology, 52*, 141–166.

Ryan, R. M., Huta, V., & Deci, E. L. (2008). Living well: A self-determination theory perspective on eudaimonia. *Journal of Happiness Studies, 9*, 139–170.

Ryff, C. D. (1989). Happiness is everything, or is it? Explorations on the meaning of psychological well-being. *Journal of Personality and Social Psychology, 57*, 1069–1081.

Ryff, C. D., & Singer, B. H. (2008). Know thyself and become what you are: A eudaimonic approach to psychological well-being. *Journal of Happiness Studies, 9*, 13–39.

Schwartz, B., & Sharpe, K. (2010). *Practical wisdom: The right way to do the right thing*. New York: Riverhead Books.

Sheldon, K. M., & Kasser, T. (1995). Coherence and congruence: Two aspects of personality integration. *Journal of Personality and Social Psychology, 68*, 531–543.

Steger, M. F., Kashdan, T. B., & Oishi, S. (2008). Being good by doing good: Daily eudaimonic activity and well-being. *Journal of Research in Personality, 42*, 22–42.

Straume, L. V., & Vittersø, J. (2012). Happiness, inspiration and the fully functioning person: Separating hedonic and eudaimonic well-being in the workplace. *The Journal of Positive Psychology, 7*, 387–398.

Taylor, C. (1989). *Sources of the self*. Cambridge, MA: Harvard University Press.

Terman, L. M. (1954). The discovery and encouragement of exceptional talent. *American Psychologist, 9*, 221–230.

Tiberius, V. (2013). Recipes for a good life: Eudaimonism and the contribution of philosophy. In A. Waterman (Ed.), *The best within us: Positive psychology perspectives on eudaimonia*. Washington, DC: American Psychological Association.

Waterman, A. S. (2008). Reconsidering happiness: A eudaimonist's perspective. *Journal of Positive Psychology, 3*, 234–252.

Waterman, A. S., Schwartz, S. J., & Conti, R. (2008). The implications of two conceptions of happiness (hedonic enjoyment and eudaimonia) for the understanding of intrinsic motivation. *Journal of Happiness Studies, 9*, 41–79.

Waterman, A. S., Schwartz, S. J., Zamboanga, B. L., Ravert, R. D., Williams, M. K., Agocha, B., et al. (2010). The questionnaire for eudaimonic well-being: Psychometric properties, demographic comparisons, and evidence of validity. *The Journal of Positive Psychology, 5*, 41–61.

Wiggins, D. (1980). Deliberation and practical reason. In A. O. Rorty (Ed.), *Essays on Aristotle's ethics* (pp. 221–240). Berkeley, CA: University of California Press.

Conceptual Challenges for a Science of Eudaimonic Well-Being

5

Lorraine L. Besser

5.1 Introduction

The first challenge I'll consider is the most basic one and fundamental to any investigation into EWB: this is the challenge of defining EWB in a way that preserves its uniqueness as a distinctive form of well-being. Tackling this challenge, indeed, was how Aristotle first introduced the concept of eudaimonia (Aristotle, 1962). His efforts to define eudaimonia began with the process of elimination. Some people, he argues, think living well consists in a life of pleasure, or a life of wealth, or a life of honor. But these views go astray insofar as they fail to identify living well—what Aristotle takes to be our supreme good—with something that is tied to our humanity and that is a complete and self-sufficient good.

A life of pleasure, he argues, is suitable to beasts, not humans. Those who pursue it "betray their utter slavishness in their preference for a life suitable to cattle" (Aristotle, 1962, bk. I.5). A life of wealth is not complete insofar as wealth is only useful for the sake of something else. The money-maker's life "is led under some kind of constraint: clearly, wealth is not the good which we are trying to find, for it is only useful, i.e., it is a means to something else" (Aristotle, bk. I.5). A life of honor is not self-sufficient insofar as honor depends upon others bestowing it: "honor seems to depend on those who confer it rather than on him who receivers it, whereas our guess is that the good is a man's own possession which cannot easily be taken away from him" (Aristotle, bk. I.5).

Through this process of elimination, the following criteria for the good life emerge: the good life must be a life distinctive to humanity, and it must be something complete (good in itself) and self-sufficient insofar as its goodness doesn't depend on something (or someone) else. Aristotle's own construal of eudaimonia makes heavy use of the first criteria and it is here that we find the language of flourishing and well-functioning that is now commonly associated with EWB. Aristotle is drawn to this interpretation of the good life insofar as it follows from the above criteria and meshes with his teleological commitments (according to which each being has a distinctive end towards which it strives).

Reflection on what is the distinctive function of human beings leads Aristotle to focus on rationality and our capacity to use reason to think, to act, and to control how we feel. Our function consists in the exercise of rationality and well-functioning consists in the best kind of exercise of rationality, which Aristotle describes as activity in conformity with virtue:

> [I]f we take the proper function of man to be a certain kind of life, and if this kind of life is an activity of the soul and consists in actions performed in

L.L. Besser (✉)
Middlebury College, Middlebury, VT, USA
e-mail: lbesserj@middlebury.edu

J. Vittersø (ed.), *Handbook of Eudaimonic Well-Being*, International Handbooks of Quality-of-Life,
DOI 10.1007/978-3-319-42445-3_5

> conjunction with the rational element, and if a man of high standards is he who performs these actions well and properly, and if a function is well performed when it is performed in accordance with the excellence appropriate to it; we reach the conclusion that the good of man is an activity of the soul in conformity with excellence or virtue, and if there are several virtues, in conformity with the best and most complete. (Aristotle, 1962, bk. I.7)

Eudaimonia, for Aristotle, is the life of virtue. Because this life consists in the exercise of our rational faculties, it is one that is distinctive to human nature; it is self-sufficient in that it does not depend upon anything else; and, in Aristotle's eyes, it is a complete good, lacking nothing and enjoyed and valued for itself.

We see that Aristotle meets the challenge of defining EWB through a pretty rigorous formula that starts with a concrete analysis of its nature and then moves from there to determine its content. Contemporary theorists, however, tend not to take this formulaic approach. Rather, the approach seems to be a looser, less-defined project of trying to capture a state of flourishing or well-functioning. That is, rather than beginning with an analysis of the features of the good life and then moving to a focus on well-functioning, contemporary theorists begin with a focus on well-functioning, and move from there to analyze the features of this state.

While, as we'll see, this contemporary approach is not without its problems, this move away from Aristotle has its merits. While we can see quite clearly why, given his approach, Aristotle's conception of EWB favors the exercise of rationality, it isn't obvious that the description of eudaimonia we end up with from his analysis captures something that is truly a flourishing state for us. And while we can accept that living well ought to be something that is both complete and self-sufficient, it isn't clear that the fact that something is distinctive to human nature ought to be the driving factor in determining our well-being. Aristotle's methodology of defining eudaimonia in terms of that which fits certain criteria thus allows too much room for gaps to be created between that which fits the criteria and our own experiences of flourishing.[1] Starting with flourishing seems a promising route, at the very least insofar as it mitigates the potential for these kind of gaps.[2]

This method seems to be the one embraced by most psychologists. Consider Waterman, who starts with this description of "personal expressiveness", which he takes to be eudaimonia:

> [T]here are instances when an individual engaging in an activity will report one of more of the following: (a) an unusually intense involvement in an undertaking, (b) a feeling of special fit or meshing with an activity that is not characteristic of most daily tasks, (c) a feeling of being complete and fulfilled while engaged in the activity, and (d) an impression that this is what the person was meant to do. (Waterman, 1990a, p. 40)

On Waterman's approach, the first task is to outline the phenomenon; with this understanding of the phenomenon in tact, we can go on to determine the conditions underwhich individuals can experience this phenomenon.

This approach reduces the chances that we end up specifying EWB in a way that feels foreign to the individual and that might present a gap between EWB and the individual's experience of well-being. The challenge this approach introduces, however, is the challenge of specifying the phenomenon. We all have experiences of better and worse states of functioning, but what is distinctive about the state of well-functioning? And what components are requisite this state? For both philosophers and psychologists, this challenge amounts to being able to describe EWB in a way that preserves its status as a unique

[1]Haybron (2008) criticizes Aristotle along these lines, charging that because Aristotle specifies well-being in terms of the species, rather than the individual, he thereby creates the potential for a gap between his theory of well-being and well-being as it is experienced by the individual.

[2]As noted, my interpretation of Aristotle draws on Book 1 of the Nicomachean Ethics. Some interpreters (e.g. McDowell 1998) find in Aristotle's subsequent analysis of virtue a methodology more akin to the contemporary one I describe here.

form of well-being, i.e., that (a) is distinct from other recognizable forms of well-being; and (b) is nonetheless still a theory of well-being, where well-being is taken to be a prudential value—that which is good for the agent. Let's consider each of these components in turn.

In trying to describe EWB as a unique form of well-being, a central challenge is to try to describe the subjective experience of EWB in a way that does not collapse into other subjective experiences associated with well-being, such as feeling pleasure or feeling satisfaction. Traditionally EWB has been understood as an objective theory of well-being insofar as it describes a state that does not depend upon the possessor experiencing positive feelings about one's life (for discussion, see Besser-Jones, 2014). If we take its roots seriously, EWB is fundamentally a state of flourishing and well-functioning; while it typically leads to positive feelings about one's life, to truly capture the phenomenon it is important to be able to identify it independently of these positive feelings with which it is correlated. These positive feelings are associated with very different approaches to well-being: respectively, hedonism and life satisfaction. Unlike EWB, these forms of well-being describe well-being entirely in terms of these positive feelings.

Insofar as EWB is meant to capture something that is importantly different from these forms of well-being, it is important to be able to specify it in objective terms of well-functioning. But of course EWB has a subjective element—well-functioning is an experience, after all, and this makes the task of specifying EWB that much more difficult. How should the subjective element enter into the specification of EWB?

Aristotle's conception of eudaimonia is largely silent on its experiential component. Where Aristotle does describe the experiential component of eudaimonia it is in the context of the feelings that he believes ought to be associated with the exercise of virtue. The exercise of virtue, he argues, ought to be something that flows from us wholeheartedly and without reservation; the existence of conflicting desires signifies continence and a lack of full virtue. When we are fully virtuous, our desires point to the exercise of virtue without conflict and we experience a kind of pleasure that "completes" the act (Aristotle, 1962, bk. X). It is difficult to parse exactly what Aristotle is after here, and his view of pleasure is complex.[3]

Backing away from providing a full description of the experiential component of eudaimonia might have been okay for Aristotle, given his methodology; but as we move away from his methodology and towards the current approach to understanding EWB by first describing the phenomenon itself, this task becomes more pressing. And, indeed, we've seen disagreement amongst psychologists regarding how best to categorize the phenomenon of EWB.

Ryan, Huta, and Deci (2008), for example, emphasize that EWB tracks a process of living well and that this is very distinct from hedonic approaches which tend to look at the outcomes.

> [H]edonic versus eudaimonic psychologies do not in principle constitute a debate about what well-being "feels like" or what "happiness," considered as a state of mind, entails. Rather, eudaimonic conceptions focus on the content of one's life, and the processes involved in living well, whereas hedonic conceptions of well-being focus on a specific outcome, namely the attainment of positive affect and an absence of pain. (Ryan et al., 2008, p. 140)

The distinction made here between well-being considered as a "process" and well-being considered as an "outcome" is an important one and certainly mirrors Aristotle's understanding of EWB. In contrast to hedonism and other forms of well-being, EWB is an active state of well-being that requires on-going activity. As LeBar (2013) has argued, it is one that requires and highlights an individual's agency. When we experience EWB, our lives go well *because of how we have lived* and not because we are passive receptors of positive feelings.

In their efforts to uniquely identify EWB, we see Ryan, Huta, and Deci's emphasis on the *content* of one's life, and the *processes* involved in living well. As a form of life, we can thus describe EWB in terms of objective features of one's life (see also Huta, Chap. 15, this volume and Ryan & Martela, Chap. 7, this volume). But, as Ryan

[3] See Annas (2008), Besser-Jones (2012), and Curzer (2002) for discussion.

et al acknowledge, this doesn't release us from the challenges of describing the subjective experience of EWB: "The foci of eudaimonic research are to specify what living well entails and to identify the expected consequences of such living. These consequences may include hedonic satisfactions, but typically eudaimonic theorists have been especially interested in other outcomes indicative of a good life, such as vitality, intimacy, health, and sense of meaning, among others" (2008). Notice here that their efforts to describe the subjective experience of EWB takes it to be an outcome indicative of a good life, but not constitutive of a good life.

In contrast, Waterman finds it important to include the subjective experience of EWB as constitutive of it (1990b). In fact, while he stresses the importance of self-realization, in one of his most recent formulations he locates EWB as a product of self-realization, rather than as constitutive of it: "'eudaimonia' is a positive subjective state that is the product (or perhaps by-product) of the pursuit of self-realization rather than the objective being sought" (Waterman, 2007). On his analysis, the subjective experience of eudaimonia is understood in terms of personal expressiveness, and arises where there is an intense involvement with one's actions, a feeling of "special fit or meshing" with the activity along with a feeling of completeness or fulfillment and an impression that this is what one is meant to be doing (Waterman, 1990a, p. 47). These experiences of personal expressiveness are constitutive of EWB, he argues, and not the activities that give rise to them, for the activities themselves might be experienced differently between individuals. This is one reason why Waterman departs from Aristotle (and Ryan, Huta, and Deci) in his emphasis on the subjective experience of EWB.

Ryff's (1989) multi-dimensional account can be seen as a kind of balance between these two divergent approaches towards understanding the subjective experience of EWB. Her account includes some elements descriptive of the objectively construed content of one's life (e.g., positive relationships, environmental mastery) and some descriptive of one's experiences of this life (e.g., self-acceptance, autonomy), all which she takes to be constitutive of EWB (Ryff, Chap. 6, this volume).

At this point we might reasonably question whether or not it matters whether we see the typical, subjectively experienced, indicators of EWB as constitutive of EWB or as outcomes of EWB. On the one hand, it seems that in order to preserve the unique status of EWB, we need to separate the outcome from the process and focus only on the process of living well, for we otherwise risk mistaking EWB for hedonism or some other subjective form of well-being. This is certainly how the philosophical approach runs, and this seems to have influenced Ryan, Huta, and Deci in their emphasis on understanding EWB as a process that can be understood independently of subjective feelings. On the other hand, it seems as if the science of EWB depends upon our abilities to identify the experiential component of it. To study EWB, and to determine which ways of living are constitutive of it, we need to be able to identify it.

While it may be conceptually possible to separate the process of EWB from its outcome and indicators, in practice this separation seems somewhat artificial. This is increasingly clear when we realize that the very methodology by which we come to learn about the process of living well is by first identifying and reflecting on its indicators, and then understanding which ways of living correlate with those indicators. This methodology, of course, presumes that we can distinguish the subjective experience of EWB from other positive feelings, a point Vittersø (2013) emphasizes in his distinction between eudaimonic and hedonic feelings. Drawing on emotion research, Vittersø (e.g., Chap. 17, this volume) argues that the capacity to distinguish between feeling states is vital to the overall purpose of emotions, which is to prompt us towards different sorts of actions. Hedonic feelings "facility stability and adaptation", while eudaimonic feelings "facilitate growth and accommodation" (Vittersø, p. 51). We thus can distinguish between positive emotions that feel hedonic, and those that do not; according to Vittersø, eudaimonic feelings just are positive non-hedonic feelings. This emphasis on describing eudaimonic feelings in terms of their direction and purpose may help to us in our efforts to identify the subjective experience of EWB.[4]

Reaching a better understanding of the subjective experience of EWB may also help to ward off concerns regarding the normativity of EWB and so may help bring discussion of EWB into greater focus. In our discussion of Aristotle, we saw that his focus on describing the process of living well in objective terms threatens to create a gap between leading a life that fits the criteria for living well and experiencing the eudaimonic feelings correlated with that life. Diener, Saptya, and Suh (1998) raise related concerns, arguing that well-being ought to be something determined by the individual experiencing it and not by experts. They go on to question whether or not the ingredients often taken to be essential to EWB have any worth independently of their connection to subjective well-being. Attributing a great role to the experiential components of EWB will help to establish its importance in the face of these challenges.

I've argued that while it is challenging to uniquely identify the subjective experience of EWB, doing so will help to advance the study of it. Emphasizing the subjective experience may be a departure from Aristotle's original conception of eudaimonia, but from a scientific perspective, the subjective experience of EWB provides the window through which we can best understand what it means to live well, and what is involved in so doing.

A second and related conceptual challenge for the science of EWB concerns how it is that we frame and understanding the concept of "well-functioning". This component is essential to EWB, yet in many respects it may be the hardest to understand.[5] As we've seen, Aristotle reaches his understanding of eudaimonia by reflecting on what he took to be the distinctive function of human nature. This analysis flows nicely with his teleological commitments, according to which everything has some end towards which it strives. While many contemporary philosophers defend Aristotle's focus on reason and the exercise of practical rationality (LeBar, 2013; Russell, 2012), from an empirical point of view this position is relatively easy to challenge. The fact that reason may be *distinctive* to human nature does not on its own carry much normative weight. There may be many features distinctive to human nature that we do not want to highlight and frame as features that ought to be developed and pursued as part of living well. Neither, for that matter, does the fact that the exercise of reason may constitute our *function* carry much normative weight. From a scientific point of view functional analyses lead us towards thinking about what is good for the species, not the individual; there is no guarantee that a functional analysis will lead us to a way of living that is recognizable as living well for that individual.

Rather, when we reflect on EWB and in what living well consists, what seems to count is whether certain ways of living tap into features of human nature, the synthesis of which leads agents to function better in their every day tasks. This, I take it, is what many psychologists are after when they discuss EWB in terms of personal growth, personal expressivism, and need satisfaction. But it is worth noting how very different the former two construals are from the latter. Talk of personal growth and personal expressivism leads to an individualized conception of EWB. Depending upon one's individual talents and skills, what counts as living well for one may very well vary from one person to the next. This consequence is something both Ryff and Singer and Waterman embrace: Ryff and Singer describe the "essence of eudaimonia" as "the idea of striving toward excellence based on one's unique potential" (2008, p. 14), and Waterman writes that "eudaimonia is experienced only on connection with activities that advance one's highest potentialities, either in terms of aptitudes and talents and/or purposes in living" (1990b, pp. 40–41).

[4] Vittersø's own proposal is that both eudaimonic and hedonic feelings are essential to optimal functioning.

[5] Some psychological approaches take EWB to consist in more specific components of well-functioning such as a life of purpose or meaning (e.g. Steger, 2012). I worry that these formulations of EWB are misleading insofar as they focus on one specific aspect of well-functioning, as opposed to beginning with the general reflection on well-functioning that, historically, lies at the heart of EWB and allows for a more inclusive approach to determining what counts as well-functioning.

These individualized understandings of eudaimonia track a very different thing than Aristotle started with. Aristotle believed that there was a way of living well that was consistent across individuals and reflective of human nature itself, and sought to describe this in his formulation of eudaimonia. In this respect, the self-determination theoretical approach towards conceptualizing EWB in terms of the satisfaction of innate psychological needs better preserves a conception of EWB as an objective form of living well, that does not vary between individuals. And to the extent to which there is evidence supporting the positing of innate psychological needs as relatively consistent across human nature, understanding EWB in these terms seems accurate, insofar as it captures the desired kind of synthesis between features of human nature and ways of living that contribute to overall functioning. Of course, that the self-determination theoretical approach more closely approximates Aristotle's conception of eudaimonia as describing an objective form of living well does not necessarily count against the individualized interpretations of EWB. But to the extent that they end up tracking very different things, this conceptual difference in the various psychologist's interpretation of EWB is worth emphasis.

Defenders of the individualized interpretation of EWB do face some unique challenges when it comes to its study. Testing whether or not an individual is using her potential and aptitudes is tricky, as is determining which potentials and aptitudes we are comfortable including in our conception of living well. An aptitude towards aggression, for instance, does not mean that the individual lives well when she develops this aptitude, and there are many more such examples.[6] A greater awareness of these challenges, and of whether or not one is committed to an individualized understanding of EWB or an objective understanding of EWB, will help the science of EWB progress.

The third and final challenge I'll discuss is one I worry may be insurmountable in practice, and this concerns how to conceptualize EWB in a way that preserves its emphasis on living well construed as an overall phenomenon, as opposed to something that we can experience in some aspects of our lives and not others. According to almost all those who theorize about EWB, EWB describes an overall way of living well that doesn't reduce to separate components; it is a function of one's whole life. But psychological research on EWB tends to carve up EWB into separate components, as if EWB could be experienced in one aspect of one's life but not in others. Waterman (1990a) is explicit about this departure, and argues that understanding EWB in terms of different aspects of one's life allows us to better appreciate how it is that EWB can be experienced in degrees. I'm not sure why Waterman believes that understanding EWB as a function of one's whole life does not allow for the attributions of EWB to come in degrees, but it is understandable that psychological research ends up carving up EWB into separate components. Doing so makes the science and study of EWB more manageable. However, to the extent that this transforms EWB into an umbrella phenomenon, capturing a variety of different aspects, I worry that we lose sight of the central thrust of EWB.

EWB is meant to capture an entire way of living, something that infiltrates all aspects of one's life. The individual who experiences EWB doesn't just experience it in one context and not another; the fascinating thing about well-functioning is that it carries over to difference contexts and infiltrates one's life. Most of us still experience it in degrees, but to the extent there are those who enjoy a fully eudaimonic life, the experience of it infuses all of her daily activities. In my own work, I've found it helpful to understand EWB through the framework of organismic integration theory (Besser-Jones, 2014). That we strive to integrate our experiences, and that we function better when we do, explains and captures well EWB as a form of living one's whole life well.

The science of EWB has made tremendous progress and, to my mind, improvements over eudaimonia as it was initially conceived by Aristotle. The challenges I've raised are genuine

[6] Waterman (1990a) addresses some of these challenges.

ones, but are not necessarily insurmountable. More careful attention to the conceptualization of EWB would go a long way, as would greater transparency regarding the differences between one's one conception of EWB and others. EWB is, in the end, a theoretical concept and effort to understand a very real phenomenon. It is understandable that we will vary on our conceptualization of the concept; but dangers arise when we use the same concept in very different ways without acknowledgement.

References

Annas, J. (2008). The phenomenology of virtue. *Phenomenology and the Cognitive Sciences, 7*(1), 21–34.

Aristotle. (1962). In M. Oswald (Ed.), *Nicomachean ethics*. New York: MacMillan Publishing Company.

Besser-Jones, L. (2012). The motivational state of the virtuous agent. *Philosophical Psychology, 25*(1), 93–108.

Besser-Jones, L. (2014). *Eudaimonic ethics: The philosophy and psychology of living well*. New York: Routledge Press.

Curzer, H. J. (2002). Aristotle's painful path to virtue. *Journal of the History of Philosophy, 40*(2), 141–162.

Diener, E., Sapyta, J. J., & Suh, E. (1998). Subjective well-being is essential to well-being. *Psychological Inquiry, 9*(1), 33–37.

Haybron, D. M. (2008). *The pursuit of unhappiness*. New York: Oxford University Press.

LeBar, M. (2013). *The value of living well*. New York: Oxford University Press.

McDowell, J. (1998). Two sorts of naturalism. In R. Hursthouse, G. Lawrence, & W. Quinn (Eds.), *Virtues and reasons*. New York: Clarendon.

Russell, D. C. (2012). *Happiness for humans*. New York: Oxford University Press.

Ryan, R. M., Huta, V., & Deci, E. L. (2008). Living well: A self-determination theory perspective on eudaimonia. *Journal of Happiness Studies, 9*(1), 139–170.

Ryff, C. D. (1989). Happiness is everything, or is it? Explorations on the meaning of psychological well-being. *Journal of Personality and Social Psychology, 57*(6), 1069–1081.

Ryff, C. D., & Singer, B. H. (2008). Know thyself and become what you are: A eudaimonic approach to psychological well-being. *Journal of Happiness Studies, 9*, 13–39.

Steger, M. F. (2012). Experiencing meaning in life. In P. Wong (Ed.), *Human quest for meaning: Theories, research, and applications* (2nd ed., pp. 165–184). New York: Routledge.

Vittersø, J. (2013). Feelings, meanings, and optimal functioning: Some distinctions between hedonic and eudaimonic well-being. In A. S. Waterman (Ed.), *The best within us: Positive psychology perspectives on eudaimonia* (pp. 39–55). Washington, DC: American Psychological Association.

Waterman, A. S. (1990a). Personal expressiveness: Philosophical and psychological foundations. *Journal of Mind and Behavior, 11*(1), 47–74.

Waterman, A. S. (1990b). The relevance of Aristotle's conception of eudaimonia for the psychological study of happiness. *Theoretical and Philosophical Psychology, 10*(1), 39–44.

Waterman, A. S. (2007). On the importance of distinguishing hedonia and eudaimonia when contemplating the hedonic treadmill. *American Psychologist, 62*, 612.

Part II

Identifying the Elements of Psychological Eudaimonics

6 Beautiful Ideas and the Scientific Enterprise: Sources of Intellectual Vitality in Research on Eudaimonic Well-Being

Carol D. Ryff

6.1 Introduction

This chapter reviews the conceptual foundations of a model of psychological well-being (Ryff, 1989) that has, over the three past decades, become the focus of extensive scientific research. The central aim is to elaborate the rich ideas – all drawn from the works of others – that guided development of this model as well as provided the foundation for its empirical translation. These vital sources include, but are not restricted to Aristotle's timelessly insightful thoughts about eudaimonia. The other beautiful ideas in the model drew on conceptions of personal development, self-realization, and the capacity to create meaning in the face of adversity. What follows is an effort to explicate what makes these formulations compelling. Along the way, empirical findings are illustrated to underscore the critical interface between inspired ideas and subsequent scientific action. The overarching message is that great philosophical and theoretical insights and ideals are invaluable in generating meaningful new knowledge that seeks to examine their core premises and in so doing, brings intellectual beauty to empirical life.

The first section below revisits the theoretical origins of the Ryff (1989) model of well-being, focusing on the array of vital ideas, all reaching to characterize optimal human functioning, that were incorporated. The second section explicates the linkage of this model to Aristotle's eudaimonia, a connection that was formulated later in time. The third section highlights select findings from the proliferating research that has grown up around this model of well-being. Emphasis is reviewing the scientific pursuits is again on beautiful ideas, such as the proposition that well-being may nurture salubrious health and further that it may be critical in fostering resilience vis-à-vis adversity. The fourth section briefly describes ongoing efforts to promote eudaimonic well-being in clinical, educational, and community contexts. The concluding message is that whatever meritorious science has grown up around this model of eudaimonic well-being, all such advances grew out of ennobling ideas aiming to articulate ideals of human functioning. The empirical research that followed is now illuminating how these elevated ideas matter for improving human lives.

C.D. Ryff (✉)
Institute on Aging/Department of Psychology,
University of Wisconsin-Madison,
Madison, WI, USA
e-mail: cryff@wisc.edu

J. Vittersø (ed.), *Handbook of Eudaimonic Well-Being*, International Handbooks of Quality-of-Life,
DOI 10.1007/978-3-319-42445-3_6

6.2 Reaching Toward a New Conception of Human Well-Being

In the 1960s and 1970s, the field of social gerontology was replete with studies life satisfaction, conceived at the time as a marker of successful aging. However, this widely measured construct had little, if any, conceptual or theoretical foundation (Ryff, 1982). Probing people's life satisfaction offered a pragmatic and straightforward window into how they felt about their lives, but it fell short of being a beautiful idea because there was largely nothing behind it conceptually, not even a rationale for why satisfaction with life matters or is worth considering. In contrast, many other literatures from developmental and clinical psychology, existential and humanistic psychology (Allport, 1961; Bühler, 1935; Erikson, 1959; Frankl, 1959; Jahoda, 1958; Jung, 1933; Maslow, 1968; Neugarten, 1973; Rogers, 1961) had provided notable depth in trying to distill what constitutes the upside of the human experience. Undergraduates frequently read about these formulations in courses on developmental psychology or theories of personality, but that was typically the end of their exposure to such perspectives. The central problem was these varied efforts to articulate the nature of optimal human functioning were largely absent in the scientific arena. Further, what accounted for their absence was the lack of credible empirical translations.

The task of bringing these ideas to the empirical arena (Ryff, 1989) rested on several premises. First, although each formulation was interesting, none in and of itself was sufficiently compelling to serve as the central theoretical foundation. Put another way, no single perspective seemed notably better, more elegant or insightful than another. Second, the decision to focus on *points of convergence* among them offered a sort of inter-rater reliability as to what constitutes core components of optimal human functioning. Six key dimensions of well-being emerged to capture the key points of convergence. Third, the empirical translation (scale development process) followed the construct-oriented approach to personality assessment (Jackson, 1967, 1976; Wiggins 1980). The key to creating theory-driven assessment instruments is that the process begins with definitions of each dimension of well-being that are derived from the conceptual underpinnings. These theory-based definitions then serve as the basis for generating items to operationalize the separate components of well-being. In an era of proliferating tools to assess well-being, many emerging from the positive psychology movement, it is worth noting how few new instruments have clearly formulated theoretical foundations. In addition, few of these new tools have been subjected to rigorous empirical scrutiny needed to test their reliability, validity, and purported dimensional structure. The above approach (Ryff, 1989) was unique in having a strong conceptual foundation, which was accompanied by extensive psychometric evaluation, including at the level of individual items. This care in scale development likely explains why the model has withstood extensive scrutiny over time (Ryff, 2014). For present purposes, the key point is that the beautiful ideas that defined the model were pivotal in its empirical translation. Such fidelity between rich, thoughtfully formulated dimensions of well-being and subsequent empirical action is a cornerstone of high-quality science.

Figure 6.1 identifies the six key components of the model (Ryff, 1989) and below them, summarizes theoretical underpinnings. The text below further articulates how each dimension of well-being drew on multiple underlying formulations of optimal human functioning.

Autonomy Many efforts to depict key features of positive human functioning emphasized independent, self-determining, and self-regulating qualities. Self-actualizers were described as showing autonomous functioning and resistance to enculturation (Maslow). The fully functioning person was described as having an internal locus of evaluation (Rogers), such that one does not look to others for approval, but evaluates oneself by personal standards. Individuation was also described as involving a deliverance from convention (Jung). Life-span theories emphasized the importance of turning inward in later life (Erikson) and gaining a sense of freedom from the norms governing everyday life (Neugarten).

Fig. 6.1 Core dimensions of psychological well-being and their theoretical underpinnings

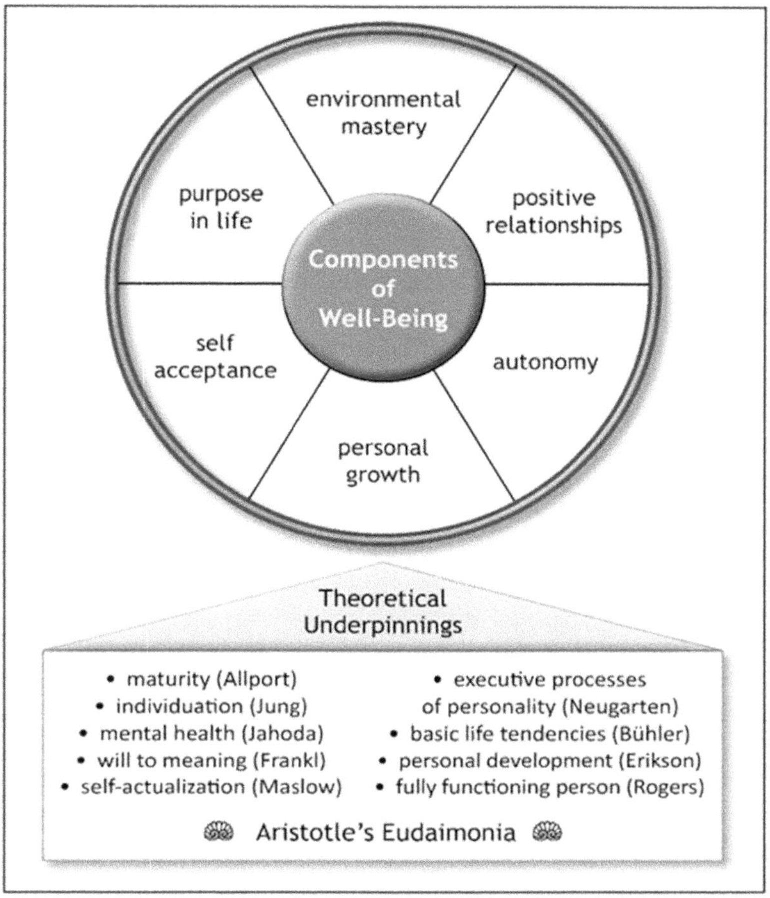

Environmental Mastery Possessing the ability to choose or create environments suitable to one's psychic needs was a key characteristic of mental health (Jahoda), which reflected a kind of fit between one's outer and inner worlds. Life-span theories described the importance of being able to manipulate and control complex environments, particularly in midlife, as well as the capacity to act on and change the surrounding world through mental and physical activities (Erikson, Neugarten). Maturity was defined as being able to extend the self into spheres of endeavor that go beyond the self (Allport). Together, these perspective conveyed that active participation in and efforts to gain mastery of one's surrounding environment are important elements in positive psychological functioning.

Personal Growth This aspect of well-being is concerned with self-realization and achieving personal potential. It is thus a dynamic aspect of positive functioning that is continually evolving through time. Self-actualization was centrally concerning with personal becoming (Maslow), as was positive mental health (Jahoda). Descriptions of the fully functioning person (Rogers, 1961) and what it means to be fully individuated (Jung) also emphasized ideas of realizing one's true self. Life-span theories, in addition, gave explicit emphasis to confronting new challenges and tasks as different periods of life (Erikson, Bühler, Neugarten).

Positive Relations with Others The ability to love was deemed a central feature of mental health (Jahoda). Self-actualizers were described as having strong feelings of empathy and affection for all human beings and the capacity for great love, deep friendship, and close identification with others (Maslow). Warm relating to others was seen as a central criterion of maturity (Allport). Adult developmental stage theories

(Erikson) emphasized the achievement of close unions with others (intimacy) as well as having a concern for guiding and directing others (generativity). It is worth noting that philosophical accounts of the criterial goods of a well-lived life (Becker, 1992) underscored the primacy of love, empathy, and affection.

Purpose in Life Having beliefs that give one a sense of purpose and meaning in life was part of positive mental health (Jahoda). The definition of maturity also included having a clear comprehension of one's purpose, which was important in contributing a sense of directedness and intentionality to life (Allport). Life-span theories depicted changing purposes or goals with different life stages, such as being creative or productive in midlife, and turning to emotional integration in later life (Erikson, Neugarten, Jung). Existential formulations, especially the search for meaning in the face of significant adversity (Frankl), were directly concerned with the challenge of finding/creating meaning amidst suffering.

Self-Acceptance Having positive self-regard is a central feature of self-actualizers (Maslow), maturity (Allport), optimal functioning (Rogers), and mental health (Jahoda). Life-span theories also emphasized the importance of acceptance of self, including of one's past life (Erikson, Neugarten). The process of individuation (Jung) added important refinements to this aspect of well-being – namely, the need to come to terms with the dark side of one's self (the shadow). This form of self-acceptance is notably richer than standard views of self-esteem because it involves awareness and acceptance of personal strengths as well as weaknesses.

6.3 The Encounter with Aristotle's Eudaimonia

At the time the above model of well-being was presented (Ryff, 1989), reference was made to Aristotle's eudaimonia via the writings of Waterman (1984), which had underscored the distinction made by the ancient Greeks between the gratification of right and wrong desires. Drawing on these past formulations, eudaimonia was formulated as "feelings accompanying behavior in the direction of, and consistent with, one's true potential (Waterman, 1984, p.16). Emphasis was given to the daimon, an ideal in the sense of an excellence, a perfection toward which one strives that gives meaning and direction to one's life. This characterization was fundamentally distinct from prevailing research approaches to happiness, which emphasized contentment or satisfaction with life.

Ryff and Singer (2008) subsequently gave serious consideration to Artistotle's *Nichomachean Ethics*, written in 350 B.C. and translated by Ross (1925). This ancient text is not easy to read, as it includes many strange terms, along with grammatical obscurities, digressions, and winding argumentative sequences. Nonetheless, sparkling insights and exquisitely distilled thoughts are also evident. Further, it is deeply evident that Aristotle was working very hard to answer the fundamental question of human existence: how should we live? He refused to rely on cant or religious dogma, and instead, sought to craft a reasoned argument with carefully articulated propositions and precise definition of terms.

For present purposes, it is important to note that Aristotle was not trying to formulate the nature of human well-being. His objective rather was to formulate an ethical doctrine that would provide guidelines for how to live. In answering the opening question, which he elaborated as "what is the highest of all human goods achievable by human action?" he stated that both the general crowd and those of superior refinement would likely answer that it is happiness. But he believed they would likely differ in what they meant by happiness. In his view, happiness was not some plain and obvious thing, like pleasure, wealth, or honor. Nor was it about the satisfying of appetites, which he likened to a life suitable to beasts. He thus challenged what the mass of mankind might construe happiness to be, and instead chose to define the highest of all human goods as activity of the soul in accord with virtue.

That definition required that he consider the nature of virtue. A first key meaning he offered was that it was a kind of mean – an aiming toward that which is intermediate. The idea of striving toward balance was applied to many domains: with regard to money, we are to avoid excess and tasteless vulgarity at one extreme, but also deficiency and niggardliness at the other. With regard to honor, too much can lead to vanity, and too little can result in undue humility. In thinking about amusement, Aristotle reminded there can be excess (buffoonery), or falling seriously short (the boor). Even pleasantness to others could involve the obsequious flatterer at one extreme, or the quarrelsome, surly person at the other. Across these wonderfully rich examples, Aristotle's message was to emphasize the virtue of choosing for deliberate actions that avoided excess or deficiency.

However, the highest of all human goods, according to Aristotle, involved more than achieving balance in diverse modes of conduct. It was in elaborating the *highest of all virtues* that Aristotle got to the heart of eudaimonia, which he formulated as "the best thing in us" (p. 263). Embedded within this idea was a strongly teleological perspective – namely, that the highest human good involves activities that are goal-directed and have purpose. The essential telos (end point) for eudaimonia is to achieve the best that we are capable of. Paraphrased by Johnston (1997), "The excellence of the human being is thus going to be associated with growth towards some final realization of his or her true and best nature" (p.6). Norton's (1976), *Personal Destinies: A Philosophy of Ethical Individualism*, further elaborated eudiamonism as an ethical doctrine in which each person is obliged to know and live in truth to his daimon, a kind of spirit given to all persons at birth. It is a journey of progressively actualizing an excellence (from the Greek *arête*) that is consistent with innate potentialities. Eudaimonia thus embodies the great Greek imperatives of self-truth (know thyself) and self-responsibility (become what you are).

Other observations about Aristotle's formulation must be acknowledged. Regretfully, his view was unequivocally elitist – several classes of humanity (slaves, women) were not seen to be invested with potential excellences. Second, not all daimons had equivalent worth; rather they were arranged hierarchically, with the final perfection of some seen to be superior to others. These less ennobling ideas were partially offset by Aristotle's awareness that basic needs (food, good health, some level of prosperity) are required to achieve the best within one's self. That is, he recognized the need to have a decent life in pursuing one's daimon. Further, he reminded that "we can do noble acts without ruling earth and sea; for even those with moderate advantages can act virtuously" (p. 268), and relatedly, underscored the important of action, not just abstract ideas. Finally, most of the *Nichomachean Ethics* was not about elaborating the meaning of eudaimonia; rather it involved Aristotle's efforts to distill a diverse array of virtues (e.g., justice, intellectual virtues, friendship). These worthwhile topics are not elaborated here.

Reflecting on the ideas covered in the first section above, which post-dated Aristotle by 2000+ years, unmistakable parallels are evident in formulations of developmental, humanistic, existential, and clinical psychology with Aristotle's eudaimonia. That is, his articulation of the highest human good was, in fact, a kind of self-realization, played out individually, each according to personal dispositions and talents. Interestingly, none of the later psychological efforts to formulate the meaning of personal development, self-actualization, maturity, individuation, fully functioning, and good mental health drew on Aristotle. Nonetheless, his thinking was there implicitly. That is, these twentieth century perspectives seeking to elaborate components of what such self-realization entails were vital in bringing multiple guiding ideas to the scientific arena, but their overarching efforts were undeniably in the spirit of Aristotle's eudiamonism.

Before turning to empirical research on eudaimonia well-being, beautiful and related ideas from two great utilitarian philosophers are noted. The first is John Stuart Mill (1893/1989, p. 117) who offered one of the most trenchant insights ever regarding human happiness:

> Those only are happy, I thought, who have their minds fixed on some object other than their own happiness, on the happiness of others, on the improvement of mankind, even on some art or pursuit, followed not as a means, but as itself as an ideal end. Aiming thus at something else, they find happiness by the way.

This view of human happiness as a by-product of other more noble deeds also harkens back to Aristotle in emphasizing that the true path to feeling happy requires living a virtuous life. Second, Bertrand Russell (1930/1958) added another key insight: happiness is not something that just happens to us, like having ripened fruit fall effortlessly into our mouths; rather it is something for which we must strive and work hard, hence his title, *The Conquest of Happiness*. Russell's efforts to elaborate the importance of zest (active interest in and engagement in life) and affection (having meaning bonds of love with significant others) in finding happiness were also richly aligned with Aristotle's eudaimonism, conceived as striving to realize personal potentialities via virtuous living.

6.4 Empirical Highlights: Eudaimonia and Health

Assessments scales from the Ryff (1989) model of well-being have been translated to more than 30 languages and have resulted in more than 500 publications, some of which were recently reviewed (Ryff, 2014). It is beyond the scope of this chapter to consider the larger array of scientific findings that have been generated across multiple topical areas. Instead, illustrative research will be considered that show the relevance of eudaimonic well-being for human health as well as its significance for understanding resilience in the face of adversity. Building scientific connections between well-being and health is worthy as a beautiful pursuit because it has challenged the pervasive and longstanding bias toward disease, disability, and dysfunction in more than a half century of research on human health. Greatly needed are studies that construe health as health, as in the distant WHO (World Health Organization, 1948) declaration, which defined health as a "state of complete physical, mental, and social well-being and not merely the absence of disease or infirmity" (p. 28). The formulation of salutogenesis (Antonovsky, 1979, 1987) further exemplifies the idea of people staying healthy and well, even in the face of stress. Human resilience thus embodies another beautiful idea in that it investigates the presence of well-being and good health in confrontations with marked life challenges. Ironically, encounters with adversity often fuel deepened experiences of personal growth and self-realization.

These brief highlights of empirical findings begin with what has been learned about age differences in components of eudaimonic well-being (Ryff, 1989). This question has been of interest since the initial cross-sectional studies revealed that the most existential and humanistic aspects of well-being (i.e., purpose in life, personal growth) appeared to decline from midlife to old age. Subsequent longitudinal evidence from large national studies verified that such decline in purpose and growth was, in fact, evident among U.S. adults (Springer, Pudrovska, & Hauser, 2011). Such decline with age offered a novel angle for investigating links between well-being and health, which was built around the notable variability among older adults in reported levels of well-being. That is, although the overall profile showed decrementing profiles of purpose in life with aging, some older adults were decidedly above the average for their age group. Their capacity to maintain high levels of well-being was, in a series of investigations, linked with multiple benefits for health and longevity.

For example, a community-based epidemiological study known as MAP (Rush Memory and Aging Project) showed, after controlling for numerous covariates, that older adults with higher levels of purpose in life at baseline had reduced risk of death 6 years later (Boyle, Barnes, Buchman, & Bennett, 2009) as well as reduced risk of Alzheimer's disease and mild cognitive impairment (Boyle, Buchman, Barnes, & Bennett, 2010). More remarkably, post-mortem analyses of brain pathology (e.g., plaques and tangles) from participants who had died showed that purpose in life moderated links between brain-based pathology and levels of cognitive function while respondents were still alive. That is, among those showing high levels of brain pathology, higher levels of cognitive function were evident among those who reported higher levels of purpose in life compared to those with comparable brain pathology but with lower levels of purpose in life (Boyle et al., 2012).

Another major national longitudinal study known as HRS (Health and Retirement Study) provided prospective evidence that older adults with higher levels of purpose in life had reduced risk of stroke (Kim, Sun, Park, & Peterson, 2013a) as well as myocardial infarction among those with coronary heart disease (Kim, Sun, Park, Kubzansky, & Peterson, 2013b). This same study also found that older adults with higher levels of purposeful engagement were more likely to engage in preventive health behaviors, such as cholesterol tests and cancer screenings (Kim, Strecher, & Ryff, 2014) relative to age peers with lower levels of purposeful in life. Findings from another major national longitudinal study known as MIDUS (Midlife in the U.S.) corroborated the evidence that purpose in life reduces risk of mortality across adult life (Hill & Turiano, 2014).

Viewed collectively, these results across major longitudinal aging studies were notably significant on two levels. First, their inquiries were accompanied by scientific evidence that certain aspects of eudaimonic well-being (purpose in life, personal growth) showed later life vulnerabilities – that is, losses were evident. These declines may reflect the "structural lag" problem described by sociologists (Riley, Kahn, & Foner, 1994). The assertion is that many adults are now living longer, but the added years are not accompanied by opportunities for meaningful roles and activities. Effectively, the surrounding social structures (in work, family, and community life) lag behind the added years of life that many now experience. Thus, key changes in later life eudaimonic well-being were implicated in major demographic transitions occurring at a societal level. Second, the evidence of later life decline in purposeful engagement has been accompanied by another set of intriguing findings based on the notable variability in reported well-being among older adults. Elders who maintain with high levels of purpose in life have been shown to experience an array of health benefits (reduced risk for multiple disease outcomes) as well as increased longevity. The key point is this: none of these scientific advances could have occurred without the guiding eudaimonic model of well-being (Ryff, 1989) and an accompanying commitment to bring it into the empirical arena.

Still other studies have probed eudaimonic well-being as a moderating factor that may afford protection of good health in the face of challenge. For example, Friedman and Ryff (2012) showed the buffering effects of two aspects of well-being (purpose in life and positive relations) vis-à-vis the problem of later-life comorbidity (having multiple chronic conditions). Such incrementing profiles of health problems (e.g. hypertension, arthritis) are not uncommon with aging. However, because many of these conditions fuel inflammation, they add yet further risk for subsequent health difficulties. But not for everyone: among older adults with higher levels of chronic conditions, those reporting high purposeful engagement and positive relations were protected against elevated levels of inflammatory markers (interleukin-6, IL-6, and C-reactive protein, CRP) compared to other elders also dealing with comorbidity but lacking high well-being. Similarly, sleep problems are known to increase with aging, but older women reporting higher levels of eudaimonic well-being (all dimensions except autonomy) reported lower levels of disrupted sleep (Phelan, Love, Ryff, Brown, & Heidrich, 2010).

Beyond the challenges of aging, protective benefits of eudaimonic well-being have been examined in contexts of social inequality. Those with lower socioeconomic standing (educational attainment, occupational status, income level) are known to increase risk for diverse health problem (Adler, Marmot, McEwen, & Stewart, 1999; Marmot, 2005). However, a study (Morozink, Friedman, Coe, & Ryff, 2010) linking educational status to interleukin-6 (IL-6), which is an inflammatory marker implicated in multiple health problems (cardiovascular disease, cancer,

Alzheimer's disease, osteoporosis), showed protective benefits of high eudaimonic well-being. That is, although lower levels of educational attainment predicted higher levels of IL—6 (thereby replicating prior findings), those with limited education who reported higher levels of multiple aspects of well-being had lower levels of IL-6 compared to their same education counterparts who reported lower well-being. Another study (Tsenkova, Love, Singer, & Ryff, 2007) showed links between income and cross-time changes in glycosylated hemoglobin (HbAlc), a marker of glycemic control connected to Type 2 diabetes. Higher income predicted lower cross-time profiles of HbAlc, but measures of well-being (purpose in life, personal growth, positive affect) moderated these relationships. Numerous other life challenges, such as being a cancer survivor, or a life-long parent of a child with developmental disabilities, or losing a spouse, or dealing with race-related inequality, have been examined in the MIDUS study with a focus on documenting profiles of resilience (Ryff et al., 2012).

The neural correlates of eudaimonic well-being are also receiving scientific attention. An initial study using electrophysiological indicators showed that adults reporting higher levels of eudaimonic well-being showed greater left than right superior frontal activation in response to emotion stimuli (Urry et al., 2004), after adjusting for reported levels of hedonic well-being. Another study used functional magnetic resonance imaging to examine amygdala activation in response to negative (compared to neutral) stimuli (van Reekum et al., 2007). Those who were faster to evaluate negative information showed increased left and right amygdala activation, but these patterns varied depending on composite profiles of eudaimonic well-being. Those with higher overall well-being were slower to evaluate such information, and they showed reduced amygdala activation as well as increased ventral anterior cingulate cortex activity, possibly recruited in response to aversive stimuli. More recently, neural responses to positive stimuli were examined (Heller et al., 2013) with findings showing that links between sustained activity in reward circuitry (ventral striatum and dorsolateral prefrontal cortex) and higher eudaimonic well-being (composite) as well as lower diurnal cortisol output. Eudaimonic well-being (personal growth, positive relations, purpose in life) has also been linked with insular cortex volume (Lewis, Kanai, Rees, & Bates, 2014) – positive links were evident between these aspects of well-being and right insular cortex grey matter volume, which is involved in a variety of higher-order functions. Another study showed that those with higher levels of purpose in life had more rapid brain-based emotional recovery from negative stimuli (Schaefer et al., 2013). Together, these brain-based inquiries have begun to explicate underlying neural mechanisms involved in psychological experiences of eudaimonia.

A final area of recent inquiry pertains to links between eudaimonic well-being and gene expression. Of interest is the conserved transcriptional response to adversity (CTRA), which is characterized by up-regulated expression of pro-inflammatory genes and down-regulated expression of antibody synthesis genes. A first study (Fredrickson et al., 2013) showed divergent transcriptome profiles for hedonic versus eudaimonic well-being. Specifically, high hedonic well-being was associated with upregulated expression of pro-inflammatory genes and decreased expression of antibody synthesis genes. In contrast, those high in eudaimonic well-being showed CTRA down regulation (i.e., decreased expression of pro-inflammatory genes and increased expression of antibody synthesis genes). These patterns were independent of demographic, health, and behavioral risk factors. Eudaimonia thus appeared to convey health-related benefits for gene expression that were not evident for hedonia. A subsequent study, using more detailed measures of eudaimonic well-being (Fredrickson et al., 2015, see also Fredrickson, Chap. 12, this volume), showed reduced CTRA expression for all but one of the six dimensions of well-being, again after adjusting for demographic characteristics, health-related confounders, and RNA indicators of leukocyte subset distribution. Another recent investigation (Cole et al., 2015) found CTRA expression to be up-regulated in association with loneliness, but again, down-regulated in association with eudaimonic well-being. Such findings suggest the potential utility of targeting health risks associated with social isolation by promoting meaning and purpose in life.

The preceding summary of select scientific research makes clear that eudaimonic well-being has become a tractable topic in basic science research. That is, thanks to the availability of conceptually-grounded, quantitative assessment tools, meaningful links of well-being with diverse biological and brain-based processes as well as with genetics have been documented. This emerging body of research, and more (summarized in Ryff, 2014) has import for public policy, including allocation of resources to improve the human condition. Arguably, the promotion of well-being to improve health and quality of life is no less needed or promising than the development of pharmaceuticals to advance the nation's health. As such, the final section below summarizes ongoing intervention efforts to promote eudaimonic well-being.

6.5 The Promotion of Eudaimonia to Improve Lives

Growing evidence suggests that eudaimonic well-being is modifiable (Ruini & Ryff, 2016; Ryff, 2014). Before considering relevant examples, it is important to underscore that the lack of well-being increases subsequent risk for mental illness (Keyes, 2002), and further that cross-time gains in well-being have been shown to predict cross-time declines in mental illness (Keyes, Dhingra, & Simoes, 2010). Thus, there is growing awareness that promoting positive mental health has notable public health significance. In treating mental health problems, it has also become clear that full recovery involves more than the reduction of symptoms or absence of psychological distress. Importantly, it must also include the promotion of experiences of well-being (Fava, Ruini, & Belaise, 2007; Ruini & Fava, 2012; 2014).

One prominent example is "well-being therapy" (Fava, 1999; Fava, Rafanelli, Cazzaro, Conti, & Grandi, 1998), which makes explicit use of eudaimonic well-being, conceived as an addition to cognitive behavioral therapy, in treating major depression. The overarching goal is to promote positive psychological experiences for patients' as a way of preventing relapse. The intervention requires keeping daily diaries of positive happenings, which then become the focus of therapy wherein patients learn how to prevent premature curtailment of such experiences as well as how to enrich and extend them. Initial finds documented improved remission profiles among those who received well-being therapy, and longitudinal follow-up further showed that relapse was prevented over a 6 year period (Fava et al., 2004). Well-being therapy was also found to be effective in treating anxiety disorders (Fava et al., 2005; Ruini, Albieri, & Vescovelli, 2015; Ruini & Fava, 2009), again with long-lasting effects.

Outside the clinical context, promoting eudaimonia may play an important role in prevention mental illness and psychological distress in the broader population. A promising context for such efforts in adolescence is the school. Ruini, Belaise, Brombin, Caffo, and Fava (2006) adapted well-being therapy for school settings with the goal of preventing the development of depression (especially among girls) during adolescence. Comparison of students receiving the intervention with an attention-placebo group revealed significant improvements in personal growth, along with reductions in distress (Ruini et al., 2009). Another controlled investigation in schools showed that well-being therapy produced significant improvements in autonomy and friendliness, whereas an anxiety management intervention ameliorated anxious and depressive symptoms (Tomba et al., 2010). Further school interventions are summarized in Ruini and Ryff (2016).

At the other end of the life course, a group intervention for promoting eudaimonia among older adults in the community has been developed (Friedman et al., 2015). Because later life comes with many challenges (loss of roles, loss of significant others, health events), individuals can be vulnerable to depression. This program, conducted over a period of 8 weeks, involves discussion of the importance of well-being in later life, the sharing of positive memories, and engagement in exercises designed to promote eudaimonia as well as to deal with difficult life challenges. Pre-post comparisons showed gains in most aspects of eudaimonic well-being as well as life satisfaction as well as reductions in depressive and physical symptoms and sleep complaints. Such improvements were particularly evident among individuals with lower levels of eudaimonic well-being prior to the intervention. This work has been expanded to include further groups of older adults in multiple community contexts.

More interventions, in clinical and community contexts, are detailed in Ryff (2014). Collectively, such work supports the idea that eudaimonic well-being can be promoted. These initiatives thus constitute important new directions in research translation and public health education. It is worth noting that none of the conceptual formulations drawn on to create the model of eudaimonic well-being described herein (Ryff, 1989) were explicitly concerned with how to promote such positive functioning; rather they were striving to articulate what are the defining features of optimal human functioning. Similarly, Aristotle's writings were not a treatise in how to promote virtuous living; rather his aim was to articulate what are the varieties of virtue. Nonetheless thanks to contemporary science and practice, the possibility of promoting ever wider experiences of eudiamonia for larger segments of society is becoming a reality.

6.6 Concluding Points

The primary contribution of this volume is to depict diverse perspectives on eudaimonia. The formulation covered in this chapter represents but one approach, which emerged from the synthesis of multiple formulations, all concerned with articulating the nature of positive human functioning. Their visions were decidedly in the spirit of Aristotle's eudaimonia, as each sought to characterize how individuals can make the most of their unique talents and capacities. What makes these ideas beautiful is the undeniable power they have to help us find our way, individually and collectively, on the journey of becoming the best that we can be. Such high-minded ideals are fundamentally needed in all periods of human history, but they are particularly critical in our own era (Edmundson, 2015), which is beset by technological distractions, growing problems of inequality, climate problems, and endless strife in certain parts of the world.

Beautiful ideas may emerge from philosophy or insightful scholarship across the disciplinary spectrum, including the humanities. But where they are critically needed is in the scientific arena, which sometimes suffers from the misguided view that what happens in science should be value free. On the on contrary, what may matter the most in generating scientific advances that have real potential improve the human condition is that the work be guided by ennobling ideas. Summarized above has been a model of well-being that encompasses multiple components of what it means to be well and function optimally. These ideas required operational definitions and accompanying assessment tools so that they could be quantified and empirically investigated. No such instruments are perfect – rather they are approximations of the beautiful ideas from which they emanated.

Despite their imperfections, much useful knowledge has been gained from bringing these beautiful but empirically tractable ideas into scientific research. Illustrative findings showed how certain aspects of eudaimonic well-being decline with aging but also how the maintenance of well-being in later life matters for diverse health outcomes as well as intervening physiological and brain-based processes. Overall, emerging evidence documents the life enhancing qualities of eudaimonic well-being, especially purposeful life engagement. These advances constitute major transformations in health research, where deeply entrenched biases have, for decades, restricted scientific inquiry to explicating pathways to illness, disease, disability, and death. The presence of eudaimonic measures of well-being, in contrast, has led to an emphasis on promotion of longer, high quality lives, and importantly, growing understanding of how well-being matters for physiology, brain-based processes, and gene expression.

Building on such work, still further endeavors are actively seeking to enhance well-being via clinical interventions, school programs, and community initiatives. Much future potential revolves around the use of eudiamonic well-being for preventive purposes, including in contexts of significance life adversity. All of these efforts are motivated by the beautiful idea that people, at all periods in the life course, can learn skills and insights for increasing their supply of eudaimonic well-being. Such nurturing of human talents and capacities, was recognized over 2000 years ago by Aristotle as the key thing we should all be about. His amazing wisdom is no less true today.

References

Adler, N. E., Marmot, M. G., McEwen, B. S., & Stewart, J. (1999). *Socioeconomic status and health in industrialized nations: Social, psychological, and biological pathways* (Vol. 896). New York: New York Academy of Sciences.

Allport, G. W. (1961). *Pattern and growth in personality*. New York: Holt, Rinehart, & Winston.

Antonovsky, A. (1979). *Health, stress, and coping* (1st ed.). San Francisco: Jossey-Bass.

Antonovsky, A. (1987). *Unraveling the mystery of health*. San Francisco: Jossey-Bass.

Aristotle. (1925). *The Nicomachean ethics* (W. D. Ross, Trans.). New York: Oxford University Press.

Becker, L. C. (1992). Good lives: Prolegomena. *Social Philosophy & Policy, 9*, 15–37. doi:10.1017/S0265052500001382.

Boyle, P. A., Barnes, L. L., Buchman, A. S., & Bennett, D. A. (2009). Purpose in life is associated with mortality among community-dwelling older persons. *Psychosomatic Medicine, 71*(5), 574–579. doi:10.1097/PSY.0b013e3181a5a7c0.

Boyle, P. A., Buchman, A. S., Barnes, L. L., & Bennett, D. A. (2010). Effect of a purpose in life on risk of incident Alzheimer disease and mild cognitive impairment in community-dwelling older persons. *Archives of General Psychiatry, 67*(3), 304–310. doi:10.1001/archgenpsychiatry.2009.208.

Boyle, P. A., Buchman, A. S., Wilson, R. S., Yu, L., Schneider, J. A., & Bennett, D. A. (2012). Effect of purpose in life on the relation between Alzheimer disease pathologic changes on cognitive function in advanced age. *JAMA Psychiatry, 69*(5), 499–506. doi:10.1001/archgenpsychiatry.2011.1487.

Bühler, C. (1935). The curve of life as studied in biographies. *Journal of Applied Psychology, 43*, 653–673. doi:10.1037/h0054778.

Cole, S. W., Levine, M. E., Arevalo, J. M. G., Ma, J., Weir, D. R., & Crimmins, E. M. (2015). Loneliness, eudaimonia, and the human conserved transcriptional response to adversity. *Psychoneuroendocrinology, 62*, 11–17. doi:10.1016/j.psyneuen.2015.07.001.

Edmundson, M. (2015). *Self and soul: A defense of ideals*. Cambridge, MA: Harvard University Press.

Erikson, E. H. (1959). Identity and the life cycle: Selected papers. *Psychological Issues, 1*, 1–171.

Fava, G. A. (1999). Well-being therapy: Conceptual and technical issues. *Psychotherapy and Psychosomatics, 68*, 171–179. doi:10.1159/000012329.

Fava, G. A., Rafanelli, C., Cazzaro, M., Conti, S., & Grandi, S. (1998). Well-being therapy: A novel psychotherapeutic approach for residual symptoms of affective disorders. *Psychological Medicine, 28*(2), 475–480.

Fava, G. A., Ruini, C., Rafanelli, C., Finos, L., Conti, S., & Grandi, S. (2004). Six-year outcome of cognitive behavior therapy for prevention of recurrent depression. *American Journal of Psychiatry, 161*(10), 1872–1876.

Fava, G. A., Ruini, C., Rafanelli, C., Finos, L., Salmaso, L., Mangelli, L., et al. (2005). Well-being therapy of generalized anxiety disorder. *Psychotherapy and Psychosomatics, 74*(1), 26–30. doi:10.1159/000082023.

Fava, G. A., Ruini, C., & Belaise, C. (2007). The concept of recovery in major depression. *Psychological Medicine, 37*(3), 307–317. doi:10.1017/s0033291706008981.

Frankl, V. E. (1959). *Man's search for meaning: An introduction to logotherapy*. Boston: Beacon Press.

Fredrickson, B. L., Grewen, K. M., Algoe, S. B., Firestine, A. M., Arevalo, J. M. G., Ma, J., et al. (2015). Psychological well-being and the human conserved transcriptional response to adversity. *Plos One, 10*(3), 17. doi:10.1371/journal.pone.0121839.

Fredrickson, B. L., Grewen, K. M., Coffey, K. A., Algoe, S. B., Firestine, A. M., Arevalo, J. M. G., et al. (2013). A functional genomic perspective on human well-being. *Proceedings of the National Academy of Sciences, 110*, 13684–13689.

Friedman, E. M., & Ryff, C. D. (2012). Living well with medical comorbidities: A biopsychosocial perspective. *Journals of Gerontology Series B, Psychological Sciences and Social Sciences, 67*(5), 535–544. doi:10.1093/geronb/gbr152.

Friedman, E. M., Ruini, C., Foy, R., Jaros, L., Sampson, H., & Ryff, C. D. (2015). Lighten up! A community-based group intervention to promote psychological well-being in older adults. *Aging and Mental Health.*

doi:10.1080/13607863.2015.1093605. Advance online publication.
Heller, A. S., van Reekum, C. M., Schaefer, S. M., Lapate, R. C., Radler, B. T., Ryff, C. D., et al. (2013). Sustained ventral striatal activity predicts eudaimonic well-being and cortisol output. *Psychological Science, 24*(11), 2191–2200. doi:10.1177/0956797613490744.
Hill, P. L., & Turiano, N. A. (2014). Purpose in life as a predictor of mortality across adulthood. *Psychological Science, 25*(7), 1482–1486. doi:10.1177/0956797614531799.
Jackson, D. N. (1967). *Personality research form manual*. Goshen, NY: Research Psychologists Press.
Jackson, D. N. (1976). *Jackson personality inventory manual*. Goshen, NY: Research Psychologists Press.
Jahoda, M. (1958). *Current concepts of positive mental health*. New York: Basic Books.
Johnston, I. (1997). *Lecture on Aristotle's Nicomachaean ethics*. Retrieved from http://records.viu.ca/~johnstoi/introser/aristot.htm
Jung, C. G. (1933). *Modern man in search of a soul* (W. S. Dell & C. F. Baynes, Trans.). New York: Harcourt, Brace & World.
Keyes, C. L. M. (2002). The mental health continuum: From languishing to flourishing in life. *Journal of Health & Social Behavior, 43*(2), 207–222.
Keyes, C. L. M., Dhingra, S. S., & Simoes, E. J. (2010). Change in level of positive mental health as a predictor of future risk of mental illness. *American Journal of Public Health, 100*(12), 2366. doi:10.2105/AJPH.2010.192245.
Kim, E. S., Sun, J. K., Park, N., & Peterson, C. (2013). Purpose in life and reduced stroke in older adults: The health and retirement study. *Journal of Psychosomatic Research, 74*(5), 427–432. doi:10.1016/j.jpsychores.2013.01.013.
Kim, E. S., Sun, J. K., Park, N., Kubzansky, L. D., & Peterson, C. (2013). Purpose in life and reduced risk of myocardial infarction among older U.S. Adults with coronary heart disease: A two-year follow-up. *Journal of Behavioral Medicine, 36*(2), 124–133. doi:10.1007/s10865-012-9406-4.
Kim, E. S., Strecher, V. J., & Ryff, C. D. (2014). Purpose in life and use of preventive health care services. *Proceedings of the National Academy of Sciences of the United States of America, 111*(46), 16331–16336. doi:10.1073/pnas.1414826111.
Lewis, G. J., Kanai, R., Rees, G., & Bates, T. C. (2014). Neural correlates of the "good life": Eudaimonic well-being is associated with insular cortex volume. *Social Cognitive and Affective Neuroscience, 9*(5), 615–618. doi:10.1093/scan/nst032.
Marmot, M. (2005). Social determinants of health inequalities. *Lancet, 365*(9464), 1099–1104. doi:10.1016/s0140-6736(05)71146-6.
Maslow, A. H. (1968). *Toward a psychology of being* (2nd ed.). New York: Van Nostrand.
Mill, J. S. (1989). *Autobiography*. London: Penguin (Original work published 1893).
Morozink, J. A., Friedman, E. M., Coe, C. L., & Ryff, C. D. (2010). Socioeconomic and psychosocial predictors of interleukin-6 in the MIDUS national sample. *Health Psychology, 29*(6), 626–635. doi:10.1037/a0021360.
Neugarten, B. L. (1973). Personality change in late life: A developmental perspective. In C. Eisodorfer & M. P. Lawton (Eds.), *The psychology of adult development and aging* (pp. 311–335). Washington, DC: American Psychological Association.
Norton, D. L. (1976). *Personal destinies: A philosophy of ethical individualism*. Princeton, NJ: Princeton University Press.
Phelan, C. H., Love, G. D., Ryff, C. D., Brown, R. L., & Heidrich, S. M. (2010). Psychosocial predictors of changing sleep patterns in aging women: A multiple pathway approach. *Psychology and Aging, 25*(4), 858–866. doi:10.1037/a0019622.
Riley, M. W., Kahn, R. L., & Foner, A. (1994). *Age and structural lag*. New York: Wiley.
Rogers, C. R. (1961). *On becoming a person*. Boston: Houghton Mifflin.
Ruini, C., & Fava, G. A. (2009). Well-being therapy for generalized anxiety disorder. *Journal of Clinical Psychology, 65*(5), 510–519. doi:10.1002/jclp.20592.
Ruini, C., & Fava, G. A. (2012). Role of well-being therapy in achieving a balanced and individualized path to optimal functioning. *Clinical Psychology & Psychotherapy, 19*(4), 291–304. doi:10.1002/cpp.1796.
Ruini, C., & Fava, G. A. (2014). The individualized and cross-cultural roots of well-being therapy. In G. A. Fava & C. Ruini (Eds.), *Increasing psychological well-being in clinical and educational settings: Interventions and cultural contexts* (Vol. 8, pp. 21–39). New York: Springer Science+Business Media.
Ruini, C., & Ryff, C. D. (2016). Using eudaimonic well-being to improve lives. In A. M. Wood & J. Johnson (Eds.), *The Wiley handbook of positive clinical psychology: An integrative approach to studying and improving well-being*. Hoboken, NJ: Wiley-Blackwell.
Ruini, C., Belaise, C., Brombin, C., Caffo, E., & Fava, G. A. (2006). Well-being therapy in school settings: A pilot study. *Psychotherapy and Psychosomatics, 75*(6), 331–336. doi:10.1159/000095438.
Ruini, C., Ottolini, F., Tomba, E., Belaise, C., Albieri, E., Visani, D., … Fava, G. A. (2009). School intervention for promoting psychological well-being in adolescence. *Journal of Behavior Therapy and Experimental Psychiatry, 40*(4), pp. 522–532. doi:10.1016/j.jbtep.2009.07.002.
Ruini, C., Albieri, E., & Vescovelli, F. (2015). Well-being therapy: State of the art and clinical exemplifications. *Journal of Contemporary Psychotherapy, 45*, 129–136. doi:10.1007/s10879-014-9290-z.
Russell, B. (1958). *The conquest of happiness*. New York: Liveright (Original work published 1930).
Ryff, C. D. (1982). Successful aging: A developmental approach. *The Gerontologist, 22*, 209–214. doi:10.1093/geront/22.2.209.

Ryff, C. D. (1989). Happiness is everything, or is it? Explorations on the meaning of psychological well-being. *Journal of Personality and Social Psychology, 57*(6), 1069–1081. doi:10.1037/0022-3514.57.6.1069.

Ryff, C. D. (2014). Psychological well-being revisited: Advances in the science and practice of eudaimonia. *Psychotherapy and Psychosomatics, 83*(1), 10–28. doi:10.1159/000353263.

Ryff, C. D., & Singer, B. H. (2008). Know thyself and become what you are: A eudaimonic approach to psychological well-being. *Journal of Happiness Studies, 9*(1), 13–39. doi:10.1007/s10902-006-9019-0.

Ryff, C., Friedman, E., Fuller-Rowell, T., Love, G., Miyamoto, Y., Morozink, J., ... Tsenkova, V. (2012). Varieties of resilience in MIDUS. *Social and Personality Psychology Compass, 6*(11), pp. 792–806. doi:10.1111/j.1751-9004.2012.00462.x.

Schaefer, S. M., Boylan, J. M., van Reekum, C. M., Lapate, R. C., Norris, C. J., Ryff, C. D., et al. (2013). Purpose in life predicts better emotional recovery from negative stimuli. *PLoS One, 8*(11), e80329. doi:10.1371/journal.pone.0080329.

Springer, K. W., Pudrovska, T., & Hauser, R. M. (2011). Does psychological well-being change with age? Longitudinal tests of age variations and further exploration of the multidimensionality of Ryff's model of psychological well-being. *Social Science Research, 40*(1), 392–398. doi:10.1016/j.ssresearch.2010.05.008.

Tomba, E., Belaise, C., Ottolini, F., Ruini, C., Bravi, A., Albieri, E., ... Fava, G. A. (2010). Differential effects of well-being promoting and anxiety-management strategies in a non-clinical school setting. *Journal of Anxiety Disorders, 24*(3), pp. 326–333. doi:10.1016/j.janxdis.2010.01.005.

Tsenkova, V. K., Love, G. D., Singer, B. H., & Ryff, C. D. (2007). Socioeconomic status and psychological well-being predict cross-time change in glycosylated hemoglobin in older women without diabetes. *Psychosomatic Medicine, 69*(8), 777–784. doi:10.1097/PSY.0b013e318157466f.

Urry, H. L., Nitschke, J. B., Dolski, I., Jackson, D. C., Dalton, K. M., Mueller, C. J., ... Davidson, R. J. (2004). Making a life worth living: Neural correlates of well-being. *Psychological Science, 15*(6), pp. 367–372. doi:10.1111/j.0956-7976.2004.00686.x.

van Reekum, C. M., Urry, H. L., Johnstone, T., Thurow, M. E., Frye, C. J., Jackson, C. A., ... Davidson, R. J. (2007). Individual differences in amygdala and ventromedial prefrontal cortex activity are associated with evaluation speed and psychological well-being. *Journal of Cognitive Neuroscience, 19*(2), pp. 237–248. doi:10.1162/jocn.2007.19.2.237.

Waterman, A. S. (1984). *The psychology of individualism.* New York: Praeger.

Wiggins, J. S. (1980). *Personality and prediction: Principles of personality assessment.* Menlo Park, CA: Addison-Wesley.

World Health Organization. (1948). Constitution of the World Health Organization. Basic documents. Geneva, Switzerland: Retrieved from http://www.who.int/about/mission/en/

Eudaimonia as a Way of Living: Connecting Aristotle with Self-Determination Theory

7

Richard M. Ryan and Frank Martela

Eudaimonia, although an ancient concept, has reemerged in modern psychology for clear reasons. Across the globe the spread of market capitalism and consumer-based economies has led to increasing material wealth, without necessarily yielding expected rises in happiness or well-being (see Clark, Frijters, & Shields, 2008; Easterlin, 1995; Kasser, Cohn, Kanner, & Ryan, 2007). Moreover, changes in societal structures in more economically advanced cultures have allowed many (though far from all) people more choice and leeway in choosing the pathways of their lives, while at the same time traditional sources of guidance and belief are diminished. This leaves open the question of what is good and worthwhile to pursue in life. For individuals, both of these trends raise concerns about the qualities of a good life that comprise and give rise to fulfillment and well-being (Ryan & Deci, 2001; Waterman, 2013). Many people have become disillusioned by the materialistic life and its capability to produce happiness, but have a hard time identifying the alternative way of living that would be more worthwhile. Eudaimonia, as a psychological concept and a target of research, presents for many the hope of finding something beyond hedonistic happiness worth striving for.

Despite its currency, eudaimonia is also a widely misunderstood concept, particularly within the discourse of positive psychology. The main issue is a tendency for some theorists to construe eudaimonia as a specific type of happiness or subjective experience, one that sits alongside other experiences like pleasure or engagement. In contrast, when relying on the fundamental roots of the concept in Aristotelian philosophy, one would not construe eudaimonia as a psychological state, or a kind of happiness (see e.g., Bartlett & Collins, 2012). Rather it is understood as a good and fulfilling way of life, the ingredients of which then contribute to happiness and thriving. This latter view is embraced within the *self-determination theory* (SDT) approach to this concept (see Niemiec & Ryan, 2013; Ryan, Curren, & Deci, 2013; Ryan, Huta, & Deci, 2008).

In this chapter we describe both ancient and modern views of eudaimonia, and why we have highlighted the eudaimonic tradition as critical for current empirical work in the psychology of well-being. We also review some specific research findings relevant to these ideas, and that concern people's ability to experience happiness and thriving in the context of the modern social forces affecting us all. Throughout our thesis and findings are guided by our overarching theoretical

R.M. Ryan (✉)
Institute for Positive Psychology and Education, Australian Catholic University, Sydney, NSW, Australia
e-mail: Richard.Ryan@acu.edu.au

F. Martela
University of Helsinki, Helsinki, Finland

J. Vittersø (ed.), *Handbook of Eudaimonic Well-Being*, International Handbooks of Quality-of-Life,
DOI 10.1007/978-3-319-42445-3_7

and empirical framework of SDT (Deci & Ryan, 2000; Ryan & Deci, 2000).

7.1 Aristotle, Eudaimonic Thinking and Positive Psychology

The pre-philosophical history of eudaimonia in ancient Greece saw the concept to denote a "broad idea of a life's going well" (Annas, 1995, p. 44). Eudaimonia was the word used to describe the kind of life all people sought to live, but there were many contradictory ideas about what this optimal way of life included. Some emphasized material prosperity, others living honorably, still others health, pleasure, or living according to virtues (see Aristotle, 2012). Yet what eudaimonia was not was a mere subjective feeling.[1] It was an evaluation of life as a whole to see whether the good things were present in that life, with the discussion focusing on what exactly the relevant good things should be.

Of different ancient views on eudaimonia, it was Aristotle who laid out the first systematic work on eudaimonia in particular and ethical theory in general, and subsequent Greek schools of philosophy walked in his footprints (Annas, 1995). Aristotle is also the figure on which contemporary discussions of eudaimonia within psychology focus, and whose views we see as resembling many views of SDT. Thus it is on Aristotle's view on eudaimonia that we concentrate.

Aristotle's view was that every living being has a *telos*, some good that it naturally strives to actualize (Aristotle, 2012). Aristotle saw that what was especially unique to our human nature (and what separates us from animals) was our ability to live in accord with reason, and the most complete way to live according to reason was to live virtuously. Thus Aristotle arrived at his famous conclusion that eudaimonia is about a "certain activity of soul in accord with complete virtue" (Aristotle, p. 23). The virtues and excellences specific to human beings included living in a reflective way that embraced our best values and engaged our highest talents and civic concerns. They also included other-oriented virtues such as friendship, justice and truthfulness. Accordingly, a person could be more or less characterized as person who lives (or has lived) a good life, insofar as that individual pursued or lived in accordance with the specific human virtues. By engaging in these personal and civic virtues and excellences, and when conditions allow, actualizing them, Aristotle expected persons to be most fulfilled. Happiness, being a reflection of that fulfillment, was also a likely outcome of living in a eudaimonic manner.

Aristotle of course had his own quite historically defined, and in some ways culturally circumscribed view of the features and characteristics of such an ideal or fulfilling human life. For him, for example, the pinnacle of human excellences was the philosophical or contemplative life, which just happened to be his own profession (he notes that "philosophy seems to have pleasures that are wondrous in purity and stability" Aristotle, 2012, p. 224). He also had ideas about who was most apt at eudaimonic living (e.g., men rather than women). Also valuing civic engagement, he considered this the domain of citizens rather than slaves. Yet acknowledging such historically conditioned limitations to his ideas does not demean the many qualities he did highlight that still pertain in our modern world. Specifically, he saw the excellent life as one in which a person lived virtuously, and in all endeavors living up to his or her potential by pursuing, in a reflective and chosen manner, one's best competencies and talents.

In providing a contemporary application of eudaimonic thinking, we draw from Aristotle's several central points. One is that there are certain ways of living that are more conducive to, and reflective of a good life and a well person (Ryan,

[1] This is perhaps most strikingly demonstrated when Solon claims that the eudaimonia of a man can only be settled after his death (Herodotus 1.32), and when Aristotle ponders whether a dishonor befalling a dead person can still alter that person's eudaimonia (Aristotle, 2012, pp. 18–19). These remarks would be very strange to make about eudaimonia as a fleeting subjective state, but make more sense when we see eudaimonia as an evaluation of one's life as a whole.

Huta, & Deci, 2008; Huta, Chap. 15, this volume). Second, when these qualities are embraced and lived, a common result is happiness in the fullest of senses understood as subjective well-being. Thus a person pursuing virtuous living is expected to feel fulfilled and satisfied with his or her life, including not only positive affect, but also a sense of meaning, connection, and depth. Importantly, happiness and well-being are for Aristotle not the primary aims of living (that is, in fact, an hedonic view). Rather these subjective experiences are byproducts of living well.

These claims are of course not merely philosophical in nature—they are also speculative and psychological. That is, whether a life of virtue and reflective engagement in one's activities leads to happiness and thriving more than, for example, a life of hedonic pursuits, selfishness or materialist excess (which would not express virtuous ideals) is an empirical question. For indeed it is plausible, and not uncommonly expressed, that it is not virtue that makes us happy, but achievement, economic success and self-interest in the narrow sense. We do not have to look far for exemplars of this alternative philosophy; they surround us in the modern media, which contains both implicit and explicit messages that money, fame and image are the royal roads to happiness (Kasser et al., 2007). It is thus important that we investigate whether indeed there are certain sensibilities and aims that more readily facilitate human thriving and wellness, and others whose pursuit, even when successful, do not yield these benefits.

In the few paragraphs above our attempt has been to characterize the Aristotelian view on eudaimonia, going back directly to his own writings. Our discussion has been brief and is not reflective of all the nuances in Aristotle's view, but nevertheless aims to highlight the main thrusts of his theses. For further discussion of these ideas, we refer the reader to a discussion by Ryan et al. (2013) as well as to even the greater exactingness of philosophers such as Annas (1995) and Curren (2014). Such careful specificity has an important place in this tradition, especially because of how readily eudaimonic thinking has at times been mischaracterized or misunderstood, perhaps especially within the fast moving positive psychology movement.

In fact, it seems important from the outset of our discussion to highlight one specific misunderstanding in modern applications of eudaimonic thinking within positive psychology, namely the idea that the specific experience or quality of happiness and affect derived from eudaimonic endeavors is different in kind from the happiness or elation one might experience through other positive events. Eudaimonia, that is, is not a special type of immediate experience, or necessarily a deeper, richer feeling of happiness. Instead eudaimonia is rather a depiction of the kinds of pursuits and a manner of living that would most reliably give rise to a life accompanied by a sense of wellness, vitality and thriving. This does not mean that one cannot look to eudaimonic living for more frequent experiences of awe, meaning, or deep fulfillment or the like (Huta & Ryan, 2010). Yet one can also be awed or struck by meaning or feel temporarily fulfilled even when not living eudaimonically.

We thus emphasize that eudaimonia is defined by a way of living that is likely to produce many beneficial outcomes like greater happiness and integrity than other pathways in life, such as non-virtuous living, hedonism, or indolence (Ryan & Huta, 2009). Therefore we see it as incorrect to put eudaimonia alongside other forms of happiness (Seligman, 2002) or to imagine that there is a specifically distinct eudaimonic experience of wellness. Instead, eudaimonic philosophy argues that a life of virtue and a pursuit of excellences leads more frequently to fulfillment and happiness. Other forms of "success" (dominance, greed, acquisition, hedonism for example) should, on average, not. It is this question that can be pursued using modern empirical methods. We thus separate eudaimonic way of living as referring to certain practices and pursuits from happiness and other subjective experiences of well-being. A eudaimonic way of living may *cause* subjective well-being, but it is not a *type* of subjective experience.

We will also revisit an even more speculative idea within Aristotle's framework, namely the proposition that eudaimonic living produces these outcomes *because it reflects our human nature*. Virtue was a central part of eudaimonia for Aristotle because it presented "the activity and hence the way of life that are best for human beings as such, as the kind of beings we are" (Bartlett & Collins, 2012, p. *x*). Some of the virtues Aristotle saw as natural for humans were other-oriented: for example friendliness and goodwill toward others. Yet in what ways can we argue that being virtuous, caring for others, and developing our excellences is *natural* to humanity, any more than the obvious selfishness, cruelty or avarice people so often display? This question of human nature, being clearly complex, is also worth pursuing, especially given that we now have new methods to examine these issues using developmental and evolutionary psychology, both of which can offer more definitive answers than one might expect (Ryan & Hawley, in press).

Thus in what follows we shall tackle both of these speculative questions raised by the eudaimonic tradition and see what answers, and remaining questions, can be identified. We thus first discuss the relations of eudaimonic living to happiness and wellness outcomes; and then we consider the topic of human nature, and evidence that Aristotelian goodwill and caring for others represents a natural proclivity, especially under nurturing conditions of development.

7.2 Does Eudaimonic Living Make Us Happy?

Insofar as eudaimonia concerns a way of living rather than merely the subjective outcomes of a life, one must have a model of what such a life entails. As we said, Aristotle, particularly in his *Nichomachean Ethics* (2012), had his own list of virtues and excellences that comprised the good life, just as do some modern eudaimonic philosophers (e.g., Nussbaum, 2001). As it turns out, in reading Aristotle's views we see many parallels with the tenets of a good life specified within our more contemporary (and more pedestrian) views in self-determination theory (SDT; Deci & Ryan, 1985; Ryan & Deci, 2000).

Previous papers within SDT have specifically argued that certain principle elements of Aristotle's view are modeled in SDT (Ryan et al., 2008; Ryan et al., 2013). More generally, SDT has aimed to find those elements of human experience that are in accordance with human nature and thus intimately connected with human thriving, and thus could be seen as modern answers to the Aristotle's call to find ways of living through which to actualize the human *telos*.

These include: (1) pursuing intrinsic goals such as intimate relationships, benevolence and community, and personal growth rather than extrinsic goals such as image, popularity or material acquisitions and success; and (2) regulating behavior autonomously rather than being controlled or being a pawn to forces alien to one's sensibilities and values, and (3) living a reflective, mindful and aware life, rather than an unreflective life or one comprised of defensiveness or avoidance of conscious living. SDT argues that these qualities of awareness, intrinsic pursuits and autonomous regulation in turn fulfill very basic human psychological needs. Thus a fourth aspect of SDT is its prediction that these qualities of living lead one to experience a greater sense of autonomy and integrity, a greater sense of competence and effectiveness; and a greater sense of connectedness to others. As basic psychological needs the fulfillment of these three needs is an experiential sign that the person in question has been able to create a life yielding the nutrients most required by human nature (Deci & Ryan, 2000). These basic need fulfillments of autonomy, competence and relatedness in turn are predictive of subjective happiness and positive experience, including more stable senses of vitality and thriving.

Before examining the empirical evidence that eudaimonic living indeed makes us happier, it must be noted that happiness and similar positive feelings by no means are the only outcomes that should be used when evaluating whether a certain form of living is eudaimonic. They indeed are merely one of the better things to which eudaimonic living should lead. In fact, eudaimonia as a broad notion of a good life allows us to consider other criteria as well. For example, Haybron (2008) has argued that a life can be good in (at least) three different ways: It can be good for the well-being of the person living that life, it can be good in a moral sense, and might also be evaluated as better or worse in aesthetic terms (see also Haybron, Chap. 2, this volume).

Moreover, a life of excellence and virtue can, in some circumstances, lead to less day-to-day positive affect and even a premature death (e.g. when a person is fighting an oppressive political system instead of supporting it). However, from a moral point of view the person living that life could choose not to live in any other way and thus might feel that despite the sacrifices, it is the only virtuous way of living in that particular situation. Of course, even in that situation, although the person might experience less joyous feelings, the person might still have more of other positive states such as a sense of autonomy and integrity. We will not delve into these complexities more here, but just want to remind the reader that in addition to happiness, there are other things that should be considered when evaluating a life as more or less eudaimonic. For example, in the future it would be interesting to see more research on what conditions and strivings increase people's sense of meaning in life and having a life worth living (Weinstein, Ryan, & Deci, 2012; Martela & Steger, 2016; Steger, Chap. 11, this volume).

7.2.1 The Empirical Case for SDT's Eudaimonic Model

As it turns out there is quite a bit of emerging evidence supporting the four empirically testable ideas about happiness and well-being we outlined above. In what follows we review some of the empirical contributions supporting the idea that these elements of living well indeed predict positive outcomes associated with truly thriving.

7.2.2 Pursuing More Intrinsic Versus Extrinsic Goals in Life

Aristotle made a distinction between two forms of action: *praxis*, which refers to action that is virtuous and an end in itself; and *poiesis*, which means production that has only an end beyond itself (Aristotle, 2012, p. 120). Echoing this distinction, Ryan, Sheldon, Kasser, and Deci (1996) proposed that all life goals are not created equal when it comes to fulfillment and happiness. In arguing this they built upon studies by Kasser and Ryan (1996), who found that the goals of financial success, becoming socially recognized, and having an attractive image loaded together on a factor they labeled extrinsic aspirations, whereas personal growth, meaningful relationships, and community contribution loaded on a factor they called intrinsic aspirations. Kasser and Ryan further showed that a stronger relative focus on intrinsic aspirations was positively correlated to well-being indicators such as self-actualization, self-worth, and vitality, and negatively related with negative indicators such as symptoms of anxiety and depression. The opposite pattern was observed when people gave greater weight to extrinsic goals.

This general pattern has been widely replicated using varying methods and measures. For example, evidence also shows that among adolescents, those with stronger materialist tendencies show lower vitality and self-esteem, and more symptoms of depression and anxiety, just as adults do (Kasser & Ryan, 1993). Materialism has also been related to higher narcissism and behaviors that reflect stress such as substance abuse. Echoing this, a recent longitudinal study by Ku, Dittmar, and Banerjee (2014) showed that students who were higher in materialism reported lower levels of mastery goals, and higher levels of both approach and avoidance forms of performance goals, which concern comparisons with others. They also showed worse school performance. There is in fact a growing body of evidence around the globe indicating that materialism and well-being are negatively related (e.g., Ahuvia & Friedman, 1998; Kim et al., 2003;

Ryan et al., 1999; Saunders & Munro, 2000; Schmuck, Kasser, & Ryan, 2000).

In addition, emphasis on extrinsic goals tends to be associated with a number of "non-eudaimonic" attitudes and beliefs. For example Duriez, Vansteenkiste, Soenens, and De Witte (2007) showed in both cross-sectional and longitudinal studies that those with stronger extrinsic goals also evidenced more interest in social dominance, and expressed more racial and ethic prejudices.

Niemiec, Ryan, and Deci (2009) examined such positive and negative effects in a longitudinal study, including the issue of the extent to which people not only valued, but actually attained, intrinsic or extrinsic aspirations. They found that over a 2-year study period well-being was increased to the extent that intrinsic goals were desired and met. Conversely, even when extrinsic aspirations were successfully attained, well-being was not significantly increased, whereas symptoms of ill-being were. Thus, as Aristotle might have predicted, placing importance on, and even attaining extrinsic life goals did not necessarily lead to greater well-being. Important for SDT, Niemiec et al. also showed that this pattern of effects was mediated by satisfaction of basic psychological needs for autonomy, competence and relatedness. Intrinsic pursuits yielded greater need satisfaction, in turn fostering greater well-being.

In SDT people's investment in materialism is seen in part as a byproduct of insecurities, stemming in part from earlier frustrations of basic psychological needs. Conversely, when in nurturing and supportive environments, SDT predicts people grow to focus more on intrinsic goals, and thus to move in even greater directions of actualization and wellness. For example, in a study of adolescents and their mothers, Kasser, Ryan, Zax, and Sameroff (1995) showed that mothers of materialistic teenagers showed a more cold and controlling parenting style. In contrast adolescents who were oriented towards more prosocial and eudaimonic values were more likely to have a more autonomy-supportive, warm and democratic parenting style. Kasser et al. (1995) argued, accordingly, that a parenting environment that nurtures essential psychological needs fosters more prosocially oriented and psychologically thriving adolescents.

Researching high school students, Williams, Cox, Hedberg, and Deci (2000) found that the less autonomy support teenagers reported receiving from parents, the more they placed value on extrinsic, relative to intrinsic aspirations. This in turn was associated with more tobacco, alcohol, and marijuana use. It seems that social contexts that thwart young people's basic psychological need satisfaction can turn them toward compensatory goals and activities that pose serious risks for psychological and physical health. More recently, Chaplin and John (2010) reported that more supportive parents had less materialistic children, a relation that was in part mediated by self-esteem, consistent with Kasser et al.'s (1995) insecurity hypothesis (see also Grolnick, 2003). In sum, such empirical findings support the SDT view that the pursuit of extrinsic goals – such as acquiring money, image and fame – does not lead to wellness, but instead to ill-being.

Parenting contexts that thwart satisfaction of basic psychological needs are more likely to result in children developing desires for wealth, fame, and image, or the most visible indicators of worth, presumably, to compensate for the low personal worth that stems from basic need thwarting.

7.2.3 Why Autonomy Is Important to Eudaimonia

Aristotle maintained that eudaimonia involved being able to live according to the virtues that are inherent to one's nature. A general principle within SDT is that when people are afforded autonomy they are more able to fulfill all of their basic needs. Autonomy is in a sense architectonic, in the sense that it represents an affordance of selection in the direction of greater fulfillments. It is thus not surprising that when people have opportunities to act with autonomy they tend to show more eudaimonic qualities. They show more propensities to act toward intrinsic values (Sheldon, Ryan, Deci, & Kasser, 2004) and more propensity to give to and help others (Weinstein & Ryan, 2010). In contrast, heteronomous or controlling forces often push people away from their core values, as they attempt to meet the demands or pressures put on them from others.

Indeed, it is a long standing theme within SDT that controlling rewards contingencies, contingent approval, and ego-related pressures often drive people away from their interests, and give external impetus to behaviors that may not be in accord with their moral or social values. Thus athletes who are ego involved are more likely to cheat or treat opponents as objects (Vansteenkiste, Mouratidis, Lens, 2010). Teachers under pressure of high stakes tests, and executives under constraints of contingent bonus systems often act in ways that, even as they may successfully reach their goals, lead to less satisfaction and congruence (Ryan & Brown, 2005).

An excellent example of this was recently reported by Sheldon and Krieger (2014). They studied a large sample of lawyers across the US, and divided them into: money lawyers who were primarily seeking wealth and financial gain; social advocates who were attempting to use their profession to do good; and a middle group that was mixed or indeterminate. As it turned out, even when controlling for income (or not) the money lawyers were less satisfied and happy than the social advocates. This effect was in part mediated by their lower autonomy. In their pursuit of extrinsic rewards they were on a day-to-day basis less able to do things that they found of interest or personal value. Instead they did "what they had to" to get ahead (see also Sheldon, Chap. 36, this volume).

When one acts with autonomy, one by definition is acting in ways that are truly self-endorsed. As we shall argue, when people really get to act in accord with what they endorse, they are more likely to appear benevolent, moral and to pursue a life that can be characterized as eudaimonic.

7.2.4 Evidence on Mindful Living

Aristotle (2012, p. 13) argues that eudaimonia entails living "in accord with reason" and being considerate in approaching one's actions and pursuits. Although these sentiments advocate a contemplative life, the nature of that contemplation is quite open. Around the same time in the Buddhist tradition, the idea of mindfulness, or being open and receptive to, and aware of what is occurring in present moments (Brown & Ryan, 2003), was born. This concept of mindfulness has in recent years attracted significant scientific attention in the Western world (see Brown, Crewell, & Ryan, 2015). In our contemporary view, mindfulness allows an individual to authentically experience what is occurring, and thus is central to a self-regulated, and well-chosen life path. In order to live according to reason one has to be aware of what is occurring both internally and externally, and accordingly mindfulness could be seen as one aspect of such a reflective life. When more mindful, people are able to more fully observe and less defensively cope with the various demands that face them (Weinstein, Brown, & Ryan, 2009). Mindfulness also facilitates more openness towards both pleasant and unpleasant experiences, helping individuals to work through life difficulties, and to integrate their lessons (Weinstein, Deci, & Ryan, 2011).

7.2.5 Mindfulness and Autonomous Regulation

There is additionally an empirical connection between mindfulness and more autonomous self-regulation. For example, early in their work on measuring mindfulness Brown and Ryan (2004) reported that both autonomous regulation and the satisfaction of the basic psychological needs were related to greater mindfulness. In fact, evidence showed that mindfulness, assessed as both a general individual difference and as a state measure, was reliably associated with more autonomous functioning. In studies with both student and adult samples it was shown that greater mindfulness at both between- and within-person levels predicted more autonomy in everyday activities as well as less negative affect.

7.2.6 Mindfulness and Intrinsic Aspirations

A greater focus on intrinsic aspirations is positively linked to being mindful. Both Brown and Ryan (2004) and Brown and Kasser (2005) reported positive relations of mindfulness to people's ratings of the importance of intrinsic (relative to extrinsic) aspirations. Still other research demonstrates that people high in mindfulness are more likely to act in ways that are congruent with the intrinsic aspirations. For example, Brown and Kasser reported that people high in mindfulness were higher in their endorsement of intrinsic aspirations and were more ecologically responsible in their behaviors. Brown, Kasser, Ryan, Linley, and Orzech (2009) also found that people higher in mindfulness were less vulnerable to consumerist messages, more likely to savor their experiences, and were significantly more accepting of their life circumstances. In fact, those higher in mindfulness showed lower discrepancy between their current financial situation and their desired income. In turn, this lower discrepancy was predictive of higher subjective well-being.

7.2.7 Mindfulness and Virtue

Also consistent with a eudaimonic portrait of friendliness as one of the main virtues, mindfulness is related to greater compassion and empathy for others (see Beitel, Cecero, & Ferrer, 2005; Brown, Ryan, & Creswell, 2007. Shapiro et al. (1998) showed medical students trained in mindfulness displayed higher empathy over time when compared to a control group. Thus it appears that mindfulness may reduce people's susceptibility to the seductive power of extrinsic rewards and materialistic goals, resulting in more autonomous self-regulation and higher well-being (Brown et al., 2009; Schultz, Ryan, Niemiec, Legate, & Williams, 2014).

7.2.8 Basic Psychological Need Satisfaction as Central to a Good Life

One of the common pathways through which both more intrinsic goal pursuits and mindful living positively affect well-being is through their facilitation of people's basic psychological need satisfactions. In fact, as we have cited, research shows that people experience more autonomy, relatedness to others, and competence when they pursue intrinsic goals and live mindfully.

In fact SDT has a long history of showing that social supports for, and experiences of basic psychological need satisfactions predict greater well-being (Deci & Ryan, 2000) and vitality (Ryan & Deci, 2008). What is most interesting is that these need satisfactions, as we have reviewed, rise with more intrinsic pursuits, more mindful living, and with prosocial behaviors (Weinstein & Ryan, 2010).

New evidence also suggests that basic psychological needs at least partially mediate the negative effects of poor economic conditions on people's flourishing. Gonzalez, Swanson, Lynch, and Williams (2014) found in a sample of U.S. workers that basic need satisfactions mediated the relations between their socioeconomic status (SES), evaluated in terms of occupational status indicators, and both physical and mental health. Di Domenico and Fournier (2014) similarly examined relations between socioeconomic status and well-being, and whether these were mediated by SDT's basic need satisfactions. They specifically assessed the relations between self-reported SES, household income, and the degree of socioeconomic inequality in one's surroundings as predictors of health and wellness. In this work, all three of these indicators were related to greater self-reported health and wellness, and importantly, SDT's basic need satisfactions mediated these relations.

Martha Nussbaum (2001), a philosopher who has made conditions for eudaimonia a central focus of her work, provided a list of ten specific capabilities understood as providing the necessary foundations upon which a good life can be established (see Anand, Hunter, & Smith, 2005).

Her list included: (1) a reasonable life expectancy; (2) ability to have bodily health; (3) ability for bodily integrity, including freedom of movement and freedom from fear of violence; (4) ability to use one's senses, imagination, and thought; (5) ability and freedom to experience and express emotions, including love; (6) ability to exercise practical reason; (7) ability to experience affiliation, including freedom to live with others, and to have the respect of others; (8) ability to have an appreciation of and contact with other species; (9) opportunities for play; and (10) ability to have control over the environment, both political and material. DeHaan, Hirai and Ryan (2015), examining adult samples from both the USA and India, applied a capability indicator tapping the attributes specified by Nussbaum. They found as expected that the capability indicator was highly positively correlated with well-being, and negatively with ill-being. Also consistent with extensive previous work in SDT (Vansteenkiste & Ryan, 2013), basic psychological need satisfaction was highly positively correlated to well-being, and highly negatively related to ill-being whereas basic psychological need frustration was highly positively correlated to ill-being, and negatively correlated to well-being. Finally, consistent with their hypotheses, DeHaan et al. found that basic psychological needs were both related to and partially accounted for the positive effects of Nussbaum's capabilities list.

7.3 Is Aristotelian Goodwill or Benevolence Part of Human Nature?

Eudaimonic ideas rest on the view that when we actualize the best of our human natures this results in both happiness and in living virtuously. The idea that people inherently strive to be both virtuous and benevolent and to grow and develop their talents has been doubted by many. Indeed, it is not hard to find authors and theorists who depict human nature in the most negative of terms. Rather than virtuous and self-cultivating some see humans as selfish and hedonically inclined.

Yet the more closely we look at the evidence the more it seems that humans indeed do have a positive proclivity—if they are positively nurtured. In contrast, when people grow up under circumstances where they are deprived or thwarted in their basic psychological needs they do show another nature. For example, they become concerned with image, ego and self over others.

Recently Ryan and Hawley (in press) addressed the issue of whether humans are good and benevolent by nature looking through the lens of both SDT and evolutionary psychology. They reviewed a number of experiments showing that even early in development humans show propensities toward helping others, including strangers. In fact, rewarding them for doing so even undermines this intrinsic propensity (see Warneken & Tomasello, 2008). Moreover there is a general finding that when people are given opportunities to autonomously help others, as opposed to doing it because of social rewards, approval or pressure, they derive greater positive feelings as a result (Weinstein & Ryan, 2010). Ryan and Hawley thus argue that these positive feelings resulting from truly being giving or altruistic in a phenomenal sense, reflect a design feature of humanity. Insofar as we find satisfaction in giving and helping we are more prone to do so, and this likely has its ultimate sources in the selective advantages associated with more giving and cooperative behaviors.

Naturally, this doesn't mean that humans wouldn't be interested in their own well-being and survival. Seeing humans as either totally egoistic or totally altruistic ignores the fact that humans can have many traits and tendencies that can sometimes contradict each other. We are thus not arguing that humans are not egoistic. Rather we are arguing that in addition to egoistic dispositions, humans are also equipped with other-oriented and benevolent dispositions, which both have adaptive advantages and are proximately accompanied by inherent satisfactions. Indeed, the very existence of proximal satisfactions for prosocial and benevolent behaviors helps ensure that these adaptive human attributes will be expressed (Ryan & Hawley, on press).

Modern evolutionary theories include several mechanisms that separately or together can explain how proximally other-oriented behavior could be ultimately beneficial for the individual's evolutionary fitness (see e.g. Fehr & Fischbacher, 2003; West, El Mouden, & Gardner, 2011). Inclusive fitness or kin selection (Hamilton, 1964) explains why it is beneficial to help kin, but because our ability to recognize kin is probabilistic and based on cues, rather than absolute (Lieberman, Tooby, & Cosmides, 2007), this care for one's kin can 'spill over' to non-kin as well. Reciprocal altruism (Trivers, 1971), where we help those who help us, is another mechanism explaining selective helping, and its explanatory power is increased when indirect reciprocity (Alexander, 1987; Nowak & Sigmund, 1998), where we help those who have a reputation of being helpers, and strong reciprocity (Fehr, Fischbacher, & Gächter, 2002; Gintis, 2000), where we punish those who don't reciprocate, are also taken into account. Multi-level selection processes (D.O. Wilson, 2012; D.S. 2003) have also been suggested as explanations, although their explanatory power beyond other mechanisms continues to be debated (e.g. Gardner & Grafen, 2009; Henrich, 2004). The more general point about the discussion around modern evolutionary theories is that the question is usually not whether human prosocial tendencies *can be explained*, but rather about the relative merits of the different existing explanations (e.g. West et al., 2011).

This nod to natural goodness in no way denies that violence and aggression are often developmental trajectories, but this is by far more frequently the case for children who have been need thwarted rather than well-nurtured (e.g., Joussemet et al., 2008). In addition violence is at times culturally sanctioned, and so-called "virtuous violence" behaviors are not uncommon (Fiske & Rai, 2015). Yet even the occurrence of these communal and/or compliant acts of violence does not typically yield need satisfaction or enjoyment (e.g., see Legate, De Haan, Weinstein, & Ryan, 2013). In short, violence, prejudice and malevolence do occur, but they are more often outcomes of threat, maltreatment and pathology than expressions of our human nature under positive conditions. The fact that we have both bright and dark sides to our human nature makes it important to understand the contingencies that evoke one over the other, and SDT argues that these contingencies are largely explained by basic psychological need supports versus thwarting.

It thus may be that Aristotle, in discussing the natural virtues of friendliness and goodwill, was onto something. People may be prone toward benevolence, and "designed" therefore to feel happier when being so. This has adaptive consequences for both individuals and the groups in which they reside, even though such advantages are not (and could not be) the proximal reasons why they act so.

A recent experiment by Martela and Ryan (2015) illustrates well this propensity to feel positively following benevolence. They argued that although many past studies have shown that prosocial behavior is associated with enhanced well-being, most all of these prior experimental studies have involved face-to-face contact with the beneficiary. Martela and Ryan wanted to examine whether it is prosocial behavior *itself*, and not only an increased sense of social relatedness to the recipient that improves well-being. Accordingly they invited participants to play a computer game in which successful performance could lead to anonymous donations to needy people. Yet they only allowed half of the participants to be aware of this anonymous impact. The other half only played the game for high scores. As compared to the control (unaware) condition, the group who knew their success produced prosocial outcomes experienced more positive affect, interest, and meaningfulness, and less negative affect. Beyond these self-reported outcomes, this benevolent group also demonstrated greater post-game vitality, and better performance on a subsequent Stroop task, providing evidence for the positive energetic effects of prosocial behavior. Interestingly, and consistent with SDT, these positive effects of prosocial behavior on well-being were mediated by subjectively assessed beneficence, which in turn produced heightened autonomy, competence, and relatedness need satisfactions. In other studies using cross-sectional and daily diary methods, Martela and Ryan (2016), showed that when people feel that they have a positive impact on others – what they called beneficence –they report an increased sense of subjective well-being and vitality.

In sum Aristotle assumed that it is by actualizing the best in our natures that we would have the best of lives, including a higher likelihood of happiness and a fuller sense of satisfaction. One particular virtue or excellence for human beings was according to Aristotle friendliness and goodwill toward others. Evidence from SDT and related perspectives supports both that there are indeed positive well-being and happiness outcomes from striving toward and enacting more caring and benevolent values. Moreover it may very well be that nature has crafted us to find such satisfactions in such behaviors, fitting with Aristotle's notion that in living eudaimonically we are living in accord with our natures.

7.4 Conclusion

Finding out the constituting elements of intrinsically worthwhile human ends and a good way of living is according to Aristotle of great practical importance: Equipped with this knowledge "would we not, like archers in possession of a target, better hit on what is needed?" (Aristotle, 2012, p. 2). In addition to the individual level importance of research on eudaimonia, Aristotle also emphasized its societal importance. He saw that the proper aim of a society and its institutions is to ensure the virtuousness and eudaimonia of its citizens (e.g. Aristotle; Curren, 2010). The more we know about the good way of living, the more we are in a position to build a society that can be supportive and offer opportunities for such a way of living for all of its citizens. Moving toward asking the eudaimonistic question therefore has crucial implications for behavioral sciences as well. It pushes researchers to "critically evaluate and compare lifestyles, organizations, and cultures in terms of their support for the good life and the outcomes that accompany it", as we have argued before (Ryan et al., 2013, p. 69).

In this article we have aimed to empirically examine certain Aristotelian propositions about what living a good life would involve. Based on research on SDT we have aimed to show that a way of living characterized by intrinsic goals, autonomy, mindfulness, and benevolence indeed seems to lead to enhanced wellness for human beings. We invite more researchers to engage in this task of aiming to find the ways of living that are both in accordance with the inherent human nature and supportive of human wellness, growth and thriving.

References

Ahuvia, A. C., & Friedman, D. C. (1998). Income, consumption, and subjective well-being: Toward a composite macromarketing model. *Journal of Macromarketing, 18*, 153–168. doi:10.1177/027614679801800207.

Alexander, R. D. (1987). *The biology of moral systems*. New York: Aldine de Gruyter.

Anand, P., Hunter, G., & Smith, R. (2005). Capabilities and well-being: Evidence based on the Sen-Nussbaum approach to welfare. *Social Indicators Research, 74*, 9–55.

Annas, J. (1995). *The morality of happiness*. New York: Oxford University Press.

Aristotle. (2012). *Nicomachean ethics* (trans: Bartlett, R. C., & Collins, S. D.). Chicago: University of Chicago Press.

Bartlett, R. C., & Collins, S. D. (2012). Introduction. In Aristotle (Ed.), *Nicomachean ethics* (pp. vii–xiv). Chicago: University of Chicago Press.

Beitel, M., Cecero, J. J., & Ferrer, E. (2005). Psychological mindedness and awareness of sell and others. *Journal of Clinical Psychology, 61*(6), 739–750.

Brown, K. W., & Kasser, T. (2005). Are psychological and ecological well-being compatible? The role of values, mindfulness, and lifestyle. *Social Indicators Research, 74*, 349–368.

Brown, K. W., & Ryan, R. M. (2003). The benefits of being present: Mindfulness and its role in psychological well-being. *Journal of Personality and Social Psychology, 84*, 822–848.

Brown, K. W., & Ryan, R. M. (2004). Perils and promise in defining and measuring mindfulness: Observations from experience. *Clinical Psychology: Science and Practice, 11*(3), 242–248. doi:10.1093/clipsy.bph078.

Brown, K. W., Ryan, R. M., & Creswell, J. D. (2007). Mindfulness: Theoretical foundations and evidence for salutary effects. *Psychological Inquiry, 18*, 211–237.

Brown, K. W., Kasser, T., Ryan, R. M., Linley, P. A., & Orzech, K. (2009). When what one has is enough: Mindfulness, financial desire discrepancy, and subjective well-being. *Journal of Research in Personality, 43*, 727–736.

Brown, K. W., Crewell, J. D., & Ryan, R. M. (2015). Introduction: The evolution of mindfulness science. In K. W. Brown, R. M. Ryan, & J. D. Creswell (Eds.), *Handbook of mindfulness* (pp. 245–265). New York: Guilford Press.

Chaplin, L. N., & John, D. R. (2010). Interpersonal influences on adolescent materialism: A new look at the role of parents and peers. *Journal of Consumer Psychology, 20*(2), 176–184.

Clark, A. E., Frijters, P., & Shields, M. A. (2008). Relative income, happiness, and utility: An explanation for the Easterlin paradox and other puzzles. *Journal of Economic Literature, 46*(1), 95–144.

Curren, R. (2010). Aristotle's educational politics and the Aristotelian renaissance in philosophy of education. *Oxford Review of Education, 36*, 543–559.

Curren, R. (2014). A Neo-Aristotelian account of education, justice, and the human good. In K. Meyer (Ed.), *Education, justice, and the human good* (pp. 80–99). London: Routledge.

Deci, E. L., & Ryan, R. M. (1985). The general causality orientations scale: Self-determination in personality. *Journal of Research in Personality, 19*, 109–134.

Deci, E. L., & Ryan, R. M. (2000). The "what" and the "why" of goal pursuits: Human needs and the self-determination of behavior. *Psychological Inquiry, 11*, 227–268.

DeHaan, C. R., Hirai, T., Ryan, R. M. (2015). *Nussbaum's capabilities and self-determination theory's basic psychological needs: Relating some fundamentals of human wellness* (under review).

Di Domenico, S. I., & Fournier, M. A. (2014). Socioeconomic status, income inequality and health complaints: A basic psychological needs perspective. *Social Indicators Research, 119*, 1679–1697.

Duriez, B., Vansteenkiste, M., Soenens, B., & De Witte, H. (2007). The social costs of extrinsic relative to intrinsic goal pursuits: Their relation with social dominance and racial and ethnic prejudice. *Journal of Personality, 75*(4), 757–782.

Easterlin, R. A. (1995). Will raising the incomes of all increase the happiness of all? *Journal of Economic Behavior & Organization, 27*(1), 35–47.

Fehr, E., & Fischbacher, U. (2003). The nature of human altruism. *Nature, 425*, 785–791.

Fehr, E., Fischbacher, U., & Gächter, S. (2002). Strong reciprocity, human cooperation, and the enforcement of social norms. *Human Nature, 13*(1), 1–25.

Fiske, A. P., & Rai, T. S. (2015). *Virtuous violence*. Cambridge, UK: Cambridge University Press.

Gardner, A., & Grafen, A. (2009). Capturing the superorganism: A formal theory of group adaptation. *Journal of Evolutionary Biology, 22*(4), 659–671.

Gintis, H. (2000). Strong reciprocity and human sociality. *Journal of Theoretical Biology, 206*(2), 169–179.

Gonzalez, M. G., Swanson, D. P., Lynch, M., & Williams, G. C. (2014). Testing satisfaction of basic psychological needs as a mediator of the relationship between socioeconomic status and physical and mental health. *Journal of Health Psychology, 61*(6), 739.

Grolnick, W. S. (2003). *The psychology of parental control: How well-meant parenting backfires*. Mahwah, NJ: Erlbaum.

Hamilton, W. D. (1964). The genetical evolution of social behaviour. *Journal of Theoretical Biology, 7*, 1–52.

Haybron, D. (2008). *The pursuit of unhappiness: The elusive psychology of well-being*. New York: Oxford University Press.

Henrich, J. (2004). Cultural group selection, coevolutionary processes and large-scale cooperation. *Journal of Economic Behavior & Organization, 53*(1), 3–35.

Huta, V., & Ryan, R. M. (2010). Pursuing pleasure or virtue: The differential and overlapping well-being benefits of hedonic and eudaimonic motives. *Journal of Happiness Studies, 11*, 735–762. doi:10.1007/s10902-009-9171-4.

Joussemet, M., Vitaro, F., Barker, E. D., Cote, S., Nagin, D., Zoccolillo, M., et al. (2008). Controlling parenting and physical aggression during elementary school. *Child Development, 79*, 411–425.

Kasser, T., & Ryan, R. M. (1993). A dark side of the American dream: Correlates of financial success as a central life aspiration. *Journal of Personality and Social Psychology, 65*, 410–422.

Kasser, T., & Ryan, R. M. (1996). Further examining the American dream: Differential correlates of intrinsic and extrinsic goals. *Personality and Social Psychology Bulletin, 22*, 280–287.

Kasser, T., Ryan, R. M., Zax, M., & Sameroff, A. J. (1995). The relations of maternal and social environments to late adolescents' materialistic and prosocial values. *Developmental Psychology, 31*, 907–914.

Kasser, T., Cohn, S., Kanner, A. D., & Ryan, R. M. (2007). Some costs of American corporate capitalism: A psychological exploration of value and goal conflicts. *Psychological Inquiry, 18*(1), 1–22.

Kim, Y., Kasser, T., & Lee, H. (2003). Self-concept, aspirations, and well-being in South Korea and the United States. *The Journal of Social Psychology, 143*(3), 277–290.

Ku, L., Dittmar, H., & Banerjee, R. (2014). To have or to learn? The effects of materialism on British and Chinese children's learning. *Journal of Personality and Social Psychology, 106*(5), 803–821.

Legate, N., De Haan, C. R., Weinstein, N., & Ryan, R. M. (2013). Hurting you hurts me too: The psychological costs of complying with ostracism. *Psychological Science*. doi:10.1177/0956797612457951.

Lieberman, D., Tooby, J., & Cosmides, L. (2007). The architecture of human kin detection. *Nature, 445*(7129), 727–731.

Martela, F., & Ryan, R. M. (2015). *Prosocial behavior increases well-being and vitality even without contact with the beneficiary: Causal and behavioral evidence* (under review).

Martela, F., & Ryan, R. M. (2016). The benefits of benevolence: Basic psychological needs, beneficence, and the enhancement of well-being. *Journal of Personality*. Advance online publication. doi: 10.1111/jopy.12215.

Martela, F., & Steger, M. F. (2016). The three meanings of meaning in life: Distinguishing coherence, purpose, and significance. *The Journal of Positive Psychology, 11*(5), 531–545. doi:10.1080/17439760.2015.1137623.

Niemiec, C. P., & Ryan, R. M. (2013). What makes for a life well lived? Autonomy and its relation to full functioning and organismic wellness. In S. David, I. Boniwell, & A. Conley Ayers (Eds.), *Oxford handbook of happiness* (pp. 214–226). Oxford, UK: Oxford University Press.

Niemiec, C. P., Ryan, R. M., & Deci, E. L. (2009). The path taken: Consequences of attaining intrinsic and extrinsic aspirations in post-college life. *Journal of Research in Personality, 43*, 291–306.

Nowak, M. A., & Sigmund, K. (1998). Evolution of indirect reciprocity by image scoring. *Nature, 393*(6685), 573–577.

Nussbaum, M. C. (2001). *The fragility of goodness: Luck and ethics in Greek tragedy and philosophy*. New York: Cambridge University Press.

Ryan, R. M., & Brown, K. W. (2005). Legislating competence: The motivational impact of high stakes testing as an educational reform. In A. J. Elliot & C. S. Dweck (Eds.), *Handbook of competence* (pp. 354–374). New York: Guilford Press.

Ryan, R. M., & Deci, E. L. (2000). Self-determination theory and the facilitation of intrinsic motivation, social development and well-being. *American Psychologist, 55*, 68–78.

Ryan, R. M., & Deci, E. L. (2001). To be happy or to be self-fulfilled: A review of research on hedonic and eudaimonic well-being. In S. Fiske (Ed.), *Annual review of psychology* (Vol. 52, pp. 141–166). Palo Alto, CA: Annual Reviews.

Ryan, R. M., & Deci, E. L. (2008). From ego depletion to vitality: Theory and findings concerning the facilitation of energy available to the self. *Social and Personality Psychology Compass, 2*(2), 702–717. doi:10.1111/j.1751-9004.2008.00098.x.

Ryan, R. M., & Hawley, P. (in press). Naturally good? Basic psychological needs and the proximal and evolutionary bases of human benevolence. In M. Leary and K. W. Brown (Eds.), *The psychology of hypoegoic behavior*. New York: Guildford Press.

Ryan, R. M., & Huta, V. (2009). Wellness as healthy functioning or wellness as happiness: The importance of eudaimonic thinking (response to the Kashdan et al. and Waterman discussion). *The Journal of Positive Psychology, 4*, 202–204.

Ryan, R. M., Sheldon, K. M., Kasser, T., & Deci, E. L. (1996). All goals are not created equal: An organismic perspective on the nature of goals and their regulation. In P. M. Gollwitzer & J. A. Bargh (Eds.), *The psychology of action: Linking cognition and motivation to behavior* (pp. 7–26). New York: Guilford.

Ryan, R. M., Chirkov, V. I., Little, T. D., Sheldon, K. M., Temoshina, E., & Deci, E. L. (1999). The American dream in Russia: Extrinsic aspirations and well-being in two cultures. *Personality and Social Psychology Bulletin, 25*(12), 1509–1524.

Ryan, R. M., Huta, V., & Deci, E. L. (2008). Living well: A self-determination theory perspective on eudaimonia. *Journal of Happiness Studies, 9*(1), 139–170. doi:10.1007/s10902-006-9023-4.

Ryan, R. M., Curren, R. R., & Deci, E. L. (2013). What humans need: Flourishing in Aristotelian philosophy and self-determination theory. In A. S. Waterman (Ed.), *The best within us: Positive psychology perspectives on eudaimonic functioning* (pp. 57–75). Washington, DC: American Psychological Association Books.

Saunders, S., & Munro, D. (2000). The construction and validation of a consumer orientation questionnaire (scoi) designed to measure fromms (1955) marketing character in Australia. *Social Behavior and Personality: An International Journal, 28*(3), 219–240.

Schmuck, P., Kasser, T., & Ryan, R. M. (2000). The relationship of well-being to intrinsic and extrinsic goals in Germany and the U.S. *Social Indicators Research, 50*, 225–241.

Schultz, P., Ryan, R. M., Niemiec, C., Legate, N., & Williams, G. C. (2014). Mindfulness, work climate, and psychological need satisfaction in employee well-being. *Mindfulness 6*, 971–985

Seligman, M. E. P. (2002). *Authentic happiness: Using the new positive psychology to realize your potential for lasting fulfillment*. New York: Free Press.

Shapiro, S. L., Schwartz, G. E., & Bonner, G. (1998). Effects of mindfulness-based stress reduction on medical and premedical students. *Journal of Behavioral Medicine, 21*(6), 581–599. doi:10.1023/A:1018700829825.

Sheldon, K. M., & Krieger, L. (2014). Walking the talk: Value importance, value enactment, and well-being. *Motivation and Emotion, 38*, 609–619.

Sheldon, K. M., Ryan, R. M., Deci, E. L., & Kasser, T. (2004). The independent effects of goal contents and motives on well-being: It's both what you pursue and why you pursue it. *Personality and Social Psychology Bulletin, 30*, 475–486.

Trivers, R. L. (1971). The evolution of reciprocal altruism. *Quarterly Review of Biology, 46*, 35–57.

Vansteenkiste, M., & Ryan, R. M. (2013). On psychological growth and vulnerability: Basic psychological need satisfaction and need frustration as a unifying principle. *Journal of Psychotherapy Integration, 23*(3), 263–280.

Vansteenkiste, M., Mouratidis, A., Lens, W., et al. (2010). Detaching reasons from aims: Fair play and well-being in soccer as a function of pursuing performance-approach goals for autonomous or controlling reasons. *Journal of Sport & Exercise Psychology, 32*(2), 217–242.

Warneken, F., & Tomasello, M. (2008). Extrinsic rewards undermine altruistic tendencies in 20-month-olds. *Developmental Psychology, 44*(6), 1785–1788.

Waterman, A. (2013). *The best within us: Positive psychology perspectives on eudaimonia*. Washington, DC: American Psychological Association.

Weinstein, N., & Ryan, R. M. (2010). When helping helps: Autonomous motivation for prosocial behavior and its influence on well-being for the helper and recipient. *Journal of Personality and Social Psychology, 98*, 222–244.

Weinstein, N., Brown, K. W., & Ryan, R. M. (2009). A multi-method examination of the effects of mindfulness on stress attribution, coping, and emotional well-being. *Journal of Research in Personality, 43*, 374–385.

Weinstein, N., Deci, E. L., & Ryan, R. M. (2011). Motivational determinants of integrating positive and negative past identities. *Journal of Personality and Social Psychology, 100*, 527–544.

Weinstein, N., Ryan, R. M., & Deci, E. L. (2012). Motivation, meaning, and wellness: A self-determination perspective on the creation and internalization of personal meanings and life goals. In P. T. Wong (Ed.), *The human quest for meaning: Theories, research, and applications* (2nd ed., pp. 81–106). New York: Routledge.

West, S. A., El Mouden, C., & Gardner, A. (2011). Sixteen common misconceptions about the evolution of cooperation in humans. *Evolution and Human Behavior, 32*(4), 231–262.

Williams, G. C., Cox, E. M., Hedberg, V., & Deci, E. L. (2000). Extrinsic life goals and health risk behaviors in adolescents. *Journal of Applied Social Psychology, 30*, 1756–1771.

Wilson, D. S. (2003). *Darwin's cathedral: Evolution, religion, and the nature of society*. Chicago: University of Chicago Press.

Wilson, E. O. (2012). *The social conquest of earth*. London: W.W. Norton.

Internal Motivation, Instrumental Motivation, and Eudaimonia

8

Barry Schwartz and Amy Wrzesniewski

8.1 Introduction

> Every art and every inquiry, and similarly every action and pursuit, is thought to aim at some good, and for this reason the good has rightly been declared to be that at which all things aim…Now, as there are many actions, arts, and sciences, their ends are also many; the end of the medical art is health, that of shipbuilding a vessel, that of strategy victory, that of economics wealth.
>
> —Aristotle, *Nicomachean Ethics*, I.1

In the golden era of learning theory in psychology, in the middle of the twentieth century, research methods were developed for studying the behavior of rats and pigeons that were meant to produce general principles that applied to the instrumental, goal-directed behavior of all organisms (Schwartz, 1978; Skinner, 1953). Rats would press levers, run down alleys, and negotiate mazes, for food or water. Pigeons would peck at illuminated disks, or keys. The central idea behind these methods was that since the relation between the response and the reward—the means and the end—was completely arbitrary, it would be representative of all instrumental, goal-directed activity. Rats pressing levers for food could be a stand-in for people working in factories or offices for their paychecks.

An assumption that helped justify these methods was that the purely instrumental relation between means and ends is what characterized most human activity. Yes, some means might be more pleasant than others (rats seemed to "enjoy" running in exercise wheels, for example), but this was an incidental fact, a mere detail, that got in the way of understanding the far more general relation between means and ends. Without a paycheck, people wouldn't work. With a paycheck, it hardly mattered what work people did. In making this assumption, learning theorists were following in the hallowed tradition of Smith (1776), the father of modern economics, and Frederick Winslow Taylor (1911/1967), the father of what came to be called "scientific management" (see Schwartz, Schuldenfrei, & Lacey, 1978 for elaboration).

We think this view of the relation between means and ends continues to dominate modern thinking about human motivation. To get CEOs to serve the interests of the company, give them company shares as a significant part of compensation. To get students to work hard in school, give them frequent tests and grades—and even better, rewards like pizza parties—if they do well. To get car salespeople to put all their effort into closing deals, pay them commissions. And to get

B. Schwartz (✉)
Psychology, Swarthmore College,
Swarthmore, PA, USA
e-mail: bschwar1@swarthmore.edu

A. Wrzesniewski
Yale School of Management, New Haven, CT, USA
e-mail: amy.wrzesniewski@yale.edu

J. Vittersø (ed.), *Handbook of Eudaimonic Well-Being*, International Handbooks of Quality-of-Life,
DOI 10.1007/978-3-319-42445-3_8

doctors to do all, and only, what is necessary for high-quality patient care, pay them bonuses for good, but efficient, medical outcomes.

There is little doubt that much human activity is instrumental in just the way that rat lever-pressing and pigeon key-pecking is. But pure, arbitrary instrumentality is not the only possible relation between means and ends. Aristotle, for example, had quite a different view, as evidenced by the quote that opens this chapter, taken from the very beginning of his masterwork of moral philosophy, *Nicomachean Ethics*. Aristotle thought that most human activities had ends, or goals, that were specific to them. It was the human *telos* to pursue excellence, and what "excellence" meant was very much specific to the activity in question. The *telos* of the builder was to produce excellent buildings. The *telos* of the doctor was to cure disease. The *telos* of the athlete was to produce outstanding athletic performances. Of course, in each of these cases, the performer might earn a livelihood, but it was earning a livelihood that was incidental, and achieving the activity-specific *telos* that was central to human activity, at least among people who rightly understood the point of their activities.

In *Nicomachean Ethics*, Aristotle identifies happiness as the final *telos* of all human activity. But what he means by happiness is not pleasure, or material acquisition, but flourishing—*eudaimonia*. And eudaimonia, he says, derives from—indeed, *is*, "good activity" or excellence, rather than amusement. The happy life, Aristotle tells us, is the virtuous life, and the virtuous life requires exertion, the strenuous pursuit of excellence, and does not consist in amusement. Yes, many of the things that people do are instrumental. They are means to an end. But the ultimate end to which all activities lead is *eudaimonia*, and that requires excellences that are intimately related to the activities that pursue them.

Aristotle's teleological framework for understanding human nature is probably foreign to most modern students of human behavior. But with a little bit of translation, his ideas can be related to modern conceptions. In this chapter, we will try to do the translation, specifically in relation to human motivation. Partly in response to the instrumentalist assumptions of learning theory, it has become a commonplace to distinguish between "intrinsic" and "extrinsic" motivation. Extrinsically motivated activity is directed to some other end. It is a means to that end. It is instrumental, like the rat's lever press. Intrinsically motivated activity is an end in itself. Extrinsically motivated behavior is work; intrinsically motivated behavior is play. Extrinsically motivated behavior is all about achieving some instrumental goal; intrinsically motivated behavior *is* the goal (see Deci, 1975; Deci & Ryan, 1985; Lepper, Greene, & Nisbett, 1973; Pink, 2011).

We believe that while the above distinction between intrinsic and extrinsic motivation offers a much richer view of human motivation than the purely instrumental view that it replaced, it fails to capture important distinctions that should be made between various types of relations between motives, actions, and consequences. In this chapter, we will try to make some of these distinctions and to clarify what the terms "intrinsic" and "extrinsic" ought to mean.

Psychologists have long realized that to understand human behavior, we need to know not only what someone does, but why he or she does it. Motives matter. Different types of motives have different effects on behavior even when the motives seem to point in the same direction. For example, Lepper et al. (1973) showed that giving nursery school children awards for drawing made them less interested in drawing, which they liked to do, and led them to draw less interesting pictures than if they weren't given awards. And Deci (1971, 1975) showed that giving college students money for solving puzzles made them less interested in working on such puzzles, which they enjoyed, later on, when money was not available. Similarly, Gneezy and Rustichini (2000) showed that adding a fine to the social sanctions already associated with parents coming late to pick up their children from nursery school weakened those social sanctions and increased lateness rather than strengthening those social sanctions and reducing lateness. In the first two cases, it might be said that the rewards that were added to the already enjoyable activities of drawing and puzzle-solving instrumentalized the activities, turning "play into work," and thus made the activities less enjoyable. Analogously, the fine for lateness instrumentalized that activity and thus gave parents permission to come late, since they were "paying" for it.

What *should* happen to the performance of demanding, effortful activities when intrinsic and extrinsic motives are combined? Logic would suggest that if you have one reason for doing something, adding a second reason to do the same thing would be even better, rendering motivation more tenacious, follow-through stronger, and outcomes better (see Cerasoli, Nicklin, & Ford, 2014, for a meta-analysis of this very question). Schools and workplaces are full of systems that attempt to tap people's intrinsic motives to act (e.g., because engaging in the activity is the moral, interesting, or meaningful thing to do) while also providing rewards intended to spark extrinsic motives to pursue the same acts (e.g., grades, bonuses, promotions, etc.). Yet, as shown by the studies of nursery-school children's drawing and nursery-school parents coming to fetch their kids, and in a direct challenge to this assumption, a substantial body of research suggests that far from boosting motivation, holding extrinsic motives can undermine whatever intrinsic motives may have been operating, leading to drops in overall motivation, persistence and performance (Deci, Koestner, & Ryan, 1999; Frey & Oberholzer-Gee, 1997; Frey, 1994; Kiviniemi, Snyder, & Omoto, 2002; and see Murayama, Matsumoto, Izuma, & Matsumoto, 2010 for evidence on the neural basis of this undermining effect). In short, this work suggests that salient instrumental incentives trigger extrinsic motives, which act to undermine motivation that would otherwise be based in the value and reward of doing the activity or engaging in the act for the sake of objectives that are intimately connected to the act itself. This effect, labeled the "motivational crowding out effect" by economists (Frey, 1994) and the "overjustification effect" by psychologists (Lepper et al., 1973), has been demonstrated across a range of experimental contexts (Deci et al., 1999), though there are some arguments that question both the reliability and the interpretation of such studies (Cerasoli et al., 2014; Eisenberger & Cameron, 1996; Lacetera, Macis, & Slonim, 2012).

Much of the existing literature in the psychology of motivation treats intrinsic and extrinsic motivation as if there is a stark categorical distinction between them (but see Gerhart & Fang, 2015). Behavior is either intrinsically motivated or extrinsically motivated. In addition, intrinsic motivation is usually associated with the pleasure that derives from simply engaging in the activity, as if the consequences don't matter. That is, the nursery school kids love to draw whether or not the end result is a nice picture. It is worth noting that this definition of intrinsic motivation rules out the possibility of being intrinsically motivated to do anything that is *not* pleasurable; an untenable definitional state of affairs to which we will return. What is more, researchers also often use the consequences of behavior as an indication of what motivates the behavior (e.g., if a student gets an "A" on an exam, she is assumed to be motivated by the grades). So, for example, an instrumental consequence may be added to a situation in an effort to improve performance (e.g., a gift certificate for high scores on a standardized test). If that consequence influences behavior (e.g., students do better on the test), researchers conclude that instrumental incentives work, and infer (since the incentives worked) that the behavior was instrumentally motivated in the first place. This presumption renders impossible the ability to discern intrinsic motives in cases where actions have produced any sort of instrumental outcome. Finally, it is generally assumed that intrinsic motivation leads to better performance than extrinsic, though interestingly, nearly every intervention designed to increase motivation focuses on the extrinsic. Though a recent meta-analysis suggests that extrinsic rewards can boost performance even when intrinsic motivation is present (Cerasoli et al., 2014), whether rewards *increase* intrinsic motivation (unlikely, in our view, as suggested by Deci, Koestner, & Ryan, 1999) or act as a supplementary boost to action is still somewhat uncertain.

We think that each of these assumptions is mistaken in ways that lead to oversimplification of what is an extremely complex relation between motives, actions, and consequences. In this chapter we attempt to clarify some of these relations and delineate some important distinctions, leading to a series of questions for both theoretical and empirical analysis.

Let us begin our discussion with a prototypical example. Imagine a second-grade teacher who enjoys her work and is good at it. Her work produces a family of consequences for her. She gets pleasure from the minute-to-minute, day-to-day character of her job, and from interacting with young kids. She gets satisfaction from knowing that she is an excellent teacher—that she does the job well. She gets satisfaction from evidence that kids are learning and are enthusiastic. She enjoys respect and admiration from her peers. She enjoys respect and admiration from parents. She enjoys respect and admiration from society at large. She appreciates her nice salary and benefits as well as her job security. She is pleased that she can leave her workplace at three in the afternoon. She likes that she has lots of vacation days and the entire summer off.

Thus, this teacher's work has multiple consequences. Which of them are also motives? We can identify several possibilities: pleasure in the activity, pursuit of excellence, status and acclaim, salary, job security, and benefits, and the desire to have a positive impact on others. Which of these motives count as "intrinsic"? And what are the criteria for establishing a motive as intrinsic?

8.2 A Conceptual Framework for Understanding Intrinsic Motivation

We think the questions above can be profitably addressed from an Aristotelian framework, or more specifically, from a framework developed by neo-Aristotelian philosopher Alasdair MacIntyre. In *After Virtue* (1981), MacIntyre introduces the idea of a "practice," which he defines as "any coherent and complex form of socially established cooperative human activity through which goods internal to that form of activity are realized in the course of trying to achieve those standards of excellence which are appropriate to, and partially definitive of, that form of activity, with the result that human powers to achieve excellence, and human conceptions of the ends and goods involved, are systematically extended" (p. 175).

This definition is complex, and has several important features that we will try to elucidate. Complexity is one feature. The game of chess is a practice, whereas tic-tac-toe is not. The game of football is a practice, whereas throwing a football accurately is not. Farming is a practice, whereas planting turnips is not.

The pursuit of excellence is a second feature. People who engage in practices strive to be good at them. Moreover, what constitutes excellence is itself defined by standards internal to the practice, largely established by practitioners themselves. Thus, one is perfectly free to say something like "I don't know much about art, but I know what I like." But one is not entitled to expect that anyone (especially artists) will care what you like or interpret your likes and dislikes as an indication of the quality of the art.

The concept of excellence is necessarily imprecise. First, if MacIntyre is right, excellence is a moving target, since as practices develop, the standards of excellence among practitioners change. And second, each practice has standards of excellence that are peculiar to it. There is no abstract standard of excellence that unites instances of excellence across different practices. Moreover, there is room for disagreement, both among practitioners and between practitioners and non-practitioners, about what excellence means. Nonetheless, however imprecise "excellence" may be, in MacIntyre's (and Aristotle's) telling, only activities that have standards of excellence can be practices.

A third feature of practices, most important for purposes of this chapter, is that practitioners pursue goods or ends that are internal to the practice itself. In other words, there is an intimate relation between the ends of the practice and the means to achieve those ends. For our hypothetical second-grade teacher, educating students and engendering in them enthusiasm for learning are internal to the practice. Salary and benefits, job security, and summers off are not. These ends could be achieved in other ways, through any number of other occupations; the relations between her teaching and these ends are purely instrumental. Not even praise and admiration from parents and peers is unambiguously internal to the practice. Perhaps praise for excellence *as a teacher* is; praise for excellence more generally is not.

Finally, in MacIntyre's conception, practices and the goods toward which they are aimed develop. As people continue to practice—as farmers, chess players, biologists, or psychologists—standards of excellence change. What it means to be an excellent psychologist in 2015 is likely quite different from what it meant to be an excellent psychologist in 1965. The line between what is and is not a practice is sometimes fuzzy, and some activities may be practices at one point in their development but not at another. But we think the differences between prototypical practices and mere instrumental activities are clear. And we also think MacIntyre's framework enables us to discern whether a given participant in a practice is a true practitioner or not.

It is worth noting that there is no mention of pleasure in MacIntyre's account of practices. Of course, our second-grade teacher may derive pleasure from her day-to-day activities, but that is just icing on the cake. As Aristotle (1988, p. X.3) writes, "there are many things that we would be keen about even if they brought no pleasure… [And] we should choose these even if no pleasure resulted." Nussbaum (1990) observes in commenting on this passage that, "even if in fact pleasure is firmly linked to excellent action as a necessary consequence, it is not the end *for which* we act" (p. 57). In other words, not every consequence of an act is a motive for the act. What makes the second-grade teacher's activities "intrinsically motivated" is that she is pursuing aims that are internally and intimately related to teaching—aims that cannot be achieved in any other activity. The crucial point here is that participation in a practice is not aimless. It is not "play." Results matter. Indeed, results matter critically. But the route to achieving those results also matters, as much if not more. As we pointed out recently (Wrzesniewski et al., 2014), a committed gardener pursues a beautiful and bountiful garden, but will not hire someone else to produce and maintain that garden. The painter pursues a striking work of art, but will not hire someone else to paint it. The doctor wants to be the one who cures disease and eases suffering, the teacher wants to be the one who opens up and inspires young minds, and so on.

Competitive games have winners and losers, and people who love the games want to win. Indeed, if they are practitioners pursuing excellence, they *should* want to win. But they should not want to win by cheating. If they cheat, they are treating the ends as external to the activities that produce them. As practitioners pursuing excellence, the cheaters are cheating themselves. One of us (B.S.) discovered the difference between playing a game for amusement and distraction and playing a game to pursue excellence when he taught his 7-year-old granddaughter to play rummy. Rummy is a rather simple game, but playing it well requires that you notice which cards have been discarded and which have been picked up by your opponent, in an effort to construct your opponent's unseen hand, so you can avoid discarding cards that will improve that hand. When granddad pointed this out to granddaughter, by showing her cards he had withheld that she needed, she asked how he knew she needed those cards. He explained, thinking that her development as a rummy player was about to accelerate. She threw down her cards exclaiming that "I thought we were playing a game, not thinking." Thus ended her career as a rummy player.

It is perhaps an unfortunate accident that early research on intrinsic motivation focused on the drawings of 4-year-olds and the puzzle-solving of college students. Neither of these activities is a practice, and both are rather effortless. Thus, the focus was on pleasure in the activity—engaging in the activity "for its own sake," rather than on pursuit of excellence in the activity. But even in these cases, we doubt that the pre-schooler would be pleased if we did the drawing and handed it to her, or the college student would be pleased to get handed already-solved puzzles. Pre-schoolers want pleasing pictures *that they drew*, and college students want solved puzzles *that they solved*. In other words, we think that the framework of means and ends is as characteristic of "intrinsically" motivated behavior as it is of "extrinsically" motivated behavior. The critical distinction between these two categories of means-ends relation is in the connection between means and ends. With so-called "intrinsically motivated" behavior, the relation between means and ends is anything but arbitrary.

For this reason, to focus on the relation between means and ends, we prefer the term "internal" to "intrinsic" and the term "instrumental" to "extrinsic" (Wrzesniewski et al., 2014). Both of our terms acknowledge that consequences matter, and focus on the relation between the consequences that matter and the activities that produce them. An instrumental relation means that it is a mere matter of contingency that a particular act produces a particular consequence. The instrumentally motivated actor is after the consequence and will presumably choose whatever route to that consequence is most efficient and convenient. The internally motivated actor cares about both the activity and the consequence as well as the relation between them.

We believe that our suggestion that consequences also matter to internally motivated activities calls attention to the most salient characteristics of those activities while at the same time honoring the distinction that previous researchers have made between intrinsic and extrinsic motivation. In reality, the pursuit of excellence in many, if not most, activities involves long periods of intense training that is often anything but pleasurable. Learning anatomy is not fun for most medical students. Weight training is not fun for most competitive athletes. If one takes "pleasure in the activity" as the hallmark of intrinsic motivation, then it is implausible to imagine, given the perseverence in the face of obstacles and challenges, and often the sheer boredom that accompanies some of what it takes to achieve excellence, that any pursuit of excellence could be regarded as intrinsically motivated. Young people searching for their "calling" (see Wrzesniewski, McCauley, Rozin, & Schwartz, 1997) may use the pleasure they get from pursuing various activities as diagnostic of whether they are "called" to them, and may thus reject many activities that demand high effort at not especially pleasurable tasks as not right for them. Duckworth's concept of "grit" captures well the point we are after (Duckworth & Gross, 2014; Duckworth, Kirby, Tsukayama, Berstein, & Ericsson, 2010; Duckworth, Peterson, Matthews, & Kelly, 2007; Duckworth & Seligman, 2005). Grit, Duckworth tells us, has two components. One is perseverance—commitment for the long haul. The second is engagement. Engagement will not always be pleasurable, but it will keep people working at things that are hard. Grit turns out to predict success in a wide variety of domains better than various kinds of aptitude tests that are typically used. The reason why, we suspect, is that grit is what enables people to withstand the countless hours of deliberate practice, much of it focused on aspects of the activity that people do poorly, that are a key ingredient in the development of expertise (Ericcson, Krampe, & Tesch-Romer, 1993).

As currently discussed, grit is viewed as a personality variable. That is, some people are "grittier" than others. But it seems possible that individuals will be gritty with regard to some tasks but not others, or even, within a task, individuals will be gritty on some occasions but not others. We have no view on these issues. Our point in invoking grit is that it highlights the importance of perseverance even in activities that are internally motivated. Our view is that pleasure should not be seen as the hallmark of whether motivation is internal or instrumental. Rather, we see pleasure as an affective state that often accompanies engaging in activities that are internally motivated, but that needn't. Nor do we think that experiencing pleasure disqualifies an activity as internally motivated (e.g., "she gardens because it gives her pleasure. Therefore, gardening is instrumental in the pursuit of pleasure.") We think a focus on pleasure distracts us from the main point, which is a distinction between behavior whose motivating consequences are intimately related to the acts and behavior whose motivating consequences are arbitrarily related to the acts.

8.3 What Motivates the Second-Grade Teacher?

With the distinction between internal and instrumental and MacIntyre's conception of practices in mind, let us revisit our second-grade teacher. As we said above, she appreciates interacting with and inspiring her students, seeing evidence that they are learning, gaining the approval of parents and peers, and having a nice salary and benefits, job security, and ample time off. Her work provides her with many attractive consequences. But which of them are motives? And which of the motives are internal to the activities?

It is obvious that the development of her students is internal to the practice of teaching. What else could excellence in pursuit of the *telos* of education mean if not this. And it is equally obvious that her salary, benefits, etc. are instrumental. She certainly appreciates all these features of her job, but would she continue to do her job if they disappeared? And would she willingly switch jobs if she found another occupation that provided similar salary and benefits?

The matter of status and approval from colleagues and parents is less clear cut. Does she want status, or *status as an educator*? If the former, then she might switch jobs if something became available that offered higher status. If the latter, then arguably what she wants is excellence as a teacher, and the acclaim she gets is just a by-product of her pursuit of the *telos* of education. The distinction here may be subtle, but we think it is a key to understanding the distinction we made some years ago between attitudes toward work as a "career" and attitudes toward work as a "calling" (Wrzesniewski et al., 1997). People with careers are interested in rising in the hierarchy and attaining the status that comes with advancement. But they are interested in advancement per se, rather than advancement that is simply a by-product of excellent practice in their particular chosen occupation. People with callings, in contrast, certainly appreciate recognition, but they want recognition for excellence in the particular work they have chosen to do.

To illustrate this subtle distinction, imagine that the school in which the teacher we are describing works, influenced by the No Child Left Behind (NCLB) Act, adopts a set of standardized tests that assess student progress. Imagine further that status and acclaim will come to teachers whose students do best on these tests. Finally, imagine that our teacher believes that these tests as metrics are misguided, both as ways to measure educational attainment and as goals for teachers to strive to achieve. What will this teacher do? If she is motivated by status and the prospects for advancement (i.e., she has a "career"), she will play by the new rules and do whatever she can to help her students excel on the tests. If she is motivated by the *telos* of education, (i.e., she has a "calling") she will continue teaching as before, even if it means foregoing the opportunity to achieve the respect and approval of peers and parents.[1] Indeed, she might even agitate to get the school to abandon these tests, suggesting that in relying on them, the school is losing sight of the true *telos* of the practice of education.

Our analysis of the second-grade teacher suggests some of the complexity in assessing the nature of the motivation underlying job performance, and the difficulty of identifying motives as internal or instrumental. We think it is more realistic to imagine the distinction between internal and instrumental as a continuum rather than as categorical. Praise from parents and peers is less "instrumental" than salary and benefits. Moreover, some aspects of the teacher's work

[1] But not all parents. One of us (A.W.) was thrilled when her daughter's veteran kindergarten teacher – with more than 25 years of experience honing her craft –explained at back to school night that she had little interest in the regimented, test-directed instructional system at use in the school, and instead planned to teach as she always had, with a single goal to guide her. That goal? "To make your children love learning." She assured us that all the rest would follow, which it did, in abundance, that year. Here was, quite clearly, a teacher dedicated to the *telos* of her practice.

that may seem quite instrumental may not be. She may value the time off she has for the opportunities it gives her to develop lesson plans and become an even better teacher. Does this make the school calendar less instrumental? We think probably it does.

More generally, it seems clear to us that some goods are only attainable through the particular activity, some are attainable through the activity but also some others (they are internal to success at a practice, but not unique to it), and some are completely arbitrary in their relation to a practice—a rule imposed from without rather than a connection that is built in.

8.4 Why and When Internal Motives Are Better Than Instrumental Motives

There is a widely held belief—almost a presumption—that internal motives will produce better performance than instrumental motives. How could this not be true? Internal motives drive people to achieve excellence in the activity. Instrumental motives will only yield this result if the instrumental outcomes depend on excellence. If a teacher is working principally for salary, benefits and time off, she will only be an excellent teacher if these aspects of her job depend on it.

We think this view is true in general, but not universally. We think that for certain kinds of work, instrumental motives may be just as powerful as internal ones. If the work involves relatively simple, routinized tasks, in which performance is easily assessed, instrumental motives will probably do the job (see Cerasoli et al., 2014). In Adam Smith's (1776) famous pin factory, the example with which he celebrates the productive efficiency that accompanies the division of labor, work is structured in exactly this way. The tasks are simple, repeated over and over, easily monitored, and with little training required. One might say that the division of labor was invented with an eye toward economizing on the need for employees who had a *telos*. For complex jobs that required flexibility and discretion, internal motives might be needed, or at least be very helpful. Deskilling the task also decreases the need for workers with such motives. And it has the added benefit of putting control of the work in the hands of the manager, who organizes the instrumental incentives, instead of in the hands of the worker, who may or may not have the needed internal motives (Marglin, 1976).

We think Aristotle would be less impressed with the pin factory than Smith was. For Aristotle, excellence required doing the right thing, at the right time, in the right way, for the right reasons. Nussbaum (1990) calls this "the priority of the particular." Can all this "rightness" be measured and quantified in a way that enables one to reward good performance with instrumental incentives? If the work is simple, we think the answer is probably yes. If the work is complex, then no. Under complex conditions that require flexibility, internal motives will almost always lead to better performance than instrumental ones. Someone motivated to be excellent will be sensitive to feedback during execution of the task and continue to monitor and improve performance (see Deci & Ryan, 2014, for a review suggesting that feedback of this sort can boost intrinsic motivation). Instrumental incentives can't match this exquisitely detailed feedback loop between performance and outcomes. Someone motivated to be excellent will be responsive to unexpected obstacles and opportunities in a way that instrumental incentives can't match. And even in the simplest work, unexpected obstacles, challenges, and opportunities to act with excellence abound. One of us (A.W.) has shown that even in situations that require relatively simple and well-defined work (as in the case of hospital janitors) those employees who seem guided by the *telos* of hospital work grasp opportunities to step outside their well-defined occupational role to do what is needed, or would be helpful, in unforeseen circumstances. Employees who work with this *telos* in mind end up sounding a lot like someone striving to become excellent in a practice and develop complex systems for discerning what kind of response is needed, and when (see Schwartz, 2015).

We think that even rather simple and easily measured work benefits from what are sometimes called "incomplete contracts." Few work contracts specify precisely what is to be done and how it is to be done. The contracts leave room for people to use their discretion when a situation calls for it. Incomplete contracts may be inevitable, and trying to make them complete almost always results in reduced employee effectiveness (Hirsch, 1976). But it is worth pointing out that there is much less danger in relying on incomplete contracts if employees are guided by internal motives than if they are guided by instrumental ones. Indeed, some of the research we described above on how "extrinsic motives" can undermine "intrinsic motives" (Deci, 1975; Lepper et al., 1973), or as economists prefer to describe it, how extrinsic motives can crowd out moral motives (Frey & Oberholzer-Gee, 1997), may suggest that the more complete one makes an employee contract, the more one threatens the aim of employees to pursue the *telos* of their occupation. We see this when dedicated teachers start "teaching to the test" as their employment status comes to depend more and more on student test performance. The problem with standardized tests is probably not the tests themselves, but the uses to which the test results are put, i.e., the outcomes that depend on student test performance.

Testing the assumption that the pursuit of *telos* in an activity can be undermined by the presence of more instrumental motives was our aim when we embarked, some years ago, on a study that assessed the long-term impact of different types of motives on outcomes in a real-world setting. We wanted to find a setting in which both internal and instrumental motives were possible, and where the outcomes at stake were of great significance to the lives of participants and to the wider world as well. And so we studied West Point cadets, chosen because they voluntarily undertake a grueling 9-year commitment when they matriculate at the United States Military Academy at West Point (Wrzesniewski et al., 2014). West Point has traditionally been the preeminent training ground for military leadership in the United States. After 4 years of undergraduate and military leadership education, involving a difficult physical component, graduates of West Point become commissioned military officers—second lieutenants—with a 5-year commitment of military service. It is a significant undertaking, and one that requires a great deal of motivation and effort. It was the structure of the motivation of cadets, and their impact on the outcomes the cadets experienced, to which we turned our attention.

While one might expect that all West Point cadets matriculate out of a motivation to serve their country as military leaders—an internal motive, impossible to separate from the activity itself—it is also true that a West Point education and military officership can yield better career opportunities later —an instrumental motive. We followed 10,238 West Point cadets from ten consecutive entering classes for periods of up to 14 years to learn what happens to them as a function of their original motives to attend. The strength of their various motives was measured twice upon entry to West Point, and fell into categories reflecting internal and instrumental motives, among other types. We found that for key educational and career outcomes, those with stronger internal motives, who were there because they deeply desired training as a military leader who would serve the country, were more likely to graduate from West Point and become commissioned officers, to be identified as eligible for early promotion in their first 5 years as a military officer, and to remain in the military up to 6 years (the end of the window we measured) after their commitment to the country was fulfilled. In contrast, those with stronger instrumental motives were less likely to be identified as eligible for early promotion or to remain after their mandatory military service period was up.

Most striking, however, were our findings regarding the combined effects of internal and instrumental motives. For every outcome—graduation, early promotion eligibility, and remaining in the military—instrumental motives weakened the positive effects of internal motives. The undermining of internal motives by instrumental motives significantly hurt cadets' chances of ever graduating from West Point and becoming military officers. Even when cadets who had successfully become military officers were internally motivated, the mere presence of instrumental motives made consideration for early promotion and the likelihood of staying in the military less probable. While our results could be interpreted to mean that internal motives can help to dampen the negative effects of instrumental motives, the story here is clear—salient instrumental motives, either on their own or in combination with internal motives, harm individual and institutional outcomes.

While the example of West Point cadets is rather specific, other evidence from individuals drawn from a range of occupations suggests that seeing work as a calling, in which the internal aims of the work are ends in and of themselves, corresponds with higher job and life satisfaction, as well as more time spent at work and fewer days of work missed (Wrzesniewski et al., 1997). Others find that those who see work a calling—whether they be classical musicians, zookeepers, or administrative assistants—are more engaged with, involved in, and motivated to stay in their jobs, even if they are no longer paid (see Bunderson & Thompson, 2009; Dobrow, 2013; Wrzesniewski et al., 1997). Indeed, people who find that the internal aims of their job are their motives for working are also more identified with and attached to the organizations in which they work (Cardador, Dane, & Pratt, 2011). Finally, while evidence on whether those with callings are better performers on the job is still thin, data showing a positive (and predictive) effect of callings on performance is growing (see Hall & Chandler, 2005; Wrzesniewski, Berg, Grant, Kurkoski, & Welle, 2015).

8.5 Conclusion: Instrumental Motivation, Internal Motivation and Eudaimonia

Research on the contrast between hedonic and eudaimonic experience suggests that while the former focuses on happiness and pleasure, the latter concerns well-being rooted in personal growth and development (Waterman, 1993). In this chapter, we have argued that engaging in and pursuing excellence in activities for reasons that underscore the purpose of the activities themselves marks a meaningful departure from the instrumental reasons so often assumed to be driving activities. What is more, to be internally motivated to pursue an activity need not be based in the pleasure that activity brings. Indeed, the opportunity to develop and grow in that activity can be an even more powerful and long-lasting motive (Ryan & Deci, 2001, Ryan & Martela, Chap. 7, this volume; Wrzesniewski et al., 2014).

This has important implications for how we understand well-being. Rather than well-being resulting from the pursuit of pleasure, or pleasurable ends—the focus of hedonic approaches to well-being, we align with a view of well-being that is based in the pursuit of excellence in the practices one undertakes. The depth, range, and nature of the well-being that results from deep engagement in activities for ends that are inextricably connected to the activities themselves is apparent in studies of work as a calling. In callings, as in any practice undertaken for the sake of the *telos* of the practice itself, well-being results from its pursuit, as well as its ends. The stability of well-being that depends not on the fleeting pleasure gotten from instrumental outcomes, but rather resides in the activity itself, makes all the difference in understanding what it is that makes work, play, or any other activity worth doing. It is possible that current efforts to measure well-being that are deployed by psychologists and other social scientists have the hedonic (rather than the eudaimonic) framework built into them, with their focus on the experience of positive and negative affect, so that pleasure seems even more important to well-being than it would if measures of well-being were differently constructed. This is so even in the face of evidence that well-being rooted in the eudaimonic framework (rather than the hedonic) is associated with better immune response at the cellular level (Fredrickson et al., 2013, Fredrickson, Chap. 12, this volume). Thus, a different set of tools for measuring well-being might provide even more impressive evidence for a eudaimonic conception of a life well-lived than is presently suggested by the evidence, though the importance to well-being of the sorts of experiences we have focused on in this chapter is impressive, even with the deck stacked against it.

References

Aristotle. (1988). *The nicomachean ethics* (trans: D. Ross). Oxford, UK: Oxford University Press.

Bunderson, J. S., & Thompson, J. A. (2009). The call of the wild: Zookeepers, callings, and the double-edged sword of deeply meaningful work. *Administrative Science Quarterly, 54*, 32–57.

Cardador, M. T., Dane, E., & Pratt, M. G. (2011). Linking calling orientations to organizational attachment via organizational instrumentality. *Journal of Vocational Behavior, 79*, 367–378.

Cerasoli, C. P., Nicklin, J. M., & Ford, M. T. (2014). Intrinsic motivation and extrinsic incentives jointly predict performance: A 40-year meta-analysis. *Psychological Bulletin, 140*, 980–1008.

Deci, E. L. (1971). Effects of externally mediated rewards on intrinsic motivation. *Journal of Personality and Social Psychology, 18*, 105–115.

Deci, E. L. (1975). *Intrinsic motivation*. New York: Plenum Press.

Deci, E. L., Koestner, R., & Ryan, R. M. (1999). A meta-analytic review of experiments examining the effects of extrinsic rewards on intrinsic motivation. *Psychological Bulletin, 125*, 627–668.

Deci, E. L., & Ryan, R. M. (1985). *Intrinsic motivation and self-determination in human behavior*. New York: Plenum.

Deci, E. L., & Ryan, R. M. (2014). The importance of universal psychological needs for understanding motivation in the workplace. In *The Oxford handbook of work engagement, motivation, and self-determination theory* (pp. 13–32). New York: Oxford University Press.

Dobrow, S. R. (2013). Dynamics of calling: A longitudinal study of musicians. *Journal of Organizational Behavior, 34*, 431–452.

Duckworth, A. L., & Gross, J. J. (2014). Self-control and grit: Related but separable determinants of success. *Current Directions in Psychological Science, 23*, 319–325.

Duckworth, A. L., Kirby, T., Tsukayama, E., Berstein, H., & Ericsson, K. (2010). Deliberate practice spells success: Why grittier competitors triumph at the National Spelling Bee. *Social Psychological and Personality Science, 2*, 174–181.

Duckworth, A. L., Peterson, C., Matthews, M. D., & Kelly, D. R. (2007). Grit: Perseverance and passion for long-term goals. *Journal of Personality and Social Psychology, 92*, 1087–1101.

Duckworth, A. L., & Seligman, M. E. P. (2005). Self-discipline outdoes IQ predicting academic performance in adolescents. *Psychological Science, 16*, 939–944.

Eisenberger, R., & Cameron, J. (1996). Detrimental effects of reward: Reality or myth? *American Psychologist, 51*, 153–1166.

Ericcson, K. A., Krampe, R. T., & Tesch-Romer, C. (1993). The role of deliberate practice in the acquisition of expert performance. *Psychological Review, 100*, 363–406.

Fredrickson, B. L., Grewen, K. M., Coffey, K. A., Algoe, S. B., Firestine, A. M., Arevalo, J. M., et al. (2013). A functional genomic perspective on human well-being. *Proceedings of the National Academy of Sciences, 110*, 13684–13689.

Frey, B. S. (1994). How intrinsic motivation is crowded out and in. *Rationality and Society, 6*, 334–352.

Frey, B. S., & Oberholzer-Gee, F. (1997). The cost of price incentives: An empirical analysis of motivation crowding out. *American Economic Review, 87*, 746–755.

Gerhart, B., & Fang, M. (2015). Pay, intrinsic motivation, extrinsic motivation, performance, and creativity in the workplace: Revisiting long-held beliefs. *Annual Review of Organizational Psychology and Organizational Behavior, 2*, 489–521.

Gneezy, U., & Rustichini, A. (2000). A fine is a price. *Journal of Legal Studies, 29*, 1–17.

Hall, D. T., & Chandler, D. E. (2005). Psychological success: When the career is a calling. *Journal of Organizational Behavior, 26*, 155–176.

Hirsch, F. (1976). *Social limits to growth*. Cambridge, MA: Harvard University Press.

Kiviniemi, M. T., Snyder, M., & Omoto, A. M. (2002). Too many of a good thing? The effects of multiple motivations on task fulfillment, satisfaction, and cost. *Personality and Social Psychology Bulletin, 28*, 732–743.

Lacetera, N., Macis, M., & Slonim, R. (2012). Will there be blood? Incentives and displacement effects in pro-social behavior. *American Journal of Economic Policy, 4*, 186–223.

Lepper, M. R., Greene, D., & Nisbett, R. E. (1973). Undermining children's intrinsic interest with extrinsic rewards: A test of the "overjustification hypothesis". *Journal of Personality and Social Psychology, 28*, 119–137.

MacIntyre, A. (1981). *After virtue*. Notre Dame, IN: University of Notre Dame Press.

Marglin, S. (1976). What do bosses do? In A. Gorz (Ed.), *The division of labour* (pp. 13–54). London: Harvester Press.

Murayama, K., Matsumoto, M., Izuma, K., & Matsumoto, K. (2010). Neural basis of the undermining effect of extrinsic reward on intrinsic motivation. *Proceedings of the National Academy of Sciences, 107*, 20911–20916.

Nussbaum, M. (1990). *Love's knowledge*. Oxford, UK: Oxford University Press.

Pink, D. H. (2011). *Drive: The surprising truth about what motivates us*. New York: Penguin.

Ryan, R. M., & Deci, E. L. (2001). On happiness and human potentials: A review of research hedonic and eudaimonic well-being. *Annual Review of Psychology, 52*, 141–166.

Schwartz, B. (1978). *The psychology of learning and behavior*. New York: Norton.

Schwartz, B. (2015). *Why we work*. New York: Simon & Schuster.

Schwartz, B., Schuldenfrei, R., & Lacey, H. (1978). Operant psychology as factory psychology. *Behaviorism, 6*, 229–254.

Skinner, B. F. (1953). *Science and human behavior*. New York: Macmillan.

Smith, A. (1776/1937). *The wealth of nations*. New York: Modern Library.

Taylor, F. W. (1911/1967). *Principles of scientific management*. New York: Norton.

Waterman, A. S. (1993). Two conceptions of happiness: Contrasts of personal expressiveness (eudaimonia) and hedonic enjoyment. *Journal of Personality and Social Psychology, 64*, 678–691.

Wrzesniewski, A., Berg, J. M., Grant, A. M., Kurkoski, J., & Welle, B. (2015). Dual mindsets at work: Achieving long-term gains in happiness. Working paper.

Wrzesniewski, A., McCauley, C. R., Rozin, P., & Schwartz, B. (1997). Jobs, careers, and callings: People's relations to their work. *Journal of Research in Personality, 31*, 21–33.

Wrzesniewski, A., Schwartz, B., Cong, X., Kane, M., Omar, A., & Kolditz, T. (2014). Multiple types of motives don't multiply the motivation of West Point cadets. *Proceedings of the National Academy of Sciences, 111*, 10990–10995.

Eudaimonia and Wisdom

9

Alan Law and Ursula M. Staudinger

Wisdom has long been considered an ideal endpoint of human development, attracting the attention of scholars for thousands of years, with the result that our thinking remains heavily influenced by the ideas of ancient Greek philosophers in particular. In more recent times psychologists, especially those interested in individual development across the lifespan, have ventured into empirical investigation of wisdom. This has been a rather courageous undertaking given the fact that there is probably no phenomenon richer in associations and ideational history. Although there has been general agreement that wisdom is not easily attained, there remains some disagreement about what wisdom is and how it should be studied.

In this chapter we outline psychological approaches to investigating wisdom and its development. We review findings relating to a view of wisdom as the perfect integration of mind and virtue: it is highly relevant to any discussion of ideal human development. Indeed it has been discussed as an important outcome of the good life (eudaimonia) and also as a means to achieve a good life (e.g., Baltes, 2004; Brugman, 2006; Schwartz & Sharpe, 2006; Schwartz & Wrzesniewski, Chap. 8, this volume). We understand eudaimonia as the kind of well-being that arises when practicing wisdom (phronesis) to solve the existential conflicts and dilemmas that occur in everyday life and thus leading a "good life" irrespective of the emotional states coming with it (e.g., Baltes, 2004; Höffe, 2007; Staudinger, 1999a). This chapter is presented in light of the challenges put forward by Nussbaum (2008), who argues that psychology has paid too little attention to eudaimonia in particular, and in general to subjective states relating to well-being: we contend that the psychological study of wisdom has already garnered a range of findings that address many of her concerns.

In psychological terms, eudaimonia may be described as productive self-actualization, as growth towards an ideal kind of mental health. In this tradition, Ryff and Singer (2008) defined eudaimonia as "self-realization, played out individually, each according to his or her own disposition and talent" (p. 17). This is in line with the earlier understanding of good psychological health as consisting in more than just the absence of symptoms of psychological ill-health (e.g., Jahoda, 1958; Maslow, 1954; Rogers, 1962). It is also understood as the feelings experienced alongside personal expressiveness (in the sense of expressing one's true self) by Waterman (1993).

A. Law (✉)
Bremen International Graduate School of Social Sciences, Bremen, Germany
e-mail: law@bigsss-bremen.de

U.M. Staudinger
Columbia Aging Center, Columbia University, New York, NY, USA
e-mail: umstaudinger@columbia.edu

J. Vittersø (ed.), *Handbook of Eudaimonic Well-Being*, International Handbooks of Quality-of-Life,
DOI 10.1007/978-3-319-42445-3_9

Similar ideas are discussed in relation to Csikszentmihalyi's "flow," which focuses specifically on subjective states experienced during rewarding activities (see Csikszentmihalyi, 1999; Waterman, 1990).

While these approaches tend to emphasize a flourishing that is individualistic and autonomous in nature, this is different from our understanding of eudaimonia, which combines this notion of ideal self-actualization with a striving towards the practice of virtues (e.g., honesty, concern for others, justice). It further involves bringing to bear our mind, in the sense of moral-practical judgment and prudence, when we attempt to solve the fundamental issues of our lives to reach the ultimate good, which we define as reaching beyond the individual and including the good of others. Balancing individual goals with a concern for the greater good and the good of others in our view is the essence of eudaimonia as it relates to wisdom (see Staudinger & Glück, 2011; Sternberg, 1998). Such balance is a lofty goal, often requiring transcendence of social constraints, and resistance to self-actualization in the more limited sense of hedonic satisfaction.

To elucidate our view of wisdom, we first present findings clarifying its definition and psychometric location and then explore its relation to the good life. Next we consider the path of normative human development through the lens of psychological conceptions of person maturation and present a model of positive person development that positions wisdom as separate from such typical lifespan developmental trajectories.

9.1 Recent Developments in the Psychological Definition and Study of Wisdom

One of the most important recent developments in the increasing body of literature regarding the psychological study of wisdom is the demarcation of more specific fields of inquiry. Defining two subtypes of wisdom, general and personal (Staudinger, 2013), has helped to reconcile some of the inconsistencies in earlier research. Personal wisdom refers to knowledge, judgment and insight relating to one's own life, while general wisdom is focused on the lives of others and life in general.

Personal wisdom was first investigated by asking laypeople to rate adjectives as to their relevance for wise persons, revealing some broad agreement: in 1976, Clayton found that wise people are typically considered to be relatively strong on affective characteristics such as empathy and compassion, reflective processes such as intuition and introspection, and cognitive capacities such as experience and intelligence (see Sternberg, 1990). Further work summarized in a review by Bluck and Glück (2005) shows that lay conceptions can be captured by five subcomponents: cognitive ability, insight, reflective attitude, concern for others and real-world skills.

In actually measuring personal wisdom, researchers such as Ardelt and Webster (e.g., Ardelt, 2003; Webster, Taylor, & Bates, 2011) have emphasized the personality and attitudinal components of wisdom identified by laypeople and have used those to construct self-report scales of personal wisdom. Such measures have yielded contradictory findings in comparison with the performance-related approach to personal wisdom, which involves the rating of verbal responses to fictitious or personal life dilemmas in an interview situation (e.g., Mickler & Staudinger, 2008). For example, measures of subjective well-being appear to be have a relationship with self-reported wisdom (e.g., Ardelt, 1997; Bergsma & Ardelt, 2012) while no relationship was found with a performance measure of wisdom (Mickler & Staudinger, 2008). As such, a research focus on an inward-turning reflection and the development of affective skills in support of mastering one's environment and a positive attitude towards one's own experience, as captured variously by Ardelt's Three Dimensional Wisdom (e.g., Ardelt, 2003), Whitbourne's Ego-integrity, based on Erikson's maturational theory (e.g., Whitbourne & Waterman, 1979), Wink and Helson's transcendent wisdom (1997), Ryff's personal growth dimension (e.g., Ryff, 1989, this volume) and Webster's Self-Assessed Wisdom Scale (e.g., Webster, 2003), yields information about personal wisdom (Staudinger & Glück, 2011).

In contrast, general wisdom is defined in terms of the knowledge, insight, and judgment a person has about life in general. General wisdom has been studied using the Berlin Wisdom paradigm, originating from the Max Planck Institute in Berlin (e.g., Pasupathi, Staudinger, & Baltes, 2001; Smith & Baltes, 1990; Staudinger, Lopez, & Baltes, 1997), and also by Sternberg (1998) and Neo-Piagetian researchers who have focused on the development of advanced forms of adult thought (e.g., Kramer, 1983). To date, there is only one performance-based measure of general wisdom, that of the Berlin paradigm. In this case, participants are asked to respond verbally to the challenging life situations of a fictitious character (for example, *a 15-year-old girl* wants to get married right away. What should one/she consider and do?), and their response is coded by trained laypeople according to five criteria of general wisdom: factual knowledge, procedural knowledge, lifespan contextualism, value relativism, and awareness and management of uncertainty. A participant's mean score for the five criteria across all tasks is referred to as his or her wisdom-related performance (WRP). Note that there is no attempt to measure whether such performance is also evidenced in actions, as discussed in Staudinger, Dörner and Mickler (2005), and the criteria are assumed to be domain-general rather than variant across domains. Reliabilities of these ratings have been found to be surprisingly high, across five criteria around 0.98 and for individual criteria ranging between 0.7 and 0.85 (Baltes & Staudinger, 2000; Staudinger, 1999b). Research using the Berlin Wisdom Interview has found wisdom to be an advanced integration of cognitive and personality characteristics with characteristics at their interface playing a major role: while crystallized and fluid intelligence both are necessary but not sufficient, the Big 5 personality characteristic of openness to experience, as well as social intelligence, thinking style (judiciousness) and creativity as well as life experiences contribute uniquely to the overall variance in WRP scores (Pasupathi & Staudinger, 2001; Staudinger et al., 1997; Staudinger, Maciel, Smith, & Baltes, 1998; Staudinger & Pasupathi, 2003). While there is a relationship between age and WRP from early adolescence to young adulthood, there is no relationship thereafter (Pasupathi et al., 2001; Staudinger, 1999b). Thus in adolescence, aging plays an important role, as it is typically accompanied by physiological and psychological changes such as increases in empathy and the ability to think abstractly and show reflective judgment (see Brugman, 2006). These may set important foundations for the development of skills in life review, which are, in the Berlin model, considered crucial for the development of wisdom. While exploration and internal conflicts are to some extent expected and encouraged for young people in their journey towards becoming contributing members of society, continued developments in such insightful thinking are non-normative (i.e., rare). It can be argued that while a socially constrained self is ideal for the pursuit of one's own subjective well-being, it is only by transcending that self that we can evidence higher levels of wisdom. Below we address the importance of such transcendence for our conception of wisdom.

9.2 The Importance of Self-Transcendence for the "Good Life"

While much of the psychological work on eudaimonia mentioned above is implicitly connected to concepts of individual flourishing or self-actualization, psychologists studying wisdom have tended to include some component of other-directedness in their conceptions of a good life, whether this involves compassion (e.g., Bergsma & Ardelt, 2012), or both interpersonal and extra-personal interests (Sternberg, 1998). What role such orientations have in wisdom has been an important question for philosophers. John Kekes, for example, emphasizes that wisdom allows for the prioritization of ideals, and that the good life will become possible from following some paths and rejecting others according to their perceived appropriateness for meeting one's goals (1983).

As it does not specify the nature of these goals, this position appears to relate more to the self-actualization notion of eudaimonia than our notion of personal wisdom. Kunzmann (2007) notes, however, that Kekes in his later writings refers to the importance of developing in this way without violating others' rights and with a concern for encouraging others to develop. Although there is a strong tradition of associating wisdom with the practice of other virtues (Baltes, 2004), there are challenges to this position, such as Whitcomb's proposition that an evil person can be wise (see S. Ryan, 2014). Obviously such a notion of wisdom is at odds with our approach, which requires that wisdom by definition is oriented towards balancing one's own good with that of others. If one has brought to bear their knowledge of how to act, with the limitations of the human condition in mind, but acts without compassionate consideration of others, this cannot be considered wise action but rather clever at best. It is clear therefore that in order to develop wisdom, it is not sufficient either to build a body of theoretical knowledge about how best to act, nor to act only towards self-actualization goals irrespective of what they are. It is only with a highly developed appreciation of the needs of others and a strong understanding of the contexts (e.g., temporal, cultural) in which actions might occur that one might show wisdom.

It can be expected that insight into the difficult and uncertain matters of life in general is more easily developed by those who are exposed to certain professional contexts, such as family judges, ministers or priests, and clinical psychologists, as they are more exposed to the fundamental challenges of other people's lives and receive training and mentorship in dealing with them, and indeed there is empirical evidence that this is so (Smith, Staudinger, & Baltes, 1994). Of course it may be the case that such professional contexts are sought out by individuals with a predilection for intense scrutiny of the lives of others, but regardless, certain professional contexts provide fertile grounds for developing theoretical knowledge. Similarly, in a nomination study in which journalists, using a delphi technique, were asked to nominate contemporary public figures whom they considered wise, and who were then interviewed according to the Berlin Paradigm, an emergent pattern in the biographies of the higher scoring nominees was a series of challenges and threats that contribute to nominees' life experience. In particular, the older wisdom nominees faced these challenges and threats within a context that appears to have been conducive to wisdom development: life under the Third Reich in Germany preceding and during World War Two, many having faced the threat of imprisonment for their actions to benefit others (Staudinger, 1999a). If professional and historical contexts can provide the opportunities (direct or vicarious) for growth that increase life insight among those who have the personal orientation to learn from them, then, as Staudinger (1999a) suggests, there may be an increased potential for high levels of wisdom in younger people of recent generations as technological advances increase our exposure to life and life problems, through the proliferation of the internet and various uses of social media. Whether the increased accessibility of such information alongisde the availability of a range of new social tools amounts to a new historical context conducive to the development of wisdom or not remains to be seen.

This is not to say that learning what is necessary to display wisdom is a satisfying process. Similarly to the subject of Wordsworth's happy warrior, from whom Nussbaum (2008) draws inspiration for her critical challenge to psychology, or more particularly to Kahneman's approach to subjective well-being (e.g., Kahneman & Krueger, 2006), among participants in studies using the Berlin paradigm, attaining high levels of insight into life is clearly not associated with high levels of hedonic satisfaction (e.g., Staudinger et al., 1997; Wink & Staudinger, 2015). Later we address some reasons for the absence of subjective well-being as a correlate of wisdom by later life but first review findings we associate with a more typical understanding of maturation.

9.3 Sad But True: Wisdom Is Not a Result of Typical Maturation

In the early days of a developmental psychology considering the whole life span, the study of the maturation of a person was most notably addressed by Erik Erikson (e.g., Erikson & Erikson, 1997). Erikson placed wisdom as a possible outcome attainable in the last phase of human development: within his framework of person development as a sequence of psychosocial crises, wisdom and integrity (vs. despair) would be achieved only after successful resolution of the conflicts of earlier stages in life and under appropriate social conditions. As such, it reflected an adaptive maturation within the confines of one's own culture and was associated with an ability to integrate one's past life and, in acknowledgement of the approaching end of one's lifetime, a sense of satisfaction with one's role in what has already happened. His alternative outcome in the eighth stage of a person's life, despair, occurs with the realization that, as the end of life approaches, one's goals from younger days are left unachieved and are now rendered unachievable. The pursuit of hedonic and eudaimonic forms of well-being in later life now can be seen as quite distinct activities: on one hand, we may attempt to adapt to increasing losses, by seeking to feel satisfied with what is left after we discard goals that are no longer possible; and on the other hand we may maximize gains, by refreshing our sense of purpose in life and being open to new experiences. Not only are these distinct activities, but pursuing Erikson's notion of integration may actually undermine progress in personal wisdom as a recent study suggests (Mickler & Staudinger, 2008).

Although there has not been a great deal of empirical work to support Erikson's ideas, other work seeks to look beyond dichotomous outcomes (i.e., integration, despair) in the manner of Marcia's (1966) identity status approach to adolescent identity outcomes. In this framework, a bipolar conception of outcomes in later life is as insufficient as in adolescence (Hearn et al., 2012). Marcia's approach to identity formation in adolescence identifies four categories to account for the different types of progress that has been made towards the achievement of identity. The basic distinction between identity achievement and diffusion is bolstered by the alternatives of moratorium and foreclosure, and there is by now a large body of evidence that supports such differentiation both in the structure of outcomes and in terms of the processes by which these are achieved (see Luyckx et al., 2008). Recent work describes four types of later-life Integrity: *integrated* persons are socially mature, open to experience, and tolerant of ambiguity (reflective of wisdom as previously discussed), and *despairing* persons do not share such characteristics and are more prone to negative emotions. *nonexploring* persons are high on social maturity and emotional positivity (reflective of hedonic pursuits), and *pseudointegrated* persons are low in social maturity and well-being but fairly high in openness to experience (Hearn et al., 2012). Also studying identity development through adulthood, Helson and Srivastava (2001) found that their sample could be categorized as *achievers*, high in personal growth and environmental mastery, *depleted*, with low scores on both dimensions, *conservers*, with high environmental mastery but low personal growth, or *seekers*, with high personal growth but low environmental mastery. While achievers appeared to be higher in terms of two typical indicators of maturity, the Competence scale of the California Personality Inventory and Peterson and Klohnen's measure of generativity (1995), only seekers showed high levels of intrapsychic differentiation as demonstrated in their scores on a composite wisdom scale.

Employing a combined neo-Piagetian and psychodynamic perspective, Gisela Labouvie-Vief has reached complementary conclusions in the affective domain. By categorizing individuals as high or low on two separate dimensions referred to as affect optimization and affect complexity, she describes four "personality" types. Affect optimization involves the automatic deployment of skills to limit individual emotional experience to the positive in order to maintain well-being, while affect complexity rather involves being able to postpone positive emotions to allow for differentiation and coordination of one's own current feelings and synchronization with those of others (Labouvie-Vief & Medler, 2002; Labouvie-Vief, Diehl, Jain, & Zhang, 2007). Those who are *integrated* in this typology are also functioning optimally, open to experience and socially mature, with high levels of positive affect, but such individuals are contrasted with a *dysregulated* group, who show low levels of both positive affect and complexity, a *defended* group, who use denial and repression to maintain positive affect with low complexity, and a *complex* group, who are open and tolerant but not experiencing high levels of well-being.

That identity development, cognitive-affective development and personality development have been found to vary each along at least two dimensions in a compellingly similar manner suggests that there are indeed latent trajectories guiding adult development. In addition, such differentiation of pathways through development makes it problematic to designate one or other as, in and of itself, leading to an ideal form of maturation, even if a typical pattern of maturation can be observed. In particular, the groups labelled above as complex, pseudointegrated and seeker are of special interest in the context of wisdom development because of their close associations with openness to experience. As explained earlier, this personality characteristic is one of the strongest unique contributors to wisdom-related performance in the Berlin Paradigm (Staudinger & Pasupathi, 2003). Although openness alone is not sufficient for the development of wisdom, we must recognize its role in orienting individuals towards more differentiated life experiences. The existence in typologies of groups that are not well adjusted but who seek new experiences is no surprise, but the possibility that the outcome of developing in this way is not always suboptimal has seldom been acknowledged.

Thus, we maintain that the typical kind of person maturation can be described to incorporate elements of identity, cognition and affect, and this is generally targeted towards hedonic well-being at the exclusion of eudaimonia-related development. This is not always associated with happiness, which is one of Nussbaum's (2008) key criticisms of psychological approaches to studying well-being. However, the psychological study of wisdom as an optimal outcome of an atypical developmental trajectory has addressed many of the characteristics of eudaimonia that Nussbaum calls attention to. Proceeding from the understanding that there is more than one form of positive person development, below we consider two such pathways, the more typical, adjustment, and the atypical trajectory, growth, which encourages the development of wisdom. In contrast to Nussbaum, we do not bemoan the fact that maturation towards adjustment and well-being exist. Rather, we even argue that this developmental trajectory serves important functions for the functioning of a given human collective.

9.4 Growth and Adjustment as Two Trajectories of Positive Person Development

Drawing on such developmental traditions as outlined above, Staudinger and colleagues (e.g., Staudinger & Kessler, 2009; Staudinger & Kunzmann, 2005) have distinguished between two types of positive personality development they have labelled as *adjustment* and *growth*: the former comprises elements of social maturity and competence, while the latter is associated with progress towards personal wisdom.

The first trajectory, adjustment, results in mastery of "the demands of everyday life and its various roles (work, family), that is, social and practical competences, reliability, and emotional stability" (Dörner, Mickler, & Staudinger, 2005, p. 279). It is one of few areas of human competence that show age-related increase, rather than decline. Adjustment reflects a prioritization of developing skills to develop and then maintain subjective well-being in the face of age-related increases in constraints, such as difficulties with movement, hearing, or finances and social status. The typical personal resources accrued include professional skills and increasing competence in everyday problem-solving, emotional balance, or social relations (Dörner et al., 2005). The related concept of social maturity (Helson & Wink, 1987) has been described in terms of "outward orientation" implying that both the demands and successes are primarily experienced socially, by means of the prescribed roles and norms for behavior present in one's socio-cultural environment (Dörner et al., 2005). By their very nature, societies depend on a rather high "prevalence" of adjustment as one means of maintaining themselves (e.g., in the conservation of values). Thus, progress towards social maturity or adjustment is reinforced and guided by social institutions, such as education and legal systems (e.g., Staudinger & Kessler, 2009; Staudinger & Kunzmann, 2005). Although in the earlier stages of life, socially determined, age- and history-graded goals seem to be the motivation for individuals to make progress towards reaching adjustment, in later life, roles and expectations are less clear and developed. It may be that an awareness of the finitude of life is a prime motivator for further adjustment-related progress in the later stages of life (Staudinger & Kunzmann, 2005).

The normative trend towards adjustment is reflected in the developmental patterns of the Big 5 personality model (Costa Jr., McCrae, & Dye, 1991): emotional stability increases (the reverse pole of neuroticism), as do conscientiousness and agreeableness (Costa Jr., McCrae, & Dye, 1991). Usually this pattern is combined with high levels of environmental mastery, positive relations with others, and self-acceptance, which are dimensions of Carol Ryff's (1989) Psychological Well-being Scale (Staudinger & Kunzmann, 2005).

In contrast, the second trajectory, growth, is characterized by the employment of critical self-reflection, complex emotion regulation, and a striving towards transcending constraints, whether social, psychological, or biological (Dörner et al., 2005). Personal growth, in this sense, however, reaches beyond the individual and includes the goal to balance one's own good with the good of others.

More specifically, three facets characterize this notion of growth: firstly, it involves cognitive insight into oneself, others and the world; secondly, it requires complex emotion regulation as indexed by a tolerance of ambiguity, and thirdly, a motivation that transcends self-interest and is focused on the well-being of others (Staudinger & Kessler, 2009). Despite the possibility that subjective well-being can be experienced alongside gains on a growth trajectory, achieving subjective well-being or hedonic happiness is not the target; instead, the ideal endpoint of progress on the growth trajectory is high levels of personal wisdom. Personality growth is not typical: it is rare, and will frequently put individuals at odds with their social context as they emancipate themselves in thinking and feeling and transcend the social structures and constraints that are embraced by those pursuing adjustment (Dörner et al., 2005; Staudinger & Kessler, 2009; Staudinger & Kunzmann, 2005).

Thus, personality growth is prototypically indicated by a high level of openness to new experience, and high scores on the Ryff scales of personal growth and purpose in life (Staudinger & Kessler, 2009). Autonomy is also an indicator of growth as it is likely to be required to transcend the given social structures (e.g., Wink & Staudinger, 2015). Although Ryff's Psychological Well-being Scale is intended to capture the eudaimonic side of well-being, at least in later life, we suggest that only these three scales are truly indicative of the kind of eudaimonia we associate with wisdom, and there is empirical evidence for this (Wink & Staudinger, 2015).

9.5 Growth, Adjustment, and Subjective Well-Being

Research has demonstrated that age-related increase in indicators of personality adjustment is typical (e.g., Field & Millsap, 1991), reflecting an increasing importance up to mid-life in finding an acceptable role and fitting in to one's social milieu. Thus, higher levels of adjustment are accompanied by high levels of hedonic well-being, reflecting satisfaction at mastering the developmental tasks largely prescribed by the given socio-historical setting: empirical evidence supports this association (Seiffge-Krenke & Gelhaar, 2008; Staudinger & Kessler, 2009).

The search for personality growth and eudaimonia, in contrast, cannot be reduced to the quest for hedonic happiness, as Nussbaum (2008) suggests. Rather, a certain amount of subjective well-being seems a necessary precondition to provide the motivational energy to venture on the pathway towards personal wisdom. Hedonic well-being may be experienced along this pathway, but probably at different times than during adjustment-related progress, and it is itself not the motivating goal (Staudinger & Kunzmann, 2005). That meeting different kinds of goals results in different emotional experience appears at first to sit neatly with Ryan and Deci's (2000) suggestion that hedonic experiences occur in response to achieving relatedness and competence, while autonomous, self-determined goals are eudaimonic (see also Ryff & Martela, this volume). However, one of the key features of our notion of growth that distinguishes it from self-determination theory or Ryff's notion of personal growth is that following this trajectory leads towards the development of personal wisdom, which entails that self-determined goals are aimed to balance the needs of the self and others and aim to increase the greater good (Staudinger & Kunzmann, 2005).

Thus, personal wisdom is not synonymous with successful maturation, in the sense of adjustment, nor necessarily accompanied by high levels of subjective well-being, nor directly linked with the achievement of self-related goals. Indeed, following a growth trajectory, transcending extant societal demands (if needed) and seeking the kind of challenges that seem necessary for making progress on the wisdom pathway will frequently be linked with challenging experiences and negative emotions. This supports Nussbaum's (2008) assertion that she would report dissatisfaction with her life as a whole if she caught herself experiencing satisfaction (like Aristotle's dumb grazing animals), because she attaches value to "striving, longing, and working for a difficult goal" (p. 587). Although Nussbaum presents this as something of a paradox, it is less of a contradiction than she suggests if we consider a distinction between growth and adjustment as outlined above: the reflective dissatisfaction of being confined to adjustment-related goals that she describes, in fact may be important in promoting the quest for growth-related goals. Such dissatisfaction with hedonic outcomes has been discussed in other literature as well (e.g., Kringelbach & Berridge, 2009; Vittersø & Søholt, 2011; Vittersø, this volume), and it may be the case that such dissatisfaction is one motivator for new goals and activities that might later contribute to the development of wisdom. The consideration of emotions experienced during certain kinds of activities, whether these are pleasurable and satisfying or challenging and interesting, is clearly important for drawing a distinction between eudaimonic and hedonic well-being. However in the broader timeframe of a whole life, we would argue that it is not that which is experienced at the time, but rather one's interpretation of these after the fact that is important for one's cognitive and affective experience of living a good life. We consider the process of life review to be essential for the development of wisdom (Staudinger, 2001), and it is partly because of the inherent temporal distance between event and review that the subjective state at the time of the event becomes less salient in our perspective.

9.6 Life Review: A Crucial Social-Cognitive Process on the Road to Wisdom and Eudaimonia

Life review, constructing, reconstructing, interpreting and evaluating an individual's life course (whether one's own or someone else's) is a process that we engage in across the lifespan (Staudinger, 2001). The ability to engage in life reflection or life review emerges in adolescence (Habermas & Bluck, 2000), as we become aware of ourselves and the gestalt of our lives. Life review is a crucial social-cognitive process when it comes to making sense of our experiences and potentially transforming them into insights into life, and therefore this social-cognitive process is at the heart of the development of wisdom (Staudinger, Smith, & Baltes, 1992). Butler's early work on life review (1963), in line with Erikson, suggested that life review was a process through which one could develop both negative (e.g., terror and suicide) and positive (e.g., serenity) outcomes. Research into life review has shown that it is no more difficult for older people than younger: indeed it may be an important skill developed over the lifespan to assist in preventing negative outcomes and maintaining subjective well-being, used by some but not by others (see Wink & Schiff, 2002) as a way of coping. In fact older adults may be better able than others to find meaning through review of personal experiences (Pasupathi, 2001). Like other skills, these may be facilitated through traning interventions, as findings from early studies involving intervention suggest that there is significant plasticity, for example in terms of increased scores when knowledge relevant to value relativism is activated, and when dyads can work on tasks (Böhmig-Krumhaar, Staudinger & Baltes, 2002; Staudinger & Baltes, 1996).

Work on *autobiographical memory* and *reminiscence* (Bluck & Levine, 1998) suggests that there are two distinct outcomes of reconstructing memories of one's life: self-acceptance, which we have associated above with adjustment and subjective well-being in a more hedonic sense; and self-change, which Bluck and Levine (1998) define as changes to one's self-concept. Looking back on one's life experiences with a goal of self-change may be associated with eudaimonic well-being, for example in the case of eudaimonic resilience. Eudaimonic resilience is a response after a difficult event that involves an exercise in meaning-making and thereby growth, not only a return to baseline levels of affect, as is typically the result of resilience (Bauer & Park, 2010; Bauer, Chap. 10, this volume). The process of review inherently involves evaluation, and here we are reminded of Erikson's (e.g., Erikson & Erikson, 1997) concept of integrity in the final stage of life: it is not an objective goodness of action throughout one's life that is indicative of wisdom: successfully navigating through the conflicts of prior stages equips one with the ability to make sense of previous experience in a manner supportive of continued mental health. Rumination, for example, as opposed to reflection, consists in passive dwelling on subjectively negative aspects and may be both a cause and a consequence of lower levels of well-being (Staudinger, 2001). An ability to actively review lives with sufficient emotional detachment to engage with previously experienced emotions without being consumed by them should be considered a necessary condition for development along a growth trajectory towards wisdom. This resonates with Nussbaum's reminder of the Socratic suggestion that happiness requires self-examination, which she claims is missing from contemporary subjective-state psychology (2008): we consider such skills in reflection to be more characteristic of growth towards wisdom rather than towards happiness per se. As stated earlier, in our view, both hedonic and eudaimonic well-being can be experienced along the path towards wisdom. However neither hedonic nor eudaimonic well-being, experienced separately or together, is sufficient for the development of wisdom. On the contrary, at least as far as hedonic satisfaction is concerned, the pursuit of well-being may well interfere with a person's development towards wisdom.

9.7 Conclusion

In this chapter, we have used the psychological study of wisdom to demonstrate that, in contrast to Nussbaum's (2008) assertions, there is a substantial body of psychological literature that, for quite some time, has looked beyond the simplistic notions of happiness limited to hedonic pursuits (cf., Diener, 2000; Kahneman & Krueger, 2006). In presenting a definition of wisdom that is heavily dependent on an understanding of the good life as involving self-transcendence and a concern for the good of others, we hope we have shown the depth of investigation already available to review. Although there remains disagreement about how to define and measure wisdom (Staudinger & Glück, 2011), the increasingly comprehensive body of work associated with these endeavours has indeed provided substantial reason for the consideration of eudaimonic pursuits as, at the very least, worthy of more attention. In particular, we have addressed a distinction between two trajectories of person development, adjustment and growth. Although adjustment is the more typical pathway and is strongly associated with the pursuit of hedonic satisfaction in life, it certainly does not encompass the full range of positive outcomes available and in this sense we agree with the criticism that an attempt to measure well-being only with indicators of adjustment will fall short. However, we have also illustrated through our presentation of findings in wisdom research that the growth trajectory, while bearing many similarities to eudaimonia, is not synonymous with it. This is in particular because the typical psychological understanding of eudaimonia tends to emphasize the pursuit of self-related, self-actualizing goals, while growth towards wisdom is charaterized by a balance of such goals with a concern for the welfare of other people and society as a whole.

References

Ardelt, M. (1997). Wisdom and life satisfaction in old age. *The Journals of Gerontology Series B: Psychological Sciences and Social Sciences, 52B*(1), P15–P27.

Ardelt, M. (2003). Empirical assessment of a three-dimensional wisdom scale. *Research on Aging, 25*(3), 275–324. doi:10.1177/0164027503025003004.

Baltes, P. B., & Staudinger, U. M. (2000). Wisdom: A metaheuristic (pragmatic) to orchestrate mind and virtue toward excellence. *American Psychologist, 55*(1), 122–136.

Baltes, P. B. (2004). *Wisdom: Orchestrating mind and virtue.* Manuscript in preparation.

Bauer, J. J., & Park, S. W. (2010). Growth is not just for the young: Growth narratives, eudaimonic resilience, and the aging self. In P. S. Fry & C. L. M. Keyes (Eds.), *New frontiers in resilient aging: Life-strengths and well-being in late life* (pp. 60–89). Cambridge, UK: Cambridge University Press.

Bergsma, A., & Ardelt, M. (2012). Self-reported wisdom and happiness: An empirical investigation. *Journal of Happiness Studies, 13*(3), 481–499. doi:10.1007/s10902-011-9275-5.

Bluck, S., & Glück, J. (2005). From the inside out: People's implicit theories of wisdom. In R. J. Sternberg & J. Jordan (Eds.), *A handbook of wisdom* (pp. 84–109). New York: Cambridge University Press.

Bluck, S., & Levine, L. J. (1998). Reminiscence as autobiographical memory: A catalyst for reminiscence theory development. *Ageing and Society, 18*(02), 185–208.

Böhmig-Krumhaar, S. A., Staudinger, U. M., & Baltes, P. B. (2002). Mehr toleranz tut not: Lässt sich wert-relativierendes wissen und urteilen mit hilfe einer wissensaktivierenden gedächtnisstrategie verbessern? [In search of more tolerance: Testing the facilitative effect of a knowledge-activating mnemonic strategy on value relativism]. *Zeitschrift Für Entwicklungspsychologie Und Pädagogische Psychologie, 34*(1), 30–43. doi:10.1026//0049-8637.34.1.30.

Brugman, G. M. (2006). In J. E. Birren & K. W. Schaire (Eds.), *Wisdom and aging* (pp. 445–475). Amsterdam, The Netherlands: Elsevier. doi:10.1016/B978-012101264-9/50023-9.

Butler, R. N. (1963). The life review: An interpretation of reminiscence in the aged. *Psychiatry, 26*, 65–76.

Costa, P. T., Jr., McCrae, R. R., & Dye, D. A. (1991). Facet scales for agreeableness and conscientiousness: A revision of the NEO personality inventory. *Personality and Individual Differences, 12*(9), 887–898. doi:10.1016/0191-8869(91)90177-D.

Csikszentmihalyi, M. (1999). If we are so rich, why aren't we happy? *American Psychologist, 54*(10), 821–827. doi:10.1037/0003-066X.54.10.821.

Diener, E. (2000). Subjective well-being: The science of happiness and a proposal for a national index. *American Psychologist, 55*(1), 34–43.

Dörner, J., Mickler, C., & Staudinger, U. M. (2005). Self-development at midlife. Lifespan perspectives on adjustment and growth. In S. L. Willis & M. Martin (Eds.), *Middle adulthood: A lifespan perspective* (pp. 277–317). Thousand Oaks, CA: Sage.

Erikson, E. H., & Erikson, J. M. (1997). *The life cycle completed.* New York: W.W. Norton.

Field, D., & Millsap, R. E. (1991). Personality in advanced old age: Continuity or change? *Journal of Gerontology, 46*(6), P299–P308. doi:10.1093/geronj/46.6.P299.

Habermas, T., & Bluck, S. (2000). Getting a life: The emergence of the life story in adolescence. *Psychological Bulletin, 126*(5), 748. doi:10.1037/0033-2909.126.5.748.

Hearn, S., Saulnier, G., Strayer, J., Glenham, M., Koopman, R., & Marcia, J. (2012). Between integrity and despair: Toward construct validation of Erikson's eighth stage. *Journal of Adult Development, 19*(1), 1–20. doi:10.1007/s10804-011-9126-y.

Helson, R., & Srivastava, S. (2001). Three paths of adult development: Conservers, seekers, and achievers. *Journal of Personality and Social Psychology, 80*(6), 995–1010. doi:10.1037/0022-3514.80.6.995.

Helson, R., & Wink, P. (1987). Two conceptions of maturity examined in the findings of a longitudinal study. *Journal of Personality and Social Psychology, 53*(3), 531–541. doi:10.1037/0022-3514.53.3.531.

Höffe, O. (2007). *Lebenskunst und moral [Art of Living and Morals].* Munich, Germany: C.H. Beck.

Jahoda, M. (1958). *Current concepts of positive mental health.* New York: Basic Books.

Kahneman, D., & Krueger, A. B. (2006). Developments in the measurement of subjective well-being. *Journal of Economic Perspectives, 20*(1), 3–24. doi:10.1257/089533006776526030.

Kekes, J. (1983). Wisdom. *American Philosophical Quarterly, 20*, 277–286.

Kramer, D. A. (1983). Post-formal operations? A need for further conceptualization. *Human Development, 26*(2), 91–105. doi:10.1159/000272873.

Kringelbach, M. L., & Berridge, K. C. (2009). Towards a functional neuroanatomy of pleasure and happiness. *Trends in Cognitive Sciences, 13*(11), 479–487. doi:10.1016/j.tics.2009.08.006.

Kunzmann, U. (2007). Wisdom: Motivational and emotional dynamics in old age. In R. Fernández-Ballesteros (Ed.), *Geropsychology: European perspectives for an ageing world* (pp. 224–238). Gottingen, Germany: Hogrefe & Huber.

Labouvie-Vief, G., Diehl, M., Jain, E., & Zhang, F. (2007). Six-year change in affect optimization and affect complexity across the adult life span: A further examination. *Psychology and Aging, 22*(4), 738–751. doi:10.1037/0882-7974.22.4.738.

Labouvie-Vief, G., & Medler, M. (2002). Affect optimization and affect complexity: Modes and styles of regulation in adulthood. *Psychology and Aging, 17*(4), 571–588.

Luyckx, K., Seiffge-Krenke, I., Schwartz, S. J., Goossens, L., Weets, I., Hendrieckx, C., et al. (2008). Identity development, coping, and adjustment in emerging adults with a chronic illness: The sample case of type 1 diabetes. *Journal of Adolescent Health, 43*(5), 451–458. doi:10.1016/j.jadohealth.2008.04.005.

Marcia, J. E. (1966). Development and validation of ego identity status. *Journal of Personality and Social Psychology, 3*(5), 551–558. doi:10.1037/h0023281.

Maslow, A. H. (1954). *Motivation and personality*. Oxford, UK: Harpers.

Mickler, C., & Staudinger, U. M. (2008). Personal wisdom: Validation and age-related differences of a performance measure. *Psychology and Aging, 23*(4), 787–799. doi:10.1037/a0013928.

Nussbaum, M. C. (2008). Who is the happy warrior? Philosophy poses questions to psychology. *The Journal of Legal Studies, 37*, S81–S113. doi:10.1086/587438.

Pasupathi, M. (2001). The social construction of the personal past and its implications for adult development. *Psychological Bulletin, 127*(5), 651. doi:10.1037/0033-2909.127.5.651.

Pasupathi, M., & Staudinger, U. M. (2001). Do advanced moral reasoners also show wisdom? Linking moral reasoning and wisdom-related knowledge and judgement. *International Journal of Behavioral Development, 25*(5), 401–415. doi:10.1080/016502501316934833.

Pasupathi, M., Staudinger, U. M., & Baltes, P. B. (2001). Seeds of wisdom: Adolescents' knowledge and judgment about difficult life problems. *Developmental Psychology, 37*(3), 351–361. doi:10.1037/0012-1649.37.3.351.

Peterson, B. E., & Klohnen, E. C. (1995). Realization of generativity in two samples of women at midlife. *Psychology and Aging, 10*(1), 20–29. doi:10.1037/0882-7974.10.1.20.

Rogers, C. R. (1962). Toward becoming a fully functioning person. In A. W. Combs (Ed.), *Perceiving, behaving, becoming: A new focus for education* (pp. 21–33). Washington, DC: National Education Association. doi:10.1037/14325-003.

Ryan, S. (2014). *Wisdom*. Retrieved from http://plato.stanford.edu/archives/win2014/entries/wisdom/

Ryan, R. M., & Deci, E. L. (2000). Self-determination theory and the facilitation of intrinsic motivation, social development, and well-being. *American Psychologist, 55*(1), 68. doi:10.1037/0003-066X.55.1.68.

Ryff, C. D. (1989). Happiness is everything, or is it? Explorations on the meaning of psychological well-being. *Journal of Personality and Social Psychology, 57*(6), 1069–1081. doi:10.1037/0022-3514.57.6.1069.

Ryff, C. D., & Singer, B. H. (2008). Know thyself and become what you are: A eudaimonic approach to psychological well-being. *Journal of Happiness Studies, 9*(1), 13–39. doi:10.1007/s10902-006-9019-0.

Schwartz, B., & Sharpe, K. E. (2006). Practical wisdom: Aristotle meets positive psychology. *Journal of Happiness Studies, 7*(3), 377–395. doi:10.1007/s10902-005-3651-y.

Seiffge-Krenke, I., & Gelhaar, T. (2008). Does successful attainment of developmental tasks lead to happiness and success in later developmental tasks? A test of Havighurst's (1948) theses. *Journal of Adolescence, 31*(1), 33–52.

Smith, J., & Baltes, P. B. (1990). Wisdom-related knowledge: Age/cohort differences in response to life-planning problems. *Developmental Psychology, 26*(3), 494–505. doi:10.1037/0012-1649.26.3.494.

Smith, J., Staudinger, U. M., & Baltes, P. B. (1994). Occupational settings facilitating wisdom-related knowledge: The sample case of clinical psychologists. *Journal of Consulting and Clinical Psychology, 62*(5), 989–999. doi:10.1037/0022-006X.62.5.989.

Staudinger, U. M. (1999a). Social cognition and a psychological approach to the art of life. In F. Blanchard-Fields & T. Hess (Eds.), *Social cognition and aging* (pp. 343–375). New York: Academic.

Staudinger, U. M. (1999b). Older and wiser? Integrating results on the relationship between age and wisdom-related performance. *International Journal of Behavioral Development, 23*(3), 641–664. doi:10.1080/016502599383739.

Staudinger, U. M. (2001). Life reflection: A social–cognitive analysis of life review. *Review of General Psychology, 5*(2), 148–160. doi:10.1037/1089-2680.5.2.148.

Staudinger, U. M. (2013). The need to distinguish personal from general wisdom: A short history and empirical evidence. In M. Ferrari & N. Westrate (Eds.), *The scientific study of personal wisdom* (pp. 3–19). Dordrecht, The Netherlands: Springer.

Staudinger, U. M., & Baltes, P. B. (1996). Interactive minds: A facilitative setting for wisdom-related performance? *Journal of Personality and Social Psychology, 71*(4), 746–762. doi:10.1037/0022-3514.71.4.746.

Staudinger, U. M., Dörner, J., & Mickler, C. (2005). Wisdom and personality. In R. J. Sternberg & J. Jordan (Eds.), *A handbook of wisdom* (pp. 191–219). New York: Cambridge University Press.

Staudinger, U. M., & Glück, J. (2011). Psychological wisdom research: Commonalities and differences in a growing field. *Annual Review of Psychology, 62*(1), 215–241. doi:10.1146/annurev.psych.121208.131659.

Staudinger, U. M., & Kessler, E. M. (2009). Adjustment and growth: Two trajectories of positive personality development across adulthood. In M. C. Smith & N. DeFrates-Densch (Eds.), *Handbook of research on adult learning and development* (pp. 241–268). New York: Routledge.

Staudinger, U. M., & Kunzmann, U. (2005). Positive adult personality development. *European Psychologist, 10*(4), 320–329. doi:10.1027/1016-9040.10.4.320.

Staudinger, U. M., Lopez, D. F., & Baltes, P. B. (1997). The psychometric location of wisdom-related performance: Intelligence, personality, and more? *Personality and Social Psychology Bulletin, 23*(11), 1200–1214. doi:10.1177/01461672972311007.

Staudinger, U. M., Maciel, A. G., Smith, J., & Baltes, P. B. (1998). What predicts wisdom-related performance? A first look at personality, intelligence, and facilitative experiential contexts. *European Journal of Personality, 12*(1), 1–17.

Staudinger, U. M., & Pasupathi, M. (2003). Correlates of wisdom-related performance in adolescence and adulthood: Age-graded differences in "Paths" toward desirable development. *Journal of Research on Adolescence, 13*(3), 239–268. doi:10.1111/1532-7795.1303001.

Staudinger, U. M., Smith, J., & Baltes, P. B. (1992). Wisdom-related knowledge in a life review task: Age differences and the role of professional specialization. *Psychology and Aging, 7*(2), 271–281. doi:10.1037/0882-7974.7.2.271.

Sternberg, R. J. (Ed.). (1990). *Wisdom: Its nature, origins, and development*. New York: Cambridge University Press.

Sternberg, R. J. (1998). A balance theory of wisdom. *Review of General Psychology, 2*(4), 347–365. doi:10.1037/1089-2680.2.4.347.

Vittersø, J., & Søholt, Y. (2011). Life satisfaction goes with pleasure and personal growth goes with interest: Further arguments for separating hedonic and eudaimonic well-being. *The Journal of Positive Psychology, 6*(4), 326–335. doi:10.1080/17439760.2011.584548.

Waterman, A. S. (1990). Personal expressiveness: Philosophical and psychological foundations. *Journal of Mind and Behavior, 11*(1), 47–73.

Waterman, A. S. (1993). Two conceptions of happiness: Contrasts of personal expressiveness (eudaimonia) and hedonic enjoyment. *Journal of Personality and Social Psychology, 64*(4), 678. doi:10.1037/0022-3514.64.4.678.

Webster, J. D. (2003). An exploratory analysis of a self-assessed wisdom scale. *Journal of Adult Development, 10*(1), 13–22. doi:10.1023/A:1020782619051.

Webster, J. D., Taylor, M., & Bates, G. (2011). Conceptualizing and measuring wisdom: A reply to Ardelt. *Experimental Aging Research, 37*(2), 256–259. doi:10.1080/0361073X.2011.554514.

Whitbourne, S. K., & Waterman, A. S. (1979). Psychosocial development during the adult years: Age and cohort comparisons. *Developmental Psychology, 15*(4), 373. doi:10.1037/0012-1649.15.4.373.

Wink, P., & Helson, R. (1997). Practical and transcendent wisdom: Their nature and some longitudinal findings. *Journal of Adult Development, 4*(1), 1–15. doi:10.1007/BF02511845.

Wink, P., & Schiff, B. (2002). To review or not to review? The role of personality and life events in life review and adaptation to older age. In J. D. Webster & B. K. Haight (Eds.), *Critical advances in reminiscence work: From theory to application* (pp. 44–60). New York: Springer.

Wink, P., & Staudinger, U. M. (2015). Wisdom and psychosocial functioning in later life. *Journal of Personality*. doi:10.1111/jopy.12160.

10 Eudaimonic Growth: The Development of the Goods in Personhood (or: Cultivating a Good Life Story)

Jack J. Bauer

That eudaimonia develops is hardly debated. No one is born with eudaimonic well-being. However, eudaimonic models of a good life, from Aristotle to the present day, in both philosophy and psychology, typically do not examine the processes and contexts of development. Eudaimonic models must assume that eudaimonia develops somehow, but in the end most models define and measure eudaimonia by whether a person's life, at one point in time, has eudaimonic qualities or not, without much regard to the developmental factors that yield such a life. This chapter is about how the goods in life develop. I call this process *eudaimonic growth*.

One might ask: Who cares? What does it matter *how* the person comes to a good life, so long as he or she does? Even I agree that, for the purpose of this or that research study, the processes of eudaimonic growth may be of no legitimate concern. But such an approach, as a model of a good life, is likely to neglect key factors in both what might constitute a good life and what makes a good life possible in the first place. Without considering the dynamic ways in which a life unfolds over time, we can be easily misled into thinking that the good in life can and should be modeled in simple ways—perhaps more for the desire of parsimonious modeling than for the endeavor to understand individuals' lives.

The term *good life* has two words. Almost all the debate on the topic revolves around the first word, good. The question of what makes a good life is almost always interpreted to mean, "What is the good?" But I prefer to start with the second word, life. "What is life?" asks George Kelly in laying the groundwork for his theory of personal constructs (1955, p. 7). "There are some parts of the universe which make a good deal of sense even when they are not viewed in the perspective of *time*. But there are other parts which make sense only when they are plotted along a time line. Life is one of the latter. …[L]ife has to be seen in the perspective of time if it is to make any sense at all" (emphasis added). Similarly, I take a good life to mean more than just an evaluation of the person at a single point in time, and certainly more than just an evaluation of one or two features of the person (say, pleasure or meaning) at a single point in time. As I see it, a claim about a good *life* is a claim about the individual person over time, about personhood over time, and about the goods within personhood that develop over time.

J.J. Bauer (✉)
University of Dayton, Dayton, OH, USA
e-mail: jack.bauer@udayton.edu

J. Vittersø (ed.), *Handbook of Eudaimonic Well-Being*, International Handbooks of Quality-of-Life,
DOI 10.1007/978-3-319-42445-3_10

10.1 Overview of this Chapter

This chapter addresses two primary questions. The first section of the chapter asks: What is the good of personhood? The second and third chapters ask: How does it develop?

The first section of the chapter outlines a model of the varied goods of personhood—a personological model of eudaimonia. This model integrates eudaimonics and hedonics; I argue that meaning and pleasure are two, irreducible goods of personhood. Furthermore, I provide a framework of philosophically subjectivist and objectivist approaches to the good in which just about every measure of eudaimonia and hedonia can be mapped. Again, the aim here is to understand personhood in terms of the good. From this perspective, well-being becomes a matter not of simply either pleasure or meaningfulness but rather of the *wellness of one's being*. One's being surely includes pleasure but not exclusively or ultimately. Wisdom, moral virtues, meaningfulness, and growth all obtain as well.

Following from that model, the second section of the chapter examines the idea of eudaimonic growth. Of particular focus is the distinction between eudaimonic, humanistic, and organismic perspectives on growth. Also of focus is the distinction between growth attained and growth valued, both of which are essential considerations.

The third section of the chapter considers the relation between eudaimonic growth and self-identity. The person who identifies with the idea of eudaimonic growth has what I call a *transformative self* (Bauer, 2016). The idea of growth serves as a central feature of this person's mental model of self—and as a central theme in this person's life story. I focus on *narrative* self-identity, an approach that is especially well suited for studying self-identity in relation to cultural concepts of a good life. Life stories and a good life shed light on each other, theoretically and empirically. A life story is an attempt to construct a story of a good life (Taylor, 1989). Conversely, the features of a good life gain their meaning—indeed, become good—in the context of stories. The words "good life story" in the title of this chapter refer to a story of a good life. The person with a transformative self draws on cultural master narratives of a good life.

To give an overview of the various concepts in this chapter, Table 10.1 shows how the varied goods in life can be divvied into five umbrella categories and how these five categories map reasonably well onto five features of life stories, respectively. The five umbrella categories of a the goods in life are hedonic happiness, love (which includes communal love for others, agentic love for activities, and a sense of meaningfulness), wisdom, and growth. The five narrative features are affective tone, motivational theme, organizational structure, and temporal development. This chapter is an exercise in explaining this table. By way of introduction, this table compares concepts that focus on similar kinds of goods in life. For example, affective tones in a personal narrative deal with the positive or negative assessments in a narrative, but not the specific value orientations or motivations of the narrative. Similarly, hedonia as a model of a good life deals with the positive or negative assessments of a life, but not the specific value orientations or motivations in the

Table 10.1 How theoretical features of narrative self-identity and a good life reflect each other to form a model of personhood and its goods

Features of narrative self-identity	Features of meaning-making	The good in life/personhood	Model of a good life
Plot	Facts	Basic needs	Assumed conditions for a good life
Tone	Affective valence	Happiness	Hedonia
Theme	Value and motive	Love	Eudaimonia
Structure	Perspectivity	Wisdom	
Time	Development	Growth	

person's life. In contrast, the narrative features of value-laden themes, structural perspectivity, and development over time all map onto primary goods in eudaimonic models of a good life.

10.2 The Big Umbrella of Eudaimonia

One of the problems of eudaimonia is that it means so many things (Kashdan, Biswas-Diener, & King, 2008; Ward & King, Chap. 35, this volume). Each eudaimonist has his or her own list of candidate goods in life. Furthermore, many if not most measures of eudaimonic well-being correlate with measures of hedonic happiness, most notably subjective well-being as defined by pleasure and satisfaction (Diener, Lucas, & Scollon, 2006; Haybron, 2008, this volume; Sheldon, 2013, this volume). As a result, some have claimed that it makes sense to drop the term *eudaimonia* altogether and simply focus on subjective well-being and the many correlates and contributors of it. However, I advocate using the terms *eudaimonia* and *eudaimonic well-being* if only because they remind us that well-being can mean something broader that merely pleasure and satisfaction (while simultaneously acknowledging their importance). Hedonic happiness is not the only worthwhile good. Furthermore, it is not the ultimate outcome; hedonic judgments of good or bad only seem to be the "bottom line," and then only from subjectivist and non-organismic perspectives on personhood.

If I had to choose a single word to represent the many facets of eudaimonia as it is typically studied, I would choose *meaning*. Naturally a single term is unsatisfactory. But meaning serves as a handy contrast to the term *pleasure*, which is commonly used as a defining characteristic of hedonia (even if hedonia is more aptly summarized as the combination of pleasurable experience and satisfaction—Haybron, 2008). The term *meaning*, as I interpret it, refers to all qualities of the good in life besides hedonic pleasure and satisfaction, such as wisdom, moral virtues, self-actualizing, a sense of meaningfulness or fulfillment, and other canonical qualities of eudaimonia.

In this section of the chapter we first consider how pleasure and meaning are two, irreducible goods of personhood. Then we examine subjectivist and objectivist approaches to the measurement of the goods of personhood, the combination of which offers a more comprehensive model of a good life. Finally I organize all those measures into five umbrella categories of a good life—basic-need fulfillment, happiness, love, wisdom, and growth—that I view as helpful to the study of well-being generally and to the study of it in relation to self-identity.

10.2.1 How Eudaimonia Can Encompass Pleasure and Meaning

Eudaimonia is typically contrasted with hedonia, but several models allow for a more compatibilist view (e.g., Bauer & McAdams, 2010; Huta, 2013, this volume; Keyes, Schmotkin, & Ryff, 2002; Sheldon, 2013). What matters for hedonic theories of a good life is the focus on pleasure and satisfaction (Haybron, 2008). In contrast, what matters for eudaimonic theories is a focus on meaning (Wolf, 2010), by which is meant an umbrella term for any of the kinds of things that might bring about enduring pleasures or enduring satisfaction—and that might be valuable for other purposes as well. Meaning in this broad sense is well-suited as an overarching, single term to capture the qualities of eudaimonia that can be differentiated from hedonia (Steger, Yeon Shin, Shim, & Fitch-Martin, 2013; Steger, Chap. 11, this volume). In this section I wish to present the case that pleasure and meaning are two, irreducible goods in life. Between hedonia and eudaimonia, only eudaimonia allows for such a view, since the hedonic argument is one of exclusivity. To the question, "What makes a good life?" the hedonist answers, "Pleasure, period." The eudaimonist typically answers, "Meaning, period." I wish to argue that the eudaimonist answer can be "Pleasure plus meaning." Put another way, pleasure is necessary but not sufficient *as a candidate good* for a good life.[1]

Is Pleasure Necessary as a Candidate Good? Yes

Pleasure is important on its own. No, pleasure is not a uniquely human quality and is certainly not virtuous in itself. But yes, pleasure is universally (or nearly universally) desired. Soon into this discussion we see that pleasure can have several meanings, e.g., as an experience, an attitude, or a positive feeling that has more to do with the feeling of knowing that one acted virtuously or even experienced virtue (Vittersø, 2013, this volume). Still, I am claiming that pleasure in the hedonic sense can be valued in its own sake. Now, intrinsically motivated activities—that is, actions done for the pleasure of doing them—have specifically eudaimonic qualities (Waterman, Schwartz, & Conti, 2008; Schwartz & Wrzesniewski, Chap. 8, this volume). But it is a strong argument that pleasure or satisfaction (either for oneself or someone else, either intense or subtle) is the ultimate aim for action (Sheldon, 2013). On a more simplistic level, the word good can mean "pleasurable" or "virtuous." A life with pleasure is more full and simply better in subjectively experienced ways than a life without pleasure, other things equal. A person whose life has virtue but lacks pleasure may certainly be said to have a good life, but try asking that person who lacks pleasure whether something significant in life is missing. For these reasons I view pleasure, on its own, to be a candidate good in life (and thereby claim that moral goods are not the only goods worth considering in a good life). However, arguments for the universality and even primacy of pleasure do not legitimize the argument for the exclusivity of pleasure.

[1] Here I am presenting a case for what goods (like pleasure and meaning) are on the list for a good life. A good life may have pleasure but not virtuous meaning. A good life may have virtuous meaning but not pleasure. A good life need not have both.

Is Pleasure Sufficient as a Candidate Good? No

I have three problems with the purely hedonic position. First is that it is too selfish. Hedonists have always had to battle this criticism. Their solutions, short of collapsing into solipsism, invariably involve the qualification of pleasures. Few models of hedonia claim that any form of pleasure counts for a good life (Flanagan, 2011). Selfishness and hurtful hedonic activity are generally out of bounds. Hedonic models of a good life often include *some* consideration of others, as in Bentham's notion of the greatest good for the greatest number of people. Problems of overindulgence are tempered by beliefs in balance, such as Aristotle's golden mean, Buddha's middle way, or (from a more hedonic perspective) Epicurus' equanimity, which derives from an equilibrium between excess and deficiency (Warren, 2009). The perils of advocating "pleasure, period" have also been tempered by qualifications that hedonic happiness be grounded in authenticity (Sumner, 1996), which is in most cases a eudaimonist concern and requires elaborate contortions to be rendered hedonic. In any case, it is clear that pleasure needs to be qualified in some context—which is to say, by this or that source of meaning.

My second reason why pleasure is not sufficient has to do with what I call the "negativity paradox." If pleasure is good and pain is bad, then it is impossible to explain a great deal of research showing that there is such a thing as too much pleasure. For instance, when adjusting to difficult life circumstances, the exclusive, subjective focus on positive experiences actually predicts poorer adjustment than a "mostly positive, some negative" focus, or a ratio of 3:1 or 5:1 positive-to-negative evaluations (Bauer & Bonanno, 2001; Fredrickson, 2013; Pennebaker & Seagal, 1999). When considering life in general, cultural ideals for a good life story are not exclusively positive but instead call for a transition from bad to good, which Dan McAdams (2006) calls "the redemptive self." As the old saying in journalism goes, no one wants to read a headline like "Millions Happy in Kansas Sunshine."

Third, hedonia is too simple. Valerie Tiberius (2013) notes that hedonists criticize eudaimonists for having too variable and too long a list of "ingredients" for a good life (see also Tiberius, Chap. 38, this volume). But she criticizes hedonists for having too short a list—a list of one item, which is to say, pleasure. Subjectively, most people value both pleasure and meaning (Baumeister, Vohs, Aaker, & Garbinsky, 2013; King & Napa, 1998). People do not want simply to feel good. The philosopher Robert Nozick's (1983) experience machine gets at this question: If you could be hooked up to a machine that makes you feel good no matter what suffering might otherwise surround you, would you choose to be hooked up? (Or, would you take the blue pill in *The Matrix*?) The fact is that truth matters for people, and the search for truth is not all roses. Then there are the evolutionary arguments for our basic need for a concern for others, which is to say, that moral behavior is an inherent good for persons (Keltner, 2010). Hedonic models simply exclude too much of what makes a life good.

Pleasurable Experience and the Slippery Slope Toward Eudaimonia

Pleasurable experience is generally the domain of hedonists. Yet intrinsically motivated activities—those done for the sheer pleasure or enjoyment of the activity itself—are closely tied to self-realization, flow experiences, and other sources of eudaimonic meaning in life (Waterman et al., 2008). Experiential rather than material purchases yield enduring effects of happiness—which is to say, *meaningful* effects (Van Boven & Gilovich, 2003). Experiential purchases foster reminiscence, particularly of experiences shared with close others, and guard against the rumination and counterfactual thinking that come with material purchases (Carter & Gilovich, 2010). The link between experiences of pure pleasure and meaning is important. The hedonist might argue that pleasure is what makes the experience important, and the eudaimonist might argue for the meaning of that pleasurable event. The pleasure of pursuing virtuous activities, as distinct from purely hedonic experience (which is to say, non-eudaimonic), plays a critical role in understanding pleasure and eudaimonia (Vittersø, 2013). However, I wish to take things a bit further to claim that hedonic pleasure on its own, regardless of whether it is tied to a virtuous context (either by the individual subjectively or by objective assessment), should serve as a candidate good in the eudaimonic list. What makes this position eudaimonic rather than hedonic is that I am also claiming that hedonic pleasure is not enough. It must be balanced, as must all candidate goods—for the same reason that any one virtuous act can do harm to someone—within the broader context of the person, in the context of situations, within the broader context of the person's development over time within a social ecology. In other words, I'm targeting the wellness of one's being, broadly construed. As for the rationale, I look to the meeting of pleasure and meaning in the concept of value.

10.2.2 Value as the Nexus of Pleasure and Meaning

Value has facets of thinking and feeling. Schwartz and Bilsky (1990) define a value as a concept or belief that has a desirable end state or behavior (note the implication of pleasure) and that endures beyond the immediate moment, among other qualities. Values represent what people (with an emphasis on persons) feel and think are important or meaningful over time. Here I argue that values are an *enduring pleasure* that is defined in terms of the specific context of that pleasure, which is to say, a *meaning*.

Any one meaning involves a sense of desirability or pleasure at its core. Yet a fleeting pleasure is itself not meaningful unless a set of fleeting pleasures are strung together conceptually into a meaning—and unless a person finds the strung-together meaning pleasing. Value is *felt* as the pleasure of a specific source or context of a pleasing or satisfying experience. Value is *thought* as the specific meaning or context of that pleasing or satisfying experience. In other words, values link together conceptual meanings and felt affects. Thus values are at the heart of meaning;

they make a conceptual meaning *meaningful*. But as to whether felt pleasure or conceptual meaning takes center stage, I am hard pressed to say. Value exists as pleasure and meaning co-arise in a context of persons, situations, personal development, and the social ecology of each.

In the context of a good life, a meaning is a conceptual knowledge structure that holds personal value; it is personally *meaningful*. Such meanings come in many forms, such as wisdom, virtue, friendship, etc. Meaning from this perspective is a *context* (Baumeister, 1991). For instance, a pleasurable experience becomes meaningful upon thinking about the experience in terms of its context: Watching a sunset, playing with a friend, or enduring a hardship becomes meaningful upon thinking about the activity in terms of the people in it (who are personally meaningful and endure over time; this might include the self), the place (which is personally meaningful and endures over time), particular ideals or values themselves (such as fairness or care), and the like.

10.2.3 Orientations, Fulfillments, and Structures of Value

Values are measured in psychology in three general ways, in terms of their orientation, fulfillment, and structure. Psychological measures of value orientation include measures that assess whether or how much a person is oriented toward particular *types* of meaning. Measures of values and motivation—but not motivation fulfillment—fall into this category (e.g., growth motivation—Bauer, Park, Montoya, & Wayment, 2015; achievement motives of mastery, performance, approach, and avoidance—Elliot & McGregor, 2001; moral foundations of justice, care, authority, loyalty, and purity—Graham et al., 2011; eudaimonic and hedonic motives—Huta & Ryan, 2010; self-determined and controlled motives—Deci & Ryan, 2000; various values like universalism, benevolence, power, security, and stimulation—Schwartz, 2007).

Measures of value fulfillment assess any form of meaningfulness, whether in general or in a specific context or domain of life. The term *meaningfulness* is the evaluation and experience that a particular value or meaning has been fulfilled. By meaningfulness I mean a value fulfillment (Baumeister, 1991; Tiberius, 2014; Wolf, 2010), which, when studied as central values to one's selfhood can include self-fulfillment (Haybron, 2008). When one assesses one's own life as meaningful, one is likely drawing on the feeling that a particular meaning or value orientation has been fulfilled to a personally satisfying degree—that a need for meaning (Baumeister, 1991) has been met. Here we see the primary difference between hedonia and eudaimonia. From the perspective of meaningfulness just described, life satisfaction can be viewed as a form of meaningfulness. Because life satisfaction does not take into consideration a specific context of meaning but rather one's life in general, life satisfaction is among the most general and abstract forms of meaningfulness, having much more in common with the context-free assessments of affectivity and global self-esteem than with the context-specific assessments of various forms of meaning in life (e.g., meaningful relationships or a sense or environmental mastery—Ryff & Singer, 2008). Life satisfaction correlates with meaningfulness in life (Steger, Frazier, Oishi, & Kaler, 2006), but life satisfaction itself is a global assessment that a life is satisfying, without reference to the varied sources (that is, the context, the meaning) of that satisfaction. It is the source or context of an assessment of pleasure or satisfaction that reflects meaningfulness and is of concern for eudaimonists (e.g., Wolf, 2010; not that meaningfulness is of universal concern for eudaimonists). As soon as an assessment involves the consideration of specific sources of meaning—love, work, personal mastery, etc.—we have an assessment of meaningfulness. Thus I have claimed that Ryff's measure of psychological well-being is a measure of meaningfulness: It assesses six domains of meaning in life, with an emphasis on the degree to which one feels that those values in life have been satisfied or fulfilled (Bauer et al., 2015; Bauer, McAdams, & Pals, 2008). Similarly, the Meaning in Life Questionnaire—Presence subscale (Steger et al., 2006) measures the degree to which a person claims to "have" meaning in life, which is to say, to have certain valued meanings relatively fulfilled in life. However, unlike Ryff's measure, Steger's measure targets meaningfulness in general, rather than specific contexts of it.

Finally, measures of value structure focus on neither the type nor the fulfillment of values but rather on the *organizational structure* of the meanings of those values. Value structure is measured as degrees of integrative complexity, perspective-taking, or differentiation and integration in a research participant's thinking about the self and others (Kegan, 1982; Labouvie-Vief, 2006; Loevinger, 1976; Suedfeld & Bluck, 1993; Tadmor, Tetlock, & Peng, 2007). Whereas most psychological measures of value orientations and value fulfillments are subjectively assessed (via self-report), measures of value structure are more objectivist: External researchers identify the degree of complexity, integration, or perspectivity of a person's subjective responses to an open-ended question. Many of (though not all) these measures derive from developmental theory—and a Piagetian, structural-developmental theory in particular. Higher capacities to take multiple perspectives are characterized by higher degrees of psychosocial maturity and wisdom (Staudinger, Dörner, & Mickler, 2005; Law & Staudinger, Chap. 9, this volume).

10.2.4 Subjective and Objective: How We Measure Personhood and a Good Life

I am especially interested in the idea of a reasonably comprehensive model of eudaimonia that is empirically measurable, even if its measurement is not possible in a single set of studies. One of the more divisive issues deals with how we know the good: subjectively or objectively. I see no compelling reason why we cannot study eudaimonia from both subjectivist and objectivist perspectives. I start from the perspective that a good life—if we consider the whole person and indeed the varieties of personhood that might be good—is multifaceted, some of it known to the individual person and some of it not known to the person, or at least not reliably so. The pluralist, radical empiricism of William James (1907, 1909) strikes me as the sensible course if our objective is to come to as comprehensive understanding as possible of a good life. To map out the territory without taking up much space, we can consider the subjectivist–objectivist debate in a 2×4 table that maps the individual person and others onto qualities of the good, such as its beneficiary, criteria, and evaluations (see Table 10.2).

Whose Well-Being? Internalist Versus Externalist Perspectives

One form of the subjectivist-objectivist debate is more precisely about internalist versus externalist perspectives (Haybron, 2008). These perspectives belong to Source 1 in Table 10.2 and address

Table 10.2 Internalist, externalist, subjectivist, and objectivist assumptions in any measure of personhood and its goods

	Sources of information in measuring a person's well-being			
	Source 1	Source 2	Source 3	Source 4
	Beneficiary of the good	Criterion of the good	Description of the Person/well-being	Evaluation of the Person/well-being
	Whose well-being?	Who sets criteria for well-being?	Who describes the person?	Who evaluates the person?
Individual	Internalist participant	Subjectivist participant	Subjectivist participant	Subjectivist participant
Other(s)	Externalist other people	Objectivist researcher(s)	Objectivist other person(s)[a]	Objectivist other person(s)

[a]The other person may be the researcher, a team of researchers, or other research participants

the question: Whose welfare is being taken into consideration—other people's (externalism) or just the individual's (internalism)? Measures that include concern for others' welfare are externalist (e.g., Keyes, 1998; Ryff & Keyes, 1995), noting (and this is important) that they may also include concerns for the individual's own welfare (Haybron, 2008). Measures that include concern for the individual's own welfare (and not explicit concern for others' welfare) are internalist, whether hedonic or (e.g., subjective well-being—Diener et al., 2006) or eudaimonic (meaning in life—Steger et al., 2006). Notably, externalist models of the good may be measured by either subjective (Keyes, 1998; McAdams & de St. Aubin, 1992; Ryff & Keyes, 1995) or objective assessments (Labouvie-Vief, 2006; Loevinger, 1976). What matters is whether the measure asks the assessor to consider the welfare of others.

Whose Criteria for Well-Being?

The question for Source 2 is: Who sets the criteria on which the participants will be measured? I mention Source 2 only for pedagogical purposes, because it is not an issue for scientific measures (and because sometimes this source is mistaken for the other sources). Virtually no scientific research allows the research participants themselves to *define the criteria* of the good for any particular measure. Only the researcher designs the measure. Of course participants can assess themselves in scientific measures via self-report, thereby determining whether a particular characteristic of self is relatively good or bad. But that deals with Sources 3 and 4, not 2.

Who Assesses Well-Being? Subjectivist Versus Objectivist Perspectives

The next two questions are more relevant for scientific measures—particularly Source 4, which is the one that deals with the production of most data in psychological research on well-being, namely self-report. Sources 3 and 4 deal with the description (Source 3) and evaluation (Source 4) of the person's well-being, characteristics, or other qualities. For most research on well-being, which is self-report, Sources 3 and 4 are the same: the individual person who makes the subjective self-report. However, some research methods distinguish the two. For example, narrative research often involves subjective descriptions of the self (Source 3) that are only converted into data by objective (i.e., researcher-rated or computer-rated) assessments of those subjective descriptions (Source 4). Almost always, Source 4 refers to the numerical data of well-being that are used in statistical analyses.

Considering the Combinations

Let's consider how these categories can be used to organize just about any measure of personhood or well-being. Table 10.3 draws on the framework of Table 10.2 to organize measures of hedonia and eudaimonia, including measures of well-being (as typically studied) and measures of motives and values. Measures are first classified by subjectivist versus objectivist evaluations (Source 4) in the top and bottom halves of the table, respectively. Measures are then classified in terms of whose welfare is to be considered (individuals or others too), as defined by the measure that instructs those people in the research study who are making the evaluations of the person. Internalist measures consider the welfare of the individual person alone, whereas externalist measures consider the welfare of other people as well as the individual person (definition of internalism versus externalism from Haybron, 2008). Sources 2 and 3 in Table 10.2 are not considered here. Table 10.3 further differentiates measures according to what they measure: value orientations, value fulfillments, value structure, or time. Finally, Table 10.3 shows how these measures align with umbrella categories of the good in life (happiness, love, wisdom, growth), which is explained in the next section.

To start wading through Table 10.3, let's consider as an example hedonic measures of subjective well-being (e.g., Diener et al., 2006) as well as eudaimonic measures of value orientations (e.g., values—Schwartz, 2007; self-determination theory motives—Deci & Ryan, 2000) and value fulfillments (e.g., presence of meaning in life—Steger et al., 2006; psychological well-being—Ryff & Keyes, 1995). For any of these measures, Source 1 is expressly internalist, because the

Table 10.3 Sample measures of hedonic and eudaimonic well-being, as organized according to internalist, externalist, subjectivist, and objectivist measures

		Source 4: subjectivist evaluation (*all are self-report measures*)					
			Hedonic pleasure	Eudaimonic meaning			
			Happiness	Love		Wisdom	Growth
		Basic needs	VO & VF[a]	Value orientation	Value fulfillment	Value structure	Time
Source 1: beneficiary of the Good	**Internalist**	Self-report on food, survival, health, etc.	Positive and negative affect	Explicit agentic motives and values	Psychological well-being–all but positive relations	Self-described coherence of self, goals, etc.	Self-described improvement in self or agentic concerns
			Life satisfaction	Intrinsic/extrinsic motivation	Presence of meaning in life	Self-rated discrepancy in actual v. ideal, ought, undesired etc. selves	Psychological well-being–personal growth
			Self-esteem	Self-rated agentic narrative themes	Satisfaction of agentic needs		Post-traumatic growth attained
			Hedonic motives	Identity status–exploration	Authenticity (indiv.)		
				Curiosity	Flow experienced		
				Savoring anticipated	Savoring done		
				Eudaimonic motives	Self-efficacy		
					Self-Concept Clarity		
	Externalist			Explicit communal motives and values	Psychological well-being–positive relations	Self-described positioning of self and others	Self-reported improvement in relation-ships or communal concerns
				Generativity	Social well-being		
				Growth motivation	Flourishing		
				Prejudice/group identity	Satisfaction of communal needs		
				Self-actualization	Authenticity (incl. others welfare)		
				Moral foundations	Adult attachment		
				Explicit motives Self-rated comm. narrative themes	Identity status–commitment		

(continued)

Table 10.3 (continued)

		Source 4: objectivist evaluation (*all are non-self-report measures*)					
			Hedonic pleasure	Eudaimonic meaning			
			Happiness	Love		Wisdom	Growth
		Basic needs	VO & VF[a]	Value orientation	Value fulfillment	Value structure	Time
Source 1: beneficiary of the good	**Internalist**	Medical records	Physiologi-cal stress etc.	Implicit agentic motives and values	Researcher-rated, agentic fulfillment	Self-rated coherence of self, goals, etc.	Objective changes over time, agentic
			Targeted marketing in business	Researcher-rated agency-motive themes in narratives[b]	Clinician-rated agentic, healthy functioning	Narrative integrative complexity	Researcher-rated growth attained
				Targeted marketing			
	Externalist	Socio-economic status		Implicit communal motives and values	Researcher-rated relatedness or communal fulfillment	Narrative positioning analysis	Changes over time, communal
				Researcher-rated communion-motive themes in narratives[b]	Clinician-rated, communally healthy functioning	Psychosocial perspective-taking	Loevinger ego development
							Kohlberg moral reason
							Kegan subject-object dev't

[a]VO & VF: Value orientation and value fulfillment. Measures of pleasure (and satisfaction) may be either value orientations of fulfillments. Most measures deal with fulfillment, i.e., *having* pleasurable experiences or satisfaction in life. Some measures deal with value orientations for seeking pleasure (e.g., hedonic motives) or seeking specific forms of it (e.g., others' approval social status, power, money, etc.). I compressed what should be two columns (for value orientations and fulfillments) into one for the sake of space

[b]Narrative measures: When coded by researchers or software, narrative measures are objective assessments, not subjective. When participants code their own narrative measures, it's subjective. Coded narratives are more common, at least when it comes to studying value and meaning. However, just as participants may rate their own personal strivings in terms of value (e.g., intrinsic versus extrinsic motivation; Sheldon & Kasser, 1995), narratives may also be rated in this way. Typically, however, one strength of narrative measures is that they are not mere self-reports

measures do not ask one to rate one's life in terms of the welfare of others. As with all scientific measures, Source 2 is expressly objective: The measure by design forces the person to define the good in terms of pleasure and satisfaction. Sources 3 and 4 are both subjective: In taking the questionnaires, the participant mentally generates a description of his or her life (Source 3) and then also generates an evaluative assessment (e.g., a series of 1–7 ratings) of that description (Source 4). Now consider a measure that is subjectivist for Sources 3 and 4 but is externalist, not internalist, for Source 1: Any measure that asks participants to rate how much they are concerned for others (e.g., social well-being—Keyes, 1998; generative concern—McAdams & de St. Aubin, 1992). As for narratives, we have already considered research-rated personal narratives, which may be either internalist or externalist for Source 1, subjectivist for Source 3, but objectivist for Source 4. Finally, some measures in Table 10.3 have subscales that appear in different cells. Within a measure, one subscale may assess value orientation or motivation (e.g., the anticipation subscale of savoring—Bryant, 2003), while another may assess value fulfillment (e.g., routine savoring experienced in life). As another example, one subscale may assess internalist concerns (e.g., five of the six subscales of psychological well-being—Ryff & Keyes, 1995), while another subscale may assess externalist concerns (e.g., the positive relations subscale of psychological well-being). Still other measurement constructs have both subjective and objective approaches, as with explicit and implicit motives (Schultheiss, Yankova, Dirlikov, & Schad, 2009; Thrash, Elliot, & Schultheiss, 2007), where explicit motives are self-reported and implicit motives are researcher-assessed.

When it comes to measuring personhood and its goods, we might employ any of these approaches: internalist subjective (e.g., Subjective Well-Being—Diener; Meaning in Life Questionnaire), internalist objective (e.g., heart rate; narrative coding of personal achievements), externalist subjective (e.g., Psychological Well-Being or the Loyola Generativity Scale), or externalist objective (e.g., Ego Development or the narrative coding of generativity). Is a subjective or objective definition of the good in life better? I reject the question; both are helpful in our collective project of understanding the fullness of personhood and flourishing. We turn now to that fullness—and the myriad measures of it.

10.2.5 Umbrella Categories: Happiness, Love, Wisdom, Growth

This model of measuring personhood and its goods is complex. Yet all those measures fit more or less squarely within five umbrella categories of a good life.

Basic Needs and Other Constraints to Flourishing

The development of a good life requires a fertile ground of leisure and luck, as Aristotle put it. Leisure is shorthand for the resources that allow a person both not to worry about basic needs like food and shelter and to have enough time to think deeply about life. These are questions about one's life in the context of biological affordances and resources available in one's social ecology. The important empirical issue as I see it is whether leisure makes eudaimonia more likely. As a survey of more than 60,000 people from more than 120 countries has shown, personal concerns for things like one's sense of competence and relatedness are significantly (and overwhelmingly) less likely if one's basic needs for food and the preservation of one's life are in question (Tay & Diener, 2011). Nussbaum's (1998, 2011) model of a good life in philosophy, the Capabilities Approach, is greatly concerned with the role of basic-need satisfaction in the development of human flourishing. It is no coincidence that her model takes a decidedly developmental approach. The following goods (below) are more akin to psychological needs (Deci & Ryan, 2000) and largely rest on the satisfaction of more basic needs. As for limitati, life in the margins of society poses significant threats to the very possibility of living out one's cultural ideals for eudaimonic growth. The margins are set in various ways, owing to race, ethnicity, sexual orientation, and gender (Bhatia, 2007; DesAutels, 2009; Hammack, Thompson, & Pilecki, 2009).

Happiness

By happiness I mean appraisals of self or of a person as satisfied or fulfilled (either by subjective or objective appraisals). Hedonic appraisals of happiness or subjective well-being (Diener et al., 2006) are viewed in terms of cognitive appraisals of either satisfaction or pleasure in life as well as in terms of pleasurable experience itself, i.e., the experiencing of pleasure rather than mere appraisals of pleasurable experience (Haybron, 2008). Happiness is a form of fulfillment. What distinguishes happiness from meaningfulness is simply a matter of whether one considers only the affective evaluation or one also considers the contexts of meaning in which affective evaluations are made. (Again, just because affective evaluations coincide with all assessments of meaningfulness does not mean that pleasure is primary.) The umbrella of eudaimonia can cover important qualities of hedonia as they are—without reducing them to meaning. However, the term *happiness* can also involve more enduring or deeper forms of happiness, which I call *meaningfulness* and categorize under "love," which is next. However, following Haybron (2008), I use the term *happiness* to mean *hedonic happiness*, and well-being to mean the wellness of one's being, including happiness but much more besides.

Love

The umbrella category of love captures elements of eudaimonia that do not easily fit into the categories of either happiness or wisdom but that deal with the enactment of personally meaningful passions. These passions may be directed communally or agentically: Love for another person is communal ("I love you"); love for an activity is agentic ("I love to do…"). Furthermore, measures of love can be value orientations or value fulfillments (see Table 10.4). Communal *values* of love include the interests and capacities for friendship and intimacy (McAdams, 1993), generativity (i.e., concern for the welfare of future generations; Erikson, 1950; McAdams & de St. Aubin, 1992), and compassion (Crocker & Canevello, 2008). Agentic values of love include capacities for activities about which one is passionate—activities that one loves to do—such as harmonious passion (Vallerand, 2008, this volume), vitality and vital engagement (Nakamura & Csikszentmihalyi, 2003; Ryan & Frederick, 1997), and various humanistically or intrinsically motivated activities (Kasser, 2002; Kasser & Ryan, 1996). Communal and agentic *fulfillments* of love include any communal and agentic forms of well-being as commonly measured (e.g., Diener et al., 2006; Ryff & Keyes, 1995). To feel good about (i.e., happiness or well-being about) one's interpersonal relationships is a form of fulfillment of the communal value of love. To feel good about one's personally meaningful activities (versus just valuing or wanting to do them) is a form of fulfillment of the agentic value of love.

Table 10.4 Expressions of love as communal and agentic orientations and fulfillments of value

	Love as value orientation (love desired)	Love as value fulfillment (love attained)
Communal	"I love you"	"Our relationship is good"
Agentic	"I love to play baseball"	"I'm a good baseball player"

Wisdom

By wisdom I mean a heightened capacity for thinking about the self and others, along the lines of Aristotle's practical wisdom, or psychosocial wisdom (Staudinger et al., 2005), or wisdom defined by the capacity to think complexly and integratively about the self and others. Forms of this kind of wisdom deal with reflective or conceptual understandings of how the self and others function in terms of values and virtues, including empirically measurable terms like expert reasoning, psychosocial maturity, ego development, integrative complexity, perspective-taking, and self-actualization (e.g., Ardelt, 2003; Labouvie-Vief, 2003; Loevinger, 1976; Maslow, 1968; Staudinger et al., 2005; Tiberius, 2008). To no small degree, wisdom is a matter of value structure—the organizational framing and perspectivity than one brings to bear on any one thought about the self and others. Thus I argue that other, more experiential forms of wisdom (e.g., affective in Ardelt, 2003) are more precisely value orientations (or sometimes fulfillments, to the degree the measure taps into "wisdom demonstrated") overlaid with value structure.

This kind of wisdom is squarely on canonical lists of virtues in a good life. In fact, I argue that wisdom in this sense is more in line with Aristotle's criterion of *arete* or excellence in practical wisdom, because these measures of wisdom are largely objectivist (see Table 10.3). Still, some subjective measures fit the category of wisdom, provided that they do not in fact assess the participant's sense of "feeling wise" or "feeling self-actualized," which I argue is more about fulfillment than about the capacity to exercise wisdom. The view that wisdom means heightened capacities for perspectivity is of course a limited view of wisdom. But it also helps differentiate objective and subjective facets of the good, when both are legitimate approaches to defining the good. Furthermore, this view of wisdom is not typically viewed as a component of well-being. Indeed, this kind of wisdom (e.g., Loevinger's ego development) does not even correlate with hedonic happiness, let alone reduce to it (Flanagan, 1991; for a review, see Bauer, & McAdams, 2004a).[2] However, if we define well-being as the wellness of one's being, certainly the capacity to take others' perspectives is one among the many markers of wellness.

Growth

The fifth umbrella category of eudaimonia—growth—cuts across the other three. Where eudaimonic growth is attained, that growth comes in the form of patterned increases in happiness, love, or wisdom over time. The other three are about the feeling and thinking of the self—measured subjectively and objectively—but without regard to time. Growth is about time. Growth may also be measured subjectively or objectively—and then as an attainment or as a value (Bauer & McAdams, 2010). Subjectively, growth may be measured as an attainment (i.e., *growth attained*; e.g., as self-assessments that one has grown) or as a desire, value, or motive (i.e., *growth valued*; e.g., as self-reported motives to grow). Objectively, growth may be measured as growth attained (e.g., demonstrated increases in eudaimonic measures over time) or as growth valued (e.g., as researcher-rated, implicit motives for growth). We will cover this topic in more depth next. For now it is important to note that growth has many meanings and forms that involve different mechanisms, principles, and paths of development (Bauer & McAdams, 2004a, 2010; Bauer, McAdams, & Sakaeda, 2005). Thus the project of eudaimonic growth is expansive.

10.3 Eudaimonic Growth

The idea of growth is central to eudaimonia, as noted earlier. In this section, we first differentiate three value orientations of eudaimonic growth and then differentiate the value (and motive) of growth from the attainment of growth.

10.3.1 Growth as Eudaimonic, Humanistic, and Organismic

Growth can mean many things—anything from mere gain across two points in time to the development over long spans of time of personally meaningful characteristics, and from purely self-focused improvements to generative concern for the development of future generations. Eudaimonic growth is, to start, eudaimonic rather than hedonic (but including some hedonic concerns, as outlined earlier). In a nutshell, eudaimonic growth is about the development of happiness, love, and wisdom. Cutting across these types of growth are three value orienta-

---

[2] I wish to thank Jeff Webster for his insightful remarks about the breadth of the construct of wisdom, some conceptions of which do correspond to subjective well-being, such as those dealing with what I am calling qualities of "meaningfulness." For an empirical measure of cognitive, affective, and reflective dimensions of wisdom, see Ardelt (2003).

tions: eudaimonic, humanistic, and organismic. These three are generally grouped together, but I wish to elaborate on their non-overlapping qualities.

Humanistic concerns focus on personally meaningful, internally motivated, subjective *experiences*, whereas materialistic or egoistic concerns focus on concerns like self-image, social status, and appearances (Kasser, 2002). Whereas humanistic concerns place value on the self as a person who experiences, materialistic concerns place value on the self more as a product or commodity to be evaluated, whose value is determined in terms of those external evaluations rather than the person's experiences. Humanistic concerns also focus on the development of the person and his or her experiences (Rogers, 1961), but we return to that idea in terms of the organismic perspective.

Eudaimonic concerns are generally considered to be humanistic, but there is a sense of humanistic concern that focuses on personal, subjective experience that is not necessarily the case with all eudaimonic concerns, especially from an objectivist, Aristotelian perspective. For example, eudaimonic concerns (e.g., for wisdom and virtue) can be framed in materialistic context of social status or notions of psychological perfectionism.[3] As an example of materialistic eudaimonia, merely consider the academic's pride in his or her C.V., which is more likely about egoistic status than about the humanistic cultivating or exercising of wisdom. My research team and I recently expanded the Hedonic and Eudaimonic Motives for Activities scale (Huta & Ryan, 2010), which assesses individual differences in hedonic and eudaimonic value orientations, to include humanistic versus materialistic/egoistic motives in a 2×2 framework. Early studies suggest that materialistic eudaimonia correlates significantly with undesirable forms of perfectionism (Chang, 2009) and obsessive but not harmonious passion (Vallerand, 2008), whereas humanistic eudaimonic correlates significantly with harmonious passion and well-being (Bauer et al., in preparation).

Organismic theory takes a whole-person approach to human development (Goldstein, 1939). Despite the seemingly abstract focus on the whole person as a system, the organismic perspective is grounded in and focuses on action—on activity. In contrast to the organismic perspective is the mechanistic perspective, which focuses not on the system but rather on its component parts. Whereas the organismic perspective focuses on process, the mechanistic perspective focuses on product. Where a person's development is concerned, the organismic perspective views the person primarily in terms of the person's process of becoming, whereas the mechanistic perspective views the person as a product. The organismic perspective also holds that the individual person (as a self-organizing system) makes a contribution to his or her own development (e.g., McAdams, 2006; Murray, 1938; Sheldon, 2004), which sounds eudaimonic but can be framed in terms of hedonically positive-and-negative affect and approach-versus-avoidance motives (e.g., Brandtstadter, 1999). Just as the organismic focus on the person as process lends itself (although not uniformly) to the humanistic focus on experience to define the person, the mechanistic focus on the person as product lends itself to the materialistic/egoistic focus on evaluations of the person to define the person.

The combination of humanistic and organismic concerns is inherently eudaimonic. For example, a subjective concern for growth itself is eudaimonic (e.g., Ryan & Deci, 2001). My use of the term *eudaimonic growth* refers to the combination of eudaimonic, humanistic, and organismic value orientations. In particular, the model of eudaimonic growth focuses on self-development (McLean, Pasupathi, & Pals, 2007), which is to say, on the development of the self as a subjective understanding of one's person, but only to the degree one defines the self with a combination of eudaimonic, humanistic, and organismic value

[3]Whereas philosophical perfectionism reflects a theory's teleological aims (as with Aristotle's eudaimonia – Haybron, 2008), psychological perfectionism often has a more dire connotation, as in the personal pursuit of unrealistically or idealistically too-high expectations (even if certain forms of perfectionism can be adaptive – e.g., Chang, 2009).

orientations. We return to this idea in the section on the transformative self.

10.3.2 Growth Values and Growth Attainments

As suggested earlier, growth can be studied as a value or as an attainment (Bauer & McAdams, 2010). As a personal value, the idea of personal growth can serve as a motivation to foster personal growth (e.g., growth motivation—Bauer et al., 2015; Robitschek, 1998), a personal goal that aims to put growth motivation into action (growth goals and other types of goals that stimulate human development—Bauer & McAdams, 2004a, 2010; Sheldon & Houser-Marko, 2001), or a personal memory that uses the value of personal growth to endow past events with meaning (growth memories—Bauer & McAdams, 2004b; Bauer et al., 2005; Lilgendahl & McAdams, 2011; Pals, 2006). Growth values are not broad personality traits that can be assessed by objective or outside observers (Tackett, Herzhoff, Kushner, & Rule, 2016). Rather, growth values are at heart subjective, in that only the person who hold the growth value can be the one to say so (either characteristic adaptations or features of a life story—McAdams & Pals, 2006), even if they may be examined by objective methods (e.g., implicitly, as in the narrative research cited here). Furthermore, growth values predict growth attained, as we will see below.

As an outcome or attainment, the term *growth* characterizes a desirably patterned or generally progressive change that has been demonstrated over time, such as increases in psychosocial maturity or well-being over multiple points in time. Growth attainment may be measured objectively (by assessing people—even self-reported assessments—at multiple points in time and looking for patterns of growth) or subjectively (by asking people whether they think they grew). The distinction between growth values and growth attainments is important for the study of topics like intentional self-development (Brandtstadter, 1999), personal growth, and eudaimonic growth, because they all involve comparisons of how personally meaningful concerns (such as growth values) relate to how people's lives actually unfold over time (such as growth attainments).

The attainment of eudaimonic growth can be operationally defined as increases over time in any of the varieties of wisdom, love, or happiness. For instance, measures of psychosocial maturity, such as Loevinger's (1976) ego development, which measures how complexly and integratively one thinks about the self and others, are forms of wisdom, notably practical wisdom in the Aristotelian sense (Staudinger et al., 2005). Ego development typically increases from childhood through emerging adulthood, after which ego development either continues to rise or stays about the same until old age (depending on the study; e.g., Bauer & McAdams, 2010; Cohn, 1998; Lilgendahl, Helson, & John, 2013), toward the middle of which some declines are noted (e.g., Labouvie-Vief, 2003). However, for people who have growth values (e.g., in the form of growth memories or growth goals in their narrative self-identity), ego development is likely to increase or remain higher than average at any age (Bauer et al., 2005; Bauer & McAdams, 2004a; King & Smith, 2004; Lilgendahl et al., 2013). The eudaimonic domain of meaningfulness may be operationally defined in many ways, e.g., as increases in moral or virtuous functioning (thinking, feeling, acting), relationship functioning, or passion-laden actions and environmental mastery. To the degree those measures tap into heightened capacities to exercise or know about those kinds of functioning, these measures might overlap with notions of wisdom. To the degree the measures tap into a sense of satisfaction or fulfillment in those areas, the measures reflect a sense of meaningfulness and might overlap with happiness (although, given their focus on a specific context of satisfaction, it's eudaimonic happiness; hence "meaningfulness"). Here we see that the umbrella categories of eudaimonia are not orthogonal, which they need not be as long as they cover the conceptual space of eudaimonic well-being.

10.3.3 Eudaimonic Growth and Self-Identity

Eudaimonic identity theory (Waterman & Schwartz, 2013) is consonant with my idea of eudaimonic growth. The primary difference deals with subjectivist and objectivist perspectives and measures. (Both are externalist, as far as I can tell.) Eudaimonic identity theory starts with identity formation in adolescence, drawing on the work of Erikson (1968) and emphasizing the eudaimonic concerns with which the adolescent (and later the adult) will grapple in forming his or her own self-identity. Eudaimonic identity theory focuses on the subjective self-identity and outlines several steps and concerns on the path toward self-actualizing, with an emphasis on grounding of eudaimonic identity in activity rather than mere abstract notions of self. Among the qualities of the Personally Expressive Activities Questionnaire (PEAQ; Waterman, 2005, a measure of eudaimonic identity, are the personal sense of vitality, engagement, true self, and fulfillment. Importantly for the notion that eudaimonic functioning includes hedonic enjoyment, Waterman and colleagues have found that eudaimonic identity corresponds to experiences of flow, to intrinsic motivation, and to well-being in the form of both life satisfaction (Diener, Emmons, Larson, & Griffen, 1985), which is more hedonic (i.e., without context of meaning), and eudaimonic, psychological well-being (Ryff & Singer, 2008). Importantly for the study of eudaimonic development, eudaimonic identity theory emphasizes the tasks of recognizing and expressing one's potentials, sustained effort in activities that foster the development of those potentials, setting goals toward that aim, that drawing on social resources in doing so.

Similarly, eudaimonic growth is a model of eudaimonic personality development that focuses on subjective self-identity. However, eudaimonic growth also emphasizes objective qualities of personality and its development that lie outside subjective assessments (Bauer et al., 2005; Bauer & McAdams, 2004a, 2004b, 2010). These objective qualities include the structural features and development of self-identity, which is generally viewed from "outside" the person (e.g., ego development—Loevinger, 1976). Other objective concerns include social structures like socioeconomic status and cultural ideals for age, gender, ethnicity, and the like that affect one's personality and development (Bauer & DesAutels, in press), much in the way of the capabilities approach to eudaimonia in philosophy (Nussbaum, 2011). Also, the model of eudaimonic growth is less focused on notions of a purely subjective notion of true self. However, authenticity does play an important role, as presented later.

Finally, like eudaimonic identity theory, the self-identity component of eudaimonic growth derives from Eriksonian theory, but with two emphases. First, eudaimonic growth focuses on narrative self-identity. Second, eudaimonic growth pays special attention to Erikson' the person's social ecology. The next section considers both.

10.4 The Transformative Self as a Good Life Story

I like to keep in mind the distinction between persons and selves. Here a self or self-identity refers to a subjective, mental representation of one's own person (James, 1890; Leary & Tangney, 2005). A person *has* a self-identity. A person *constructs* (and reconstructs and co-constructs) a self-identity (McLean et al., 2007). This distinction is important for the study of how people use their life stories to construct a self-identity, which then corresponds to other measures of personhood, subjective and objective, over time. Self-identity comes in many forms, but when it comes to an understanding of what is important about one's own person to oneself over time in the big picture, nothing beats a *narrative* self-identity (McAdams, 2008). In this section, we first consider some strengths of narrative research and then move to the notion of a good life story, particularly a life story that serves as a self-identity that fosters eudaimonic growth, the transformative self.

10.4.1 Why Narratives?

Through a narrative self-identity, researchers can study how people conceptualize their lives and impute this or that kind of meaning on this or that person, activity, personal characteristic, or life circumstance. Part of the reason is that meaning-making *comes* in narrative form (Bruner, 1990). In constructing meaning in an event or about a person (whether one's own person or another person), we position the event or person with settings in time and place, actors and agents and actions, intentions and effects, associations of preferences and values, metaphors, and a host of other narrative devices or elements. Each of these elements comes to life in relation to the others in the story at hand. We can make lists of the people and places and intentions and values, but their particular arrangement in a story is what conveys the meaning of the story as well as of the events and people in that story. In this way the life story conveys the meaning or meanings of the person's life. In the case of an autobiographical life story, that meaning is the person's self-identity, writ large (McAdams, 1993, 2008).

Narratives and Personality

Narrative self-identity plays an important and unique role in the personological system, distinct from both personality traits and characteristics like motives, goals, and well-being (McAdams, 1995, 2013; McAdams & Pals, 2006). McAdams' three-domain or three-level model of the person describes "what we know when we know a person"—at the level of the actor, the agent, and the author. Broad personality traits like the Big Five convey information about the person at the level of the *actor*—a level that is abstracted from specific contexts in life and that does not require that we have much information about the person's subjective self-understanding; we can predict people's traits by observing them in action. Characteristic adaptations—the level of the *agent*—convey more information about the person's subjective self-views, such as motives, values, and ego defenses. At the level of the author, life stories convey information about how the person creates meaning among the varied and often competing motives, aims, people, life conditions, and other complexities of one's life. Past research has established that elements of life stories are related to specific traits and motives yet are independent of them in predicting well-being and personality development over time (Adler, 2012; Adler, Lodi-Smith, Philippe, & Houle, 2016; Bauer & McAdams, 2004b, 2010; Bauer et al., 2015; Dunlop & Tracy, 2013; Lilgendahl et al., 2013; Lilgendahl & McAdams, 2011; Lodi-Smith, Geise, Roberts, & Robins, 2009; McAdams et al., 2001; Pals, 2006). In other words, narrative self-identity operates as a unique, predictive feature of the personological system.

Narrative as Method

As a method for research, narratives can be studied purely qualitatively or (as in the research cited above) turned into quantitative data. In contrast to self-report surveys that tap into elements of self-identity, personal narratives and life stories are an excellent way to study how people select or generate their own topics and methods of meaning-making. Plus, when coded by trained researchers who demonstrate high levels of inter-rater reliability in their coding, those narratives yield an objective form of data, particularly compared to self-report surveys (see Table 10.3).

Facts and Meanings

Narratives are about meaning-making, and we generally assume that all meanings are interpretations of events and experiences. Still, certain facts are more objective than others, if only by consensus agreement, as when everyone comes to the same interpretation of an event. Then again, stories are about meanings, not facts (McAdams, 1993). As noted in the section on pleasure and meaning, what makes a fact meaningful is that an affect or value is associated with that fact. The general facts of a story refer to its plot (see Table 10.1), but the meaning of a story comes from the affects, values, structure, and timing involved. Furthermore, the predictive utility of personal narratives—that is, the capacity for narratives to predict objective conditions—rests not in the facts of the stories but in the meaningful interpretations of them (Bauer & McAdams, 2010; Wirtz, Kruger, Scollon, & Diener, 2003).

10.4.2 A Good Life Story

The phrase "good life story" is a double-entendre: a good life-story and a good-life story. A good life-story is a story about a life that makes for a good read. The criteria for what makes a life story good depends largely on one's culture (McAdams, 2006). Cultural master narratives—which we see every day in literature, in film, in political discourse, in advertisements—tell us what our culture values as the good in life, and thus as the basic values and storylines to be used in one's own life (Hammack, 2011; Thorne, 2004). One prominent example is the redemptive self (McAdams, 2006), a life story that moves from bad to good—perhaps from rags to riches, from ignorance to enlightenment, from depravity to salvation. The redemptive self, as McAdams portrays it, is also a story of a eudaimonically good life, particularly in the redemptive self's emphasis on generativity, or contributing to future generations.[4] In other words, a good life-story can also be a story of a good life, i.e., a good-life story.

Bildungsroman: A Cultural Master Narrative of Eudaimonic Growth

A prominent master narrative of eudaimonic growth is found in the Bildungsroman genre—stories about character development (Jeffers, 2005). Here the protagonist chooses a life of personal growth by largely following of rejecting mainstream values of status-seeking and the hedonic treadmill, seeking the margins of society to cultivate one's own talents and interests toward the eudaimonic ideal of self-actualization. In Joseph Campbell's (1948) hero story, we see the protagonist return to society with generative concerns to help. These types of stories are what mainstream, Western, industrialized culture calls "good." To the degree one's life story models such a story, one feels good about one's life because, as the one sees it, one's life matches the cultural ideal of the good. In any case, it is both a good life-story and a good-life story.

Two Paths: Upward Mobility and Personal Growth

However, not all good stories are about a good life from the eudaimonic perspective; not all good life-stories are stories about a good life. Stories of villains can make for a good story but do not necessarily portray a cultural master narrative of virtue (or even pleasure, for that matter). We can think of cultural master narratives along two paths of self-improvement, where self-improvement may be either internally or externally motivated (Sedikides & Hepper, 2009). First is the path of upward mobility, which is largely materialistic (as with the American Dream—Kasser & Ryan, 1996). Then lies the path of personal growth, which is largely about eudaimonic growth and the bildungsroman genre. The person with a transformative self constructs a narrative self-identity that is modeled on the idea of the second path. The transformative self is a good-life story. (But whether it is a good good-life story is another question.)

10.4.3 The Transformative Self

The transformative self is a self-identity that features the idea of eudaimonic growth (Bauer, 2016). A person who has a transformative self identifies with the idea (and cultural ideal) of eudaimonic growth. The person with a transformative self deeply values the idea of growth to the point that he or she interprets and plans his or her life in terms of growth: This person creates meaning in personal memories by framing them in terms of growth and does the same when setting personal goals. This person wants to grow, and much as in eudaimonic identity theory (Waterman & Schwartz, 2013), pursues activities that facilitate eudaimonic growth. As described earlier, eudaimonic growth is not just about

[4] However, any one redemptive event might be narrated in eudaimonic (e.g., selfishness to compassion) or hedonic ways (e.g., rags to riches).

attaining high levels of meaning and meaningfulness in life; eudaimonic growth is about a deepening of personal experiences. Thus the person is paradoxically less interested in the status of "having meaning" than in participating in doing the kinds of thing and pursuing the kinds of relationships that naturally yield a sense of meaningfulness.

The transformative self is not a Pollyanna idea. The fostering of growth demands critical self-reflection. Indeed, the person with a transformative self is critical of the limits of self-identity, in part because it is, in the end, a mental construct rather than an activity. And just as eudaimonic theory since Aristotle has emphasized the claim that eudaimonia is an activity, the person with a transformative self focuses on action. Furthermore, there are pitfalls to the transformative self, such as the dangers of perfectionism and trying to squeeze growth out of every situation and person in one's path (the *Growth Nazi*—Bauer, 2016). But when actions and self-identity align around the eudaimonic, humanistic, and organismic values at the root of the transformative self, on average we can expect eudaimonia and eudaimonic growth.

10.4.4 Narratives of Eudaimonic Growth

The transformative self is importantly (but not exclusively) a narrative construct. Life stories, like stories in literature, have narrative elements that are common to a culture that make the meaning of a story recognizable—elements like narrative tone and narrative theme. The transformative self is especially characterized by *narrative themes* of eudaimonic growth that tie the people and events in one's life to value orientations—namely eudaimonic, humanistic, and organismic orientations.

Growthy Tones

Narrative tone conveys the general qualities of positivity or negativity, optimism or pessimism, comedy or tragedy (McAdams, 1993). A life story that is analyzed for exclusively for narrative tone is a purely hedonic measure of narratives. Some measures of narrative tone involve changes in affectivity over time—what is called an *affective sequence* (Adler, 2012). A prominent example of affective sequence is the redemptive sequence, which involves an event that is narrated as starting off bad but ending up good (McAdams et al., 2001; Dunlop & Tracy, 2013). However, not all redemption sequences involve eudaimonic growth. Some redemption sequences are purely about material circumstances getting better. When controlling for narrative themes of eudaimonic growth (see below), these measures of tone have a markedly diminished capacity to predict measures of eudaimonic well-being (and even hedonic well-being—e.g., Bauer et al., under review). Thus I say that some narratives are *growthy* but not squarely about eudaimonic growth (Bauer, 2016).

Growth Themes

Another element is narrative theme, which conveys *not just affect but values*—and specifically, value orientations. Two prominent themes in life stories (and stories generally) are agency and communion (Bakan, 1966; McAdams, 1993). Agency involves values like power, achievement, mastery, victory, and status-seeking, whereas communion involves values like love, intimacy, sharing, and dialogue (McAdams, Hoffman, Mansfield, & Day, 1996). Caring for others involves both agency and communion (McAdams & de St. Aubin, 1992). Such themes connect the myriad people, actions, and events within a story (and episodes within a story) into a coherent sense of meaning, so much so as to define that person or event: Some characters are all about power, some about love; the more interesting characters in stories have multiple, even competing themes. So it is in the life story: We often see people telling life stories in which they wrestle with the competing desires and demands of agency and communion, power and love, independence and dependence. In this section we consider themes of eudaimonic growth—themes rooted in eudaimonic, humanistic, and organismic values—that a person with a transformative self uses to construct his or her life story (and that make that life story a transformative self).

Growth Themes and Time

Whereas themes of agency and communion position the self and others in psychosocial space, themes of eudaimonic growth ("growth themes" for short) position the self and others in psychosocial time. Narrative time unfolds and is conveyed in numerous ways (Brockmeier, 2000), but some framing of time is inherent to narratives (Riceour, 1990). The particular model of time in themes and stories of eudaimonic growth is organismically progressive (which is to say, not necessarily linearly). Growth themes convey the value for—and sometimes the attainment of—the development of deeper, broader, more adaptive capacities for experience and action over time. These developments may be agentic, communal, or both.

Experiential and Reflective Growth Themes

As two broad classes of growth themes, I have identified *experiential* growth themes and *reflective* growth themes. Experiential growth themes deal with a concern for deepening one's skills, one's experience of activities and relationships, and those of other people. Reflective growth themes deal with a concern for deeper conceptual understanding, for intellectual development, or for other forms of differentiating and integrating multiple points of view about one's life.[5] Following is an example of the personal narrative of a college student with a theme of experiential growth. This excerpt comes from a study of how people describe their "personal growth projects" in an effort to distinguish themes of eudaimonic growth from hedonic forms of self-improvement and recovery (Bauer et al., 2015).

> Developing a better relationship with my mom… My mom and myself were never close in high school and we butted heads all the time. We never really hung out together, and when she tried to talk to me I completely would just shut her off and ignore her. I decided to pursue this project because I want a great relationship with my mom for the rest of my life. I love her more than anything and she is the one person who will always be honest and there for me no matter what situation comes into my life. There are a few conflicts considering we have very different personalities and opinions on certain matters, and also trying to talk to her as much as possible when I'm away at college. My siblings and my dad have helped take part in this process by planning more family activities together as much as possible, especially stuff that my mom and me can enjoy together.

This excerpt focuses on the project of developing the experience and quality of a relationship that the narrative portrays as personal meaningful. The narrative showcases eudaimonic and humanistic ideals, specific actions taken that are necessary for organismic development, and the consideration of difficulties amid a bigger picture of optimism for growth. However, the narrative does not focus on reflective growth. Yes, it shows that reflection was done, but the cultivation of reflective growth itself is not of concern in this narrative. The following narrative, from the same study, conveys reflective growth.

> In the past two years or so I have begun to really try and understand other people and what makes them "tick" instead of jumping to conclusions and judgments. A few situations led me to launch the project. First, I was beginning to realize I was becoming very judgmental and cynical about people and the world in general. Secondly, I took a trip to Europe and met many different people, and I became fascinated with people's stories and how they got to where they are. The initial realization, and my trip to Europe caused me to become conscious of the people I interact with, and remember that everyone has a story and a purpose and I cannot be quick to judge things I do not immediately understand. I continue to work on this project by keeping that thought process, and also by reading about new people, looking at quotes, listening to different music. I think this project exposes and reflect that I am a people person and a story-teller/listener, and I want to relate to the world as best I can.

[5]Growth themes always express growth concerns (i.e., values and motives of eudaimonic growth) and sometime express growth attainments (e.g., "I grew from that event"). I am less interested in subjective assessments of growth at any one point in time and more interested in how growth concerns at one time predict subsequent increases in eudaimonic growth attained longitudinally. Still, all such research is needed and can shed light on the enormous project of studying eudaimonic development.

This narrative features not only a great deal of self-reflection but, as stated in its opening sentence, an explicit concern for *understanding* people—and not for deepening relationships with them. The focus is on understanding, realization, thought processes, and taking actions (reading, listening to music) that might expand such reflection. This narrative was also coded for experiential growth (the two growth themes are not mutually exclusive), as it also conveyed a joy in activities to promote learning and meaningful dialogue. Also, I wish to note that I have chosen two, *communal* growth themes for comparison, but either experiential or reflective growth themes may be agentic as well (Bauer & McAdams, 2004b, 2010).

Two Themes of Growth Valued, Two Paths of Growth Attained

Despite the fact that any one narrative might convey both experiential and reflective growth, these growth themes—which reflect *values* or *concerns* for growth—predict two distinct classes of growth *attainments*, notably happiness and wisdom. Experiential growth themes predict high levels of—and increases years later in—measures of happiness and well-being. Reflective growth themes predict high levels of—and increases years later in—measures of psychosocial maturity, where maturity deals with wisdom-related capacities for perspective-taking, differentiation and integration of psychosocial phenomena, and integrative complexity of thinking about the self and others (Bauer et al., 2008; Bauer & McAdams, 2010). Importantly, growth themes function these ways in good times and in bad: Whether narrating high points in life or low points in life—such as loss, trauma, and serious illness—themes of eudaimonic growth can be found (first of all) and can be found to predict maturity and well-being.

10.4.5 Young Growth, Mature Growth

The excerpts above come from college students whose ages placed them in the life period of emerging adulthood, roughly ages 18 to the mid-to-late 20s in modern societies (Arnett, 2000). From an updated Eriksonian (1950, 1968) perspective, emerging adulthood extends the period of identity versus role confusion beyond adolescence, as emerging adults engage in the process of defining the self and finding one's place in an increasingly complex society (Arnett). From a narrative perspective, emerging adulthood marks the development of the person as author of his or her own life story, defining one's life in terms of contextualized stories (McAdams, 1993, 2013; McLean et al., 2007). Growth themes can be found in the stories of both younger and older adults—which is to say, young and old can have a transformative self. Those growth themes predict measures of wisdom, love, and happiness throughout adulthood (Bauer et al., 2008).

Yet the stories of emerging adults do not deal with the same things as the stories of, say, midlife or older adults. Consonant with Eriksonian theory, younger adults focus more on concerns of identity, whereas their older counterparts focus more on concerns of generativity (Bauer et al., 2015; McAdams & de St. Aubin, 1992). Furthermore, older adults' life stories simply convey more personal meaning-making: more emotion-laden evaluations than mere descriptions, greater structural complexity, greater thematic coherence (Bauer et al., 2005, Bauer et al., 2015; Lilgendahl et al., 2013; McLean, 2008; Pasupathi, 2001; Pasupathi & Mansour, 2006). In a nutshell—and in contrast to the belief that "growth is for the young"—older adults are more likely to tell growth stories than are younger adults (Bauer & Park, 2010). The excerpts above are good examples of what I call "young growth," showing concerns for eudaimonic growth but without a lifetime of experience informing them, making the descriptions of any one person or idea more straightforward. Compare those narratives with a narrative exhibiting "mature growth" from a woman, age 62, who recalls a high point in her life:

> My granddaughter [name] was at my house. She was approx. 3 yr. old. We were lying on my bed…I suddenly felt this incredible love for her and almost simultaneously I felt a surge of deep pain and

> sadness and I became conscious, I feel, for the first time, that the price of loving so completely, so unconditionally is that the other side is that I would feel excrutiating pain if she were to die or be separated from me forever. This event is significant because I felt so alive—so capable of being loving without consciousness about acceptance/nonacceptance and other self-centered thoughts. The awareness of the other side of connection is loss—I know this and have felt this since, and the knowing has greatly enhanced my life—much more freely able to love and to understand why I have been so fearful of this kind of loving in the past.

The presence of growth themes in personal narratives (and in open-ended goals) has been shown repeatedly to explain the bivariate relation between age and well-being (citations above). In other words, older people may report higher life satisfaction (in some studies; seldom lower), but this is explained by the fact that older adults are more likely to tell growth stories; they are more likely to have a transformative self.

10.4.6 Authorship, Authenticity, and Self-Actualizing

For all the depth of meaning in narratives of mature, eudaimonic growth, they do not necessarily reveal self-actualization. Psychological science, for good reason, hardly holds the bar for eudaimonic well-being as high as Maslow's self-actualization. Self-actualizing is one of the canonical, candidate goods among the many goods of personhood and eudaimonia, as noted earlier. Furthermore, self-actualizing is an aim for the person with a transformative self. This person can be said, at any phase of development, to be aiming for a more authentic life story—a story about activities that increasingly reflect and foster authentic living. The person with a transformative self strives for heightened capacities for authentic self-authorship.

Identity Achievement Versus Self-Actualizing

When self-identity first takes its relatively adult form, sometime in late adolescence or emerging adulthood, the person can be said to first *author* his or her own self-identity as a life story (McAdams, 2013; although autobiographical reasoning is present earlier—see Dunlop & Walker, 2013). This development may well involve a push to cultivate one's "true self" (if only as subjectively perceived—Schlegel, Hicks, Arndt, & King, 2009; Schlegel, Hicks, & Christy, Chap. 14, this volume), but identity formation at this point is largely defined by various freedoms from parental or school authority and various freedoms to pursue one's own course of action and belief. The aim of identity achievement in youth, as Erikson puts it, is to find "where one stands" in a world of others. But this is a far cry from the subtler considerations of existential authenticity in the manner of Sartre or Rollo May.

Does that sound elitist? If a person is to be judgmental about the descriptive differences between young and mature self-identity, then we see elitism. Then the claims here are ageist, but with a bias against youth. Few adolescents can even conceptualize the issues of authenticity and self-actualizing within the vicissitudes of the actual, lived contexts of adult life (let alone shape their largely unconscious, personal patterns of intentions, actions, and interpretations in a way that exudes self-actualizing routinely).[6] It simply takes decades of experience in life, on average, to develop the capacities for perspective-taking that are required of Maslow's self-actualizing or Loevinger's integrated stage of development.

Now, an adolescent's self-identity can surely reflect qualities of authenticity and surely involve a focus on eudaimonic growth. But on average, the adolescent self-identity is considerably more likely than the mid-life or older-adult self-identity to be focused on extrinsically motivated concerns, such as self-image, social status, and appearances—and, conversely, less likely to be focused on internally or humanistically motivated concerns like personally meaningful activities and relationships (Bauer et al., 2005, 2015;

[6] To temper the reverse ageism, let's keep in mind that the cultivation of self-understanding toward authenticity is but one of many lines of development that constitute a good life (cf. the big umbrella of eudaimonia). One need not scale the heights of authenticity to be a good neighbor or parent etc.

Sheldon & Kasser, 2001). Such concerns are not sufficient requirements of existential authenticity, but they do seem to be necessary. So, even though adolescent self-identity may reflect authenticity, authenticity seems more likely in mature years than in youth.

Still, adolescents can act authentically or not. So I maintain that authenticity has a developmentally sliding scale. Authenticity in youth is not the same authenticity as in maturity. Similarly, the authenticity of earlier stages of ego development more simplistic understandings of self and others than does the authenticity of later stages of ego development. Authenticity at later stages is not about one's achieving an identity that is merely based on, as in youth, one's self-examination and commitments to roles and beliefs in society. In other words, mature authenticity is not just about identity achievement. Mature authenticity is more about self-actualizing.

Independence and Authenticity

Another way to oversimplify the scenario with authorship and authenticity is to view them in terms of basic notions of freedom: *freedom from* (i.e., negative freedom, which is the absence of hindrances to self-determination) and *freedom to* (i.e., positive freedom, which is the presence of self-determination; Berlin, 1969). In the course of personal development, the emergence of the adult form of authorship in adolescence or emerging adulthood is largely about *independence*, which deals largely with *freedom from* one's parents or guardians (as in adolescence) as well as *freedom to* choose one's own responsibilities and courses of action in society. In contrast, authenticity deals largely with *freedom from* society (particularly the directives and ideologies of social institutions and social roles, notably the ones that the independence-focused person so eagerly chose for him- or herself in youth) as well as *freedom to* choose among self-examined ideals. In both cases we see a development toward a "truer" self than had been known and lived prior. But whereas the earlier true self in the dawn of adult authorship deals with independence, the more mature true self deals with authenticity.

Authenticity and Self-Authorship

Authenticity can be viewed as a refined or mature form of self-authorship. Authenticity is a refined form of authorship. We often see how novelists refine their craft over the course of their career such that their earlier works come across as the work of a younger person. Similarly, individual persons—if they continue to develop—refine their capacities to author their own narrative self-identity. More mature life stories involve greater attention to multiple meanings, to greater acceptance of the good and bad in one's life as integral to one's "one and only life" (Erikson, 1968), or to the balancing of competing and underlying motives—motives that might not have even been perceived as competing or even existing in youth. Authenticity as a characteristic of a narrative self-identity is not the only way in which a life story might be refined, but it is one kind—and a kind especially relevant to the study of self-actualizing and, more broadly, eudaimonic growth. Authenticity is a way of authorship that accounts for the multifaceted, multivalenced, myriad qualities of a life with honesty, humility, a lack of defensiveness (a quiet ego—Wayment, Bauer, & Sylaska, 2015), a deep sense of connection to the people in one's life (at multiple levels of the social ecology, from immediate others to society over history—Bronfenbrenner, 1979), a deep understanding of how one's motivations and values and actions both conflict and integrate (e.g., self-concordance—Sheldon & Houser-Marko, 2001), and other qualities that acknowledge the various virtues of the fullness of one's personhood.

Authenticity, Traits, and Self-Authorship

Finally, when I say *authenticity*, I do not mean only *being true to your traits*, which is a common way of interpreting authenticity (McGregor, McAdams, & Little, 2006; Little, Chap. 19, this volume). Instead, I mean something closer to "being true to your beliefs." Both forms of authenticity are important and facilitate well-being (Sheldon, Ryan, Rawsthorne, & Ilardi, 1997). An authenticity that means nothing more than living in accord with some deeply ingrained traits—say, if one is born or raised to be hyper-aggressive or just simply a jerk—strikes me as good for little more than fostering a sense of satisfaction that might come from either self-verification or a massive dose of self-justification: "Yeah, I was a jerk. That's just me being me. Tough luck for you." Being true to one's beliefs involves at least some reflection of what is meaningful and valuable in life, ideally from a non-defensive point of view (Bauer, 2008; Wayment, Bauer, & Sylaska, 2015). The system of eudaimonic and humanistic values exists in part to guard against the more selfish impulses of human nature (that continue to exist in even the most self-actualized among us—Maslow, 1968). So authenticity involves characteristics of the person at the level of traits and characteristic adaptations, the latter of which involves subjective beliefs, values, and motivations (McAdams & Pals, 2006).

Subjectivity, Objectivity, Authenticity, and Self-Authorship

Yet even "being true to one's beliefs" is problematic, particularly in its reliance on internality The philosopher Wayne Sumner (1996) tries to get around this problem with a subjectivist notion of authentic happiness. Certain externalist criteria for the welfare of others obtain. Furthermore, we probably need stories, a narrative account of how the person weaves the various activities and people and personal beliefs in his or her life into an a sense of not merely coherence but also integrity—where one's activities and interactions in actual, lived contexts bring one's abstract values to life. As noted earlier, we see that the capacity to tell such a story increases with age but is more proximally tied to the transformative self. From a narrative perspective, this process is a matter of moving from authorship to authenticity. However, this movement does not happen overnight. Instead, authorship throughout adulthood may be viewed in terms of gradually increasing authenticity over the years, perhaps in fits and starts as one makes attempts, fails, and tries to learn from experience, but nonetheless gradually over broad spans of time. The transformative self, as a self-identity rooted in the process of eudaimonic growth, facilitates such development.

References

Adler, J. M. (2012). Living into the story: Agency and coherence in a longitudinal study of narrative identity development and mental health over the course of psychotherapy. *Journal of Personality and Social Psychology, 102*, 367–389.

Adler, J. M., Lodi-Smith, J., Philippe, F. L., & Houle, I. (2016). The incremental validity of narrative identity in predicting well-being: A review of the field and recommendations for the future. *Personality and Social Psychology Review, 20*, 142–175.

Ardelt, M. (2003). Empirical assessment of a three-dimensional wisdom scale. *Research on Aging, 23*, 275–324.

Arnett, J. J. (2000). Emerging adulthood: A theory of development from the late teens through the twenties. *American Psychologist, 55*, 469–480.

Bakan, D. (1966). *The duality of human existence: Isolation and communion in Western man*. Boston: Beacon Press.

Bauer, J. J. (2016). *The transformative self: Identity, growth, and a good life story: A theory of eudaimonic personality development*. New York: Oxford University. Manuscript in preparation.

Bauer, J. J., & Bonanno, G. A. (2001). Doing and being well (for the most part): Adaptive patterns of narrative self-evaluation during bereavement. *Journal of Personality, 69*, 451–482.

Bauer, J. J., & DesAutels, P. (in press). Eudaimonia Cosmopolitan: Toward an integrative, developmental model of a good life. In E. Nelson (Ed.), *Naturalism and Asian Philosophy: Owen Flanagan and Beyond*. Albany, NY: SUNY Press.

Bauer, J. J., & McAdams, D. P. (2004a). Growth goals, maturity, and well-being. *Developmental Psychology, 40*, 114–127.

Bauer, J. J., & McAdams, D. P. (2004b). Personal growth in adults' stories of life transitions. *Journal of Personality, 72*, 573–602.

Bauer, J. J., & McAdams, D. P. (2010). Eudaimonic growth: Narrative growth goals predict increases in ego development and subjective well-being three years later. *Developmental Psychology, 46*, 761–772.

Bauer, J. J., McAdams, D. P., & Pals, J. L. (2008). Narrative identity and eudaimonic well-being. *Journal of Happiness Studies, 9*, 81–104.

Bauer, J. J., McAdams, D. P., & Sakaeda, A. R. (2005). Interpreting the good life: Growth memories in the lives of mature, happy people. *Journal of Personality and Social Psychology, 88*, 203–217.

Bauer, J. J., & Park, S. W. (2010). Growth isn't just for the young: Growth narratives, eudaimonic resilience, and the aging self. In P. S. Frye & C. L. M. Keyes (Eds.),

Frontiers of resilient aging (pp. 60–89). Cambridge, UK: Cambridge University Press.

Bauer, J. J., Park, S. W., Montoya, R. M., & Wayment, H. A. (2015). Growth motivation toward two facets of eudaimonic self-development. *Journal of Happiness Studies, 16*, 185–210.

Baumeister, R. F. (1991). *Meanings of life*. New York: Guilford.

Baumeister, R. F., Vohs, K. D., Aaker, J. L., & Garbinsky, E. N. (2013). Some key differences between a happy life and a meaningful life. *Journal of Positive Psychology, 8*, 505–516.

Berlin, I. (1969). *Two essays on liberty*. Oxford: Oxford University.

Bhatia, S. (2007). *American karma: Race, culture, and identity in the Indian diaspora*. New York: New York University.

Brandtstadter, J. (1999). The self in action and development: Cultural, biosocial, and onogenetic bases of intentional self-development. In J. Brandtstadter & R. M. Lerner (Eds.), *Action and self-development: Theory and research through the life span* (pp. 37–66). Thousand Oaks, CA: Sage.

Brockmeier, J. (2000). Autobiographical time. *Narrative Inquiry, 10*, 51–73.

Bronfenbrenner, U. (1979). *The ecology of human development: Experiments by nature and design*. Cambridge, MA: Harvard University.

Bruner, J. (1990). *Acts of meaning*. Cambridge, MA: Harvard University.

Bryant, F. B. (2003). Savoring Beliefs Inventory (SBI): A scale for measuring beliefs about savouring. *Journal of Mental Health, 12*, 175–196.

Campbell, J. (1948/1972). *The hero with a thousand faces*. Princeton, NJ: Princeton University.

Carter, T. J., & Gilovich, T. (2010). The relative relativity of material and experiential purchases. *Journal of Personality and Social Psychology, 98*, 146–159.

Chang, E. (2009). An examination of optimism, pessimism, and performance perfectionism as predictors of positive psychological functioning in middle-aged adults: Does holding high standards of performance matter beyond generalized outcome expectancies? *Cognitive Therapy Research, 33*, 334–344.

Cohn, L. D. (1998). Age trends in personality development: A quantitative review. In P. M. Westenberg, A. Blasi, & L. D. Cohn (Eds.), *Personality development: Theoretical, empirical, and clinical investigations of Loevinger's conception of ego development* (pp. 133–143). Mahwah, NJ: Lawrence Erlbaum.

Crocker, J., & Canevello, A. (2008). Creating and undermining support in communal relationships: The role of compassionate and self-image goals. *Journal of Personality and Social Psychology, 95*, 555–575.

Deci, E. L., & Ryan, R. M. (2000). The what and why of goal pursuits: Human needs and the self-determination of behavior. *Psychological Inquiry, 11*, 227–268.

DesAutels, P. (2009). Resisting organizational power. In L. Tessman (Ed.), *Feminist ethics and social and political philosophy: Theorizing the non-ideal* (pp. 223–236). New York: Springer.

Diener, E., Emmons, R. A., Larson, R. J., & Griffen, S. (1985). The satisfaction with life scale. *Journal of Personality Assessment, 49*, 71–75.

Diener, E., Lucas, R. E., & Scollon, C. N. (2006). Beyond the hedonic treadmill: Revising the adaptation theory of well-being. *American Psychologist, 61*, 305–314.

Dunlop, W. L., & Tracy, J. L. (2013). Sobering stories: Narratives of self-redemption predict behavioral change and improved health among recovering alcoholics. *Journal of Personality and Social Psychology, 104*, 576–590.

Dunlop, W. L., & Walker, L. J. (2013). The life story: Its development and relation to narration and personal identity. *International Journal of Behavioral Development, 37*, 235–247.

Elliot, A. J., & McGregor, H. A. (2001). A 2×2 achievement goal framework. *Journal of Personality and Social Psychology, 80*, 501–519.

Erikson, E. H. (1950/1994). *Childhood and society*. New York: Norton.

Erikson, E. H. (1968/1994). *Identity: Youth and crisis*. New York: Norton.

Flanagan, O. (1991). *Varieties of moral personality: Ethics and psychological realism*. Cambridge, MA: Harvard University.

Flanagan, O. F. (2011). *The bodhisattva's brain: Buddhism naturalized*. Cambridge, MA: MIT.

Fredrickson, B. L. (2013). Updated thinking on positivity ratios. *American Psychologist*, 68, 814–822.

Goldstein, K. (1939). *The organism, a holistic approach to biology derived from pathological data in man*. New York: American Book Company.

Graham, J., Nosek, B. A., Haidt, J., Iyer, R., Koleva, S., & Ditto, P. H. (2011). Mapping the moral domain. *Journal of Personality and Social Psychology, 101*, 366–385.

Hammack, P. L. (2011). *Narrative and the politics of identity: The cultural psychology of Israeli and Palestinian youth*. New York: Oxford University.

Hammack, P. L., Thompson, E. M., & Pilecki, A. (2009). Configurations of identity among sexual minority youth: Context, desire, and narrative. *Journal of Youth and Adolescence, 38*, 867–883.

Haybron, D. (2008). *The pursuit of unhappiness*. New York: Oxford University.

Huta, V. (2013). Pursuing eudaimonia versus hedonia: Distinctions, similarities, and relationships. In A. S. Waterman (Ed.), *The best within us: Positive psychology perspectives on eudaimonic functioning* (pp. 139–158). Washington, DC: American Psychological Association.

Huta, V., & Ryan, R. M. (2010). Pursuing pleasure or virtue: The differential and overlapping well-being benefits of hedonic and eudaimonic motives. *Journal of Happiness Studies, 11*, 735–762.

James, W. (1890/1950). *Principles of psychology, vol. 2*. New York: Dover.

James, W. (1907/1909/1978). *Pragmatism and the meaning of truth* (A. J., Ayer, Ed.). Cambridge, MA: Harvard University.

Jeffers, T. J. (2005). *Apprenticeships: The bildungsroman from Goethe to Santayana*. New York: Palgrave Macmillan.

Kashdan, T. B., Biswas-Diener, R., & King, L. A. (2008). Reconsidering happiness: The costs of distinguishing between hedonics and eudaimonia. *Journal of Positive Psychology, 3*, 219–233.

Kasser, T. (2002). *The high price of materialism*. Cambridge, MA: MIT.

Kasser, T., & Ryan, R. M. (1996). Further examining the American dream: Well-being correlates of intrinsic and extrinsic goals. *Personality and Social Psychology Bulletin, 22*, 281–288.

Kegan, R. (1982). *The evolving self*. Cambridge, MA: Harvard University.

Kelly, G. A. (1955). *A theory of personality: The psychology of personal constructs*. New York: Norton.

Keltner, D. (2010). The compassionate instinct. In D. Keltner, J. Marsh, & J. A. Smith (Eds.), *The compassionate instinct: The science of human goodness* (pp. 8–15). New York: Norton.

Keyes, C. L. M. (1998). Social well-being. *Social Psychology Quarterly, 61*, 121–140.

Keyes, C. L. M., Schmotkin, D., & Ryff, C. D. (2002). Optimizing well-being: The empirical encounter of two traditions. *Journal of Personality and Social Psychology, 82*, 1007–1022.

King, L. A., & Napa, C. K. (1998). What makes a life good? *Journal of Personality and Social Psychology, 75*, 156–165.

King, L. A., & Smith, N. G. (2004). Gay and straight possible selves: Goals, identity, subjective well-being, and personality development. *Journal of Personality, 72*, 967–994.

Labouvie-Vief, G. (2003). Dynamic integration: Affect, cognition, and the self in adulthood. *Current Directions in Psychological Science, 12*, 201–206.

Labouvie-Vief, G. (2006). Emerging structures of adult thought. In J. J. Arnett & J. L. Tanner (Eds.), *Emerging adults in America: Coming of age in the 21st century*. Washington, DC: American Psychological Association.

Leary, M. R., & Tangney, J. P. (2005). The self as an organizing construct in the behavioral and social sciences. In M. R. Leary & J. P. Tangney (Eds.), *Handbook of self and identity* (pp. 3–14). New York: Guilford.

Lilgendahl, J. P., Helson, R., & John, O. P. (2013). Does ego development increase during midlife? The effects of openness and accommodative processing of difficult events. *Journal of Personality, 81*, 403–416.

Lilgendahl, J. P., & McAdams, D. P. (2011). Constructing stories of self-growth: How individual differences in patterns of autobiographical reasoning relate to well-being in midlife. *Journal of Personality, 79*, 391–428.

Lodi-Smith, J., Geise, A. C., Roberts, B. W., & Robins, R. W. (2009). Narrating personality change. *Journal of Personality and Social Psychology, 96*, 679–689.

Loevinger, J. (1976). *Ego development*. San Francisco: Jossey-Bass.

Maslow, A. H. (1968). *Toward a psychology of being*. New York: Van Nostrand Reinhold.

May, R. (1969/2007). *Love and will*. New York: Norton.

McAdams, D. P. (1993). *The stories we live by: Personal myths and the making of the self*. New York: Morrow.

McAdams, D. P. (1995). What do we know when we know a person? *Journal of Personality, 63*, 365.

McAdams, D. P. (2006). *The redemptive self: Stories Americans live by*. New York: Oxford University.

McAdams, D. P. (2008). Personal narratives and the life story. In O. P. John, R. W. Robins, & L. A. Pervin (Eds.), *Handbook of personality: Theory and research* (3rd ed., pp. 242–262). New York: Guilford.

McAdams, D. P. (2013). The psychological self as actor, agent, and author. *Perspectives on Psychological Science, 8*, 272–295.

McAdams, D. P., & de St. Aubin, E. (1992). A theory of generativity and its assessment through self-report, behavioral acts, and narrative themes in autobiography. *Journal of Personality and Social Psychology, 62*, 1003–1015.

McAdams, D. P., Hoffman, B. J., Mansfield, E. D., & Day, R. (1996). Themes of agency and communion in significant autobiographical scenes. *Journal of Personality, 64*, 339–377.

McAdams, D. P., & Pals, J. L. (2006). A new big five: Fundamental principles for an integrative science of personality. *American Psychologist, 61*, 204–217.

McAdams, D. P., Reynolds, J., Lewis, M., Patten, A. H., & Bowman, P. J. (2001). When bad things turn good and good things turn bad: Sequences of redemption and contamination in life narrative and their relation to psychosocial adaption in midlife adults and in students. *Personality and Social Psychology Bulletin, 27*, 474–485.

McGregor, I., McAdams, D. P., & Little, B. R. (2006). Personal projects, life stories, and happiness: On being true to traits. *Journal of Research in Personality, 40*, 551–572.

McLean, K. C. (2008). Stories of the young and the old: Personal continuity and narrative identity. *Developmental Psychology, 44*, 254–264.

McLean, K. C., Pasupathi, M., & Pals, J. L. (2007). Selves creating stories creating selves: A process model of self-development. *Personality and Social Psychology Review, 11*, 262–278.

Murray, H. A. (1938/2007). *Explorations in personality*. (Dan P. McAdams, Ed.). New York: Oxford University.

Nozick, R. (1983). *Philosophical explanations*. Cambridge, MA: Belknap.

Nussbaum, M. C. (1998). *Women and human development: The capabilities approach*. New York: Cambridge University.

Nussbaum, M. C. (2011). *Creating capabilities: A human development approach*. Cambridge, UK: Cambridge University.

Pals, J. L. (2006). Narrative identity processing of difficult life experiences: Pathways of personality development and positive self-transformation in adulthood. *Journal of Personality, 74*, 1079–1109.

Pasupathi, M. (2001). The social construction of the personal past and its implications for adult development. *Psychological Bulletin, 127*, 651–672.

Pasupathi, M., & Mansour, E. (2006). Adult age differences in autobiographical reasoning in narratives. *Developmental Psychology, 42*, 798–808.

Pennebaker, J. W., & Seagal, J. D. (1999). Forming a story: The health benefits of narrative. *Journal of Clinical Psychology, 55*, 1243–1254.

Riceour, P. (1990). *Time and narrative, vol. 3*. (K. Blamey & D. Pallauer, Trans.)

Robitschek, C. (1998). Personal growth initiative: The construct and its measure. *Measurement and Evaluation in Counseling and Development, 30*, 183–198.

Rogers, C. R. (1961). *On becoming a person*. Boston: Houghton Mifflin.

Ryan, R. M., & Deci, E. L. (2001). On happiness and human potentials: A review of research on hedonic and eudaimonic well-being. *Annual Review of Psychology, 52*, 141–166.

Ryff, C. D., & Keyes, C. L. M. (1995). The structure of psychological well-being revisited. *Journal of Personality and Social Psychology, 69*, 719–727.

Ryff, C. D., & Singer, B. (2008). Know thyself and become what you are: A eudaimonic approach to psychological well-being. *Journal of Happiness Studies, 9*, 13–39.

Sawyer, R. K. (2005). *Social emergence: Societies as complex systems*. Cambridge, UK: Cambridge University.

Schlegel, R. J., Hicks, J. A., Arndt, J., & King, L. A. (2009). Thine own self: True self-concept accessibility and meaning in life. *Journal of Personality and Social Psychology, 96*, 473–490.

Schultheiss, O. C., Yankova, D., Dirlikov, B., & Schad, D. J. (2009). Are implicit and explicit motive measures statistically independent? A fair and balanced test using the picture story exercise and a cue- and response-matched questionnaire measure. *Journal of Personality Assessment, 91*, 72–81.

Schwartz, S. (2007). Universalism and the inclusiveness of our moral universe. *Journal of Cross-Cultural Psychology, 38*, 711–728.

Schwartz, S. H., & Bilsky, W. (1990). Toward a theory of the universal content and structure of values: Extensions and cross-cultural replications. *Journal of Personality and Social Psychology, 58*, 678–891.

Sedikides, C., & Hepper, E. G. D. (2009). Self-improvement. *Social and Personality Psychology Compass, 3*(6), 899–917.

Sheldon, K. M. (2004). *Optimal human being*. Mahwah, NJ: Lawrence Erlbaum Associates.

Sheldon, K. M. (2013). Individual daimon, universal needs, and subjective well-being: Happiness as the natural consequence of a life well lived. In A. S. Waterman (Ed.), *The best within us: Positive psychology perspectives on eudaimonic functioning* (pp. 207–226). Washington, DC: American Psychological Association.

Sheldon, K. M., & Houser-Marko, L. (2001). Self-concordance, goal attainment, and the pursuit of happiness: Can there be an upward spiral? *Journal of Personality and Social Psychology, 80*, 152–165.

Sheldon, K. M., & Kasser, T. (1995). Coherence and congruence: Two aspects of personality integration. *Journal of Personality and Social Psychology, 68*, 531–543.

Sheldon, K. M., & Kasser, T. (2001). Getting older, getting better? Personal strivings and psychosocial maturity across the life-span. *Developmental Psychology, 34*, 491–501.

Sheldon, K. M., Ryan, R. M., Rawsthorne, L. J., & Ilardi, B. (1997). Trait self and true self: Cross-role variation in the big-five personality traits and its relations with psychological authenticity and subjective well-being. *Journal of Personality and Social Psychology, 73*, 1380–1393.

Staudinger, U. M., Dörner, J., & Mickler, C. (2005). Wisdom and personality. In R. J. Sternberg & J. Jordan (Eds.), *A handbook of wisdom: Psychological perspectives* (pp. 191–219). Cambridge, UK: Cambridge University.

Steger, M. F., Frazier, P., Oishi, S., & Kaler, M. (2006). The meaning in life questionnaire: Assessing the presence of and search for meaning in life. *Journal of Counseling Psychology, 53*, 80–93.

Steger, M. F., Yeon Shin, J., Shim, Y., & Fitch-Martin, A. (2013). Is meaning in life a flagship indicator of well-being? In A. S. Waterman (Ed.), *The best within us: Positive psychology perspectives on eudaimonic functioning* (pp. 159–182). Washington, DC: American Psychological Association.

Suedfeld, P., & Bluck, S. (1993). Changes in integrative complexity accompanying significant life events: Historical evidence. *Journal of Personality and Social Psychology, 64*, 124–130.

Sumner, L. W. (1996). *Welfare, happiness, & ethics*. New York: Oxford University.

Tackett, J. L., Herzhoff, K., Kushner, S. C., & Rule, N. (2016). Thin slices of child personality: Perceptual, situational, and behavioral contributions. *Journal of Personality and Social Psychology, 110*, 150–166.

Tadmor, C. T., Tetlock, P. E., & Peng, K. (2007). Acculturation strategies and integrative complexity: The cognitive implications of biculturalism. *Journal of Cross-Cultural Psychology, 40*, 105–139.

Tay, L., & Diener, D. (2011). Needs and subjective well-being around the world. *Journal of Personality and Social Psychology, 101*, 354–365.

Taylor, C. (1989). *Sources of the self: The making of the modern identity*. Cambridge, MA: Harvard University.

Thorne, A. (2004). Putting the person into social identity. *Human Development, 47*, 361–365.

Thrash, T. M., Elliot, A. J., & Schultheiss, O. C. (2007). Methodological and dispositional predictors of congruence between implicit and explicit need for achievement. *Personality and Social Psychology Bulletin, 33*, 961–974.

Tiberius, V. (2008). *The reflective life: Living wisely within our limits*. New York: Oxford University.

Tiberius, V. (2013). Recipes for a good life: Eudaimonia and the contribution of philosophy. In A. S. Waterman (Ed.), *The best within us: Positive psychology perspectives on eudaimonic functioning* (pp. 19–38). Washington, DC: American Psychological Association.

Tiberius, V. (2014). How theories of well-being can help us. *Journal of Practical Ethics, 2*, 1–19.

Vallerand, R. J. (2008). On the psychology of passion: In search of what makes people's lives most worth living. *Canadian Psychology, 49*, 1–13.

Van Boven, L., & Gilovich, T. (2003). To do or to have? That is the question. *Journal of Personality and Social Psychology, 85*, 1193–1302.

Vittersø, J. (2013). Feelings, meanings, and optimal functioning: Some distinctions between hedonic and eudaimonic well-being. In A. S. Waterman (Ed.), *The best within us: Positive psychology perspectives on eudaimonia* (pp. 39–56). Washington, DC: American Psychological Association.

Warren, J. (2009). Removing fear. In J. Warren (Ed.), *The Cambridge companion to epicureanism* (pp. 234–248). Cambridge, UK: Cambridge University.

Waterman, A. S. (2005). When effort is enjoyed: Two studies of intrinsic motivation for personally salient activities. *Motivation and Emotion, 29*, 165–188.

Waterman, A. S., & Schwartz, S. J. (2013). Eudaimonic identity theory. In A. S. Waterman (Ed.), *The best within us: Positive psychology perspectives on eudaimonia* (pp. 99–118). Washington, DC: American Psychological Association.

Waterman, A. S., Schwartz, S. J., & Conti, R. (2008). The implications of two conceptions of happiness (hedonic enjoyment and eudaimonia) for the understanding of intrinsic motivation. *Journal of Happiness Studies, 9*, 41–79.

Wayment, H. A., Bauer, J. J., & Sylaska, K. (2015). The quiet ego scale: Measuring the compassionate self-identity. *Journal of Happiness Studies, 16*, 999–1033.

Wirtz, D., Kruger, J., Scollon, C. N., & Diener, E. (2003). What to do on spring break? The role of predicted, on-line, and remembered experience in future choice. *Psychological Science, 14*, 520–524.

Wolf, S. (2010). *Meaning in life and why it matters*. Princeton, NJ: Princeton University.

11 Hedonia, Eudaimonia, and Meaning: Me Versus Us; Fleeting Versus Enduring

Michael F. Steger

The longing for Paradise is man's longing not to be man.
There is no perfection only life. – Milan Kundera, *The Unbearable Lightness of Being*

I study meaning in life. How silly is that? What can a flawed, capricious, short-sighted person, embalmed in his own narrative, possibly understand about what life really means? In fact, the roots of my interest in meaning rise from such human weaknesses. I grew up confounded and infuriated by the flawed, capricious, short-sighted behavior I saw in those around me, as well as by my own tendencies toward the same. In this sense—if I was to be totally honest—my first research question was not "what makes life meaningful for people?" but rather "why are people so terrible at living?" Sometimes it seems as if every turn of a street corner, flip of a page in a newspaper, or click on a hyperlink (or even worse, expedition through the junk email folder) confronts one with some awful, pathetic animal of a person committing foul, base or harmful deeds against other people, society, the planet. Each of us are so far from the ideal, can there ever be hope for us?

Thank goodness that I was not permanently transfixed by my notion of the ideal, and how far away from it we actually are. It was the science fiction writer, Samuel R. Delany, who paved the way for a release from ideological paralysis with one simple quote: "The problem isn't to learn to love humanity, but to learn to love those members of it who happen to be at hand" (Delaney, 1975). The cumulative weight of our human sins may seem too great to overcome, but those people we can see right in front of us have encouraging and inspiring qualities. Releasing the ideal of how people ought to be enabled me to work on understanding the best of how people actually are.

In some ways, psychologists who study well-being face a similar pull between the poles of the ideal and the actual. The debate over eudaimonia vs. hedonia is a compelling example of this dynamic. Whereas philosophy may have the imperative to characterize the ideal, psychology more or less has the imperative to observe the actual. In this chapter I will consider whether psychology should be concerned about succumbing to "conception confusion and normative naïveté" (Nussbaum, 2008) regarding eudaimonia and hedonia. I will offer my own interpretation of these two concepts from a psychological standpoint, and I will use the construct of meaning in life as an example of why psychology might find a third way between eudaimonia and hedonia.

M.F. Steger (✉)
Colorado State University, Fort Collins, CO, USA

North-West University, Vanderbijlpark, South Africa
e-mail: Michael.f.steger@colostate.edu

J. Vittersø (ed.), *Handbook of Eudaimonic Well-Being*, International Handbooks of Quality-of-Life,
DOI 10.1007/978-3-319-42445-3_11

11.1 Actual or Ideal?

In a nutshell, modern psychology builds models, and sometimes theories, based on observed data, then tests whether these models or theories yield observed data that comply with or contradict expected outcomes. Models and theories are then modified to better account for what was observed if there is deviation. This is ultimately a practical approach to building knowledge. We read about ideas, we synthesize them and combine them, we pore over other people's data analyses, then we make predictions based on the ideas and data we have consumed. We test our predictions and learn a little bit with each study. If we cannot turn our ideas, models, or theories into a prediction that can be tested, then we do not get very far.

Granted, simple observations tell us very little without theory to guide us in interpretation. We need theory to know what to test and how to test it, how to evaluate the quality of what is tested, how to analyze observations, and what we have learned from the endeavor. At least in this regard, philosophical objections to psychology's research into happiness are very helpful. One of the most prominent philosophers of happiness, Nussbaum (2008), argues that psychology has been misguided because of a struggle to define satisfactorily key concepts such as *pleasure*, *happiness*, and even *positive*, and a tendency to treat such constructs as unitary when they may be multidimensional. I agree with this critique, yet at the same time, its threat might be overstated for my discipline. One of the most lengthy of Nussbaum's critiques on conceptual problems concerns focuses on making a case for psychology to broaden its perspective on which emotions count as "positive," that grief, for example, may be just as positive as love. This critique has already been made numerous times (e.g., Ryan & Deci, 2001) and has been the subject of many years of research under the general name of posttraumatic growth (e.g., Tedeschi & Calhoun, 1995).

A related criticism of Nussbaum's is that psychologists, rather than trying to understand what our research participants might mean, instead resort to "bullying people into disregarding features of their own experience that reflection would quickly reveal" (p. S86). Psychologists are presumed to proceed in a way that cows our participants into coughing up artificial answers to our surveys on happiness, short-circuiting their ability consider the richness of their experience. Nussbaum argues that if notions of happiness put forth by philosophers such as Aristotle, Mill, or Gosling are correct then psychologists' methods do not yield particularly relevant knowledge. This reference to past philosophers brings to light one of the troubling aspects of philosophy from the perspective of a more empirically inclined questioner: Why can't we tell if Aristotle is correct yet? We've had more than 2000 years to decide already! When are debates settled in philosophy, and if such core controversies as the nature of happiness are not decided, how are we in psychology supposed to put key philosophical issues and concepts to use? Are we to wait another 1000 years for Aristotle's ideas to be evaluated, and another 3000 for Mill's to be mulled over? I noted above that scholars have discussed ideas about unpleasant emotions being positive and growth following trauma for decades. It is not enough in psychology to be able to conceive that people might experience such things. Instead, we need to demonstrate that they are relevant and important, and in roughly what proportion of people. For example, it is widely acknowledged that many, if not most, people report growing in some ways after a trauma, but it is still important from a psychological standpoint to question rigorously whether such growth is an illusory belief or an observable increase in capacity (e.g., Frazier et al., 2009).

Overall, Nussbaum's critique of positive psychology has quite limited relevance to our field, not because it is a critique—I am heavily in favor of that—but because it relies on such a simple, monolithic reading of the field. It is overly reliant on Seligman's (2002) popular press book and on Diener's (2000) work on subjective well-being, though she does not cite it. Even then, arguments focus on only a narrow slice of work, namely that positive emotions are preferable for happiness, and that it may be time to consider working happiness into public policy. She misses hundreds if not thousands of works related to the topic, many dozens by Seligman and Diener themselves. Essentially, the portrayal of positive psychology offered in Nussbaum's critique is a field absorbed in a simple-minded hedonistic paradigm: that happiness is no more or no less than more pleasurable emotions and less unpleasant emotions. This critique targets a position held by very few people in the world of positive psychology, to my knowledge (cf. Kahneman & Krueger, 2006). Instead, books, journals, conferences, and articles about positive psychology are filled with myriad constructs; gratitude, character strengths, curiosity, courage, self-compassion, mindfulness, authenticity, etc. I would guess that most of the people studying these constructs, as well as higher-order constructs such as happiness, quality of life, and well-being, would say that they are part of a broader endeavor to understand human flourishing on multiple levels.

11.2 Me Versus Us; Fleeting Versus Enduring

The hedonic-eudaimonic debate appears to pit pleasure against virtuous striving. I think it is pretty interesting that it is this pair that we humans have been debating for so long. Part of my intrigue is that these two ideals do not always seem to be opposites. We might just as well argue that "real" happiness is autonomy versus creativity, languor versus aesthetics, or collective effort versus ambition. But this is the debate we are stuck with. Suffice it to say that I think there are plenty of virtuous activities that yield pleasure, and plenty of pleasures that are virtuous. In the remainder of this chapter, I wish to describe an understanding of hedonia and eudaimonia that seems to make more sense for psychology, and discuss how meaning in life exemplifies key features of my revised notions of hedonia and eudaimonia.

11.2.1 The Hedonic Axiom: A Dead End?

The hedonic stance is that pleasure is the only true source of goodness (Tiberus & Hall, 2010; Tiberius, Chap. 38, this volume). In its most reduced form, if happiness is indeed a goal for societies then people should be given license to do whatever feels good regardless of costs or consequence. In a more sophisticated form, from a psychological standpoint, the hedonic axiom is essentially arguing that operant conditioning is sufficient to explain all human behavior. After all, in Skinner's (1938) elegant studies on animal (and perhaps his own children's) learning, organisms are instinctively motivated to avoid stimuli they find aversive or painful and obtain more of stimuli they find desirable or pleasurable. Punishment and reinforcement rely on these dynamics and can be deployed in a manner to shape behavior. Behavior is punished by deploying pain or removing pleasure, and reinforcement is deployed by removing pain or deploying pleasure. Humans are animals with well-evolved pleasure and pain circuits, so these operant conditioning principles work with us, too, as one can see in many behavioral psychotherapies (e.g., Barlow, Craske, Cerny, & Klosko, 1989).

From a psychological standpoint, the hedonic axiom would lead to a version of happiness resembling Skinner's fictional utopia *Walden Two* (Skinner, 1948). In his novel, Skinner describes a community in which environmental variables are dictated from on high to condition ideal behavior, leading to people living out happy productive lives because their life experience has been carefully calibrated to punish away impediments to happiness and reinforce desirable behaviors. Assuming that such control is possible and can be directed toward happiness rather than suppression, the notion of pleasure would need to expand considerably to encompass any construct that seems desirable. Setting aside for the moment the fact that people act in all manner of ways that ignores, or perhaps even contradicts, any pursuit of pleasure, critical cultural values such as social harmony, industriousness, conformity, all would need to cause pleasure in some way for the hedonic account to pertain to even this reductionistic approach to human flourishing. The problem from my perspective is, as Nussbam (2008) points out, that pleasure can be caused by or construed as being so many different things to different people that the word itself loses meaning exactly when it attempts to account for any behavior more complex that immediate gratification.

I prefer to view hedonism as being marked by two different qualities rather than simple (or omnivorously vague) pleasure. At its worst, hedonia has been depicted as vulgar or animalistic, and that it can lead people down dark alleys of selfishness, materialism, objectified sexuality, and ecological destructiveness (Ryan, Huta, & Deci, 2008; Ryan & Martela, Chap. 7, this volume; Huta, Chap. 15, this volume). These dire outcomes are facilitated by an overemphasis on an individual's self-centered pursuit of short-term gratification. Maximization of pleasure is not, in and of itself, sufficient to explain why devotion to hedonia might create individual and shared desolation (Steger, Shin, Shim, & Fitch-Martin, 2013). Instead, the true trap of hedonia is created by two qualities: the excessive priority given to one's self-centered interests and experiences and the excessive priority given to immediate experience in the limited present tense. Thus, my understanding of hedonia is that it is marked by excessive self-centered priorities and short-term gratifications.

11.2.2 The Eudaimonic Axiom: Not Helpful

The eudaimonic axiom asserts that eudaimonia is the ultimate life goal that all seek. This characterization is clearly not helpful from a psychological perspective. Defining eudaimonia as a universal striving shared by all people is not compelling because not everyone seeks the same thing, and defining it as the most important thing that individual people idiosyncratically seek is not helpful because of the boundless malleability allowed. Just as pleasure could be expanded to provide the payoff for nearly any activity or inactivity, so could an ultimate life goal. While psychology has become quite adept as studying goals and goal-setting (e.g., Brandtstädter & Rothermund, 2002), depicting eudaimonia in terms of an ultimate life goal introduces an additional difficulty. Eudaimonia is supposed to be the very thing that people strive for constantly in life, motivating their decisions, actions, and intentions. How do we measure such a construct? Are we to take it that Eudaimonia is the justification people apply to all their decisions or just some of them? Does eudaimonia inform the route they take to and from work, their preference for cherry versus vanilla yogurt, their choice of a life partner, whether they have children, whether they wear sweaters or jackets, what they want their life to count for at the end of their days? I believe we need to avoid defining happiness in terms of grand, all-encompassing justifications for people's behavior whether that be pleasure or the ultimate life goal.

Taking a further step to specify eudaimonia as an active striving toward virtuous excellence and perfection, as Aristotle seems to have done, pulls the construct closer to something that psychology can study. Rather than the broadness of an ultimate life goal, relentless and committed self-improvement is more easily operationalized. There still are questions about some of the definitional components that may stimulate controversy. What counts as virtue, or excellence? Who gets to decide, experts or individuals? Can someone be happy if they constantly fail to self-improve?

I would like to argue that my framing of hedonia sets up a much more useful contrast with eudaimonia. Rather than trying to argue pleasure versus virtuous striving, the focus shifts to identifying the extent to which a person's behavior is directed at self-centered versus collective aims or at immediate gratification versus more enduring impact. Hedonia would be actions motivated by self-centered interest in immediate gratification and eudaimonia would be effort directed at making a more enduring impact that benefits the self in the context of other people and responsibility toward the collective or community. In essence, I think it is worth considering hedonia and eudaimonia as opposite poles of the gap between acting for Me versus Us and acting for Fleeting impulse versus Enduring impact.

Next, I will contrast this characterization with other descriptions in psychology, followed by a consideration of how a dual process model of happiness supports my characterization of hedonia/eudaimonia.

11.2.3 Eudaimonia in Psychology

The most prominent approaches to eudaimonia in psychology have adopted two strategies (Deci & Ryan, 2008). The first is an overarching definition approach, similar to philosophical accounts, and the second is a list of criterial goods approach, which seeks to list characteristics the cultivation of which would satisfy eudaimonic criteria for happiness. In the first camp, Waterman (1993) understood eudaimonia in terms of *personal expressiveness* and an effort to bring to life the potential of one's true self. Ryan and Deci (2001) understood eudaimonia in Aristotelian terms, as well-being achieved through cultivation of virtue and satisfaction of universal psychological needs; both virtue and psychological needs being nutritive for human beings. Both of these efforts contrast with the understanding of eudaimonia put forth in this chapter because they emphasize self-improvement or self-enrichment, and while developing positive relationships with other people is important in these efforts, people are presumed happy in the eudaimonic sense if they are self-focused rather than focused on potential impacts on other people as well as the self. Both of these efforts emphasize the importance of enduring efforts, as cultivating virtue and potential are long-term goals.

In the second camp, the most prominent work has been done by Ryff (1989, Ryff & Singer, 1998; Ryff & Keyes, 1995; this volume), who developed a model of beneficial psychological qualities that constitute eudaimonic well-being: self-acceptance, positive relations with others, autonomy, environmental mastery, purpose in life, and personal growth. An important contrast with the approach offered in this chapter is that it is unclear what the criteria are for determining is a psychological quality if beneficial enough for inclusion in the list. Why is self-acceptance good enough but not positive affect? This approach creates the perception that there are unspoken criteria in a search for psychological constructs that are really, really, really good. One example comes from Ryan et al. (2008) who included basic psychological needs (competence, relatedness, and autonomy), intrinsic goals and values, and mindfulness among the leading indicators of eudaimonia. An additional example comes from my own research in which we asked a panel of experts to help us determine a checklist of behaviors that were prototypically eudaimonic or hedonic (Steger, Kashdan, & Oishi, 2008). The resulting checklist of eudaimonic behaviors included some really, really good things, such volunteering, generosity, cultivating relationships, persevering, and working toward valued goals. Perhaps it was just blind luck, but many of the behaviors that made that checklist are amenable to my current depiction of eudaimonia as being efforts directed at making an enduring positive impact on one's self as well as others (See also Huta & Ryan, 2010).

11.2.4 Dual Process Model of Happiness

In an effort to move away from potential traps of describing hedonia and eudaimonia in overly philosophical terms and to move toward a more psychologically measurable approach, Steger and Shin (2012) proposed a dual process model of happiness. The aim of the present chapter is not to review the substantial literature on the neurobiology of cognition, but just to offer a new perspective on hedonia and eudaimonia.

The essence of an argument for a dual process model of happiness is that people make decisions using multiple neural networks, which for convenience can be broken down into fast and automatically evaluative versus slow and intentionally deliberative. The fast system seems to rely on pleasure and pain, or at least rapid evaluations of whether a stimulus is pleasing or aversive. The slow system seems to rely on abstract thinking, examination of relevant information in light of personal values, goals, and memories, and an exertion of intentional processing and reasoning.

If we choose to link hedonia to a fast-processing evaluative system, rather than to vague notions about pleasure, we avoid depictions of hedonia as being base, craven, or animalistic. In contrast, we gain the possibility that hedonia may give rise to ethical, moral, and prosocial behavior even though such laudable behavior may be stimulated by self-gratifying impulses. In return, we gain a sense that hedonia is a heuristic mode of decision making present in all people but which may be activated or countered. We also gain a new lens to investigate hedonia, namely through the neurological correlates and substrates of fast evaluations and heuristic decision-making ("fast thinking" in the popular words of Kahneman, 2011).

If we choose to link this eudaimonia to a slow-processing deliberative system ("slow thinking," Kahneman, 2011), rather than potentially contentious ideals such as virtue, potential, and excellence, we avoid depictions of eudaimonia as being difficult, idealized, and unimpeachably noble (see also Steger & Shin, 2012; Steger et al., 2013). In return, we gain a sense of eudaimonia as an intentional mode of decision making that is present in all people but which may be distracted, diverted, or overwhelmed at times, and consciously deployed at others. We also gain a new lens for studying eudaimonia as a neurological process of interpreting information, making decisions, and motivating action on an intentional, deliberative basis, and directing those resources toward more enduring, less self-centered pursuits.

If we choose to use the notions of hedonia and eudaimonia suggested here, new lines of research would be revealed. For example, rather than weighing arguments about whether the pleasure of helping a sick child is hedonic or eudaimonic, we can assess whether people making the decision to help show signs of greater activation in areas associated with fast versus slow processing. Differential activation could be compared with self-reported well-being on a variety of indices, as well as with satisfaction with helping attempts and outcomes. Rather than argue over whether hedonia or eudaimonia is better or more true, we can examine the life outcomes of those who typically show signs of fast versus slow system activation, or we can examine outcomes related to whether people typically make decisions based on self-centered urges for immediate gratification or based on more collectively-oriented desires for long-term impact. In short, it seems that what may be needed is not to debate the accuracy or merits of Aristotle versus Bentham in determining the course of psychological research into flourishing, but rather a re-analysis of hedonia/eudaimonia in terms that are more compatible with modern scientific psychology.

11.2.5 Meaning in Life: Eudaimonic But Not Solely Eudaimonic

In classic models of hedonia and eudaimonia, meaning in life usually was placed into the eudaimonic category (e.g., Ryff, 1989) because there was a strong hint of self-improvement and virtue to meaning. If we take a step further back to the basic axiom of eudaimonia, that a life marked by meaning is also a good life spent in active pursuit of the ultimate goal for life, then meaning seems to fit most people's notions of what meaning in life is. If we examine formal definitions of meaning in life, then "meaning in life is the set of subjective judgements people make that their lives are (a) worthwhile and significant, (b) comprehensible and make sense, and (c) marked by the embrace or pursuit of one or more highly valued, over-arching purposes or missions" (Steger, in press; see also Martela & Steger, 2015; Steger, 2009). The first component, that one's life is worthwhile, that it matters, is clearly in line with what seems to be the level of gravity intended by descriptions of the eudaimonic life. Thus, even at the basic level, a life is good and worthy of one's ultimate aims if it is meaningful because that life matters and is significant. Meaning in life thus defined also fits with more specific models of eudaimonia because of the third component, pursuit of purpose, which reflects the level of virtuous striving common to classic psychological and philosophical descriptions of eudaimonia. Indeed, research evidence has been presented showing stronger relations over time of meaning with eudaimonic activity versus hedonic activity (e.g., Steger, Kashdan, Sullivan, & Lorentz, 2008).

There is another aspect of meaning that resonates with the notion of eudaimonia proposed in this chapter. People not only experience meaning in life, they also search for meaning in life. In fact, people search for meaning whether they perceive their lives to have abundant meaning or to be empty of meaning (e.g., Steger et al., 2008). On average, people searching for meaning experience greater distress than others, but they also endorse a wide range of variables that tie into deliberative cognitive processes directed toward trying to consider and understand the nature of their experiences and of life as a whole. Search for meaning, then, seems clearly eudaimonic in the present model.

At the same time, it is fairly easy to counter such classification of meaning in life as a eudaimonic variable with evidence that meaning in life has hedonic characteristics, too, primarily in terms of consistent and robust correlations with positive affect (Ryff, 1989; Steger et al., 2008; Steger, Frazier, Oishi, & Kaler, 2006). Several studies by Hicks, King, and colleagues have shown a clear influence of positive affect on improving judgments of meaning in life (e.g., King, Hicks, Krull, & Del Gaiso, 2006; Ward & King, Chap. 35, this volume). It is true that definitions of meaning in life often speak of striving and pursuit, which may be strenuous rather than pleasurable. It is also true that the historical roots of meaning grow from the observation that meaning may be particularly relevant as a source of strength in the face of suffering, and a stronger sense of meaning in life may be one of the fruits of suffering (Frankl, 1963). Nevertheless, research suggests that meaning in life is a bit promiscuous, and positively correlates with a huge array of well-being indicators, from pleasure and positive emotions to spirituality and altruism (Steger, 2012). Using the classic models, then, meaning in life would seem to be eudaimonic and even a bit hedonic (Steger et al., 2013).

11.3 Conclusion

In the view presented in this chapter, hedonia and eudaimonia are distinguished by their emphasis on Me versus Us, and Fleeting versus Durable. Within this framework, meaning in life has features, shown by empirical research, that are hedonic because non-conscious cues and short-term gratifications affect people's judgments of meaning. Meaning also can be moved convincingly into the eudaimonic camp because rather than concerning ourselves about whether people are overly interested in experiencing fun and pleasure (boo-hiss!), this new framework asks about people's intentions, motivations, and concerns for engaging in particular actions. Meaning in life is thought to be marked by a sense of mattering, a conceptualization of existence that incorporates the self and others as well as an extended world of reality, and dedication to the pursuit of a purpose or aspiration that provides direction throughout one's life. For example, the person who sings songs to entertain people in long-term care facilities is not judged then on whether she or he enjoys that activity versus whether the activity can be considered to be virtuous and self-improving. Instead, that person is judged based on whether the activity was stimulated by an interest in gratifying immediate, self-centered desires or by an interest in making a contribution to others as well as to her or his self. Everyone can have fun, or everyone can find it poignant. Neither emotional outcome is relevant to whether the action would be judged as hedonic or eudaimonic. Meaningful actions will be driven by an interest in making a difference, making a contribution, striving toward the future, and consciously incorporating experience into an understanding of the world. Meaning finds its highest expression in the transcendence (see Reker & Wong, 1988) of exactly the kinds of actions driven by a faulty field of view that stops at one's own skin and extends only to the next moment. It is through rising above what I want right now for my own sake that we find meaning.

And that seems pretty eudaimonic to me.

References

Barlow, D. H., Craske, M. G., Cerny, J. A., & Klosko, J. S. (1989). Behavioral treatment of panic disorder. *Behavior Therapy, 20*, 261–282.

Brandtstädter, J., & Rothermund, K. (2002). The life-course dynamics of goal pursuit and goal adjustment: A two-process framework. *Developmental Review, 22*, 117–150.

Deci, E. L., & Ryan, R. M. (2008). Hedonia, eudaimonia, and well-being: An introduction. *Journal of Happiness Studies, 9*, 1–11.

Delaney, S. R. (1975). *Dhalgren*. New York: Bantam.

Diener, E. (2000). Subjective well-being: The science of happiness and a proposal for a national index. *American Psychologist, 55*, 34–43.

Frankl, V. E. (1963). *Man's search for meaning: An introduction to logotherapy*. New York: Washington Square Press.

Frazier, P., Tennen, H., Gavian, M., Park, C., Tomich, P., & Tashiro, T. (2009). Does self-reported posttraumatic growth reflect genuine positive change? *Psychological Science, 20*, 912–919.

Huta, V., & Ryan, R. M. (2010). Pursuing pleasure or virtue: The differential and overlapping well-being benefits of hedonic and eudaimonic motives. *Journal of Happiness Studies, 11*, 735–762.

Kahneman, D. (2011). *Thinking, fast and slow*. New York: Macmillan.

Kahneman, D., & Krueger, A. B. (2006). Developments in the measurement of subjective well-being. *Journal of Economic Perspectives, 20*, 3–24.

King, L. A., Hicks, J. A., Krull, J., & Del Gaiso, A. K. (2006). Positive affect and the experience of meaning in life. *Journal of Personality and Social Psychology, 90*, 179–196.

Martela, F., & Steger, M. F. (2015). The three meanings of meaning in life: Distinguishing coherence, purpose and significance. *Manuscript under review*.

Nussbaum, M. C. (2008). Who is the happy warrior? Philosophy poses questions to psychology. *Journal of Legal Studies, 37*, S81–S113.

Reker, G. T., & Wong, P. T. P. (1988). Aging as an individual process: Toward a theory of personal meaning. In J. E. Birren & V. L. Bengston (Eds.), *Emergent theories of aging* (pp. 214–246). New York: Springer.

Ryan, R. M., & Deci, E. L. (2001). On happiness and human potentials: A review of research on hedonic and eudaimonic well-being. *Annual Review of Psychology, 52*, 141–166.

Ryan, R. M., Huta, V., & Deci, E. L. (2008). Living well: A self-determination theory perspective on eudaimonia. *Journal of Happiness Studies, 9*, 139–170.

Ryff, C. D. (1989). Happiness is everything, or is it? Explorations on the meaning of psychological well-being. *Journal of Personality and Social Psychology, 57*, 1069–1081.

Ryff, C. D., & Keyes, C. L. M. (1995). The structure of well-being revisited. *Journal of Personality and Social Psychology, 69*, 719–727.

Ryff, C. D., & Singer, B. H. (1998). The contours of positive human health. *Psychological Inquiry, 9*, 1–28.

Seligman, M. E. P. (2002). *Authentic happiness: Using the new positive psychology to realize your potential for lasting fulfillment*. New York: Free Press.

Skinner, B. F. (1938). *The behavior of organisms: An experimental analysis*. New York: Appleton-Century.

Skinner, B. F. (1948). *Walden two*. Indianapolis, IN: Hackett Publishing Company.

Steger, M. F. (2009). Meaning in life. In S. J. Lopez & C. R. Snyder (Eds.), *Oxford handbook of positive psychology* (2nd ed.). New York: Oxford University Press.

Steger, M. F. (2012). Experiencing meaning in life: Optimal functioning at the nexus of spirituality, psychopathology, and well-being. In P. T. P. Wong (Ed.), *The human quest for meaning* (2nd ed., pp. 165–184). New York: Routledge.

Steger, M. F., Frazier, P., Oishi, S., & Kaler, M. (2006). The meaning in life questionnaire: Assessing the presence of and search for meaning in life. *Journal of Counseling Psychology, 53*, 80–93.

Steger, M. F., Kashdan, T. B., Sullivan, B. A., & Lorentz, D. (2008). Understanding the search for meaning in life: Personality, cognitive style, and the dynamic between seeking and experiencing meaning. *Journal of Personality, 76*, 199–228.

Steger, M. F., Kashdan, T. B., & Oishi, S. (2008). Being good by doing good: Eudaimonic activity and daily well-being correlates, mediators, and temporal relations. *Journal of Research in Personality, 42*, 22–42.

Steger, M. F., & Shin, J. Y. (2012). Happiness and meaning in a technological world. In P. Brey, A. Briggle, & E. Spence (Eds.), *The good life in a technological age* (pp. 92–108). New York: Routledge.

Steger, M. F., Shin, J. Y., Shim, Y., & Fitch-Martin, A. (2013). Is meaning in life a flagship indicator of well-being? In A. Waterman (Ed.), *The best within us: Positive psychology perspectives on eudaimonia* (pp. 159–182). Washington, DC: APA Press.

Steger, F. (in press). Meaning in life: A unified model. In S. J. Lopez, L. M. Edwards, & S. C. Marques (Eds.), *Oxford handbook of positive psychology* (3rd Ed.), Oxford, UK: Oxford University Press.

Tedeschi, R. G., & Calhoun, L. G. (1995). *Trauma and transformation: Growing in the aftermath of suffering*. Thousand Oaks, CA: Sage.

Tiberus, V., & Hall, A. (2010). Normative theory and psychological research: Hedonism, eudaimonism and why it matters. *The Journal of Positive Psychology, 5*, 212–225.

Waterman, A. S. (1993). Two conceptions of happiness: Contrasts of personal expressiveness (eudaimonia) and hedonic enjoyment. *Journal of Personality and Social Psychology, 64*, 678–691.

12 The Eudaimonics of Positive Emotions

Barbara L. Fredrickson

12.1 The Eudaimonics of Positive Emotions

The science of positive psychology reveals that humans experience well-being in multiple forms. One form is hedonic, characterized by the experience of sensory pleasures or positive emotions. Another form is eudaimonic, characterized by experiences that transcend immediate sensory or emotional gratification to enable individuals to experience themselves as connected to the higher callings of purpose, meaning, contribution, and interconnectedness.

The tendency to subdivide and rank distinct constructs – philosophical, psychological, or otherwise – can be strong, especially in Western cultures (Nisbett, Peng, Choi, & Norenzayan, 2001). That tendency, coupled with caricatured depictions of the positive emotions as merely representing the pleasures of self-gratification, has sometimes led scholars and others to place eudaimonic experiences and the pursuit of them on a high pedestal, while situating hedonic experiences and their pursuit as more lowly human motivations. Others push this distinction further, by suggesting a typology, in which some individuals, for at least some of the time, are chiefly governed by hedonia, whereas other individuals are chiefly governed by eudaimonia, again, for at least some of the time.

These prevailing representations of hedonia and eudaimonia can divert scholars from investigating other, more complex and dynamic interrelationships between these two forms of well-being, and in turn, the contributions that each holds for physical health. Ultimately, how hedonia and eudaimonia interrelate is an empirical, not a philosophical question.

12.1.1 Initial Empirical Insights

Data from my team's recent research offer a few strands of evidence regarding the dynamic interconnections of hedonic and eudaimonic well-being. Ample past research had linked each form of well-being to physical health and longevity (e.g., Chida & Steptoe, 2008; Hill & Turiano, 2014). In addition, although conceptually distinct, both forms of well-being are positively correlated with one another (Keyes, Shmotkin, & Ryff, 2002; Ryff, Chap. 6, this volume; Waterman, 1993). This close association can make it a challenge to discern whether one form of well-being is more directly associated with biological health benefits.

My team's initial foray into the study of eudaimonia involved gathering self-reports of both hedonic and eudaimonic well-being, as two fac-

B.L. Fredrickson (✉)
University of North Carolina at Chapel Hill, Chapel Hill, NC, USA
e-mail: blf@unc.edu

J. Vittersø (ed.), *Handbook of Eudaimonic Well-Being*, International Handbooks of Quality-of-Life,
DOI 10.1007/978-3-319-42445-3_12

ets of the broader construct of flourishing mental health (Keyes, 2002; Keyes & Annas, 2009), using the Mental Health Continuum-Short Form (MHC-SF; Lamers, Westerhof, Bohlmeijer, ten Klooster, & Keyes, 2011). Hedonic well-being was captured by items such as, "During the past month, how often did you feel… happy? … interested in life? …satisfied with life?" Eudaimonic well-being, by contrast, was captured by items such as, "During the past month, how often did you feel… that you had something to contribute to society? …that your life has a sense of direction or meaning to it? … that you belonged to a community (like a social group, or your neighborhood)? In addition to these self-report measures, we drew a blood sample from each participant to examine profiles of gene expression within their circulating white blood cells.

This approach to using functional genomics as a window onto physical health status was inspired by the work of my colleague, Steve Cole. Across of series of studies, Cole and his collaborators have linked adverse psychological and social conditions to a pattern of altered gene expression within circulating leukocytes (Cole, 2012, 2013; Irwin & Cole, 2011). This profile, termed the *conserved transcriptional response to adversity* (CTRA), is marked by higher expression of genes involved in inflammation (e.g., pro-inflammatory cytokines such as *IL1B*, *IL6*, *IL8*, and *TNF*) and lower expression of genes involved in type I IFN antiviral responses (e.g., *IFI*-, *OAS*-, and *MX*-family genes) and IgG1 antibody synthesis (e.g., *IGJ*) (Cole, 2012, 2013; Irwin & Cole, 2011; Slavich & Cole, 2013). Studies of non-human primates show that experimental imposition of threatening or unstable social conditions can causally induce CTRA gene expression (Cole et al., 2012; Tung et al., 2012). The CTRA program is thought to have evolved to help human ancestors' immune systems anticipate and counter changing patterns of microbial threat recurrently associated with changing environmental conditions, such as increased risk of wound-related bacterial infection associated with experienced threat, social conflict, or isolation versus increased risk of socially-mediated viral infection associated with frequent and positive social contact (Cole, Hawkley, Arevalo, & Cacioppo, 2011; Irwin & Cole, 2011). In modern environments, however, chronic CTRA activation by social or psychological threats may promote inflammation-mediated chronic diseases and impair host resistance to viral infections.

Given that various forms of psychosocial adversity had been convincingly linked with the CTRA profile, together with Cole, my team and I have investigated whether either hedonia, eudaimonia, or both – either singly or in combination – would oppose the CTRA gene expression profile, as represented across a set of 53 genes selected a priori based on Cole and colleagues' past results within studies of psychosocial adversity. An opposing leukocyte gene expression profile would be marked by a *lower* expression of proinflammatory genes, coupled with a *higher* expression of antiviral and antibody synthesis genes. Such a molecular signature is arguably supportive of a healthy functioning immune system, although that assumption remains to be tested empirically.

We took this empirical approach in our first published study on hedonia and eudaimonia, which featured a sample of midlife adults from the Southeastern United States (Fredrickson et al. 2013). This initial publication met with considerable interest and also some disbelief (Brown, MacDonald, Samanta, Friedman, & Coyne, 2014). As such, we published a replication of our initial findings using the same exact measures in an independent sample of midlife adults from the same US region (Fredrickson et al., 2015), and also sought to explore more deeply the strength of the evidence. Here, in the interest of economy, I report the results for the pooled sample ($N = 198$, as presented in Fredrickson et al., 2015), which combines the participants from both our Discovery and Confirmation Studies.

We used mixed effect linear models to predict participants' CTRA gene expression profiles, as observed within their circulating white blood cells, from their self-reports of hedonic and eudaimonic well-being. Across all models, statistical evidence suggested that these two forms of well-being, although correlated, captured distinct constructs (i.e., Variance Inflation Factors, VIF, were well below the threshold that would indicate distortion by multicollinearity between predictor variables). The overall pattern of results that emerged from these mixed effect linear models suggests that, when both hedonia and eudaimonia are simultaneously entered as predictor variables (alongside an a priori set of demographic and health-related control variables), only eudaimonic well-being emerges as significantly associated with the inverse of the CTRA gene expression profile. The association for hedonic well-being, in this same analysis, is of the opposite sign (i.e., it shows a *positive* association with the adversity-related gene expression profile) although it does not achieve traditional levels of statistical significance.

We also explored alternative representations of well-being, including (a) a three-dimensional scoring of the MHC-SF, which subdivides the index of eudaimonic well-being into separate subscales for psychological and social well-being; (b) a one-dimensional scoring of the MHC-SF, which can be called total well-being, (c) a categorical scoring of the MHC-SF, that follows Keyes' criteria (Keyes, 2006) for identifying flourishing mental health, and (d) an alternative three-dimensional scoring of the MHC-SF, advanced by Brown, MacDonald, Samanta, Friedman, & Coyne (2014). Overall, these additional analyses revealed that the substantial variance shared in common by psychological and social well-being – the two sub-dimensions of eudaimonic well-being measured by the MHC-SF – carried most of the association with gene expression. Integration of the MHC-SF hedonia items (i.e., for total well-being, or for the categorical identification of flourishing mental health), tended to degrade the strength and reliability of the association between eudaimonia and CTRA gene expression.

These results lead to the conclusion that eudaimonia (but not hedonia) may be most directly related to the inverse of the adversity-related pattern of leukocyte gene expression. To test whether this inverse association between eudaimonia and CTRA gene expression generalized to a different and more robust measure of eudaimonic well-being, my team and I drew archival genomic data from a study of midlife adults in Western Canada ($N = 107$) that included the Ryff Scales for Psychological Well-Being (Ryff-PWB; Ryff, 1989). Whereas psychological well-being is assessed in the MHC-SF by 6 items, it is assessed in the Ryff-PWB by 54 items (6 subscales of 9 items each). The six targeted subdomains of eudaimonia in the Ryff-PWB include (a) *purpose in life*, (b) *environmental mastery*, (c) *self-acceptance*, (d) *autonomy*, (e) *personal growth*, and (f) *positive relations with others*. Analyses of this independent Generalization Study revealed that five of Ryff's six subdomains of eudaimonia predicted reduced CTRA gene expression when analyzed separately (i.e., all subdomains except *personal growth*), and three remained distinctly prognostic in mutually adjusted analyses (i.e., *self-acceptance*, *autonomy*, and *positive relations with others*, although it bears noting that *purpose in life* was marginally significant).

The inverse association between eudaimonic well-being and the CTRA gene expression profile has emerged in a fourth published study as well (Cole et al., 2015). Drawing on data from a nationally representative sample of US adults over the age of 50 ($N = 108$), Cole and colleagues again linked self-reports of eudaimonia (here measured with seven items from the Ryff-PWB *purpose in life* scale) to the inverse of the CTRA gene expression profile. The association between eudaimonic well-being and this (presumably beneficial) molecular signature was robust. It remained statistically significant even when other positive psychological constructs were in turn added as additional predictors within statistical models, namely positive affect, optimism and life satisfaction.

To sum, considering all the empirical evidence to date, the link between eudaimonia and this potentially health-relevant pattern of gene expression – marked by lower expression of proinflammatory genes coupled with higher expression of antiviral and antibody synthesis genes – appears robust: It is unaffected by (1) multicollinearity between measures of hedonia and eudaimonia, (2) the use of alternative analytical techniques (i.e., mixed effect linear models), (3) the use of alternative scoring systems and alternative measures of eudaimonia, and (4) the in inclusion of other positive psychological constructs in mutually-adjusted analyses.

12.1.2 A Role for Positive Emotions?

Does the finding that eudaimonia appears to have a more direct tie to an objective indicator of physical health mean that hedonia has no role to play in fostering human health and longevity? Not necessarily. Indeed, this new evidence need be interpreted in light of existing data on the relationships between hedonia and eudaimonia – or, alternatively phrased, between pleasant experiences – particularly positive emotions – and the transcendent experiences of purpose, meaning, contribution, and interconnectedness.

Those existing data suggest that hedonia and eudaimonia are not only positively correlated, but that aspects of hedonia have been found to prospectively predict and even cause increases in the eudaimonia. In particular, across a series of prospective correlational studies of daily life experience together with tightly-controlled laboratory experiments, King and her colleagues demonstrate that positive affective states forecast and cause people to be more likely to detect meaning in life (King & Hicks, 2009; King, Hicks, Krull, & Del Gaiso, 2006; see also Ward and King, Chap. 35, this volume) Moreover, this effect of hedonia on eudaimonia becomes significantly stronger when people perceive threats to their social relationships, such as loneliness (Hicks, Schlegel, & King, 2010; Schlege, Hicks & Christy, Chap. 14, this volume), or constrained future time horizons, such as perceiving the end of their lifespan as relatively near (Hicks, Trent, Davis, & King, 2012).

Further evidence that increases in hedonia produce subsequent increases in eudaimonia can be drawn from an earlier randomized controlled trial that my team and I conducted to test my broaden-and-build theory of positive emotions (Fredrickson, 1998, 2001, 2013). In brief, the broaden-and-build theory posits that pleasant emotional states (such as joy, gratitude, serenity, and the like) momentarily broaden people's mindsets in ways that, over time, incrementally build their resources and resilience. To test whether experimentally induced increases in positive emotions indeed predicted growth in resources, we conducted a longitudinal field experiment. A sample of midlife adults residing in the US Midwest ($N=202$) was randomized to one of two experimental conditions (Fredrickson, Cohn, Coffey, Pek, & Finkel, 2008). Half were taught how to self-generate more positive emotions in daily life, through the practice of loving-kindness meditation (Salzberg, 2011). The others served in a monitoring, waitlist control group. Participants' daily reports of both positive and negative emotions revealed that, among those randomly assigned to learn loving-kindness meditation, positive emotions did indeed significantly increase over the 8-week study (no significant changes emerged for negative emotions). Following from these increments in positive emotions, we observed systematic and consequential increases in four of the six subdomains of eudaimonic well-being indexed by the Ryff PWB measure (using a variant of the scale that included seven to eight items per subscale). Specifically, we found that the four eudaimonic subdomains of *purpose in life*, *environmental mastery*, *self-acceptance*, and *positive relations with others* each showed significant increases over the course of the study, and that these facets of eudaimonia, in turn, predicted increases in life satisfaction and decreases in depressive symptoms (Fredrickson et al., 2008). Eudaimonia, then, appears to be one of the many resources that positive emotions serve to build.

These clear, evidence-based prospective and causal connections between positive emotions and facets of eudaimonia are what led my colleagues and I to make a key caveat when presenting our initial findings on the genomic correlates of hedonia and eudaimonic well-being. Specifically, we cautioned:

> *In interpreting these results, it is important to note that hedonic and eudaimonic well-being are not mutually exclusive approaches to happiness, nor do they represent a simple typology or a tradeoff. Both types of well-being share some common sources (e.g., perceived social connections) and can reciprocally influence one another … As such, the current finding that a purified index of eudaimonic well-being (purged of shared variance with hedonia) predicts a more favorable pattern of gene expression than does a purified index of hedonic well-being (purged of shared variance with eudaimonia) says more about which form of well-being one would not want to do without, rather than which one would be better to avoid.* (Fredrickson et al., 2013, p. 4)

Put differently, even if the elements of hedonia that are devoid of association with the transcendent experiences of purpose, meaning, contribution, and interconnectedness may well function as "empty calories" with respect to physical health, the overall concept of hedonia need not be considered suspect or base. Indeed, the hedonic experiences of positive emotions, with their documented abilities to expand momentary awareness, may be vital contributing factors to the subsequent detection of meaning and the emergence of eudaimonic experiences more generally. If so, hedonia may well be contribute *indirectly* to a healthy pattern of gene expression as a result of its direct relationship with eudaimonia. The figure below presents this hypothesized conceptual model of mediation.

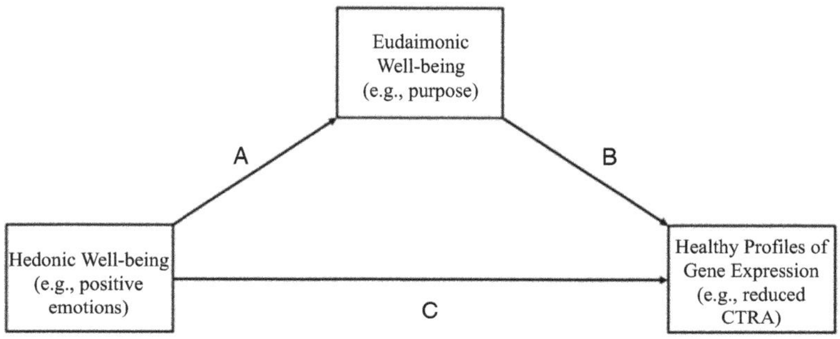

12.1.3 Further Empirical Analyses

To test the viability of this conceptual model, my colleagues and I reanalyzed and extended data from the Confirmation Study reported in our recent replication paper (i.e., Fredrickson et al., 2015). Specifically, we tested whether hedonia, as indexed by the MHC-SF, predicted the inverse of the CTRA gene expression profile. It did: When the index of hedonic well-being was the sole predictor of the CTRA profile, it shows a negative (healthy) association with this gene expression profile (supporting Path C in the above Figure). Yet further tests suggest that eudaimonia, also as indexed by the MHC-SF, accounts for (mediates) this relationship (supporting Paths A and B in the above Figure). That is, this reanalysis suggests that, to the extent that hedonic well-being is positively associated with eudaimonic well-being, hedonia is indirectly related to a (presumably) health-supportive pattern of gene expression – one marked by reduced expression of proinflammatory genes and increased expression of antiviral and antibody synthesis genes (Isgett, Boulton, Cole, & Fredrickson, 2016). It is worth noting that this same indirect path between hedonia and the inverse of the CTRA profile (mediated by eudaimonia) is implied within the latest report (Cole et al., 2015) that tested the relevant associations using a nationally representative sample reported. In this sample, hedonia was represented by positive affect as assessed from items on the PANAS (Watson, Wiese, Vaidya, & Tellegen, 1999).

It is important to recognize that assessment of hedonia using the MHC-SF is limited. The three global, retrospective items that contribute to the MHC-SF hedonia subscale ask study participants to reflect on the past week and indicate how frequently they felt "happy," "interested in life" and "satisfied." (The PANAS scale, used in Cole et al., 2015, does not go appreciably further, with the question stem: "During the last 30 days, to what degree did you feel…" and example individual items: "enthusiastic," "happy," "attentive," and "inspired.") Fortunately, the original dataset from which our Confirmation Study was drawn also included more fine-grained self-reports of positive emotions. At the end of each day, over the course of 1 week (prior to an experimental intervention), participants also completed the modified Differential Emotions Scale (mDES;

Fredrickson, 2013). Although response on the mDES are still global and retrospective, the focal period was 24 h, rather than 7 or 30 days, and the emotions assessed included 20 different emotion trios, 10 of which were positive. Specifically, study participants were asked to reflect on the past day and indicate the greatest degree that they'd experienced the following positive emotions: "amused/fun-loving/silly," "awe/wonder/amazement," "grateful/appreciative/thankful," "hopeful/optimistic/encouraged," "inspired/uplifted/elevated," "interested/alert/curious," "joyful/glad/happy," "love/closeness/trust," "proud/confident/self-assured," and "serene/content/peaceful."

We thus computed an alternative measure of hedonia for each participant by calculating the mean across these ten distinct positive emotions assessed by the mDES, both within the day, and also across the 7 days. We then tested the mediation model depicted in the figure above. Specifically, we tested whether this new index of hedonia (based on aggregated daily reports on the mDES) also predicted the inverse of the CTRA gene expression profile, as mediated by eudaimonia (indexed, as before, by the MHC-SF). We observed the same pattern of results as with the two other measures of hedonia. That is, using this more fine-grained assessment of hedonia based on daily positive emotions, we found support for an indirect path from positive emotions to a healthy pattern of leukocyte gene expression that was accounted for (mediate by) eudaimonia (Isgett et al., 2016).

12.1.4 Positive Emotions Broaden Mindsets and Build Eudaimonic Resources

Anchored as it is to the common synonyms of self-indulgence and greed, hedonia is often maligned. *Hedonia*, however, is an umbrella term that includes a large variety of pleasurable experiences that range from sensory pleasures, which often are biologically bound (Cabanac, 2010), to positive emotions, which stem from appraisals of meaning (Smith, Tong, & Ellsworth, 2014) and can be other-focused (e.g., gratitude), self-transcendent (e.g., awe), or both (e.g., elevation). The value of positive emotions cannot be dismissed: Multiple meta-analytic studies convincingly link the experience and expression of positive emotions to physical health and longevity (Boehm & Kubzansky, 2012; Chida & Steptoe, 2008; Howell, Kern, & Lyubomirsky, 2007). Consistent with these meta-analyses, the data presented here begin to illuminate the psychological and molecular pathways by which positive emotions may foster physical health.

Viewed against the backdrop of the broaden-and-build theory of positive emotions (Fredrickson, 1998, 2001, for a comprehensive review, see Fredrickson, 2013), many pleasant, uplifted emotional states are likely to broaden people's awareness (Fredrickson & Branigan, 2005; see Harmon-Jones, Gable, & Price, 2013 for important boundary conditions), enabling them to see the big picture, connect the dots, or otherwise transcend the self or the moment. Expanded mindsets like these appear to facilitate people's ability to perceive the many ways in which they contribute to, and are interconnected with others, or are otherwise called to a higher purpose or meaning. Eudaimonia, from this perspective, is one of the many durable resources that positive emotions function to build. Although eudaimonia may be more directly tied to the molecular shifts that support physical health, hedonia may be the more experience-near springboard that leads to increments in eudaimonia. It's time, then, to move beyond "either-or" thinking and suggestions of typologies or separate paths to well-being. Hedonia and eudaimonia are dynamically intertwined facets of well-being, each of which plays a vital role the overall process of human flourishing.

References

Boehm, J. K., & Kubzansky, L. D. (2012). The heart's content: The association between positive psychological well-being and cardiovascular health. *Psychological Bulletin, 138*(4), 655–691. doi:10.1037/a0027448.

Brown, N. J. L., MacDonald, D. A., Samanta, M. P., Friedman, H. L., & Coyne, J. C. (2014). A critical reanalysis of Fredrickson et al'.s study of genomics and well-being. *Proceedings of the National Academy of Sciences, 111*(35), 12705–12709.

Cabanac, M. (2010). The dialectics of pleasure. In M. L. Kringelbach & K. C. Berridge (Eds.), *Pleasures of the brain* (pp. 113–124). Oxford, UK: Oxford University Press.

Chida, Y., & Steptoe, A. (2008). Positive psychological well-being and mortality: A quantitative review of prospective observational studies. *Psychosomatic Medicine, 70*(7), 741–756. doi:10.1097/PSY.0b013e31818105ba.

Cole, S. W. (2012). Social regulation of gene expression in the immune system. In S. Segerstrom (Ed.), *Handbook of psychoneuroimmunology* (pp. 254–273). New York: Oxford University Press.

Cole, S. W. (2013). Social regulation of human gene expression: Mechanisms and implications for public health. *American Journal of Public Health, 103*(Suppl 1), S84–S92. doi:10.2105/AJPH.2012.301183.

Cole, S. W., Conti, G., Arevalo, J. M. G., Ruggiero, A. M., Heckman, J. J., & Suomi, S. J. (2012). Transcriptional modulation of the developing immune system by early life social adversity. *Proceedings of the National Academy of Sciences, 109*(50), 20578–20583. doi:10.1073/pnas.1218253109.

Cole, S. W., Hawkley, L. C., Arevalo, J. M. G., & Cacioppo, J. T. (2011). Transcript origin analysis identifies antigen-presenting cells as primary targets of socially regulated gene expression in leukocytes. *Proceedings of the National Academy of Sciences, 108*(7), 3080–3085. doi:10.1073/pnas.1014218108.

Cole, S. W., Levine, M. E., Arevalo, J. M. G., Ma, J., Weir, D. R., & Crimmins, E. M. (2015). Loneliness, eudaimonia, and the human conserved transcriptional response to adversity. *Psychoneuroendocrinology, 62*, 11–17.

Fredrickson, B. L. (1998). What good are positive emotions? *Review of General Psychology, 2*(3), 300–319.

Fredrickson, B. L. (2001). The role of positive emotions in positive psychology: The broaden-and-build theory of positive emotions. *American Psychologist, 56*(3), 218.

Fredrickson, B. L. (2013). Positive emotions broaden and build. *Advances in Experimental Social Psychology, 47*, 1–53. doi:10.1016/B978-0-12-407236-7.00001-2.

Fredrickson, B. L., & Branigan, C. (2005). Positive emotions broaden the scope of attention and thought-action repertoires. *Cognition and Emotion, 19*(3), 313–332. doi:10.1080/02699930441000238.

Fredrickson, B. L., Cohn, M. A., Coffey, K. A., Pek, J., & Finkel, S. M. (2008). Open hearts build lives: Positive emotions, induced through loving-kindness meditation, build consequential personal resources. *Journal of Personality and Social Psychology, 95*(5), 1045–1062. doi:10.1037/a0013262.

Fredrickson, B. L., Grewen, K. M., Algoe, S. B., Firestine, A. M., Arevalo, J. M. G., Ma, J., et al. (2015). Psychological well-being and the human conserved transcriptional response to adversity. *PloS One, 10*(3), e0121839.

Fredrickson, B. L., Grewen, K. M., Coffey, K. A., Algoe, S. B., Firestine, A. M., Arevalo, J. M. G., … & Cole, S. W. (2013). A functional genomic perspective on human well-being. *Proceedings of the National Academy of Sciences, 110*(33), 13684–13689. doi:10.1073/pnas.1305419110.

Harmon-Jones, E., Gable, P. A., & Price, T. F. (2013). Does negative affect always narrow and positive affect always broaden the mind? Considering the influence of motivational intensity on cognitive scope. *Current Directions in Psychological Science, 22*(4), 301–307. doi:10.1177/0963721413481353.

Hicks, J. A., Schlegel, R. J., & King, L. A. (2010). Social threats, happiness, and the dynamics of meaning in life judgments. *Personality and Social Psychology Bulletin, 36*(10), 1305–1317. doi:10.1177/0146167210381650.

Hicks, J. A., Trent, J., Davis, W. E., & King, L. A. (2012). Positive affect, meaning in life, and future time perspective: An application of socioemotional selectivity theory. *Psychology and Aging, 27*(1), 181–189. doi:10.1037/a0023965.

Hill, P. L., & Turiano, N. A. (2014). Purpose in life as a predictor of mortality across adulthood. *Psychological Science*, 1–5. doi:10.1177/0956797614531799.

Howell, R. T., Kern, M. L., & Lyubomirsky, S. (2007). Health benefits: Meta-analytically determining the impact of well-being on objective health outcomes. *Health Psychology Review, 1*(1), 83–136. doi:10.1080/17437190701492486.

Irwin, M. R., & Cole, S. W. (2011). Reciprocal regulation of the neural and innate immune systems. *Nature Reviews Immunology, 11*(9), 625–632. doi:10.1038/nri3042.

Isgett, S. F., Boulton, A. J., Cole, S. W., & Fredrickson, B. L. (2016). Coda: Positive emotions, mediated by eudaimonic well-being, predict potentially salutogenic leukocyte gene expression profiles. *In preparation.*

Keyes, C. L. M. (2002). The mental health continuum: From languishing to flourishing in life. *Journal of Health and Social Behavior, 43*(2), 207–222. doi:10.2307/3090197.

Keyes, C. L. M. (2006). The Mental Health Continuum-Short Form (MHC-SF) for adults. http://www.sociology.emory.edu/downloads/MHC-SF_Brief_Description.pdf2006

Keyes, C. L. M. & Annas, J. (2009). Feeling good and functioning well: Distinctive concepts in ancient philosophy and modern science. *Journal of Positive Psychology, 4*, 197–201.

Keyes, C. L. M., Shmotkin, D., & Ryff, C. D. (2002). Optimizing well-being: The empirical encounter of two traditions. *Journal of Personality and Social Psychology, 82*(6), 1007–1022. doi:10.1037//0022-3514.82.6.1007.

King, L. A., & Hicks, J. A. (2009). Detecting and constructing meaning in life events. *Journal of Positive*

Psychology, 4(5), 317–330. doi:10.1080/17439760902992316.
King, L. A., Hicks, J. A., Krull, J. L., & Del Gaiso, A. K. (2006). Positive affect and the experience of meaning in life. *Journal of Personality and Social Psychology, 90*(1), 179–196. doi:10.1037/0022-3514.90.1.179.
Lamers, S. M. A., Westerhof, G. J., Bohlmeijer, E. T., ten Klooster, P. M., & Keyes, C. L. M. (2011). Evaluating the psychometric properties of the Mental Health Continuum-Short Form (MHC-SF). *Journal of Clinical Psychology, 67*(1), 99–110. doi:10.1002/jclp.20741.
Nisbett, R. E., Peng, K., Choi, I., & Norenzayan, A. (2001). Culture and systems of thought: Holistic versus analytic cognition. *Psychological Review, 108*(2), 291–310. doi:10.1037//0033-295X.108.2.291.
Ryff, C. D. (1989). Happiness is everything, or is it? Explorations on the meaning of psychological well-being. *Journal of Personality and Social Psychology, 57*(6), 1069–1081. doi:10.1037/0022-3514.57.6.1069.
Salzberg, S. (2011). *Real happiness*. New York: Workman Publishing.
Slavich, G. M., & Cole, S. W. (2013). The emerging field of human social genomics. *Clinical Psychological Science, 1*(3), 331–348. doi:10.1177/2167702613478594.
Smith, C. A., Tong, E. M. W., & Ellsworth, P. C. (2014). The differentiation of positive emotional experience as viewed through the lens of appraisal theory. In M. M. Tugade, M. N. Shiota, & K. N. Kirby (Eds.), *The handbook of positive emotions* (pp. 11–27). New York: Guilford.
Tung, J., Barreiro, L. B., Johnson, Z. P., Hansen, K. D., Michopoulos, V., Toufexis, D., … & Gilad, Y. (2012). Social environment is associated with gene regulatory variation in the rhesus macaque immune system. *Proceedings of the National Academy of Sciences, 109*(17), 6490–6495. doi:10.1073/pnas.1202734109.
Waterman, A. S. (1993). Two conceptions of happiness: Contrasts of personal expressiveness (eudaimonia) and hedonic enjoyment. *Journal of Personality and Social Psychology, 64*(4), 678–691. doi:10.1037/0022-3514.64.4.678.
Watson, D., Wiese, D., Vaidya, J., & Tellegen, A. (1999). The two general activation systems of affect: Structural findings, evolutionary considerations, and psychobiological evidence. *Journal of Personality and Social Psychology, 76*, 820–838.

On the Synergy Between Hedonia and Eudaimonia: The Role of Passion

13

Robert J. Vallerand

Over the years, much discussion has taken place on the role of two perspectives on happiness. The first, hedonia, leads one to focus on positive experiences per se, while the second, eudaimonia, posits that true happiness is to be found in self-realization in line with one's true self (or daimon) (see Ryan & Deci, 2001; Waterman, 2013 for reviews). While these two positions have often been portrayed as antagonistic, my personal position is that they need not be. One reason why this is so developed in this chapter is that very often the two forms of well-being go hand in hand and can combine in a synergy that facilitates optimal functioning (Vallerand, 2013, 2015). Specifically, the position defended in this chapter is that in real life situations, experiencing positive affective experiences within the confines of a meaningful activity that one loves and is passionate about can lead one to pursue repeated engagement in this activity thereby fostering long-term self-realization and self-growth (Vallerand, 2015). Hedonia and eudaimonia can thus be seen as interacting in a synergy that fosters self-growth. Although the possibility that the two positions cohere is not necessarily new (see Huta, 2013, Chap. 15, this volume; Vitterso, 2013, Chap. 17, this volume), what is novel, however, is the role that passion can play in the hedonia-eudaimonia positive interface.

The goal of this chapter is to document the role of passion in the hedonia-eudaimonia synergy. Specifically, in this chapter, I intend to show that passion for a given activity can trigger one important type of positive hedonic experiences, namely positive emotions, that, in turn, promote eudaimonic well-being and self-growth. However, as will be seen not all passions are alike and some may be more likely than others to facilitate this adaptive function of hedonia in eudaimonia. I start by presenting important elements on the construct of passion, including the Dualistic Model of Passion (DMP; Vallerand et al., 2003; Vallerand, 2008, 2010, 2015). Then, research is reviewed that addresses the role of passion in the "Passion → Positive Emotions → Self-Growth" sequence with respect to psychological well-being[1], quality of interpersonal relationships, and societal outcomes. Finally, I conclude with some further thoughts on the role of passion in the hedonia-eudaimonia interface.

R.J. Vallerand (✉)
Laboratoire de Recherche sur le Comportement Social, Département de Psychologie, Université du Québec à Montréal, Montreal, QC, Canada

Australian Catholic University, Sydney, NSW, Australia
e-mail: Vallerand.bob@gmail.com

J. Vittersø (ed.), *Handbook of Eudaimonic Well-Being*, International Handbooks of Quality-of-Life,
DOI 10.1007/978-3-319-42445-3_13

13.1 On the Psychology of Passion

13.1.1 A Brief History on Passion

Initially, passion was first seen as maladaptive by Greek philosophers, such as Plato (427–348 BC). This was because passion was perceived as controlling the person who would eventually become a slave to his or her passion. Other influential philosophers who wrote brilliantly about the pros and cons of passion were René Descartes and Emmanuel Kant. It is only later with the Romantics that passion was fully celebrated and cast in a positive light. For instance, Hegel (1770–1831) posited that passion was highly adaptive because it generated high energy necessary for high achievement and Kierkegaard (1813–1855) posited that: "To exist, if we do not mean by that only a pseudo existence, cannot take place without passion".

Initial work in psychology started at the turn of the twentieth century in France. It did not involve experiments or research as such but some solid armchair psychology. Ribot (1907) wrote a book devoted entirely to passion called "*Essai sur les passions*" ("*Essay on passions*") where, in line with René Descartes, he defined passion as an enduring and prolonged intellectualized emotion toward an object that has gone through some transformation. According to Ribot, there are three main characteristic of passion: the "fixed" idea (or a clear and persistent goal toward an object or activity), the duration (from a few days to sometimes an entire life), and intensity (involving some form of energy deployed toward one's goal or object). Later, Joussain (1928) extended the work of Ribot by positing that passion can serve some integrative function and[1] purposeful direction in one's life. Joussain also suggested that passions interacted among themselves in at least two ways: some passions can conflict while others can peacefully coexist with other passions. Such a statement underscored that passions are not all equivalent and that some may be more adaptive than others with respect to some of the outcomes that we experience.

The construct of passion was largely ignored by psychologists for the next 50 years. It is only in the early 1970s that passion made a comeback. Theorizing and research on passion then focused on passionate love (e.g., Hatfield & Walster, 1978) and passion as a sexual drive and a component of love (e.g., Sternberg, 1986). Although such research is important, it does not deal with passion toward activities. It is only later that research on passion toward activities took place. Such research was conducted in the workplace and simply focused on passion as "love for one's work" (e.g., Baum & Locke, 2004). Such a definition of passion left the distinction between passion and intrinsic motivation unclear. Finally, Vallerand et al. (2003) presented a more precise definition of passion that, in addition to one's love for the activity, also included activity importance, regular activity engagement, and the activity being part of one's identity. It is with such a background that the first contemporary theoretical analysis of the passion construct was postulated by Vallerand et al. (2003) and Vallerand & Houlfort (2003).

13.1.2 A Dualistic Model of Passion (DMP)

In line with Self-Determination Theory (SDT; Deci & Ryan, 2000; Ryan & Martela, Chap. 7, this volume), the DMP proposes that throughout life, people engage in various activities in the hope of satisfying the basic psychological needs of autonomy (to feel a sense of personal initiative), competence (to interact effectively with the environment), and relatedness (to feel connected to significant others). With time and experience, most people eventually start to display preference for some activities, especially those that are enjoyable and allow the satisfaction of the aforementioned basic psychological needs. Of these activities, a limited few will be perceived as particularly enjoyable and important, and to have

[1]By psychological well-being, I refer to well-being at the psychological level and not to Carol Ryff's construct of "psychological well-being" (e.g., Ryff, Chap. 6, this volume). See Vallerand (2012) for more on this issue.

some resonance with our identity or how we see ourselves. These activities become passionate activities. In line with the above, passion is defined as a strong inclination toward a self-defining activity that one likes (or even loves), finds important, and in which one invests time and energy (Vallerand et al., 2003). These activities come to be so self-defining that they represent central features of one's identity. This will be the case to the extent that the activity is highly valued by the person (Aron, Aron, & Smollan, 1992), thereby leading to a passion toward that activity.

The DMP further posits the existence of two types of passion, harmonious and obsessive passion. In line with past research on the internalization of non-interesting activities, it is posited that activities that people love will also be internalized in the person's identity to the extent that these are highly valued and meaningful for the person through either a controlled or an autonomous process (see Deci, Egharri, Patrick, & Leone, 1994; Sheldon, 2002, Chap. 36, this volume; Vallerand, 1997, 2001, 2007; Vallerand, Fortier, & Guay, 1997). It is these two types of internalization processes that determine the two types of passion mentioned previously, harmonious and obsessive passion.

Obsessive passion, results from a controlled internalization of the activity that one loves into identity. Such an internalization process leads not only the activity representation to be part of the person's identity, but also to values and regulations associated with the activity to be at best partially internalized in the self, and at worse to be internalized in the person's identity but completely outside the integrative self (Ryan & Deci, 2000). A controlled internalization originates from intra and/or interpersonal pressure typically because certain contingencies are attached to the activity such as feelings of social acceptance or self-esteem (Mageau, Carpentier, & Vallerand, 2011), or because the sense of excitement derived from activity engagement is uncontrollable. People with an obsessive passion can thus find themselves in the position of experiencing an uncontrollable urge to partake in the activity they view as important and enjoyable. They cannot help but to engage in the passionate activity. Consequently, they risk experiencing conflict and other negative affective, cognitive, and behavioral consequences during and after activity engagement. For instance, if a university professor who needs to work on a research grant due the next day has an obsessive passion for playing the guitar, she might not be able to resist an invitation to play music with her friends that evening. During the jam session, she might feel upset with herself for playing music instead of working on the grant. She might therefore have difficulties focusing on the task at hand (playing the guitar), may not experience much positive affect and flow while playing the guitar, and may experience guilt and anxiety as she should be doing something else instead (i.e., working on her research grant). It is thus proposed that individuals with an obsessive passion come to display a rigid persistence toward the activity, as oftentimes they can't help but to engage in the passionate activity. This is so because ego-invested, rather than integrative, self-processes (Hodgins & Knee, 2002) are at play with obsessive passion leading the person to eventually becoming dependent on the activity. While such persistence may lead to some benefits (e.g., improved performance at the activity), it may also come at a cost for the individual, potentially leading to less than optimal functioning within the confines of the passionate activity and outside of it because of the lack of flexibility that it entails.

Conversely, harmonious passion results from an autonomous internalization of the activity into the person's identity and self. An autonomous internalization occurs when individuals have freely accepted the activity as important for them without any contingencies attached to it. This type of internalization emanates from the intrinsic and integrative tendencies of the self (Deci & Ryan, 2000; Ryan & Deci, 2003) and produces a motivational force to willingly engage in the activity that one loves and engenders a sense of volition and personal endorsement about pursuing the activity. When harmonious passion is at play, individuals do not experience an uncontrollable urge to engage in the passionate activity, but rather freely choose to do so. With this type of passion, the activity occupies a significant but not overpowering space in the person's identity and is in harmony with other aspects of the person's life. In other words, with harmonious passion the authentic integrating self (Deci & Ryan, 2000) is at play allowing the person to fully partake in the passionate activity in a mindful (Brown & Ryan, 2003) and open way (Hodgins & Knee, 2002) that is conducive to positive experiences.

In line with the above, engaging in an activity with a harmonious passion should allow people to fully focus on the task at hand and to experience positive outcomes and pleasure both during task engagement (e.g., positive affect, concentration, flow etc.) and after task engagement (general positive affect, life satisfaction etc.). Thus, there should be little or no conflict between the person's passionate activity and his/her other life activities. Furthermore, when prevented from engaging in their passionate activity, people with a harmonious passion should be able to adapt well to the situation and focus their attention and energy on other tasks that need attention. Finally, with harmonious passion flexible persistence in the activity is possible because the person is in control of the activity and can decide when to and when not to engage in the activity. For instance, to continue with the above example, if our university professor has a harmonious passion for playing the guitar, she should be able to resist playing music with her friends so as to complete the research grant that still needs work. Thus, she could readily tell her friends that she'll take a rain check on the music jam and proceed to be fully immersed in the grant without thinking about music. People with a harmonious passion are able to decide not to play on a given day if needed or even to eventually terminate the relationship with the activity if they decide that it has become a permanent negative factor in their life. Thus, behavioral engagement in the passionate activity can be seen as flexible thus leading to adaptive outcomes both within the activity and outside of it.

13.1.3 On Passion and Self-Growth

As mentioned in the introduction, one of the main tenets of the eudaimonic position is that one's happiness is to be found in trying to reach one's personal fulfillment in accordance with one's true self. That is, one's well-being is achieved through self-realization and reaching one's true potential (see Ryan & Deci, 2001; Waterman, 1993, 2013). In line with the eudaimonic position, the DMP rests on the firm assumption that people have a natural tendency toward self-growth that is experienced throughout life. That is, people seek to master both their outside and inside worlds (e.g., Deci & Ryan, 1985; Maslow, 1954; Rogers, 1963). In so doing, they grow psychologically. One of the key variables that contributes to self-growth is the activities that we are passionate about. In life, we engage in a number of activities. Typically, we are motivated for most of them and passionate only for one or two. For instance, we are motivated to go school and do chores at home but may be passionate about playing a musical instrument or playing basketball or hockey. I would like to suggest that those activities that people are passionate about have the best potential for self-growth. This is not to say that other activities that people are non passionate about do not lead to self-growth. Clearly, everything we do in life has such a potential. However, I posit that everything being equal in terms of activity complexity, and thus self-growth potential, activities that we are passionate about should contribute the most to self-growth.

There are a number of reasons why activities that we are passionate about should lead to higher levels of self-growth than those engaged in without passion. I will only mention three here (see Vallerand, 2015, Chap. 3 for a more detailed discussion). First, passion entails a powerful motivational force that is conducive to fully engaging in the activity with high levels of energy and enthusiasm. You do not have to push or force people to do the activity that they are passionate about. Quite the contrary. Sometimes, you may even be tempted to restrain people from engaging in their activity as they just can't get enough of it and may sometimes overdo it. When passionate about an activity, people engage in their beloved activity with full energy, persistently, regularly, several hours weekly (on average 8 h per week; Vallerand et al., 2003, Study 1). They put in lots of hours with a high quality engagement that is likely to promote self-growth within the purview of the activity. A second reason why passion can maximize self-growth is that it fosters mastery goals (Elliot, 1997) that are known to foster high performance on the activity (see Bonneville-Roussy, Lavigne, & Vallerand, 2011; Vallerand et al., 2007, 2008). Over time, people come to know just about everything there is to know about the activity; they become experts at their activity, thereby allowing them to psychologically grow at least within the realm of the activity.

A third and final reason why passion may lead to the highest levels of self-growth is that one's passion for a given activity can facilitate the experience of a number of positive experiences and processes during activity engagement that promote adaptive outcomes within the sphere of the activity as well as outside of it in one's life in general. One of these processes is positive emotions. These emotions are important because they are hypothesized to serve several adaptive functions. Perhaps the most vocal contemporary proponent of the adaptive function of positive emotions is Barbara Fredrickson (2001, 2009, Chap. 12, this volume). According to Fredrickson's broaden-and-build theory, positive emotions (especially, joy, interest, contentment, and love) serve to broaden the momentary thought – action repertoire. Thus, when experiencing positive emotional states, people will broaden their scope of attention and show an expanded use of information to their disposal (e.g., Fredrickson & Branigan, 2005; Johnson, Waugh, & Fredrickson, 2010). Of importance, Fredrickson posits that such momentary improvement in one's attention leads to a more permanent building of physical and psychological skills and tools that can be made available in the future when needed and that can contribute to self-growth. Furthermore, it should be underscored that emotions may also serve some social functions (Frijda & Mesquita, 1994). Indeed, much research reveals that emotions serve to communicate with others. For instance, emotional behavior seen at sporting events such as smiling, slapping hands (giving "high fives"), and talking loudly to others convey that one is experiencing intense positive emotions such as happiness and is willing to share such joy with others. Such emotions are likely to lead to more positive interactions with others both at the dyadic (Waugh & Fredrickson, 2006) and the collective level (Haidt, 2003). Thus, overall, positive emotions lead to both the broadening of attentional resources and the building of enduring resources that can contribute to self-growth.

The above discussion reveals that hedonia may actually contribute to eudaimonia. If positive emotions indeed serve such an adaptive function and contribute to self-growth, then an important question becomes: "Which factors trigger these positive emotions?" One answer is through repeated engagement in a passionate activity. Indeed, as posited by the DMP, regularly engaging in a meaningful activity that one loves and is passionate about can lead one to fully immerse in the activity and to experience positive emotions repeatedly. However, as seen above not all passions are alike and some may be more likely to facilitate this adaptive function of hedonia in eudaimonia than others. Specifically, because harmonious passion leads one to partake in the passionate activity in a mindful (Brown & Ryan, 2003) and open way (Hodgins & Knee, 2002), one is more likely to experience positive emotions and, consequently, derive self-growth and well-being. Conversely, with obsessive passion people can find themselves in the position of experiencing an uncontrollable urge to partake in the activity that they love. Consequently, they should experience conflict between activity engagement and other spheres of their lives, resulting in repeated instances of negative affect both during and after activity engagement. Self-growth is thus not optimal and if it takes place at all, it should be largely circumscribed to the passionate activity.

13.2 Research on Passion

The above position is that harmonious passion facilitates self-growth and adaptive outcomes in part through its effects on positive emotions. Conversely, the effects of obsessive passion are much less adaptive because it does not foster positive emotions as much and, in fact, can trigger negative emotions known to undermine self-growth. In this section, we review empirical support for this key hypothesis from the DMP. The adaptive outcomes reviewed are psychological well-being, interpersonal relationships, and contributions to society. However, before reviewing such research, I present the findings of some initial passion research that provide support for the concept of passion and its methodology.

13.2.1 Initial Passion Research

There were three major purposes to the initial work on passion (Vallerand et al., 2003): (1) to determine the prevalence of passion for an activity in one's life; (2) to develop the Passion Scale; and (3) to test the validity of some of the elements of the passion constructs. To that end, Vallerand et al. (2003, Study 1) had over 500 university students complete the Passion Scale with respect to an activity that they loved, that they valued, and in which they invested time and energy (i.e., the passion definition), as well as other scales leading to testing predictions derived from the DMP. A large variety of passionate activities were reported ranging from physical activity and sports to watching movies, playing a musical instrument, and reading. Participants reported engaging in their passionate activity for an average of 8.5 h per week and had been engaging in that activity for almost 6 years. Thus, clearly passionate activities are meaningful to people and are long-lasting in nature. Of importance regarding the first purpose of this research, 84 % of participants indicated that they had at least a moderate level of passion for a given activity in their lives (they scored at least 4 out of 7 on a question asking them if their favorite activity was a « passion » for them). In a similar vein, a subsequent study (Philippe, Vallerand, & Lavigne, 2009) with close to 800 participants ranging in age from 18 to 90 using a more stringent criterion of having a mean of five out of seven on the four criteria of passion (loving the activity, activity valuation, activity engagement, and perceiving the activity as a passion) revealed that 75 % of participants had a high level of passion for an activity in their life. It would thus appear that the prevalence of passion is rather high and not the exclusivity of the happy few, not only in the Province of Quebec, Canada but also in other countries (e.g., Lecoq, 2012; Liu, Chen, & Yao, 2011; Stenseng, 2008).

Second, it should be underscored that the Passion Scale, Vallerand et al. (2003, Study 1), has gone through extensive development and validation procedures. The Passion Scale consists of two subscales of six items each reflecting Obsessive (e.g., "I almost have an obsessive feeling toward this activity") and Harmonious Passion (e.g., "This activity is in harmony with other activities in my life"). For instance, the results of confirmatory factor analysis provide strong support for its bi-factorial structure in over 20 studies dealing with a number of activities and languages (see Vallerand, 2015, Chap. 4 for a review). In addition, in a study with over 3500 participants, Marsh and colleagues (2013) have shown that the scale is relatively invariant (or equivalent) both in English and French, for both men and women, across various age groups, and for a number of different activities. Furthermore, internal consistency analyses have shown that both subscales are reliable (typically 75 and above). Finally, test-retest correlations over periods ranging from 4 to 6 weeks revealed moderately high stability values (in the .80s, Rousseau, Vallerand, Ratelle, Mageau, & Provencher, 2002), thereby supporting the reliability of the scale. Thus, overall, the Passion Scale can be readily used for most if not all types of activities and populations and in several languages.

With respect to the third purpose, a series of critical findings with partial correlations (controlling for the correlation between the two types of passion) revealed that both harmonious and obsessive passions were positively associated with the passion criteria thereby providing support for the definition of passion (see Vallerand et al., 2003, Study 1; Marsh et al., 2013). In addition, both types of passion were found to relate to one's identity and obsessive passion was found to more strongly relate to a measure of conflict with other life activities than harmonious passion. These findings support the view that both harmonious and obsessive passions are indeed a "passion" as each one reflects the definition of the passion construct. Furthermore, other studies in this initial research (Vallerand et al., 2003) have also shown that obsessive (but not harmonious) passion correlated with rigid persistence in ill-advised activities such as cycling over ice and snow in winter (Vallerand et al., 2003, Study 3) and pursuing one's engagement in activities that have become negative for the person such as pathological gambling (Vallerand et al., 2003, Study 4).

Overall, initial research provided support for the concept of harmonious and obsessive passion. Since then, over 200 studies have been conducted on the concept of passion and have focused on a host of cognitive, affective, behavioral, relational, and performance outcomes experienced within the realms of hundred of activities conducted in both our own as well as other laboratories (see Curran et al., 2015; Vallerand, 2010, 2015 for a review). Below, I review research on the role of the harmonious and obsessive passions in emotions experienced within the confines of the passionate activity as well as their contribution to the "Passion → Positive Emotions → Self-Growth" sequence with respect to psychological well-being, quality of interpersonal relationships, and societal outcomes.

13.2.2 Passion and Affect

The DMP posits that harmonious passion leads people to volitionally engage in the passionate activity with an openness and a mindfulness that allow them to fully partake in the activity, and thus to experience positive affective experiences (Hodgins & Knee, 2002) during task engagement (e.g., positive affect). Furthermore, the lack of conflict with other life activities that harmonious passion entails should maximize the experience of positive affect both during and after activity engagement. Finally, because task engagement is volitional, one is unlikely to experience negative affect when unable to engage in the passionate activity (such as feelings of dependence). Conversely, with obsessive passion, one engages in the activity with a defensive, rather than an open, orientation preventing one from fully experiencing the positive emotions that should be derived from engaging in one's favorite activity. Moreover, because engagement is often out of one's control, and may be performed at ill-advised times, some conflict may thus be experienced with other life activities, thereby preventing one from fully enjoying participation in the passionate activity and leading one to experience negative affect following task engagement. (e.g., guilt, shame, anxiety). One is then likely to experience high levels of negative affect when prevented from engaging in the passionate activity because engagement in the passionate activity out of obsessive passion is experienced as an uncontrollable desire to partake in the activity. Consequently, being prevented from engaging in the passionate activity should lead to some sense of suffering.

Results from a number of studies have supported these hypotheses. For instance, Vallerand et al. (2003, Study 1) asked college students who were passionate toward an activity to complete the Passion Scale and to report the positive and negative emotions they typically experience during and after task engagement, as well as when they are prevented from engaging in their passionate activity. Results from partial correlations (controlling for obsessive passion) revealed that harmonious passion was positively associated with positive emotions during activity engagement. In addition, harmonious passion was positively related to positive emotions and the absence of negative affect following task engagement, and the absence of negative emotions when prevented from engaging in the passionate activity. On the other hand, when controlling for harmonious passion, obsessive passion was positively associated with negative emotions (especially shame) and either slightly related or unrelated to positive emotions both during and following activity engagement. Furthermore, obsessive passion was strongly related to negative affect when one was prevented from engaging in the activity.

These results have been replicated in a number of studies with a variety of designs and participants (for reviews see Vallerand, 2008, 2010, 2015). Further, in a recent meta-analysis of 94 studies, including 28 that specifically focused on passion and affect (Curran et al., 2015), it was found that harmonious passion had a moderately strong relationship to positive emotions and no significant negative relationship to negative emotions. Conversely, obsessive passion displayed a significant relationship with negative affect and no significant relationship with positive affect. Clearly, harmonious passion contributes to positive emotions whereas obsessive passion does not and rather contributes to negative affect.

13.2.3 Passion and Psychological Well-Being

The Dualistic Model of Passion predicts that engaging in a meaningful and enjoyable activity that provides with opportunities for self-improvement and actualization will maximize self-growth to the extent that one's passion for the activity is harmonious in nature. Research provides support for this hypothesis. For instance, in a study with elderly individuals, Rousseau and Vallerand (2003) showed that harmonious passion positively predicted positive indices of psychological well-being (life satisfaction, meaning in life, and vitality) but negatively predicted negative indices (anxiety and depression). Conversely, obsessive passion positively predicted anxiety and depression, was negatively related to life satisfaction, and was unrelated to meaning in life and vitality. Research with young adults and teenagers using various measures of psychological well-being has yielded similar findings. Specifically, harmonious passion is positively related to life satisfaction and vitality (Vallerand et al., 2007, Studies 1 and 2; Vallerand et al., 2008, Study 2), while obsessive passion is either negatively related (Vallerand et al., 2007, Study 2) or unrelated (Vallerand et al., 2007, Study 1; Vallerand et al., 2008, Study 2) to these indices. Of additional importance is the research of Lafrenière and colleagues (2012) that showed that experimentally inducing harmonious passion led to higher levels of life satisfaction than inductions of obsessive passion and a control group. Furthermore, in their study with over 3500 participants, Marsh et al. (2013) also found that harmonious passion positively correlated with life satisfaction while only a non significant negative correlation was obtained with obsessive passion. Finally, in their meta-analysis, Curran et al., (2015) found very similar findings to those of Marsh et al.

Clearly, the above findings reveal that harmonious (but not obsessive) passion facilitates well-being. Then, is the experience of positive emotions the mediator of the positive effects of harmonious passion on well-being as posited by the DMP? A study conducted by Rousseau and Vallerand (2008) provided support for this hypothesis. At Time 1, participants who were passionate for exercise completed the Passion Scale with respect to physical activity, as well as measures of well-being. At Time 2, immediately following an exercise session, they completed situational measures of positive and negative affect. Finally, at Time 3, they completed measures of well-being again. Results from a path analysis revealed that harmonious passion positively predicted positive affect, which led to increases in psychological well-being from Time 1 to Time 3. On the other hand, obsessive passion was unrelated to positive affect but positively predicted negative affect. The latter did not predict well-being. Obsessive passion also had a direct negative link to well-being. These basic findings were replicated in another study (Rousseau & Vallerand, 2008). Overall, these findings provide strong support for the role of situational positive affect experienced during task engagement as a mediator of the effect of harmonious passion on psychological well-being.

The above research suggests that harmonious passion positively contributes to well-being through the experience of situational positive affect. Because people typically spend on average 8 h per week on the activity they are passionate about, such a "Harmonious Passion → Positive Affect → Psychological Well-Being" sequence is recurrent in the person's life thereby leading to sustainable well-being through this virtuous circle (see Vallerand, 2012 on this issue). As posited by the DMP, hedonia is in the service of eudaimonia.

13.2.4 Passion and Interpersonal Relationships

The DMP posits that another dimension of optimal functioning that passion can affect is the quality of the relationships that we develop and maintain with others. Specifically, the DMP posits that having a harmonious passion for a given activity should facilitate having positive relationships with others while engaging in the passionate activity. Further, such positive effects should be mediated by the experience of positive affect. As discussed previously, positive emotions serve some social functions, including facilitating the emission of interactive cues such as smiling and positive and open non verbal behavior that are conducive to positive relationships. Because harmonious passion leads one to experience positive affect during engagement in the passionate activity, one would then predict that it should therefore indirectly lead to high quality relationships within the passionate activity. If positive emotions should facilitate quality relationships with others, negative emotions should do the opposite because the person is then defensive and inclined to stay to him or herself. Instead of connecting with others, the person is then likely to remain aloof, to shy away from others, and to look unhappy. And if we look unhappy, we may keep others at bay, as people typically do not want to interact with unhappy people (Fowler & Christakis, 2008). Thus, because it is typically unrelated to positive affect and generally positively related to negative affect, obsessive passion should not facilitate quality of relationships and may even negatively affect relationships.

First, does passion predict the quality of relationships? The answer is a resounding yes. A number of studies (e.g., Jowett, Lafrenière, & Vallerand, 2013; Lafrenière, Jowett, Vallerand, Donahue, & Lorimer, 2008; Philippe, Vallerand, Houlfort, Lavigne, & Donahue, 2010; Utz, Jonas, & Tonkens, 2012) have shown that harmonious passion promotes positive relationships during engagement in the passionate activity whereas obsessive passion does not. Further, research reveals that these findings hold for relationships with collaborators of equal status (e.g., work colleagues) as well as in "one-up" relationships between supervisors and supervisees such as coaches and athletes (Jowett et al., 2013; Lafrenière et al., 2008, Studies 1 and 2). In addition, the positive contribution of harmonious passion to positive relationships also takes place with respect to both new relationships and those that already exist (see Philippe et al., 2010, Studies 1–4). For instance, passion for one's studies measured at the beginning of a 15-week semester allowed predicting the quality of friendships that developed over the duration of semester within university study groups (Philippe et al., 2010, Study 4). Finally, research also reveals that the perception of relationship quality does not only take place in the passionate person's head but also in that of others who witness interactions between the passionate individual and other people in the activity. For instance, in the study group experiment discussed above, all members of the study group were asked to assess the quality of relationships that other members developed over the semester. Results revealed that these ratings agreed with those of the members' self-report (Philippe et al., 2010, Study 3; see also Study 4). Overall, passion, and especially harmonious passion, for a given activity contributes to the development and maintenance of quality relationships within the purview of this activity.

The second issue of importance here, with respect to the present position, deals with the mediating role of positive emotions in the positive effects of harmonious passion on relationship quality. In their series of studies on passion and relationships, Philippe et al. (2010) tested the proposed processes in all four studies. Because all four studies yielded the same findings, only one is summarized here. In this study (Philippe et al., 2010, Study 3), teen basketball players participating in a 1-week basketball camp were asked early in the camp to complete the Passion Scale for playing basketball. Then, toward the end of the basketball camp, athletes were asked to report on the positive and negative emotions experienced during camp as well as complete a measure of quality of relationships with their new teammates. In addition, the coach of each team was asked to complete the same relationship quality measure for each of his or her player. As hypothesized, harmonious passion was found to positively predict positive, but negatively predict negative, affect experienced over the week. Conversely, obsessive passion was weakly related to positive affect and positively related to negative affect. In turn, positive affect positively, while negative affect negatively, predicted the quality relationship assessments completed by both the athletes and their coaches (see Philippe et al., 2010 for other studies supporting the present perspective). Once more, hedonia facilitates eudaimonia.

13.2.5 Passion and Societal Contributions

The third and final adaptive outcome to be discussed in this chapter is that of contributing to society. Although this dimension is much less discussed in positive psychology, it nevertheless requires our attention. Indeed, as posited by Vallerand (2013), individuals who aspire to be fully functioning within society should not only display high levels of individual functioning but also be contributing to that of others. Doing so allows them to display high levels of "optimal functioning in society" (Vallerand, 2013). Once more, the first question here deals with establishing the role of passion. The well known environmentalist David Suzuki wrote "Without passion, change is not possible" (2002, p. 3). Is this true? Is passion necessary to contribute to society? One way to find out is to determine if people who engage in activities that promote the welfare of society are passionate or not. If they are, then this would provide support for the role of passion in contributing to society. In a series of three studies on passion for the environmental cause, Gousse-Lessard, Vallerand, Carbonneau, and Lafrenière (2013) assessed the passion of over 400 workers, members, and volunteers actively engaged in the environmental cause through their involvement in environmental organizations in the Province of Québec. Participants in all three studies completed the Passion Scale, including the passion criteria (love, valuation, and regularly engagement in the activity, as well as the activity being part of one's identity). Taking the usual cut-off point of four and above on the mean of the passion criteria (see Mageau et al., 2009; Vallerand & Houlfort, 2003), it was found that over 93 % of the participants reached this criterion and displayed a passion for the environment. Similar findings were obtained in a series of three studies conducted with people who engaged in humanitarian causes for associations such as the Red Cross and Doctors without Borders (St-Louis, Carbonneau, & Vallerand, 2016) where 89 % of those who espoused the humanitarian cause were found to be passionate. Finally, similar numbers were obtained for those pursuing a political cause (79 %; Rip et al., 2012, Study 1).

If passion contributes to society, then is affect involved once more? Specifically, it should be recalled that in the Philippe et al. (2010) series of studies on the role of passion in interpersonal relationships, positive affect facilitated, while negative affect undermined, high quality relationships. Are the two types of affect also at play in mediating the adaptive and less adaptive effects of harmonious and obsessive passion, respectively, on environmental behavior? In Study 3 of their series of studies on passion and the environment, Gousse-Lessard and colleagues (2013, Study 3) asked environmental activists to complete the Passion Scale for the environment and a measure of positive and negative affect generally experienced when engaging in environmental behavior. Further, they also measured both mainstream activist behavior (e.g., educating the general population on the environment) and radical activism (e.g., using violence to protect the environment). The authors reasoned that harmonious passion would strongly and positively predict positive emotions while obsessive passion would positively predict negative emotions and perhaps positive emotions to a lesser degree. In turn, positive emotions should positively predict mainstream activist behaviors whereas negative emotions were expected to predict radical forms of activist behavior.

Overall, the results of Study 3 supported the hypotheses. First, results of a path analysis revealed that the association between the two types of passion and adaptive mainstream behaviors was totally mediated by the experience of positive emotions experienced when engaged in activist behaviors. Further, as expected the link from harmonious passion to positive emotions was statistically stronger than that involving obsessive passion. Thus, once more hedonia served eudaimonia as adaptive activist behavior was facilitated by the experience of positive affect. Second, results showed that the association between obsessive passion and radical behaviors was mediated by the experience of negative emotions. Finally, harmonious passion negatively predicted negative affect, thereby showing that harmonious passion provides some protection against the negative effects of negative emotions on radical activist behavior. Thus, just as it was the case with the first two adaptive outcomes, positive emotions experienced within the purview of the activity that one is passionate about mediated the positive effects of harmonious passion on optimal functioning behavior toward society. Once more, hedonia was found to contribute to eudaimonia.

13.3 Conclusion

For centuries, two positions of happiness have been pitted against each other. Specifically, hedonia and eudaimonia have often been seen as antagonistic entities (see Ryan & Deci, 2001; Waterman, 2013). The position defended in this chapter is that hedonia and eudaimonia do not always clash. In fact, when people engage regularly in a meaningful activity that they love with full volition and in a mindful and open fashion, then hedonia and eudaimonia cohere and lead to self-growth and optimal functioning (Vallerand, 2013). Specifically, the DMP posits that engaging in an activity out of harmonious passion allows one to experience positive emotions that, in turn, promote adaptive outcomes and self-growth. However, such should not be the case with obsessive passion because activity involvement becomes largely out of the person's control thereby minimizing the experience of positive affect and facilitating negative emotions that curtail self-growth and adaptive functioning.

Research reviewed herein provided strong support for the position of the DMP as pertains to two elements. First, harmonious passion does promote the experience of positive emotions whereas obsessive passion facilitates negative affect and is either unrelated or only slightly related to positive affect. Second, strong support has been found for the mediating role of positive affect in the harmonious passion-adaptive outcomes relationship as pertains to three types of outcomes: psychological well-being, high relationship quality, and contributions to society. Thus, impressive support was obtained for the "Passion → Positive Affect → Adaptive Outcomes" sequence. Conversely, obsessive passion does not contribute to this adaptive sequence and may even detract from it through its impact on negative emotions. In sum, when one engages regularly in a meaningful activity out of harmonious (but not obsessive) passion, self-growth is achievable and the pleasure experienced during activity engagement is one of the psychological mechanisms that makes it happen: Hedonia can contribute to eudaimonia.

In closing, it should be mentioned that in this chapter, I have focused on only one type of positive hedonistic experiences, namely positive emotions. Other types of positive experiences exist such as pleasant sensory stimulations (see Carbonneau & Vallerand, 2012) and even cognitive states such as flow. These other positive hedonic states may also mediate the impact of passion on self-growth. In fact, past research has shown that harmonious passion contributes to flow that, in turn, prevents the experience of burnout (e.g., Lavigne, Forest, & Crevier-Braud, 2012). Although such research underscores the preventive role of flow in maladaptive outcomes, it does not show that flow is a key mediator in the passion-self-growth relationship. Future research is needed to test this hypothesis.

Over the past 15 years or so, positive psychologists have tried to answer the question "How people's lives can be most worth living" (Seligman & Csikscentmihalyi, 2000). Some have proposed that hedonia provides one answer while others suggest that eudaimonia is the key. As was shown in the present paper, when harmonious passion is at play, one needs not choose between the two positions as hedonia and eudaimonia synergistically integrate in providing the elements of a rich life definitely worth living for. The concept of passion would thus appear to be of great relevance in an analysis in which hedonia and eudaimonia combine in contributing to happiness and optimal functioning.

References

Aron, A., Aron, E. N., & Smollan, D. (1992). Inclusion of other in the self scale and the structure of interpersonal closeness. *Journal of Personality and Social Psychology, 63*, 596–612.

Baum, J. R., & Locke, E. A. (2004). The relationship of entrepreneurial traits, skill, and motivation to subsequent venture growth. *Journal of Applied Psychology, 89*, 587–598.

Bonneville-Roussy, A., Lavigne, G. L., & Vallerand, R. J. (2011). When passion leads to excellence: The case of musicians. *Psychology of Music, 39*, 123–138.

Brown, K. W., & Ryan, R. M. (2003). The benefits of being present: Mindfulness and its role in psychological well-being. *Journal of Personality and Social Psychology, 84*, 822–848.

Carbonneau, N., & Vallerand, R. J. (2012). Toward a tripartite model of intrinsic motivation. *Journal of Personality, 80*, 1147–1178.

Curran, T., Hill, A. P., Appleton, P. R., Vallerand, R. J., & Standage, M. (2015). The psychology of passion: A meta-analytical review of a decade of research on intrapersonal outcomes. *Motivation and Emotion, 39*, 631–655.

Deci, E. L., Egharri, H., Patrick, B. C., & Leone, D. R. (1994). Facilitating internalization: The self-determination perspective. *Journal of Personality, 62*, 119–142.

Deci, E. L., & Ryan, R. M. (1985). The general causality orientations scale: Self-determination in personality. *Journal of Research in Personality, 19*(2), 109–134.

Deci, E. L., & Ryan, R. M. (2000). The "what" and "why" of goal pursuits: Human needs and the self-determination of behavior. *Psychological Inquiry, 11*, 227-268.

Elliot, A. J. (1997). Integrating "classic" and "contemporary" approaches to achievement motivation: A hierarchical model of approach and avoidance achievement motivation. In P. Pintrinch & M. Maehr (Eds.), *Advances in motivation and achievement* (Vol. 10, pp. 143–179). Greenwich, CT: JAI Press.

Fowler, J. H., & Christakis, N. A. (2008). Dynamic spread of happiness in a large social network: Longitudinal analysis over 20 years in the Framingham Heart Study. *BMJ [British Medical Journal], 337*, 1–9.

Fredrickson, B. L. (2001). The role of positive emotions in positive psychology: The broaden-and build theory of positive emotions. *American Psychologist, 56*, 218–226.

Fredrickson, B. L. (2009). *Positivity*. New York: Three Rivers Press.

Fredrickson, B. L., & Branigan, C. (2005). Positive emotions broaden the scope of attention and thought-action repertoires. *Cognition and Emotion, 19*, 313–332.

Frijda, N. H., & Mesquita, B. (1994). The social roles and functions of emotions. In S. Kitayama & H. R. Markus (Eds.), *Emotion and culture: Empirical studies of mutual influence* (pp. 51–87). Washington, DC: American Psychological Association.

Gousse-Lessard, A.-S., Vallerand, R. J., Carbonneau, N., & Lafrenière, M.-A. K. (2013). The role of passion in mainstream and radical behaviors: A look at environmental activism. *Journal of Environmental Psychology, 35*, 18–29.

Haidt, J. (2003). The moral emotions. In R. J. Davidson, K. R. Scherer, & H. H. Goldsmith (Eds.), *Handbook of affective sciences* (pp. 852–870). New York: Oxford University Press.

Hatfield, E., & Walster, G. W. (1978). *A new look at love*. Reading, MA: Addison-Wesley.

Hodgins, H. S., & Knee, R. (2002). The integrating self and conscious experience. In E. L. Deci & R. M. Ryan (Eds.), *Handbook on self-determination research: Theoretical and applied issues* (pp. 87–100). Rochester, NY: University of Rochester Press.

Huta, V. (2013). Pursuing eudaimoniaVersus hedonia: Distinctions, similarities, and relationships. In A. S. Waterman (Ed.), *The best within us: Positive psychology perspectives on eudaimonic functioning* (pp. 139–158). Washington, DC: APA Books.

Johnson, K. J., Waugh, C. E., & Fredrickson, B. L. (2010). Smile to see the forest: Facially expressed positive emotions broaden cognition. *Cognition and Emotion, 24*(2), 299–321.

Joussain, A. (1928). *Les passions humaines (The human passions)*. Paris: Ernest Flammarion.

Jowett, S., Lafrenière, M.-A. K., & Vallerand, R. J. (2013). Passion for activities and relationship quality: A dyadic approach. *Journal of Social and Personal Relationship, 30*, 734–749.

Lafrenière, M.-A., Jowett, S., Vallerand, R. J., Donahue, E. G., & Lorimer, R. (2008). Passion in sport: On the quality of the coach-player relationship. *Journal of Sport and Exercise Psychology, 30*, 541–560.

Lafrenière, M.-A. K., St-Louis, A. C., Vallerand, R. J., & Donahue, E. G. (2012). On the relation between performance and life satisfaction: The moderating role of passion. *Self and Identity, 11*, 516–530.

Lavigne, G., Forest, J., & Crevier-Braud, L. (2012). Passion at work and burnout: A two-study test of the mediating role of flow experiences. *European Journal of Work and Organizational Psychology, 21*, 518–546.

Lecoq, J. (2012). *La passion: Aspects émotionnels, sociaux et existentiels* (The passion: Emotional, social, and existential aspects). Doctoral thesis, Université Catholique de Louvain, Belgique.

Liu, D., Chen, X. P., & Yao, X. (2011). From autonomy to creativity: A multilevel investigation of the mediating role of harmonious passion. *Journal of Applied Psychology, 96*, 294–309.

Mageau, G. A., Carpentier, J., & Vallerand, R. J. (2011). The role of self-esteem contingencies the distinction between obsessive and harmonious passion. *European Journal of Social Psychology, 41*, 720–729.

Mageau, G. A., Vallerand, R. J., Charest, J., Salvy, S., Lacaille, N., Bouffard, T., et al. (2009). On the development of harmonious and obsessive passion: The role of autonomy support, activity valuation, and identity processes. *Journal of Personality, 77*, 601–645.

Marsh, H. W., Vallerand, R. J., Lafreniere, M. A. K., Parker, P., Morin, A. J. S., Carbonneau, N., … & Paquet, Y. (2013). Passion: Does one scale fit all? Construct validity of two-factor passion scale and psychometric invariance over different activities and languages. *Psychological Assessment, 25*, 796–809.

Maslow, A. H. (1954). *Motivation and personality*. Oxford, UK: Harpers.

Philippe, F. L., Vallerand, R. J., Houlfort, N., Lavigne, G. L., & Donahue, E. G. (2010). Passion for an activity and quality of interpersonal relationships: The mediating role of emotions. *Journal of Personality and Social Psychology, 98*, 917–932.

Philippe, F. L., Vallerand, R. J., & Lavigne, G. L. (2009). Passion does make a difference in people's lives: A look at well-being in passionate and non-passionate individuals. *Applied Psychology: Health and Well-Being, 1*, 3–22.

Ribot, T. (1907). *Essai sur les passions (Essay on passions)*. Paris: Alcan.

Rip, B., Vallerand, R. J., & Lafrenière, M.-A. K. (2012). Passion for a cause, passion for a creed: On ideological passion, identity threat, and extremism. *Journal of Personality, 80*(3), 573–602.

Rogers, C. (1963). The actualizing tendency in relation to "motives" and to consciousness. In M. R. Jones (Ed.), *Nebraska symposium on motivation* (Vol. 11). Lincoln, OR: University of Nebraska Press.

Rousseau, F. L., & Vallerand, R. J. (2003). Le rôle de la passion dans le bien-être subjectif des aînés [The role of passion in the subjective well-being of the elderly]. *Revue Québécoise de Psychologie, 24*, 197–211.

Rousseau, F. L., & Vallerand, R. J. (2008). An examination of the relationship between passion and subjective well-being in older adults. *International Journal of Aging & Human Development, 66*, 195–211.

Rousseau, F. L., Vallerand, R. J., Ratelle, C. F., Mageau, G. A., & Provencher, P. (2002). Passion and gambling: On the validation of the Gambling Passion Scale (GPS). *Journal of Gambling Studies, 18*, 45–66.

Ryan, R. M., & Deci, E. L. (2000). Self-determination and the facilitation of intrinsic motivation, social development, and well-being. *American Psychologist, 55*, 68–78.

Ryan, R. M., & Deci, E. L. (2001). On happiness and human potentials: A review of research on hedonic and eudaimonic well-being. *Annual Review of Psychology, 52*, 141–166.

Ryan, R. M., & Deci, E. L. (2003). On assimilating identities to the self: A self-determination theory perspective on internalization and integrity within cultures. In M. R. Leary & J. P. Tangney (Eds.), *Handbook of self and identity* (pp. 253–272). New York: Guilford.

Seligman, M. E. P., & Csikscentmihalyi, M. (2000). Positive psychology: An introduction. *American Psychologist, 55*, 5–14.

Sheldon, K. M. (2002). The self-concordance model of healthy goal-striving: When personal goals correctly represent the person. In E. L. Deci & R. M. Ryan (Eds.), *Handbook of self-determination research* (pp. 65–86). Rochester, NY: The University of Rochester Press.

Stenseng, F. (2008). The two faces of leisure activity engagement: Harmonious and obsessive passion in relation to intrapersonal conflict and life domain outcomes. *Leisure Sciences, 30*, 465–481.

Sternberg, R. J. (1986). A triangular theory of love. *Psychological Review, 93*, 119–153.

St-Louis, A. C., Carbonneau, N., & Vallerand, R. J. (2016). Passion for a cause: How it affects health and well-being. *Journal of Personality, 84*, 263–276.

Suzuki, D. (2002). http://www.davidsuzuki.org/.

Utz, S., Jonas, K. J., & Tonkens, E. (2012). Effects of passion for massively multiplayer online role-playing games on interpersonal relationships. *Journal of Media Psychology: Theories, Methods, and Applications, 24*, 77–86.

Vallerand, R. J. (1997). Toward a hierarchical model of intrinsic and extrinsic motivation. *Advances in Experimental and Social Psychology, 29*, 271–360.

Vallerand, R. J. (2001). A hierarchical model of intrinsic and extrinsic motivation in sport and exercise. In G. Roberts (Ed.), *Advances in motivation in sport and exercise* (pp. 263–319). Champaign, IL: Human Kinetics.

Vallerand, R. J. (2007). A hierarchical model of intrinsic and extrinsic motivation for sport and physical activity. In M. S. D. Hagger & N. L. D. Chatzisarantis (Eds.), *Self-determination theory in exercise and sport* (pp. 255–279). Champaign, IL: Human Kinetics.

Vallerand, R. J. (2008). On the psychology of passion: In search of what makes people's lives most worth living. *Canadian Psychology, 49*, 1–13.

Vallerand, R. J. (2010). On passion for life activities: The dualistic model of passion. In M. P. Zanna (Ed.), *Advances in experimental social psychology* (pp. 97–193). New York: Academic.

Vallerand, R. J. (2012). The role of passion in sustainable psychological well-being. *Psychological Well-Being: Theory, Research, and Practice, 2*, 1–21.

Vallerand, R. J. (2013). Passion and optimal functioning in society: A eudaimonic perspective. In A. S. Waterman (Ed.), *The best within us: Positive psychology perspectives on eudaimonic functioning* (pp. 183–206). Washington, DC: APA Books.

Vallerand, R. J. (2015). *The psychology of passion: A dualistic model*. New York: Oxford.

Vallerand, R. J., Blanchard, C. M., Mageau, G. A., Koestner, R., Ratelle, C. F., … & Léonard, M. (2003). Les passions de l'âme: On obsessive and harmonious passion. *Journal of Personality and Social Psychology, 85*, 756–767.

Vallerand, R. J., Fortier, M. S., & Guay, F. (1997). Self-determination and persistence in a real-life setting: Toward a motivational model of high school dropout. *Journal of Personality and Social Psychology, 72*, 1161–1176.

Vallerand, R. J., & Houlfort, N. (2003). Passion at work: Toward a new conceptualization. In S. W. Gilliland, D. D. Steiner, & D. P. Skarlicki (Eds.), *Emerging perspectives on values in organizations* (pp. 175–204). Greenwich, CT: Information Age Publishing.

Vallerand, R. J., Mageau, G. A., Elliot, A. J., Dumais, A., Demers, M. A., & Rousseau, F. (2008). Passion and performance attainment in sport. *Psychology of Sport and Exercise, 9*, 373–392.

Vallerand, R. J., Ntoumanis, N., Philippe, F. L., Lavigne, G. L., Carbonneau, N., Bonneville, A., … Maliha, G. (2008). On passion and sports fans: A look at football. *Journal of Sports Sciences, 26*, 1279–1293.

Vallerand, R. J., Salvy, S. J., Mageau, G. A., Elliot, A. J., Denis, P. L., Grouzet, F. M. E., et al. (2007). On the role of passion in performance. *Journal of Personality, 75*, 505–533.

Vitterso, J. (2013). Feelings, meaning, and optimal functioning: Some distinctions between hedonic and eudaimonic well-being. In A. S. Waterman (Ed.), *The best within us: Positive psychology perspectives on eudaimonic functioning* (pp. 39–55). Washington, DC: APA Books.

Waterman, A. S. (1993). Two conceptions of happiness: Contrasts of personal expressiveness (eudaimonia) and hedonic enjoyment. *Journal of Personality and Social Psychology, 64*(4), 678–691.

Waterman, A. S. (Ed.). (2013). *The best within us: Positive psychology perspectives on eudaimonia*. Washington, DC: APA Books.

Waugh, C. E., & Fredrickson, B. L. (2006). Nice to know you: Positive emotions, self-other overlap, and complex understanding in the formation of new relationships. *Journal of Positive Psychology, 1*, 93–106.

The Eudaimonics of the True Self

14

Rebecca J. Schlegel, Joshua A. Hicks,
and Andrew G. Christy

14.1 The Eudaimonics of the True Self

This chapter will explore our growing program of research that examines the meaning-making function of the true self-concept, as well as existing theory and empirical research on the importance of the true self. We argue that the true self plays a critical role in one's ability to experience eudemonic well-being. More specifically, we argue that behaviors people perceive to be consistent with their true self enhance the experience of meaning. In our research, we further argue that the true self-concept itself (i.e. a person's avowed true self) serves as a hub of meaning by guiding decision-making and serving as a justification for one's choices that needs no further justification. We argue that this allows people to imbue their life activities with subjective meaning.

14.2 The True Self

What is the true self? Historically, the true self was characterized as a set of innate characteristics that each person is born with and must discover within his or her self (e.g. (Horney, 1950; Miller, 1979; Rogers, 1959). By comparison, contemporary psychological theorists have tended to take a more fluid approach to defining the true self. For example, self-determination theory (SDT) argues that the true self is not a static set of traits or tendencies, rather it is any self-aspect that feels autonomous, internally caused, personally meaningful, and self-determined (DeCharms, 1968; Deci, 1980; Deci & Ryan, 1985, 1991; Ryan, 1993). Of course even a fluid approaches to the true self may still be influenced by innate characteristics. What feels autonomous to one person may not feel autonomous to another and those differences may be explained, in part, by differences in innate characteristics.

While debates about the "true" nature of the true self are intellectually interesting, it is equally important to consider what laypeople think about the true self. This is because the true self may be similar to other psychological constructs such as free will (Vohs & Schooler, 2008; Wegner, 2002) in that it is the *perception* of reality that matters as much, if not more, than the actual reality (particularly given that the "actual reality" may be impossible to determine!). Such "phenomenological realties" need not actually exist to have important psychological consequences (Gergen, 1977, 1985). To the extent that people believe they have a true self, it is likely that the perceived true self will influence other important domains of their lives. Thus our research has largely taken a lay theories approach (e.g., Molden & Dweck, 2006) to addressing the issue of the true self.

R.J. Schlegel (✉) • J.A. Hicks • A.G. Christy
Texas A&M University, College Station, TX, USA
e-mail: beccaschlegel@tamu.edu

J. Vittersø (ed.), *Handbook of Eudaimonic Well-Being*, International Handbooks of Quality-of-Life,
DOI 10.1007/978-3-319-42445-3_14

Interestingly, laypeople's beliefs about the true self seem to correspond more with the historical, essentialist conception of the true self as a static set of traits than with the more contemporary, fluid definitions (Christy, Schlegel, & Cimpian, 2015; Schlegel, Vess, & Arndt, 2012). Consistent with an essentialist view of the true self, people perceive the true self as something that is "inside" the person (Baumeister, 1987). That is, the true self is seen as who someone "really is" inside when they are stripped of their outward social masks (e.g., Harter, 2002; Jung, 1953; Kernis & Goldman, 2006; Rogers, 1959; Rosenberg, 1979; Winnicott, 1960). Consistent with this idea, people tend to believe that private aspects of the self (i.e., thoughts and feelings) are more diagnostic of the true self than public behaviors (Andersen, 1984; Andersen, Lazowski & Donisi, 1986; Andersen & Ross, 1984; Andersen & Williams, 1985; Johnson, Robinson, & Mitchell, 2004). When people believe behavior stems from the true self, they refer to that behavior as "authentic" (Kernis & Godlman, 2006; Wood, Linley, Maltby, Baliousis, & Joseph, 2008). The very idea that some behavior is authentic and other behavior is inauthentic (i.e. emanating from the true self versus not) entails that a person may be different on the inside than they seem on the outside (e.g., Baumeister, 1987). In cases where the two differ, people clearly regard the part on the inside as the "true" self.

In addition to its internality, the true self seems to be highly related to morality. Two investigations by Strohminger and Nichols (2014, 2015), demonstrate that a person's moral traits and characteristics are perceived as central to who they are. In these studies, participants perceived the identity of either a hypothetical or real target (i.e. a family member with a neurodegenerative disorder) as most profoundly changed when the target's moral traits changed. This was relative to other kinds of personal characteristics (e.g. personality traits, desires/preferences, memories/knowledge), leading Strohmingor and Nichols to conclude that "moral capacities are the most central part of identity" (p. 1). Not only are true selves perceived as the "home" of morality, people tend to further believe all true selves are morally good. Research by Newman, Knobe, and colleagues (Newman, Bloom, & Knobe, 2014; Newman, De Frietas, & Knobe, 2014) has shown that people selectively attribute behaviors they deem to be morally good as representative of another person's true self. For example, political conservatives believe someone who becomes more patriotic over time is becoming more like their true self. Bench, Schlegel, Davis, and Vess (2015) found similar patterns for any change perceived as good or bad (regardless of whether it was morally relevant), further suggesting that people believe all true selves are good.

In sum, the true self may best be defined as the version of the self that represents who a person really is, regardless of their outward behavior. It is the part of the self that is genuine and uninfluenced by context or outside factors (e.g., social norms, pressures, societal demands). Of interest, people see this genuine self as morally and generally good (an idea consistent with Carl Roger's theorizing). A variety of empirical approaches in psychology have argued for the importance of the true self in eudaimonia.

14.3 The True Self and Eudaimonia: Theory and Past Research

There are a number of other broad theoretical perspectives that suggest that the true self is important to eudaimonic well-being. Indeed, eudaimonia is sometimes defined as "fulfilling or realizing one's *daimon* or true nature" (Deci & Ryan, 2008; p. 2) and the true self is either explicitly or implicitly invoked in much of the theorizing in Self-Determination Theory. Similarly, Carol Ryff has suggested that the importance of fulfilling one's unique potential (and the value of that above and beyond simple happiness) is what motivated her efforts to develop her highly influential conception of Psychological Well-Being (Ryff, 1989, this volume; Ryff & Singer, 2008). Narrative approaches to identity (McAdams, 1985) similarly emphasize that a rich and complex understanding of the self as an important part of eudaimonia (Bauer, McAdams, &

Pals, 2008) and research suggests that the extent to which life stories involve deeper understanding and integration (i.e., integrative growth) predicts self-reports of purpose in life and personal growth (Bauer & McAdams, 2004; Bauer, McAdams, & Sakaeda, 2005; Bauer, this volume). Finally, Waterman's Eudaimonic Identity Theory (1990, 2011, 2013) and Waterman, Schwartz, & Conti, (2008) very clearly and squarely places the true self at the heart of eudaimonia. Waterman's (1993) Personally Expressive Activities Questionnaire (PEAQ) distinguishes eudaimonic from hedonic activities with items such as "This activity gives me my strongest feeling that this is who I really am". Our work in this area is consistent with these broader approaches and aims to specifically explicate the role of feelings of true self-knowledge and true self-expression in the achievement of eudaimonic well-being.

To further consider the role the true self might play in the eudaimonic life we believe it is worth considering two examples that highlight the distinction between hedonia and eudaimonia (though we agree with Waterman (1993) and others that the two typically co-occur). On the one hand, there may be activities in life that are more characterized more by hedonia (pleasure) than eudaimonia, such as eating ice cream. On the other hand, there may be activities in life that are more characterized by eudaimonia than hedonia. For example, One might consider the "parenthood paradox" (Baumeister, 1991), which suggests that parenting may make day to day life more stressful and less pleasurable, but often makes people's lives feel more meaningful.

To best understand these distinctions, we are particularly appreciative of recent theorizing by Baumeister, Vohs, Aaker, & Garbinsky (2013). These authors argue that "Happiness may be rooted in having one's needs and desires satisfied, including being largely free from unpleasant events. Meaningfulness may be considerably more complex than happiness, because it requires interpretive construction of circumstances across time according to abstract values and other culturally mediated ideas" (p. 505; see also Maslow's theorizing on b-needs and d-needs; Maslow, 1971). They go on to cite concerns about personal identity and self-expression as one of the key factors that distinguishes the two, going so far as to suggest that "doing things that express the self is about meaning, not happiness" (p. 513). This is not to say that expressing the self cannot be both meaningful and pleasurable, of course, but suggests that meaning may be the primary motivator when it comes to self-expression. In other words, hedonia is about satisfying universal reward mechanisms, whereas eudaimonia requires a match between the activity and the individual. This theorizing is consistent with classic research done by McGregor and Little (1998) demonstrating that the extent to which personal projects are judged to be self-expressive predicts the perceived meaningfulness of those projects.

Consistent with Baumesiter and colleagues' contention (and McGregor and Little's work, see for instance Little, this volume), we suggest that considering the role of the true self in these two examples helps highlight the nature of the difference between hedonia and eudaimonia. The pleasure derived from eating ice cream likely has more to do with the positive feelings that surround the immediate experience of one's desires and less to do with the pursuit of understanding, expressing and realizing one's true self (e.g., McGregor & Little, 1998; Waterman et al., 2008). By comparison, parenting is tough work that is not always pleasurable, but it offers a variety of opportunities to learn about and express one's true self in personally meaningful ways (Baumeister et al., 2013). In this way, we see the pursuit of understanding, expressing and realizing one's true self as the fundamental key to eudaimonia.

These examples highlight another observation made by Baumeister and colleagues (2013) – self-expressive activities aren't necessarily pleasurable activities. While self-expressive activities are typically going to promote both meaning and happiness (e.g. Waterman et al., 2008), some activities are simply unrelated to happiness and others may even detract from it (e.g. standing up for one's ideals at the cost of social exclusion or even punishment).

This is consistent with Nussbaum's (2008) discussion of "good pains". As argued by Nussbaum, Aristotle believed that pleasure does not always go along with eudaimonia, "only most of the time" (p. 597). Nussbaum goes on to note that pains can be good specifically because they deepen one's self-knowledge by helping us grapple with our weaknesses, fears, and insecurities. Kernis and Goldman (2006) make similar points in their theoretical account of authentic functioning. Kernis and Goldman argue that the unbiased processing of one's strengths and weaknesses is one of the four primary components of authenticity.

Another way the true self is relevant in the distinction between hedonia and eudaimonia is considering the fact that the hedonic value of a particular activity is fairly similar across individuals. That is, hedonia relies on the gratification of basic biological drives that are shared by all humans and many non-human species. In contrast, the path to eudaimonia (or at least experienced eudaimonia) may be far more individualized; there is more inter-individual variability in a given activity's eudaimonic value compared to its hedonic value. In other words, hedonia is more about satisfying these universal reward mechanisms, whereas eudaimonia requires a match between the activity and the true self-concept of the individual. This idea is consistent with the contention we have made in previous work (Schlegel, Hicks, Davis, Hirsch, & Smith, 2013) that the true self-concept helps each person form their own unique "life philosophy" about what is worth pursuing. While one person might see great personal meaning in becoming an accountant, another person may not see any personal meaning or intrinsic value in that career.

14.4 Our Empirical Approach: The True Self-Concept and Meaning in Life Judgments

To hone in on the role of the true self in eudaimonia, our research has focused specifically on judgments of meaning in life (e.g., indicating agreement with statements such as "I understand my life's meaning," Steger, Frazier, Oishi, & Kaler, 2006). Although there is no universal agreement on exactly how eudaimonia should best be operationalized and measured, we believe that feelings of meaning should be one clear "flagship indicator" (Steger, Shin, Shim, & Fitch-Martin, 2013; Steger, this volume). Indeed, we know almost intuitively the importance that meaning has in our lives and many people are familiar with the experience of searching for meaning. Of course, asking people to judge the meaningfulness of their lives, on aggregate, is less than ideal. As Nussbaum (2008) notes, people may feel very differently about different aspect of their lives, and asking for a single judgment of the meaningfulness of something as vast and varied as a life loses much of this nuance. However, global judgments of meaning are associated with many important subjective outcomes such as life satisfaction (Steger & Kashdan, 2007; Zika & Chamberlin, 1992), quality of life (e.g., Krause, 2007), and depression (e.g., Mascaro & Rosen, 2005), as well as more "objective" outcomes such as alcohol and drug use (e.g., Lecci, MacLean, & Croteau, 2002), suicidal ideation (e.g., Heisel & Flett, 2004) and even mortality rates (Boyle, Barnes, Buchman, & Bennett, 2009; Hill & Turiano, 2014; Krause, 2009). Thus, we believe that self-reported global judgments of meaning in life are incredibly valuable, despite their limitations, as they offer scientific insight into questions that may otherwise not be empirically accessible.

Operationalizing the true self for the purposes of empirical research is a thorny issue. Indeed, Waterman (1984) suggested that the true self is an abstraction that can never be observed or measured directly. Thus, our research focuses on people's subjective beliefs about who their true selves are, what we have termed their "true self-concepts". In a growing line of research, we have demonstrated that in a variety of ways, the true self-concept serves as a hub of meaning. This research continually shows that "being in touch" with one's true self-concept consistently predicts judgments of meaning in life.

14.4.1 Cognitive Accessibility

Our first demonstration of the relationship between the true self-concept and meaning involved a set of five studies that examined how the cognitive accessibility of the true self-concept predicted judgments of meaning in life. Cognitive accessibility refers to how easily or quickly something can be retrieved from long term memory (e.g. Rholes & Pryor, 1982). Given previous research that had shown the cognitive accessibility of other meaning sources (e.g., religion, personal relationships) predicts meaning judgments (e.g., Hicks & King, 2008, 2009a, 2009b; Hicks, Schlegel, & King, 2010; King, Hicks, Krull, & Del Gaiso, 2006; Ward & King, this volume), we reasoned that the simple activation of the true self-concept itself should be sufficient to elicit a corresponding increase in meaning in life, even in the absence of the phenomenological experience or actual expression of one's true self-concept.

To test this idea, we asked participants to provide words that they felt best described both their true and actual selves (Schlegel, Hicks, Arndt, & King, 2009). The true self was defined to participants as "*who you believe you really are, even if you sometimes act in different ways*" and the actual self was defined as "*who you are during most of your daily activities, even if these traits don't reflect who you really are*." The words the participants generated served as stimuli in a reaction time task designed to measure the cognitive accessibility of one's true self-concept (e.g., Bargh & Chartrand, 2000) or as stimuli in a priming task that manipulated cognitive accessibility of the true self. The reaction time task was a "me/not me" task (Markus, 1977) in which participants were asked to decide as quickly as they could whether or not words on a computer screen described them or not by clicking a key labled "me" or a key labled "not me". The task was programmed to include the words participants had previously judged (or generated) as descriptive of the true or actual self-concept. The latencyfor responding served as an indicator of the relative accessibility of self-concepts, such that faster reaction times indicate greater accessibility (Bargh & Chartrand, 2000). In the priming studies, participants were asked to make non self-judgments (i.e. word/non-word decisions) and were flashed true or actual self descriptos for a very brief amount of time (e.g. 400 ms) between trials (e.g., Friedman, McCarthy, Bartholow, & Hicks, 2007 Friedman et al., 2005).

In each of five studies, true self-concept accessibility (whether measured or manipulated) predicted people's global meaning in life judgments such that the more accessible one's true self-concept, the greater one's perception that his or her life was meaningful. In contrast, accessibility of the actual self-concept (i.e. beliefs about how one behaves in everyday life) had no relationship with meaning in life, suggesting that the true self has a unique relationship with the experience of meaning over and above the self-concept more generally (in this case, the actual self).

14.4.2 Metacognitive Ease

Next, we examined how more explicit measures of perceived true self-knowledge might mirror the observed effects of true self-concept accessibility (Schlegel, Hicks, King, & Arndt, 2011). Studying the effects of accessibility required the use of relatively non-conscious and difficult to control measures and manipulations (i.e., very quick reaction times or subliminal priming). While this has the benefit of minimizing response biases, we also wanted to examine how other true self processes, particular those that participants were more aware of, might influence meaning. In this way, we wanted to more directly examine subjective experiences that people are likely to encounter in their daily lives. Thus, we utilized the metacognitive experience of ease/difficulty (Schwarz, 1998; Schwarz & Clore, 1996) in a true self description task. Because people use the metacognitive experience of ease (or difficulty) as a cue to how much they know about a topic (Schwarz, 2004), experiencing a self-description task as easy (vs. difficult) should influence the perception of possessing (or not possessing) true self-knowledge. People who experience true self description as easy should feel confident in their level of true self-knowledge, whereas those who experience it as difficult should question their level of true self-knowledge.

Across three studies, we asked participants to generate lists of words that described their true and/or actual selves and either measured perceived self-knowledge by asking participants how easy it was to complete the task or manipulated perceived self-knowledge by explicitly making the task easy or difficult by asking participants to generate either a few (8) or many words (15; adapted from Schwarz et al., 1991). Consistent with the findings for true self-concept accessibility, we found that perceived true self-knowledge positively predicted global judgments of meaning in life and that perceived actual self-knowledge was unrelated to those judgments. These studies also controlled for self-reported positive and negative affect as well as self-esteem in multiple regression analyses, revealing that the effect of metacognitive ease was over and above the influence of those factors. This further supports the strong influence of the true self-concept in meaning.

Taken together, these studies on the relationship between the true self-concept and global judgments of meaning provide compelling evidence for the role of the true self in eudaimonic functioning in general, and meaning-making specifically.

14.5 Why Is the True Self a Hub of Meaning?

Why might the true self serve as a hub of meaning? In a classic paper, Baumeister (1987) argues that over the course of history, people have looked more and more to the self for answers to the question of how to best live one's life. For example, one may wonder whether they should become a lawyer or an accountant. Society offers no answer as to which of these careers is more meaningful or satisfying. Thus, people are likely to look to the self for guidance (Baumeister, 1991; Bellah, Madsen, Sullivan, Swidler, & Tipton, 1985). Choices and actions are thus judged in terms of how self-expressive they are and those acts that are more self-expressive are deemed more valuable (e.g. being a lawyer is more consistent with who I really am inside). This is useful as Baumeister (1991) notes because "the self provides legitimacy and justification to other things without itself needing a higher source of value". That is, in the absence of clear societal or cultural guidance as to what career to pursue or who to marry, choices become personal and idiosyncratic.

When faced with such personal choices, most people explicitly believe that trusting in/following their true self is the most reliable strategy for making a good choice. Consistent with this proposition, we (Schlegel et al., 2013) asked a sample of adults to rate how likely 36 decision-making strategies were to lead to a satisfying decision. Embedded within these items were items that assessed the "true self as guide" lay theory (e.g., "People are likely to make a satisfying decision if they use their true self as a guide," "People are likely to make a satisfying decision if they follow who they really are"). The true self items were rated as the most important strategy overall, and were rated as significantly more important than all but two of the other strategies (considering what the future self would want, rational processing). This suggests that people explicitly believe that following one's true self is an important strategy for making personally satisfying decisions.

One consequence of this widely held "true self as guide" lay theory is that people use their perceived knowledge of their true selves as a means of reducing the uncertainty inherent in complex decisions and in evaluating the quality of their decisions (Nakao, Takezawa, Shiraishi, & Miyatani, 2009, 2010). That is, when people feel that they know their true self, they feel confident in their ability to make optimal decisions and this bolsters their satisfaction with those decisions. For example, in one study that manipulated perceived true self knowledge, participants in a high self-knowledge condition reported significantly greater decision satisfaction than their counterparts in a low self-knowledge condition (Schlegel et al., 2013). We suggest that when this process is applied over many life decisions, the result is a life that feels more meaningful on the whole.

Recent emerging evidence suggests another route by which the true self may confer meaning. Specifically, studies (Newman, Bloom, Knobe, 2014; Strohminger & Nichols, 2014, 2015) are starting to show the key role that morality plays in defining the true self. If morality is central to people's true self definitions, then the true self is likely a source of people's values, which are another clear source of meaning in life. Indeed, having a clear system of values is sometimes used part of the definition of meaning in life (e.g., Crumbaugh & Maholick, 1964; Krause, 2007). Further, because most people seem to operate on the assumption that their own true self (Bench et al., 2015) and the true selves of others are morally good (Newman, Bloom, et al., 2014; Newman, De Frietas, et al., 2014), true self-knowledge may even facilitate virtuous behavior; a pattern that would clearly be consistent with much of humanistic psychology (e.g., Maslow, 1962; Rogers, 1961).

14.6 Conclusions

While other factors may foster purpose and meaning (e.g., flow experiences), we believe that the subjective experience of knowing one's core self is a primary contributor to eudaimonia. When people feel the know who they truly are, they are in a better position to pursue satisfying and meaningful endeavors, and that metacognitive feeling itself engender the perception that life is meaningful. We are encouraged by the variety of approaches aimed at understating this elusive topic and look forward to future research that continues to elucidate the role of the true self (as well as other variables) in a life well-lived.

References

Andersen, S. M. (1984). Self-knowledge and social inference: II. The diagnosticity of cognitive/affective and behavioral data. *Journal of Personality and Social Psychology, 46*, 294–307.

Andersen, S. M., Lazowski, L. E., & Donisi, M. (1986). Salience and self-inference: The role of biased recollections in self-inference processes. *Social Cognition, 4*, 75–95.

Andersen, S. M., & Ross, L. (1984). Self-knowledge and social inference: I.The impact of cognitive/affective and behavioral data. *Journal of Personality and Social Psychology, 46*, 280–293.

Andersen, S. M., & Williams, M. (1985). Cognitive/affective reactions in the improvement of self-esteem: When thoughts and feelings make a difference. *Journal of Personality and Social Psychology, 49*, 1086–1097.

Bargh, J. A., & Chartrand, T. L. (2000). A practical guide to priming and automaticity research. In H. Reiss & C. Judd (Eds.), *Handbook of research methods in social psychology* (pp. 253–285). New York: Cambridge University Press.

Bauer, J. J., & McAdams, D. P. (2004). Personal growth in adults' stories of life transitions. *Journal of Personality, 72*, 573–602.

Bauer, J. J., McAdams, D. P., & Pals, J. L. (2008). Narrative identity and eudaimonic well-being. *Journal of Happiness Studies, 9*, 81–104.

Bauer, J. J., McAdams, D. P., & Sakaeda, A. R. (2005). Interpreting the good life: Growth memories in the lives of mature, happy people. *Journal of Personality and Social Psychology, 88*, 203–217.

Baumeister, R. F. (1987). How the self became a problem: A psychological review of historical research. *Journal of Personality and Social Psychology, 52*, 163–176.

Baumeister, R. F. (1991). *Meanings of life*. New York: Guilford.

Baumeister, R. F., Vohs, K. D., Aaker, J. L., & Garbinsky, E. N. (2013). Some key differences between a happy life and a meaningful life. *Journal of Positive Psychology, 8*, 505–516.

Bellah, R. N., Madsen, R., Sullivan, W. M., Swidler, A., & Tipton, S. M. (1985). *Habits of the heart: Individualism and commitment in American life*. Berkeley, CA: University of California Press.

Bench, S., Schlegel, R. J., Davis, W. E., & Vess, M. (2015). Thinking about change in the self and others: The role of self-discovery metaphors and the true self. *Social Cognition, 33*, 169–185.

Boyle, P. A., Barnes, L. L., Buchman, A. S., & Bennett, D. A. (2009). Purpose in life is associated with mortality among community-dwelling older persons. *Psychosomatic Medicine, 71*, 574–579.

Christy, A. G., Schlegel, R. J., & Cimpian, A. (2015). Essentialism and the true-self-concept. *Unpublished Manuscript*.

Crumbaugh, J. C., & Maholick, L. T. (1964). An experimental study in existentialism: The psychometric approach to Frankl's concept of noogenic neurosis. *Journal of Clinical Psychology, 20*(2), 200–207.

DeCharms, R. (1968). *Personal causation*. New York: Academic.

Deci, E. L. (1980). *The psychology of self-determination*. Lexington, MA: Heath.

Deci, E. L., & Ryan, R. M. (1985). *Intrinsic motivation and self-determination in human behavior*. New York: Plenum Press.

Deci, E. L., & Ryan, R. M. (1991). A motivational approach to self: Integration in personality. In R. A. Dienstbier & R. A. Dienstbier (Eds.), *Nebraska symposium on motivation, 1990: Perspectives on motivation* (pp. 237–288). Lincoln, NE: University of Nebraska Press.

Deci, E. L., & Ryan, R. M. (2008). Hedonia, eudaimonia, and well-being: An introduction. *Journal of Happiness Studies, 9*, 1–11.

Friedman, R. S., McCarthy, D. M., Förster, J., & Denzler, M. (2005). Automatic effects of alcohol cues on sexual attraction. *Addiction, 100*, 672–681.

Friedman, R. S., McCarthy, D. M., Bartholow, B. D., & Hicks J. A. (2007). Interactive effects of alcohol outcome expectancies and suboptimal alcohol cues on non-consumptive behavior. *Experimental and Clinical Psychopharmacology, 15*, 102–114.

Gergen, K. J. (1977). The social construction of self-knowledge. In T. Mischel (Ed.), *The self: Psychological and philosophical issues* (pp. 139–169). Blue Ridge Summit, PA: Rowman & Littlefield.

Gergen, K. J. (1985). The social constructionist movement in modern psychology. *American Psychologist, 40*, 266–275.

Harter, S. (2002). Authenticity. In C. R. Snyder & S. J. Lopez (Eds.), *Handbook of positive psychology* (pp. 382–394). Oxford, UK: Oxford University Press.

Heisel, M. J., & Flett, G. L. (2004). Purpose in life, satisfaction with life, and suicide ideation in a clinical sample. *Journal of Psychopathology and Behavioral Assessment, 26*, 127–135.

Hicks, J. A., & King, L. A. (2008). Religious commitment and positive mood as information about meaning in life. *Journal of Research in Personality, 42*, 43–57.

Hicks, J. A., & King, L. A. (2009a). Positive mood and social relatedness as information about meaning in life. *Journal of Positive Psychology, 4*, 471–482.

Hicks, J. A., & King, L. A. (2009b). Meaning in life as a subjective judgment and lived experience. *Social and Personality Psychology Compass, 3*, 638–653.

Hicks, J. A., Schlegel, R. J., & King, L. A. (2010). Social threats, happiness, and the dynamics of meaning in life judgments. *Personality and Social Psychology Bulletin, 36*, 1305–1317.

Hill, P. L., & Turiano, N. A. (2014). Purpose in life as a predictor of mortality across adulthood. *Psychological Science, 25*, 1482–1486.

Horney, K. (1950). *Neurosis and human growth: The struggle toward self-realization*. Oxford, UK: Norton.

Johnson, J. T., Robinson, M. D., & Mitchell, E. B. (2004). Inferences about the authentic self: When do actions say more than mental states. *Journal of Personality and Social Psychology, 87*, 615–630.

Jung, C. G. (1953). *Two essays in analytical psychology* (R. F. Hull, Trans.). New York: Pantheon.

Kernis, M. H., & Goldman, B. M. (2006). A multicomponent conceptualization of authenticity: Theory and research. In M. P. Zanna (Ed.), *Advances in experimental social psychology* (38th ed.). New York: Academic.

King, L. A., Hicks, J. A., Krull, J., & Del Gaiso, A. (2006). Positive affect and the experience of meaning in life. *Journal of Personality and Social Psychology, 90*, 179–196.

Krause, N. (2007). Self-expression and depressive symptoms in late life. *Research on Aging, 29*, 187–206.

Krause, N. (2009). Meaning in life and mortality. *The Journals of Gerontology: Series B: Psychological Sciences and Social Sciences, 64B*, 517–527.

Lecci, L., MacLean, M. G., & Croteau, N. (2002). Personal goals of predictors of college student drinking motives, alcohol use and related problems. *Journal of Studies on Alcohol, 63*, 620–630.

Mascaro, N., & Rosen, D. H. (2005). Existential meaning's role in the enhancement of hope and prevention of depressive symptoms. *Journal of Personality, 73*, 985–1014.

Maslow, A. H. (1962). *Towards a psychology of being*. D. Van Nostrand Company: Princeton.

Maslow, A. (1971). *Farther reaches of human nature*. New York: McGraw-Hill.

McAdams, D. P. (1985). *Power, intimacy, and the life story: Personological inquiries into identity*. New York: Guilford.

McGregor, I., & Little, B. R. (1998). Personal projects, happiness, and meaning: On doing well and being yourself. *Journal of Personality and Social Psychology, 74*, 494–512.

Miller, A. (1979). *The drama of the gifted child: The search for the true self*. New York: Basic Books.

Molden, D. C., & Dweck, C. S. (2006). Finding "meaning" in psychology: A lay theories approach to self-regulation, social perception, and social development. *American Psychologist, 61*, 192–203.

Nakao, T., Mitsumoto, M., Nashiwa, H., Takamura, M., Tokunaga, S., Miyatani, M., ... Watanabe, Y. (2010). Self-knowledge reduces conflict by biasing one of plural possible answers. *Personality and Social Psychology Bulletin, 36*, 455–469.

Nakao, T., Takezawa, T., Shiraishi, M., & Miyatani, M. (2009). Activation of self-knowledge reduces conflict during occupational choice: An ERP study. *International Journal of Neuroscience, 119*, 1640–1654.

Newman, G. E., Bloom, P., & Knobe, J. (2014). Value judgments and the true self. *Personality and Social Psychology Bulletin, 40*, 203–216.

Newman, G. E., De Freitas, J., & Knobe, J. (2014). Beliefs about the true self explain asymmetries based on moral judgment. *Cognitive Science, 2014*, 1–30.

Nussbaum, M. C. (2008). Who is the happy warrior? Philosophy poses questions to psychology. *Journal of Legal Studies, 37*, 81–113.

Rholes, W. S., & Pryor, J. B. (1982). Cognitive accessibility and causal attributions. *Personality and Social Psychology Bulletin, 8*(4), 719–727.

Rogers, C. R. (1959). A theory of therapy, personality, and interpersonal relationships, as developed in the client-centered framework. In S. Koch (Ed.), *Psychology: A study of a science* (pp. 184–256). New York: McGraw-Hill.

Rogers, C. (1961). *On becoming a person.* Boston: Hougton Mifflin Company.

Rosenberg, M. (1979). *Conceiving the self.* New York: Basic Books.

Ryan, R. M. (1993). Agency and organization: Intrinsic motivation, autonomy, and the self in psychological development. In J. E. Jacobs (Ed.), *Nebraska symposium on motivation, 1992: Current theory and research in motivation* (pp. 1–56). Lincoln, NE: University of Nebraska Press.

Ryff, C. D. (1989). Happiness is everything, or is it? Explorations on the meaning of psychological well-being. *Journal of Personality and Social Psychology, 57*, 1069.

Ryff, C. D., & Singer, B. H. (2008). Know thyself and become what you are: A eudaimonic approach to psychological well-being. *Journal of Happiness Studies, 9*, 13–39.

Schlegel, R. J., Hicks, J. A., Arndt, J., & King, L. A. (2009). Thine own self: True self-concept accessibility and meaning in life. *Journal of Personality and Social Psychology, 96*, 473–490.

Schlegel, R. J., Hicks, J. A., Davis, W. E., Hirsch, K. A., & Smith, C. M. (2013). Dynamic interplay between perceived true self-knowledge and decision satisfaction. *Journal of Personality and Social Psychology, 104*, 542–558.

Schlegel, R. J., Hicks, J. A., King, L. A., & Arndt, J. (2011). Feeling like you know who you are: Perceived true self-knowledge and meaning in life. *Personality and Social Psychology Bulletin, 37*, 745–756.

Schlegel, R. J., Vess, M. K., & Arndt, J. A. (2012). To discover or to create: Metaphors and the true self. *Journal of Personality, 80*, 969–993.

Schwarz, N. (1998). Accessible content and accessibility experiences: The interplay of declarative and experiential information in judgment. *Personality and Social Psychology Review, 2*, 87–99.

Schwarz, N. (2004). Metacognitive experiences in consumer judgment and decision making. *Journal of Consumer Psychology, 14*, 332–348.

Schwarz, N., Bless, H., Strack, F., Klumpp, G., Rittenauer-Schatka, H., & Simons, A. (1991). Ease of retrieval as information: Another look at the availability heuristic. *Journal of Personality and Social Psychology, 61*, 195.

Schwarz, N., & Clore, G. L. (1996). Feelings as phenomenal experiences. In E. T. Higgins & A. Kruglanski (Eds.), *Social psychology: Handbook of basic principles* (pp. 433–465). New York: Guilford.

Steger, M. F., Frazier, P., Oishi, S., & Kaler, M. (2006). The meaning in life questionnaire: Assessing the presence of and search for meaning in life. *Journal of Counseling Psychology, 53*, 80–94.

Steger, M. F., & Kashdan, T. B. (2007). Stability and specificity of meaning in life and life satisfaction over one year. *Journal of Happiness Studies, 8*, 161–179.

Steger, M. F., Shin, J. Y., Shim, Y., & Fitch-Martin, A. (2013). Is meaning in life a flagship indicator of wellbeing? In *The best within us: Positive psychology perspectives on eudaimonia* (pp. 159–182). Washington, DC: American Psychological Association.

Strohminger, N., & Nichols, S. (2014). The essential moral self. *Cognition, 131*, 159–171.

Strohminger, N., & Nichols, S. (2015). Neurodegeneration and identity. *Psychological Science, 26*, 1469–1479.

Vohs, K. D., & Schooler, J. D. (2008). The value of believing in free will: Encouraging a belief in determinism increases cheating. *Psychological Science, 19*, 49–54.

Waterman, A. S. (1984). Identity formation: Discovery or creation? *Journal of Early Adolescence, 4*, 329–341.

Waterman, A. S. (1990). Personal expressiveness: Philosophical and psychological foundations. *The Journal of Mind and Behavior, 11*, 47–74.

Waterman, A. S. (1993). Two conceptions of happiness: Contrasts of personal expressiveness (eudaimonia) and hedonic enjoyment. *Journal of Personality and Social Psychology, 64*, 678–691.

Waterman, A. S. (2011). Eudaimonic identity theory: Identity as self-discovery. In S. J. Schwartz, K. Luyckx, & V. L. Vignoles (Eds.), *Handbook of identity theory and research* (pp. 357–379). New York: Springer.

Waterman, A. S. (2013). The humanistic psychology–positive psychology divide: Contrasts in philosophical foundations. *American Psychologist, 68*(3), 124.

Waterman, A. S., Schwartz, S. J., & Conti, R. (2008). The implications of two conceptions of happiness (hedonic enjoyment and eudaimonia) for the understanding of intrinsic motivation. *Journal of Happiness Studies, 9*, 41–79.

Wegner, D. M. (2002). *The illusion of conscious will.* Cambridge, MA: MIT Press.

Winnicott, D. W. (1960). Ego distortion in terms of true and false self. In *The maturational process and the facilitating environment: Studies in the theory of emotional development* (pp. 140–152). New York: International Universities Press.

Wood, A. M., Linley, P. A., Maltby, J., Baliousis, M., & Joseph, S. (2008). The authentic personality: A theoretical and empirical conceptualization and the development of the authenticity scale. *Journal of Counseling Psychology, 55*, 385–399.

Zika, S., & Chamberlain, K. (1992). On the relation between meaning in life and psychological well-being. *British Journal of Psychology, 83*, 133–145.

15 Eudaimonic and Hedonic Orientations: Theoretical Considerations and Research Findings

Veronika Huta

15.1 Definition Categories

This chapter is organized around the structure proposed in Huta and Waterman (2014), which reviewed definitions of eudaimonia and hedonia used in psychology research. In performing the review, we realized that the definitions of different researchers fell into four somewhat distinct *definition categories*, and that findings with measures from the same given category were more similar than findings with measures from different categories. Eudaimonia and hedonia have been defined as one or more of the following:

1. *Orientations*: personal priorities, reasons, motives, values, and goals behind a person's chosen behaviors (e.g., seeking to grow and mature as a person, seeking pleasure).
2. *Behaviors*: specific behaviors a person engages in, including actions and thoughts (e.g., planning personal goals, attending big parties).
3. *Experiences*: subjective emotions, feelings, and cognitive-affective appraisals (e.g., feeling of meaning/value, feeling of positive affect).
4. *Functioning*: abilities, accomplishments, and healthy habits, often acquired after an extended period of eudaimonic/hedonic orientation and behavior (e.g., self-regulation, being good at savoring).

V. Huta (✉)
University of Ottawa, Ottawa, Canada
e-mail: Veronika.Huta@uottawa.ca

The first two categories – orientations and behaviors – might be called *ways of living*, because they can be more directly chosen and changed than the latter two categories. Experiences and functioning are often *outcomes* of ways of living. Furthermore, I associate the term *a good life* primarily with orientations (as detailed below), and the term *well-being* primarily with experiences and functioning, though on a broader level, I think both terms can lend themselves to all four definition categories.

15.2 Conceptual Definitions of Eudaimonia and Hedonia

15.2.1 Using Orientations as the Primary Definition Category

I believe that all four definition categories are needed for a complete understanding of eudaimonia and hedonia. Nevertheless, in my research, I have defined eudaimonia and hedonia primarily as orientations, for the following reasons (see Huta, 2013, 2015b; Huta & Ryan, 2010, for additional discussions of the reasons). We can choose our way of life more directly than our experiences

J. Vittersø (ed.), *Handbook of Eudaimonic Well-Being*, International Handbooks of Quality-of-Life,
DOI 10.1007/978-3-319-42445-3_15

or functioning. Good feelings tend come in their own time, as by-products of healthy choices. High levels of functioning are often outcomes as well-being achieved after long periods of a certain way of living. Thus, ways of living are more direct points of intervention than well-being outcomes. I also think it's more fair to define a good life in terms of people's efforts, rather than their successes. Furthermore, though orientations and behaviors can both be chosen more than experiences and functioning, I consider orientations more fundamental than behaviors. Two people can exhibit the same surface behavior for very different reasons, e.g., one person may donate to charity to enhance their public image, while another may do so out of genuine empathy. I believe it's the underlying reason that matters most.

15.2.2 Defining a Eudaimonic Orientation and a Hedonic Orientation

I define a eudaimonic orientation in terms of four core elements: (1) *authenticity*: clarifying one's true self and values, and acting in accord with them; (2) *meaning*: seeking what truly matters and has value, and understanding the bigger picture, aligning oneself with it, and contributing to it (note that I distinguish between meaning as an orientation – which I will simply call meaning in this chapter – and meaning as an experience, with the latter involving subjective feelings of significance, value, resonance, and broad implications); (3) *excellence*: striving for high standards and quality in one's ethics, behavior, performance, and products; and (4) *growth*: gaining knowledge, insight, and skill; actualizing one's unique potentials; and maturing as a human being (Huta, 2015b). All four elements are about striving to do what is truly, objectively, and inherently good and right and meaningful, even if it's difficult.

I define a hedonic orientation as the pursuit of two elements: (1) *pleasure*: positive emotions, pleasant sensations, and emotional/visceral satisfaction; and (2) *comfort*: relaxation, ease, and painlessness. A hedonic orientation, therefore, is the pursuit of what is subjectively pleasant.

Eudaimonia and hedonia can coexist, though they can also be at odds with each other, since they are based on different ways of evaluating what is good.

15.3 Operational Definitions of Eudaimonia and Hedonia: The HEMA Scale

The measure I developed to assess eudaimonic and hedonic orientations is the HEMA (Hedonic and Eudaimonic Motives for Activities, Huta & Ryan, 2010). It consists of the first nine items in Table 15.1, where items 1, 4, 6, 7, and 10 represent hedonia, and items 2, 3, 5, and 8 represent eudaimonia. The hedonia items reflect the concepts of pleasure (items 4, 6, and 9), and comfort (items 1 and 7). The eudaimonia items reflect the concepts of authenticity (items 3 and 8), excellence (items 5 and 8), and growth (item 2). As detailed later, an additional item has recently been added (item 10) to reflect the concept of meaning, thus forming the HEMA-R (HEMA-Revised). All research findings reported in this chapter are based on the original HEMA scale; findings with the HEMA-R are forthcoming.

Table 15.1 The HEMA questionnaire (hedonic and eudaimonic motives for activities) and the HEMA-R (HEMA- revised)

To what degree do you typically approach your activities with each of the following intentions, whether or not you actually achieve your aim?
1. Seeking relaxation?
2. Seeking to develop a skill, learn, or gain insight into something?
3. Seeking to do what you believe in?
4. Seeking pleasure?
5. Seeking to pursue excellence or a personal ideal?
6. Seeking enjoyment?
7. Seeking to take it easy?
8. Seeking to use the best in yourself?
9. Seeking fun?
10. Seeking to contribute to others or the surrounding world?
The items are rated from 1 (not at all) to 7 (very much)
Items 1–9 make up the HEMA; items 1–10 make up the HEMA-R

15.3.1 Different Adaptations of the HEMA

The HEMA can be used at different levels of measurement: the trait level, to inquire about a person's general or typical orientations to life (e.g., Huta, 2012; Huta, Pelletier, Baxter, & Thompson, 2012); the state level, to inquire about a person's orientations at a given moment or during a specific period of time (e.g., Henderson, Knight, & Richardson, 2013a, 2013b; Huta & Ryan, 2010); or the situational level, to inquire about a person's orientations toward a specific type of activity (e.g., favorite leisure activity – Anić, 2014; physical education classes – Behzadnia, 2015; leisure time physical activities – Mack et al., 2011; health-enhancing physical activity – Ferguson, Kowalski, Mack, Wilson, & Crocker, 2012). The trait level instructions are the ones shown above, but they can be adapted as needed.

The HEMA has been studied in several different languages: Japanese (Asano, Igarashi, & Tsukamoto, 2014), Croatian (Anić, 2014), Polish (Bujacz et al., 2014b; Bujacz, Vittersø, Huta, & Kaczmarek, 2014a), Persian (Behzadnia, 2015), and German, Italian, and Swedish (Bujacz, Dunne, et al., 2014b).

A youth version, the HEMAY, has recently been developed (A. Gentzler and V. Huta, October 15, 2015). The HEMAY items are adapted for children aged 7–12 years, and thus are more simple, concrete, and numerous. Nevertheless, the items are generic and comprehensive enough to be used in adolescents or even adults if age-related research is desired.

15.3.2 Psychometric Properties of the HEMA

Most studies have shown that the HEMA items (whether trait or state) form two factors (e.g., Anić, 2014; Huta, 2015a; Huta & Ryan, 2010). In nearly all studies, Cronbach alphas of the eudaimonic and hedonic scales have been above 0.80, and in no study have they dropped below 0.76.

In some studies, though, a two-factor solution did not reach adequate fit in Confirmatory Factor Analysis and a three-factor solution was required, whereby the eudaimonic items formed one factor, the hedonic pleasure items formed a second factor, and the hedonic comfort items formed a third factor (Asano et al., 2014; Behzadnia, 2015; Bujacz, Vittersø, et al., 2014a). Alphas for the hedonic pleasure scale have been above 0.80 (except in the Persian translation where alpha was 0.69, Behzadnia, 2015), whereas alphas for the hedonic comfort scale have averaged 0.73 (Asano et al., 2014; Behzadnia, 2015; reanalysis of Bujacz, Vittersø, et al., 2014a; Huta, 2015a). This suggests an additional item is warranted if the hedonic comfort scale is to be used on its own – I would suggest "Seeking to have things comfortable."

The 2-month test-retest reliability is 0.64 for HEMA eudaimonia and 0.62 for HEMA hedonia, when the instructions ask people to report their orientations during the previous week (reanalysis of 44 participants in the fourth study of Huta & Ryan, 2010).

In general, HEMA eudaimonia and hedonia have shown little relationship with gender, age, or ethnicity (Asano et al., 2014; Behzadnia, 2015; Huta, 2012; Huta & Ryan, 2010).

As shown in Table 15.2, the correlation between eudaimonic and hedonic orientations varies widely, anywhere from +0.7 to −0.3, depending on the time frame and life domain being studied. Note that, in all tables and appendices, the correlations are rounded to a single decimal, as they are intended to provide a general overview rather than precise findings. If more than one study has provided a correlation, the mean correlation across studies is shown.

As shown in Table 15.3, the eudaimonia and hedonia scales of the HEMA show good convergent and discriminant validity when correlated with other operationalizations of eudaimonic and hedonic ways of living.

Table 15.2 The correlation between HEMA eudaimonic and hedonic motives at different time spans and in different situations

	Eud. and hed. correlation	Studies
Different time spans		
When reporting on one's life in general, i.e., trait	0.3	Huta (2012); Huta et al. (2012); Huta and Ryan (2010)
When reporting on the past week	0.2	Myskiw (2014)
When reporting at bedtime on that day	0.0	Huta and Ryan (2010)
When reporting on the immediate moment	−0.3	Huta and Ryan (2010)
Different situations		
Favourite leisure activity:		Anić (2014)
Social, reading, music/media, outdoor	0.3	
Sports, dancing	0.4	
Arts	0.7	
Leisure time physical activities	0.7	Mack et al. (2011)
Health enhancing physical activities	0.7	Besenski (2009); Ferguson et al. (2012)
Physical education university classes	0.3	Behzadnia (2015)

Table 15.3 Correlations of HEMA eudaimonic and hedonic motives with other measures of eudaimonic and hedonic orientations and behaviors

	HEMA eudaimonia	HEMA hedonia	Studies
Eudaimonic orientation/behavior measure (authors in parentheses)			
OTHQ meaningful life (Peterson et al., 2005)	0.4	0.1	Henderson et al. (2013b); Huta (2015a); Huta and Ryan (2010); Pearce et al. (2015)
Peer-rated HEMA eudaimonia (Huta et al., 2012)	0.4	0.1	Huta et al. (2012)
Personal growth composite (Vittersø, Oelmann, & Wang, 2009)	0.4	0.1	Huta (2015a)
PEAQ self-realization values (Waterman, 1993)	0.4	0.1	Huta (2015a)
Intrinsic goal content (Sheldon & Kasser, 1995)	0.3	0.1	Huta (2015a)
GCOS autonomous orientation (Deci & Ryan, 1985)	0.3	0.2	Huta (2015a)
OTHQ engaged life (Peterson et al., 2005)	0.3	0.2	Henderson et al. (2013b); Huta and Ryan (2010)
Eudaimonic behavior checklist (Steger et al., 2008)	0.2	0.0	Huta (2015a)
Challenge x skill in activities (Csikszentmihalyi, 1975)	0.2	0.1	Huta (2015a)
Constitutive goals (Fowers, Molica, & Procacci, 2010)	0.2	0.2	Huta (2015a)
Hedonic orientation/behavior measure (authors in parentheses)			
OTHQ pleasurable life (Peterson et al., 2005)	0.1	0.4	Henderson et al. (2013b); Huta (2015a); Huta and Ryan (2010)
Peer-rated HEMA hedonia (Huta et al., 2012)	0.0	0.2	Huta et al. (2012)
Hedonic aspirations (Grouzet et al., 2005)	0.2	0.3	Huta (2015a)
Hedonic behavior checklist (Steger et al., 2008)	−0.1	0.1	Huta (2015a)

15.3.3 The Revised HEMA Scale: HEMA-R

I have recently added a fifth item to the HEMA eudaimonia scale: "Seeking to contribute to others or the surrounding world", as shown above in Table 15.1. I made this decision based on the review in Huta and Waterman (2014), which made it clear that most definitions of eudaimonia included the concept of meaning, i.e., caring about and contributing to the bigger picture. Though I have always seen meaning as closely related to eudaimonia, I initially hesitated to include it in my research definition because I worried about making the eudaimonia concept too broad, and because some critics suggested that a focus on personal authenticity, excellence, and growth sounded egoistic and would be negatively related, not positively related, to caring about others (see Annas, 2008; Waterman, 1981). I have come to believe that eudaimonia is and should be a broad umbrella term. I also now have evidence that eudaimonia is positively linked with caring beyond the self (Huta et al., 2012; Pearce, Huta, & Voloaca, 2015). And it is clearer to me than ever that meaning is intimately tied to authenticity, excellence, and growth. To pursue any of these three elements, a person has to care about what really matters in the broader sense.

In my lab, we have piloted the HEMA-R in one unpublished study thus far (N=342), and found that the revised eudaimonia scale coheres as a single distinct factor, has an alpha above 0.80, and correlates 0.95 with the original eudaimonia scale.

15.4 Correlates of HEMA Eudaimonic and Hedonic Orientations

15.4.1 Links with Personal Well-Being Experiences, Need Satisfaction, and Health Behaviors

When correlating the HEMA with measures of well-being experiences, need satisfaction, and health behaviors, the findings have been as follows (see Behzadnia, 2015; Besenski, 2009; Ferguson et al., 2012; Henderson et al., 2013a, 2013b; Huta, 2012, 2015a; Huta et al., 2012; Huta & Ryan, 2010; Mack et al., 2011; Myskiw, 2014; Ramirez, 2013). Eudaimonia has been the orientation more related to feelings of meaning, elevation, self-connectedness, interest/engagement/flow, accomplishment, and personal expressiveness; the satisfaction of psychological needs, especially the need for competence; and physical exercise. Hedonia has been the orientation more related to carefreeness, certain measures of positive affect (especially in the short term); getting more sleep; and consuming more alcohol. Hedonia has also had stronger negative links with most measures of negative affect and distress. Some measures of positive affect, however, have been more related to eudaimonia than to hedonia, suggesting that positive affect is a multifaceted concept that deserves finer differentiation in the future. The correlations and their references appear in Appendix A.

15.4.2 Links with Personal Well-Being Functioning

Measures intended to represent eudaimonic functioning have generally correlated more with HEMA eudaimonia than with HEMA hedonia (Besenski, 2009; Ferguson et al., 2012; Henderson et al., 2013a; Huta, 2013, 2015a). Those correlating more with eudaimonia have included the Questionnaire for Eudaimonic Well-Being (Waterman et al., 2010), the Purpose subscale of the Purpose in Life test (Crumbaugh & Maholick, 1964), the Framework subscale of the Life Regard Index (Battista & Almond, 1973), Presence of Meaning (Steger, Frazier, Oishi, & Kaler, 2006; Steger, Chap. 11, this volume), Flourishing (Diener et al., 2009), Psychological Well-Being (at least at the trait level; Ryff, 1989, Chap. 6, this volume), Social Well-Being (Keyes, 1998), Self-actualization (Jones & Crandall, 1986), and Mindfulness (Brown & Ryan, 2003). The correlations and their references appear in Appendix B.

Past research has not included operationalizations or theoretical models of healthy hedonic functioning. The focus has been only on eudaimonic functioning. To fill this gap, I recently proposed a set of variables to represent hedonic functioning (Huta, 2015c), as summarized in the last section of this chapter. I have developed a set of hedonic functioning measures and data collection is ongoing.

15.4.3 Links with Thinking and Contributing Beyond the Self, the Present Moment, and the Concrete

My students and I have also been studying the relationships of eudaimonic and hedonic orientations with contributing to the well-being of other people and the world, thinking beyond the present moment, and abstract thinking (i.e., seeing beyond the concrete features of activities to their broader implications). I refer to this set of outcomes as indices of a "broad scope of concern." We have found that HEMA eudaimonia was more linked with these indices than was HEMA hedonia, including: positively impacting the well-being of close friends and relatives (Huta et al., 2012); positively impacting one's children such that they derived greater well-being from their own eudaimonic pursuits (Huta, 2012); and altruistic behavior and values, generative behavior, pro-environmental behavior and values, abstract thinking, and thinking about the future (Pearce et al., 2015).

We have also collected some data on indices of a narrow scope of concern. The results have been mixed – HEMA hedonia related more to focusing on the present moment and valuing power and material possessions, but HEMA eudaimonia related more to valuing personal ambition and influence (Huta, 2013; Pearce et al., 2015). These initial findings suggest that eudaimonia is not exclusively about self-sacrifice and broad concerns, but rather involves a balance of self-focused and broad concerns.

15.4.4 Links with the Behavior of One's Parents

Two studies thus far have examined predictors of eudaimonic and hedonic orientations, focusing on adult participants' retrospective recollections of their parents' behavior while they were growing up (Huta, 2012). In Study 1, the results showed that parents who were both demanding and responsive had children who pursued eudaimonia as adults, whereas parenting styles were unrelated to adult children's hedonia. This suggests that the development of eudaimonia may require greater parental investment than the development of hedonia. In Study 2, adult children pursued eudaimonia whether their parents only verbally endorsed eudaimonia or actually role modeled eudaimonia; the same was true for hedonia. However, adult children only derived high levels of well-being from their eudaimonic pursuits if their parents had actually role modeled eudaimonia; again, the same was true for hedonia.

15.4.5 The Combination of Eudaimonia and Hedonia

In my work, I have hypothesized that eudaimonic and hedonic pursuits are both beneficial for personal well-being. The data support this hypothesis, in several ways. As shown in Appendix A, eudaimonic and hedonic orientations have been linked with somewhat different well-being experiences and benefits. This suggests that the combination of eudaimonia and hedonia is linked with more complete well-being than either orientation alone. This more complete well-being includes variables that fall under "eudaimonic experiences" in the factor analyses below, as well as variables that fall under "hedonic experiences."

Not only has the combination of eudaimonic and hedonic orientations been linked with more complete well-being, it has also been linked with a higher degree of well-being than either orientation alone (Behzadnia, 2015; Huta & Ryan, 2010; Peterson, Park, & Seligman, 2005).

Furthermore, findings have tentatively suggested that eudaimonic and hedonic ways of living fill different well-being niches over time, such that hedonia is more linked with well-being in the short-term, while eudaimonia is more linked with well-being in the long-term. In a 10-day intervention study where participants were randomized to increase either their eudaimonic activity or their hedonic activity, participants in the hedonic condition reported greater boosts in well-being immediately after the 10-day intervention, while participants in the eudaimonic condition reported greater boosts 3 months after the intervention (Huta & Ryan, 2010). In two daily diary studies linking eudaimonic and hedonic behavior checklists to well-being experiences, eudaimonic behaviors on a given day were more consistently linked to well-being on the following day than were hedonic behaviors (Steger, Kashdan, & Oishi, 2008). And as shown in Appendix A, the largest advantage of hedonic pursuits has been found at the state level (i.e., in the short-term), especially in the case of positive affect, carefreeness, vitality, and low negative affect. At the trait level (which to some degree reflects the longer term), these advantages of hedonia were noticeably diminished or even disappeared.

15.5 Whether Eudaimonia Is Truly Distinct from Hedonia

Some researchers have raised doubts about whether the distinction between eudaimonia and hedonia is real (Biswas-Diener, Kashdan, & King, 2009; Kashdan, Biswas-Diener, & King, 2008; Ward & King, Chap. 35, this volume; Sheldon, Chap. 36, this volume). I see a distinction on both conceptual and empirical grounds, especially when it comes to orientations. Conceptually, as detailed in Huta (2015b), eudaimonia and hedonia are based on two distinct and complementary sets of psychological processes: cognitive values vs. emotional/physical pleasure, broad focus vs. self-focus, long-term perspective vs. short-term perspective, investing vs. stocking up.

Empirically, there are at least ten published studies showing that items on measures of orientations load onto separate factors that can clearly be labeled as eudaimonic and hedonic (see the references cited earlier, as well as Peterson et al., 2005, Ruch, Harzer, Proyer, Park, & Peterson, 2010; Harzer, Chap. 20, this volume). There is also a small amount of published evidence on well-being experiences, showing that feelings of interest/engagement load on a separate factor from feelings of happiness/joy/satisfaction (Vittersø, Dyrdal, & Røysamb, 2005; Vittersø, Chap. 17, this volume).

To shed further light on the degree of distinctness between eudaimonia and hedonia, I am conducting a large ongoing study with many of the self-report scales that have been used in this literature (Huta, 2015a). As reported in more detail in Huta (2015c, 2015d), I have performed preliminary factor analyses with the first 677 participants, on trait level measures in the two definition categories where multiple measures exist – orientations and experiences. One factor analysis focused on the 12 measures of trait eudaimonic and hedonic orientations in Table 15.3, including HEMA eudaimonia and hedonia. Three factors had eigenvalues above 1. When extracting a three-factor solution (which explained 50 % of the variance) and Direct Oblimin (or Varimax) rotating it, the three hedonia measures formed a distinct factor, and the nine eudaimonia measures loaded on the other two factors. When forcing a two-factor solution (which explained 40 % of the variance) and Direct Oblimin (or Varimax) rotating it, the eudaimonia measures cleanly separated from the hedonia measures, with no cross-loadings above 0.31. In the obliquely rotated solution, the eudaimonic factor and the hedonic factor correlated only 0.35. (At the state level, there has also been a clear distinction between eudaimonic and hedonic orientations, though the correlation has been in the opposite direction – Huta and Ryan, 2010, found that HEMA eudaimonic and hedonic orientations correlated -.28 at a given moment.) I also factor analyzed trait measures of the 27 well-being experience measures in Appendix A with Huta (2015a) as a reference. Theoretically, the experiences might be expected to fall into four groups: eudaimonic experiences (all measures of meaning experience, elevation, accomplishment, self-connectedness, interest, engagement, and flow); positive hedonic experiences (all measures of positive affect, carefreeness, and emotional well-being); negative hedonic experiences (all measures of negative affect); and need satisfaction experiences (all measures of satisfaction of relatedness, competence, and autonomy). In my preliminary analysis, four factors had eigenvalues above 1, and the four-factor solution explained 64 % of the variance. Following Varimax rotation of the four factors, all the eudaimonic experiences formed one factor and all the hedonic experiences formed another factor, but a third factor represented a combination of high need satisfaction and low negative affect, and a fourth factor represented only Waterman's PEAQ Personal Expressiveness and PEAQ Hedonic Enjoyment scales (possibly because the PEAQ methodology differs from the methodology of the other experience measures). Measures which cross-loaded included PERMA relationships (loading with need satisfaction/low negative hedonic and with eudaimonic experiences); vitality (loading with eudaimonic and positive hedonic experiences; and life satisfaction (loading with eudaimonic, positive hedonic, and need satisfaction/low negative hedonic experiences). The Direct Oblimin solution was similar, except that vitality only loaded with positive hedonic experiences. In the obliquely rotated solution, the eudaimonic factor and the positive hedonic factor correlated quite strongly, at 0.54, suggesting that the difference between trait levels of the experiences was subtle. In addition, as reported in Huta (2015c), I have factor analyzed seven trait-level studies and three state-level studies which included all or most of the following well-being experiences: positive affect, negative affect, life satisfaction, carefreeness, vitality, meaning experience, elevation, and self-connectedness. In nine of the ten studies, there were two eigenvalues above 1 (in one study there was one eigenvalue above 1). In Varimax-rotated two-factor solutions, one factor consisted of meaning experience, elevation, and self-connectedness; the second factor consisted of carefreeness, positive affect (at the state level), and low negative affect; vitality and life satisfaction loaded similarly on both factors; and positive affect loaded similarly on both factors at the trait level. Recent reanalyses with oblique rotation have shown the same loading patterns; the two factors had a mean correlation of .38 at the trait level, and a correlation of .30 at the momentary state level.

Note that the experiences which loaded on "hedonic experiences" were usually, but not always, the same as the experiences which correlated primarily with a hedonic orientation. The exceptions were several positive affect and negative affect measures that correlated somewhat more with eudaimonia at the trait level (see Appendix A). The labels "hedonic experiences" and "eudaimonic experiences" are based on the factor analyses, not the correlations with orientations.

15.5.1 The Place of Life Satisfaction

I will add a note here about life satisfaction. There is little agreement on its place in the eudaimonic-hedonic distinction. Some scholars have discussed it as a hedonic concept (e.g., Ryan & Deci, 2001; Ryan & Martela, Chap. 7, this volume), some have viewed it as a final common outcome of both hedonic and eudaimonic fulfillment (e.g., Waterman, 2007), and a few have argued that it is a eudaimonic concept (Sumner, 1996). I believe that the place of life satisfaction depends very much on the wording of the instrument used to measure it. If the wording implies getting what one wants and needs, then the measure leans towards hedonic concepts; if the wording implies achieving a valued goal or achieving congruence between one's behavior and one's values, then the measure leans towards eudaimonic concepts; and if the wording is very general and does nor refer to either getting or achieving, then the measure can reflect both eudaimonia and hedonia. The measure of life satisfaction by Diener and colleagues (1985) that I have used in my research includes a blend of hedonic, eudaimonic, and general wording. This likely explains why it has correlated similarly with eudaimonic and hedonic orientations, and why it has cross-loaded with both eudaimonic and hedonic experiences in factor analysis.

15.6 Fleshing Out Eudaimonia and Hedonia in All Four Definition Categories

As discussed earlier, I consider eudaimonia and hedonia to be primarily orientations, and above I have outlined the core elements in my definition of a eudaimonic orientation (authenticity, meaning, excellence, and growth) and a hedonic orientation (pleasure and comfort). I also stated, though, that all four definition categories are needed for a full understanding of these functions. I would like to return to that statement now.

I believe that, as a field, we need to flesh out all four definition categories to clarify the correlates and consequences that can be expected of eudaimonic and hedonic orientations. In addition, our understanding of behaviors, experiences, and functioning provides a deeper understanding of orientations. The concepts of authenticity, meaning, excellence, and growth are anchor points, but they need to be embedded in a richer description if they are to be properly interpreted. The richer description also provides additional details that map the conceptual territory more fully.

In Huta (2015c), I fleshed out the sets of variables reflecting eudaimonia and hedonia in each definition category. This included healthy hedonic functioning, which has not been previously outlined – I proposed a set of abilities, achievements, and healthy habits that a hedonically oriented person could excel at. Table 15.4 summarizes the list in each definition category (the list of behaviors is from Steger et al., 2008).

15.7 What Is the Highest Good?

15.7.1 Why Is Eudaimonia Good?

Many reasons for the goodness of eudaimonia could be given. Among the more important reasons, eudaimonia builds a sense of meaning and value, it connects discrete events into a framework where the events acquire additional roles and thus additional value and vibrancy; the meaning framework promotes increasing organization and complexity, the hallmarks of evolution; eudaimonia elevates the person to a higher level of functioning, so they see farther; eudaimonia produces learning, accomplishment, progress, and skill, so that the individual comes to encompass a bigger slice of life; it leads to refinement and appreciation of things from multiple perspectives, increasing a person's ability to navigate both small nuances and large challenges; and eudaimonia is what builds community and civilization. If an individual were to focus exclusively on hedonia, they would miss opportunities to build something, and to discover just how far they can grow.

15.7.2 Why Is Hedonia Good?

Hedonia is also good for many reasons. Among other things, hedonia meets what I believe to be genuine visceral and emotional needs, like getting rest and achieving a positive mental state; hedonia serves to charge up the psychological battery, filling the person with pleasurable experiences and memories; hedonia lets the person take a break from ongoing concerns, and be able to return with a fresh perspective; it lets us acknowledge and express our primal side; and it is necessary for self-care. If an individual were to focus exclusively on eudaimonia, always investing, it would lead to exhaustion. It would also lead to a loss of perspective, a loss of intimate personal contact with the feeling that things matter. Humans need the hedonic influx of energy, and the connection to life on a more immediate emotional level.

Table 15.4 Concepts associated with eudaimonia and hedonia in each definition category

	Eudaimonia	Hedonia
As orientations (priorities, motives, values, goals)	Pursuits of authenticity, self-discovery, autonomy, identity	Pursuits of pleasure, enjoyment, fun
	Pursuits of meaning, mattering, contributing to big picture	Pursuits of comfort, ease, painlessness
	Pursuits of excellence, quality performance, virtue	
	Pursuits of growth, self-realization, maturity, learning	
As behaviors (specific behaviors engaged in)	Many possible behaviors, such as:	Many possible behaviors, such as:
	Planning personal goals	Going to a big party
	Volunteering	Having sex with a person one does not love
	Expressing gratitude	Drinking alcohol
	Listening to another person's point of view	Shopping for non-essentials
	Persevering at a specific valued goal despite obstacles	Watching a movie that is pure entertainment
As experiences (subjective emotions, feelings, cognitive-affective appraisals)	Feelings of meaning, value, purpose, broad implications	Positive affect, emotional well-being, affect balance
	Elevation, inspiration, awe, transcendence	High, moderate, and low arousal positive affect
	Feelings of self-connectedness, authenticity	Satisfaction, wants/needs are met, replenishment
	Feelings of accomplishment, progress, non-hubristic pride	Carefreeness, lightheartedness
	Engagement, immersion, interest, flow	Comfort, low negative affect, low strain, relief
	Personal expressiveness, deep fit with one's activities	
	Life satisfaction	
	Happiness	
	Vitality, feeling alive	
As functioning (abilities, accomplishments, healthy habits)	Self-realization, individuation, coming into one's own	Abilities to savor, play, prioritize enjoyment
	Maturity, wisdom, ego development, sophistication	Abilities to let go, take breaks, not worry needlessly
	Competence, excellence, insight, understanding, skill	Abilities to be here and now, be spontaneous, go with flow
	Accomplishment, achievement, progress	Healthy selfishness, ability to put self first if warranted
	Achievements of meaning, purpose, big picture framework	Habit of minimizing unnecessary effort and difficulty
	Integration, autonomy, non-conformism	Skills at things that are hands-on, practical, applied
	Ethics, morality, virtue, honesty, integrity, justice	Sensuality, physicality, sexuality, ability to be primal
	Social contribution, generativity, altruism, responsibility	
	Self-regulation, perseverance, planning, organizing	
	Abstract thinking, perspective-taking, long-term view	
	Quality relationships, social well-being	
	Resilience, active coping	

15.7.3 Which Is the Highest Good?

I believe that both eudaimonia and hedonia are important for personal well-being, and on a philosophical level, I believe we are "meant" to pursue both. But could I chose one over the other? Which is the highest good?

It depends on the exact wording. As I have argued in Huta (2013, 2015b), one orientation is not "better" than the other. Each takes priority in a certain way: eudaimonia is "higher," while hedonia is more "fundamental."

Hedonia is more necessary and pre-wired, though there is plenty of room for choice as well. Eudaimonia is less of a need and more of a bonus, but still somewhat pre-wired. Hedonia is more "pushed" by our constitution, while eudaimonia is more "pulled" by what Seligman calls *prospection* (Seligman, Railton, Baumeister, & Sripada, 2013). Eudaimonia is pulled by values, goals, ideals, inspiration, and visions of a better future, and thus makes full use of the "higher" cognitive and existential capacities that are so evolved in humans (though growth can also be forced upon us when we encounter life-shattering events). The pull is subtler than the push, more easily overlooked, unless it has become a habit; and it rests more on a mental structure of values and discipline that we first have to build. In its ultimate form, eudaimonia becomes an end in itself. The value of eudaimonia is intrinsic to the pursuit itself, and the only remaining rationales are really aesthetic ones, like beauty and rightness. It's simply beautiful to try to do the right thing, try to grow. As subtle as the pull may be, eudaimonia IS the *highest* path to personal fulfillment. It's about more than getting by, it's about getting somewhere.

Appendix A: Correlations of HEMA Eudaimonic and Hedonic Motives with Well-Being Experiences, Need Satisfaction, and Health Behaviors: Trait, Situational, State

	HEMA eudaimonia	HEMA hedonia	Studies
Well-being experience measure (authors in parentheses)			
Meaning experience (Huta & Ryan, 2010)	**0.4**	**0.2**	Huta (2012), Huta et al. (2012, and 4x Huta and Ryan (2010)
Meaning experience (Huta & Ryan, 2010)	0.4	–0.1	(Behzadnia, 2015)
Meaning experience (Huta & Ryan, 2010)	*0.5*	*0.1*	2x Huta and Ryan (2010) and Myskiw (2014)
PERMA meaning (Kern & Butler, J. (June, 2013)	**0.4**	**0.1**	Huta (2015a)
Elevating experience (Huta & Ryan, 2010)	**0.4**	**0.1**	Henderson et al. (2013a), Huta (2012), Huta et al. (2012), and 4x Huta and Ryan (2010)
Elevating experience (Huta & Ryan, 2010)	0.2	0.2	Behzadnia (2015)
Elevating experience (Huta & Ryan, 2010)	*0.4*	*0.2*	2x Huta and Ryan (2010) and Myskiw (2014)
Self-connectedness (Huta, 2012)	**0.4**	**0.1**	Huta (2012), Huta et al. (2012), and 4x Huta and Ryan (2010)
Self-connectedness (Huta, 2012)	*0.4*	*0.2*	2x Huta and Ryan (2010) and Myskiw (2014)
Interest (Vittersø et al., 2005)	**0.4**	**0.1**	Huta (2015a)
PERMA engagement (Kern & Butler, J. (June, 2013)	**0.4**	**0.1**	Huta (2015a)
Flow experience (Delle Fave & Massimini, 1988)	**0.3**	**0.0**	Huta (2015a)
PERMA accomplishment (Kern & Butler, J. (June, 2013)	**0.4**	**0.1**	Huta (2015a)
PEAQ personal expressiveness (Waterman, 1993)	**0.3**	**0.2**	Huta (2015a)
Carefreeness (Huta & Ryan, 2010)	**0.1**	**0.3**	Henderson et al. (2013a) and 4x Huta and Ryan (2010)
Carefreeness (Huta & Ryan, 2010)	0.0	0.3	Behzadnia (2015)
Carefreeness (Huta & Ryan, 2010)	*0.1*	*0.5*	2x Huta and Ryan (2010) and Myskiw (2014)
Positive affect (Diener & Emmons, 1984)	**0.3**	**0.4**	Huta (2012), Huta et al. (2012), and 4x Huta and Ryan (2010)
Positive affect (Diener & Emmons, 1984)	0.2	–0.1	Behzadnia (2015)
Positive affect (Diener & Emmons, 1984)	*0.2*	*0.6*	2x Huta and Ryan (2010) and Myskiw (2014)
PANAS positive affect (Watson, Clark, & Tellegen, 1988)	**0.3**	**0.4**	Henderson et al. (2013a)
PANAS positive affect (Watson et al., 1988)	0.5	0.5	Besenski (2009)
Bradburn positive affect (Bradburn, 1969)	**0.3**	**0.2**	Huta (2015a)
PERMA positive emotions (Kern & Butler, J. (June, 2013)	**0.3**	**0.2**	Huta (2015a)
SPANE positive experience (Diener et al., 2009)	**0.3**	**0.2**	Huta (2015a)

PEAQ hedonic enjoyment (Waterman, 1993)	**0.3**	**0.2**	Huta (2015a)
Pleasure (Vittersø et al., 2005)	**0.4**	**0.2**	Huta (2015a)
Emotional well-being (Keyes, 2002)	**0.2**	**0.1**	Huta (2015a)
Negative affect (Diener & Emmons, 1984)	**−0.1**	**−0.1**	Huta (2012), Huta et al. (2012), and 4x Huta and Ryan (2010)
Negative affect (Diener & Emmons, 1984)	−0.3	0.3	Behzadnia (2015)
Negative affect (Diener & Emmons, 1984)	*0.0*	*−0.4*	2x Huta and Ryan (2010) and Myskiw (2014)
PANAS negative affect (Watson et al., 1988)	**0.0**	**−0.2**	Henderson et al. (2013a)
PANAS negative affect (Watson et al., 1988)	−0.1	−0.2	Besenski (2009)
DASS21 depression (Lovibond & Lovibond, 1995)	**−0.1**	**−0.3**	Henderson et al. (2013a)
DASS21 stress (Lovibond & Lovibond, 1995)	**−0.2**	**−0.3**	Henderson et al. (2013a)
DASS21 anxiety (Lovibond & Lovibond, 1995)	**−0.1**	**−0.2**	Henderson et al. (2013a)
SPANE negative experience (Diener et al., 2009)	**−0.1**	**0.0**	Huta (2015a)
Bradburn negative affect (Bradburn, 1969)	**−0.2**	**0.0**	Huta (2015a)
Life satisfaction (Diener, Emmons, Larsen, & Griffin, 1985)	**0.2**	**0.2**	Henderson et al. (2013a, 2013b), Huta (2012), Huta et al.. (2012), and 4x Huta and Ryan (2010)
Life satisfaction (Diener et al., 1985)	0.3	0.2	Behzadnia (2015) and Besenski (2009)
Vitality (Ryan & Frederick, 1997)	**0.3**	**0.2**	Henderson et al. (2013a), Huta (2012), Huta et al. (2012), and 4x Huta and Ryan (2010)
Vitality (Ryan & Frederick, 1997)	0.3	−0.1	Behzadnia (2015)
Vitality (Ryan & Frederick, 1997)	*0.2*	*0.4*	2x Huta and Ryan (2010) and Myskiw (2014)
Self-esteem (Robins, Hendin, & Trzesniewski, 2001)	**0.2**	**0.2**	Huta (2012), Huta et al. (2012), and 4x Huta and Ryan (2010)
Self-esteem (Robins et al., 2001)	0.2	0.0	Behzadnia (2015)
Self-esteem (Robins et al., 2001)	*0.3*	*0.3*	Huta and Ryan (2010) and Myskiw (2014)
Need satisfaction measure (authors in parentheses)			
Competence satisfaction (Gagné, 2003)	**0.3**	**0.1**	Huta (2015a)
Competence satisfaction (Gagné, 2003)	0.5	0.4	Besenski (2009) and Mack et al. (2011)
Workplace competence satisfaction (Gagné, 2003)	**0.3**	**0.1**	(2x Ramirez, 2013)
Relatedness satisfaction (Gagné, 2003)	**0.3**	**0.2**	Huta (2015a)
Relatedness satisfaction (Gagné, 2003)	0.5	0.4	Besenski (2009) and Mack et al. (2011)
Workplace relatedness satisfaction (Gagné, 2003)	**0.2**	**0.2**	(2x Ramirez, 2013)

(continued)

	HEMA eudaimonia	HEMA hedonia	Studies
PERMA relationships (Kern & Butler, J. (June, 2013)	**0.3**	**0.1**	Huta (2015a)
Autonomy satisfaction (Gagné, 2003)	**0.2**	**0.1**	Huta (2015a)
Autonomy satisfaction (Gagné, 2003)	0.4	0.4	Besenski (2009) and Mack et al. (2011)
Workplace autonomy satisfaction (Gagné, 2003)	**0.3**	**0.2**	(2x Ramirez, 2013)
Health behavior measure (authors in parentheses)			
Physical activity (Godin & Shepard, 1985)	0.4	0.3	Mack et al. (2011)
Physical activity (Wendel-Vos, Schuit, Saris, & Kromhout, 2003)	0.2	0.1	Besenski (2009) and Ferguson et al. (2012)
Hours of exercise per week (ad hoc)	**0.2**	**0.0**	Myskiw (2014)
Hours of exercise per week (ad hoc)	*−0.1*	*0.1*	Myskiw (2014)
Hours slept per night (ad hoc)	**0.0**	**0.2**	Myskiw (2014)
Hours slept per night (ad hoc)	*0.0*	*0.4*	Myskiw (2014)
Number of alcoholic drinks per week (ad hoc)	**−0.1**	**0.1**	Myskiw (2014)
Number of alcoholic drinks per week (ad hoc)	*−0.1*	*0.2*	Myskiw (2014)

Note. Studies in parentheses are master’s or doctoral theses, forthcoming publications, or unpublished data

Appendix B: Mean Correlations of HEMA Eudaimonic and Hedonic Motives with Indices of Eudaimonic Well-Being Functioning: Trait, Situational

Eudaimonic functioning measure (authors in parentheses)	HEMA eudaimonia	HEMA hedonia	Studies
Questionnaire for eudaimonic well-being (Waterman et al., 2010)	**0.5**	**0.0**	Huta (2015a)
Purpose in life – purpose scale (Crumbaugh & Maholick, 1964)	**0.4**	**0.0**	Huta (2015a)
Life regard index – framework scale (Battista & Almond, 1973)	**0.4**	**0.1**	(2x Huta, 2013)
MLQ presence of meaning (Steger et al., 2006)	**0.4**	**0.2**	Henderson et al. (2013a) and Huta (2015a)
Flourishing (Diener et al., 2009)	**0.4**	**0.3**	Henderson et al. (2013a) and Huta (2015a)
PWB psychological well-being composite (Ryff, 1989)	**0.4**	**0.0**	Huta (2015a)
PWB psychological well-being composite (Ryff, 1989)	0.3	0.3	Besenski (2009) and Ferguson et al. (2012)
SWB social well-being composite (Keyes, 1998)	**0.3**	**0.1**	Huta (2015a)
Self-actualization (Jones & Crandall, 1986)	**0.2**	**0.1**	Huta (2015a)
Mindfulness (Brown & Ryan, 2003)	**0.1**	**0.0**	Huta (2015a)

Note. Studies in parentheses are master's or doctoral theses, forthcoming publications, or unpublished data

References

Anić, P. (2014). Hedonic and eudaimonic motives for favourite leisure activities. *Primenjena Psihologija, 7*, 5–21.

Annas, J. (2008). Virtue ethics and the charge of egoism. In P. Bloomfield (Ed.), *Morality and self-interest* (pp. 205–221). Oxford: Oxford University Press.

Asano, R., Igarashi, T., & Tsukamoto, S. (2014). Hedonic and eudaimonic motives for activities (HEMA) in Japan: The pursuit of well-being. *Japanese Journal of Psychology, 85*, 69–79.

Battista, J., & Almond, R. (1973). The development of meaning in life. *Psychiatry, 36*, 409–427.

Behzadnia, B. (2015). *The role of eudaimonic and hedonic motivation in physical education: Findings from Iran.* Manuscript in preparation.

Besenski, L. J. (2009). *Health-enhancing physical activity and eudaimonic well-being.* Unpublished master's thesis, University of Saskatchewan, Saskatoon, Saskatchewan.

Biswas-Diener, R., Kashdan, T., & King, L. (2009). Two traditions of happiness research, not two distinct types of happiness. *The Journal of Positive Psychology, 4*, 208–211.

Bradburn, N. M. (1969). *The structure of psychological well-being*. Chicago: Aldine.

Brown, K. W., & Ryan, R. M. (2003). The benefits of being present: Mindfulness and its role in psychological well-being. *Journal of Personality and Social Psychology, 84*, 822–848.

Bujacz, A., Vittersø, J., Huta, V., & Kaczmarek, L. D. (2014a). Measuring eudaimonia and hedonia as motives for activities: Cross-national investigation through traditional and Bayesian Structural Equation Modeling. *Frontiers in Psychology, Special Issue: Frontiers in Quantitative Psychology and Measurement, 5*, 984.

Bujacz, A., Dunne, S., Fink, D., Gatej, A. R., Karlsson, E., Ruberti, V., et al. (2014b). Does creativity make you happy? The influence of creative activity on hedonic and eudaimonic well-being. *Journal of European Psychology Students, 5*, 19–23. DOI: http://dx.doi.org/10.5334/jeps.by.

Crumbaugh, J. C., & Maholick, L. T. (1964). An experimental study in existentialism: The psychometric approach to Frankl's concept of noogenic neurosis. *Journal of Clinical Psychology, 20*, 200–207.

Csikszentmihalyi, M. (1975). *Beyond boredom and anxiety.* San Francisco: Jossey-Bass.

Deci, E. L., & Ryan, R. M. (1985). The general causality orientations scale: Self-determination in personality. *Journal of Research in Personality, 19*, 109–134.

Delle Fave, A., & Massimini, F. (1988). Modernization and the changing context of flow in work and leisure.

In M. Csikszentmihalyi & I. Csikszentmihalyi (Eds.), *Optimal experience: Psychological studies of flow in consciousness* (pp. 193–213). New York: Cambridge University Press.

Diener, E., & Emmons, R. A. (1984). The independence of positive and negative affect. *Journal of Personality and Social Psychology, 47*, 1105–1117. doi:10.1037/0022-3514.47.5.1105.

Diener, E., Emmons, R. A., Larsen, R. J., & Griffin, S. (1985). The satisfaction with life scale. *Journal of Personality Assessment, 49*, 71–75. doi:10.1207/s15327752jpa4901_13.

Diener, E., Wirtz, D., Tov, W., Kim-Prieto, C., Choi, D., Oishi, S., et al. (2009). New well-being measures: Short scales to assess flourishing and positive and negative feelings. *Social Indicators Research, 39*, 247–266. doi:10.1007/s11205-009-9493-y.

Ferguson, L. J., Kowalski, K. C., Mack, D. E., Wilson, P. M., & Crocker, P. R. E. (2012). Women's health-enhancing physical activity and eudaimonic well-being. *Research Quarterly for Exercise and Sport, 83*, 451–463.

Fowers, B. J., Molica, C. O., & Procacci, E. N. (2010). Constitutive and instrumental goal orientations and their relations with eudaimonic and hedonic well-being. *Journal of Positive Psychology, 5*, 139–153.

Gagné, M. (2003). The role of autonomy support and autonomy orientation in prosocial behavior engagement. *Motivation and Emotion, 27*, 199–223.

Godin, G., & Shepard, R. J. (1985). A simple method to assess exercise behavior in the community. *Canadian Journal of Applied Sport Sciences, 10*, 141–146.

Grouzet, F. M. E., Kasser, T., Ahuvia, A., Dols, J. M. F., Kim, Y., Lau, S., et al. (2005). The structure of goal contents across 15 cultures. *Journal of Personality and Social Psychology, 5*, 800–816.

Henderson, L. W., Knight, T., & Richardson, B. (2013a). An exploration of the well-being benefits of hedonic and eudaimonic behavior. *The Journal of Positive Psychology, 8*, 322–336. doi:10.1080/17439760.2013.803596.

Henderson, L. W., Knight, T., & Richardson, B. (2013b). The hedonic and eudaimonic validity of the orientations to happiness scale. *Social Indicators Research, 115*, 1087–1099.

Huta, V. (2012). Linking peoples' pursuit of eudaimonia and hedonia with characteristics of their parents: Parenting styles, verbally endorsed values, and role modeling. *Journal of Happiness Studies, 13*, 47–61.

Huta, V. (2013). Pursuing eudaimonia versus hedonia: Distinctions, similarities, and relationships. In A. S. Waterman (Ed.), *The best within us: Positive psychology perspectives on eudaimonia* (pp. 139–158). Washington, DC: APA Books.

Huta, V. (2015a). *The inter-relationships of different measures of eudaimonia and hedonia*. Data collection is ongoing; analyses are based on the first 677 participants after data cleaning.

Huta, V. (2015b). Chapter 10: The complementary roles of eudaimonia and hedonia and how they can be pursued in practice. In S. Joseph (Ed.), *Positive psychology in practice: Promoting human flourishing in work, health, education, and everyday life* (2nd ed.). Hoboken, NJ: Wiley.

Huta, V. (2015c). Chapter 2: An overview of hedonic and eudaimonic well-being concepts. In L. Reinecke & M. B. Oliver (Eds.), *Handbook of media use and well-being*. New York: Routledge. Manuscript accepted for publication.

Huta, V. (2015d, June). Introduction to symposium. In V. Huta (Chair), *Advances in research on eudaimonia*. Symposium conducted at Fourth World Congress on Positive Psychology, Orlando, FL.

Huta, V., Pelletier, L., Baxter, D., & Thompson, A. (2012). How eudaimonic and hedonic motives relate to the well-being of close others. *Journal of Positive Psychology, 7*, 399–404.

Huta, V., & Ryan, R. M. (2010). Pursuing pleasure or virtue: The differential and overlapping well-being benefits of hedonic and eudaimonic motives. *Journal of Happiness Studies, 11*, 735–762.

Huta, V., & Waterman, A. S. (2014). Eudaimonia and its distinction from hedonia: Developing a classification and terminology for understanding conceptual and operational definitions. *Journal of Happiness Studies, 15*, 1425–1456.

Jones, A., & Crandall, R. (1986). Validation of a short index of self-actualization. *Personality and Social Psychology Bulletin, 12*, 63–73.

Kashdan, T., Biswas-Diener, R., & King, L. (2008). Reconsidering happiness: The costs of distinguishing between hedonics and eudaimonia. *The Journal of Positive Psychology, 3*, 219–233.

Kern, M. L., & Butler, J. (June, 2013). *The PERMA-Profiler: A brief multidimensional measure of flourishing*. Poster presented at the Third World Congress on Positive Psychology, Los Angeles.

Keyes, C. L. M. (1998). Social well-being. *Social Psychology Quarterly, 61*, 121–140.

Keyes, C. L. M. (2002). The mental health continuum: From languishing to flourishing in life. *Journal of Health and Social Behavior, 43*, 207–222. doi:10.2307/3090197.

Lovibond, P. F., & Lovibond, S. H. (1995). The structure of negative emotional states: Comparison of the depression anxiety stress scale (DASS) with the beck depression and anxiety inventories. *Behavior Research and Therapy, 33*, 335-343. doi:10.1016/00005-7967(94)000075-u.

Mack, D. E., Gunnell, K. E., Wilson, P. M., Gilchrist, J. D., Kowalski, K. C., Crocker, P. R. E., et al. (2011). Physical activity in individuals living with osteopenia: Association with psychological need satisfaction and motives for well-being. *International Journal of Physical Education and Sports Science, 06*, 26–41.

Myskiw, K. (2014, July). Eudaimonic and hedonic motives in relation to health behaviors. In V. Huta

(Chair), *Research findings to date on hedonic and eudaimonic motivation*. Symposium conducted at the Second Canadian Conference on Positive Psychology, Ottawa, Ontario.

Pearce, K., Huta, V., Voloaca, M. (2015). *How eudaimonia and hedonia relate to thinking and contributing broadly: Seeing beyond the self, the present, and the concrete*. Manuscript in preparation.

Peterson, C., Park, N., & Seligman, M. E. P. (2005). Orientations to happiness and life satisfaction: The full life versus the empty life. *Journal of Happiness Studies, 6*, 25–41.

Ramirez, S. A. (2013). *An investigation of perceived organizational support from a self-determination theory perspective*. Unpublished master's thesis, North Carolina State University, Raleigh, NC.

Robins, R. W., Hendin, H. M., & Trzesniewski, K. H. (2001). Measuring global self-esteem: Construct validation of a single-item measure and the Rosenberg Self-Esteem Scale. *Personality and Social Psychology Bulletin, 27*, 151–161.

Ruch, W., Harzer, C., Proyer, R. T., Park, N., & Peterson, C. (2010). Ways to happiness in German-speaking countries: The adaptation of the German version of the orientations to happiness questionnaire in paper-pencil and internet samples. *European Journal of Psychological Assessment, 26*, 227–234.

Ryan, R. M., & Deci, E. L. (2001). On happiness and human potentials: A review of research on hedonic and eudaimonic well-being. *Annual Review of Psychology, 52*, 141–166. doi:10.1146/annurev.psych.52.1.141.

Ryan, R. M., & Frederick, C. (1997). On energy, personality, and health: Subjective vitality as a dynamic reflection of well - being. *Journal of Personality, 65*, 529–565. doi:10.1111/j.1467-6494.1997.tb00326.x.

Ryff, C. D. (1989). Happiness is everything, or is it? Explorations on the meaning of psychological well-being. *Journal of Personality and Social Psychology, 57*, 1069–1081.

Seligman, M. E. P., Railton, P., Baumeister, R. F., & Sripada, C. (2013). Navigating into the future or driven by the past. *Perspectives on Psychological Science, 8*, 119–141.

Sheldon, K. M., & Kasser, T. (1995). Coherence and congruence: Two aspects of personality integration. *Journal of Personality and Social Psychology, 3*, 531–543.

Steger, M. F., Frazier, P., Oishi, S., & Kaler, M. (2006). The meaning in life questionnaire: Assessing the presence of and search for meaning in life. *Journal of Counseling Psychology, 53*, 80–93. doi:10.1037/0022-0167.53.1.80.

Steger, M. F., Kashdan, T. B., & Oishi, S. (2008). Being good by doing good: Daily eudaimonic activity and well-being. *Journal of Research in Personality, 42*, 22–42.

Sumner, L. (1996). *Welfare, happiness and ethics*. Oxford: Oxford University Press.

Vittersø, J., Dyrdal, G. M., & Røysamb, E. (2005, June). *Utilities and capabilities: A psychological account of the two concepts and their relations to the idea of a good life*. Paper presented at Workshop on Capabilities and Happiness, Bicocca, Italy.

Vittersø, J., Oelmann, H. I., & Wang, A. L. (2009). Life satisfaction is not a balanced estimator of the good life: Evidence from reaction-time measures and self-reported emotions. *Journal of Happiness Studies, 10*, 1–17.

Waterman, A. S. (1981). Individualism and interdependence. *American Psychologist, 36*, 762–773.

Waterman, A. S. (1993). Two conceptions of happiness: Contrasts of personal expressiveness (eudaimonia) and hedonic enjoyment. *Journal of Personality and Social Psychology, 64*, 678–691.

Waterman, A. S. (2007). Doing well: The relationship of identity status to three conceptions of well-being. *Identity: An International Journal of Theory and Research, 7*, 289–307. doi:10.1080/15283480701600769.

Waterman, A. S., Schwartz, S. J., Zamboanga, B. L., Ravert, R. D., Williams, M. K., Agocha, V. B., et al. (2010). The questionnaire for eudaimonic well-being: Psychometric properties, demographic comparisons, and evidence of validity. *Journal of Positive Psychology, 5*, 41–61. doi:10.1080/17439760903435208.

Watson, D., Clark, L. A., & Tellegen, A. (1988). Development and validation of brief measures of positive and negative affect: The PANAS Scales. *Journal of Personality and Social Psychology, 6*, 1063–1070.

Wendel-Vos, G. C., Schuit, A. J., Saris, W. H., & Kromhout, D. (2003). Reproducibility and relative validity of the short questionnaire to assess health-enhancing physical activity. *Journal of Clinical Epidemiology, 56*, 1163–1169.

Genes, Environments and Core Features of Eudaimonic Wellbeing

16

Espen Røysamb and Ragnhild Bang Nes

16.1 Introduction: Genetics of Wellbeing

Why are some happier, more autonomous or curious than others? And why do characteristics from body height and eye colour to optimism, grit and mastery run in families? For centuries, individual differences and family resemblance have intrigued and challenged scientists, philosophers and lay people. The nature-versus-nurture debate constituted one of the most important themes of the biomedical and social sciences in the twentieth century, and proponents of the nature *or* nurture perspective stimulated ardent debate for decades. Today these competing paradigms have been integrated into a more unified approach based on numerous studies across the biomedical and social sciences showing that both nature and nurture play crucial roles, with most characteristics resulting from genetic and environmental factors that transact dynamically over time (Boomsma, Busjahn, & Peltonen, 2002; Plomin, DeFries, Knopik, & Neiderhiser, 2013; Polderman, Benyamin, de Leeuw, Sullivan, & van Bochoven, 2015).

Human wellbeing is influenced by both environmental and genetic factors (Nes, 2010; Røysamb, Nes, & Vitterso, 2014). During the last two decades, an increasing number of genetically informative studies have documented substantial genetic influences for various types of wellbeing. In one recent meta-analysis, the weighted average heritability of subjective wellbeing (SWB) was estimated to be 0.40 (Nes & Røysamb, 2015). Another meta-analysis reported a heritability of 0.36 for wellbeing in general, and 0.32 for life satisfaction (Bartels, 2015). Importantly, these meta-studies also provide strong evidence of the causal role of environmental factors in wellbeing.

Most twin- and family-studies of wellbeing have focused on SWB in general and life satisfaction in particular and until recently few have examined the role of genetic factors in eudaimonic wellbeing (Archontaki, Lewis, & Bates, 2013). The general aim of this chapter is to review some of these recent findings and to discuss implications for theory, practice and future research. Before moving into the landscape of twins, genes and DNA we will address some issues of conceptual nature.

The chapter is structured into three parts. First, we share some thoughts on the current state of construct affairs, and introduce the concept of *well-moving* as central to eudaimonic wellbeing. In the second part, we provide a review of genetically informative studies examining genetic and

E. Røysamb (✉) • R.B. Nes
Department of Psychology, University of Oslo, Oslo, Norway

Norwegian Institute of Public Health, Oslo, Norway
e-mail: espen.roysamb@psykologi.uio.no

J. Vittersø (ed.), *Handbook of Eudaimonic Well-Being*, International Handbooks of Quality-of-Life,
DOI 10.1007/978-3-319-42445-3_16

environmental influences on eudaimonic wellbeing. Finally, in the third part we discuss some implications of the genetic findings, with regard to conceptual issues and to the notion of positive interplay between genes and environment.

16.2 Conceptual Challenges: What We Talk About When We Talk About Eudaimonic Wellbeing

During the relatively brief history of wellbeing research, a number of constructs have been launched. Table 16.1 shows different types of wellbeing with selected key references.

Table 16.1 Overview of selected wellbeing constructs in use

Wellbeing construct	Key references
Subjective wellbeing	Diener et al. (1985), (1999)
Psychological wellbeing	Bradburn (1969), Ryff (1989), and Ryff and Keyes (1995)
Objective wellbeing	Muffels and Headey (2013) and Oswald and Wu (2010)
Eudaimonic wellbeing	Ryan and Deci (2001)
Hedonic wellbeing	Ryan and Deci (2001)
Personal wellbeing	Lau, Cummins, and McPherson (2005) and Tomyn, Tyszkiewicz, and Cummins (2013)
Mental wellbeing	Keyes et al. (2010)
Functional wellbeing	Vitterso (2013) and Vitterso et al. (2010)
Emotional wellbeing	Keyes (2000) and Pavot and Diener (1993)
Cognitive wellbeing	Luhmann, Hawkley, Eid, and Cacioppo (2012) and Robinson (2000)
Social wellbeing	Keyes (1998) and Shapiro and Keyes (2008)
Evaluative wellbeing	Deaton and Stone (2014) and Steptoe, Deaton, and Stone (2015)
Spiritual wellbeing	Frankenburg (2001) and Gomez and Fisher (2003)
Community wellbeing	Christakopoulou, Dawson, and Gari (2001) and Sirgy, Widgery, Lee, and Yu (2010)
Ontological wellbeing	Simsek (2009)

If these constructs were all used in a coherent and systematic fashion, life would be good (or at least easier) – for wellbeing researchers. We would have shared ideas about the content and measurement of the constructs, and we could examine and compare causes, correlates and consequences while knowing we referred to the same phenomena. But maybe life isn't just supposed to be good (or easy). Maybe we also value obstacles, problems and challenges. If so, the current state of construct affairs might give amble opportunities for growth and fulfilling of potentials – personally, but perhaps more importantly – for the field of wellbeing research.

The number and variety of constructs can be seen as a testimony to the flourishing of the wellbeing field and the innovative research involved. Yet, there are several challenges pertaining to the different terms in use. First, single terms are used with quite different meanings. For example, in the Diener tradition the term *subjective wellbeing* includes the three components of life satisfaction, positive affect and infrequent negative affect, is closely related to the hedonic perspective, and is distinguished from *psychological wellbeing*, which in turn is related to the eudaimonic perspective (Diener, Oishi, & Lucas, 2009; Diener, Suh, Lucas, & Smith, 1999; Lucas & Diener, 2008b; Ryan & Deci, 2001). Other renowned researchers sometimes use *subjective wellbeing* as a general term including both the hedonic and eudaimonic perspectives, and comprising the components of *psychological*, *social* and *emotional wellbeing* (Keyes, Kendler, Myers, & Martin, 2015).

Second, different terms are used to denote the same, or highly similar, phenomena. For example, the term *emotional wellbeing* being (Keyes, 2007, 2013; Keyes et al., 2015) includes the same triad of components (life satisfaction, positive and negative affect) as is typically comprised in the term *subjective wellbeing* (Diener et al., 1999; Lucas & Diener, 2008a).

Third, the boundaries between terms are far from clear. For example, *eudaimonic*, *functional* and *psychological wellbeing* are seen as closely connected, or partly overlapping – yet not identical terms (Huta & Waterman, 2014; Ryan, Huta,

& Deci, 2008; Ryff & Singer, 2008; Vitterso, 2013; Huta, this volume, Vittersø, this volume).

Fourth, there is no consensus as to what phenomena should represent wellbeing, in contrast to phenomena that predict, correlate with or result from wellbeing. For example, whereas some approaches conceive of social relations or support as predictors or correlates of wellbeing (Bergeman, Plomin, Pedersen, & McClearn, 1991; Brannan, Biswas-Diener, Mohr, Mortazavi, & Stein, 2013; Novin, Tso, & Konrath, 2014; Waterman, 2008) other approaches include positive social relations as part of the wellbeing phenomenon (Keyes, Myers, & Kendler, 2010; Ryff, 1989, this volume; Seligman, 2011).

Fifth, whereas hedonic wellbeing has been relatively clearly defined, eudaimonic wellbeing appears as a broad landscape yet to be delineated. *Hedonic wellbeing* is mainly seen as comprising the subjective wellbeing components of life satisfaction, positive and negative affect (Diener et al., 1999; Ryan & Deci, 2001). *Eudaimonic wellbeing* has been proposed to comprise phenomena such as psychological well-being, including self-acceptance, positive relations, personal growth, purpose in life, environmental mastery and autonomy (Ryan & Deci, 2001; Ryff & Keyes, 1995), self-realization, challenge-skill balance, personally expressive activities and pursuit of excellence (Huta & Waterman, 2014; Waterman, 2008), curiosity, engagement, preference for complexity, competence and well-functioning (Vitterso, 2013; Vitterso, Soholt, Hetland, Thoresen, & Roysamb, 2010; Vittersø, this volume), social well-being, including social acceptance, social actualization, social contribution, social coherence and social integration (Keyes, 1998, 2013), pursuit of intrinsic goals, living out potentials, autonomy, competence and relatedness (Ryan & Deci, 2001; Ryan et al., 2008; Ryan & Martela, this volume), meaning and use of virtues, strengths (Seligman, 2002, 2011), behaviors such as volunteering, expressing gratitude and persevering (Steger, Kashdan, & Oishi, 2008), orientations and motives such as striving to use and develop best self (Huta & Waterman, 2014), meaning making, and flow (Csikszentmihalyi, 2000; Fave, 2013; Seligman & Csikszentmihalyi, 2000).

Substantial variation in term usage, and unclear borders and definitions should not be seen as implying erratic researchers or unmeasurable phenomena. Rather, the dynamics of a young research field will, and should, include differences of opinion and developments in conceptual content. Yet, as the field of wellbeing research is beginning to gain scientific maturity there is an obvious need for a stringent and clear conceptual system. Eventually, there should be a high degree of shared understanding and consensus about what we talk about when we talk about eudaimonic wellbeing.

16.2.1 Lessons from the Development of DSM-5 and ICD-10

Taxonomies and diagnostic systems for mental disorders and psychopathology have a much longer history than the scientific study of wellbeing. Although the wellbeing field has developed partly as a contrast to, and a scientific revolt against, the sole focus on pathology, the field might still benefit from lessons learned during decades of developing diagnostic systems. Today two major diagnostic systems exist; the Diagnostic and Statistical Manual of Mental Disorders (APA, 2013), now in its fifth major version (DSM-5), and the International Statistical Classification of Diseases and Related Health Problems (WHO, 1992), now in its tenth version (ICD-10). Although there is no fully agreed upon definition of mental disorder, the main systems and perspectives converge on the dual notion of disorders as involving *distress and/or dysfunction* (APA, 2013; Huppert & So, 2013; Wakefield, 1992). The classification systems can be seen as evidence of the dynamic process of taxonomy development. During their existence the DSM and ICD have undergone substantial changes: we have witnessed disorders come and go, and we have seen disorders being defined and operationalized with increasing clarity.

Current classifications and structural models of mental disorders are hierarchical: At a general level there are distinctions between for example internalizing and externalizing disorders. Among the internalizing disorders there is a distinction between mood disorders and anxiety disorders, and within the latter there are distinctions between specific disorders such as Generalized Anxiety Disorder, Panic Disorder, Social Anxiety Disorder, Specific phobias and Obsessive-Compulsive Disorder (APA, 2013; Røysamb et al., 2011; WHO, 1992).

What can be learned from the development of mental disorder classifications to current attempts of identifying, defining and delineating the dimensions of wellbeing? We want to point out four noteworthy lessons:

1. Classifications develop over time and are not static – but should ideally move towards increasingly clearer and stringent systems, involving also reliable and valid methods of measurement. Such improvements go along with moving from reliance on expert opinions to stronger empirical foundations.
2. Distinctions between types and dimensions of wellbeing should be established at different levels, from the general to the more specific. Hierarchical models incorporate global dimensions and finer nuances, and we encourage increased efforts to establish such comprehensive models.
3. Whereas mental disorders have typically been defined as categories or dichotomies, a dimensional representation of wellbeing is fruitful. There is also an increasing acceptance that mental disorders have an underlying dimensional nature, and that the categorical model has several limitations (Widiger & Samuel, 2005). A new continuous approach to capturing personality disorders, the Personality inventory for DSM-5 (PID-5) has been included in Section III (APA, 2013). Although cut-offs and categories might sometimes be useful for practical purposes, we believe wellbeing – and illbeing – is often best conceptualized and measured dimensionally.
4. As mental disorders are characterized by *distress* and/or *dysfunction*, wellbeing could be seen as characterized by *feeling good* and/or *functioning well*. Positive feelings are valued and desired, have played a crucial role in our evolutionary history, are strongly connected to approach-related responses, might involve both the 'wanting' and 'liking' systems, and represent a signal that something is good for us, or that we did something right. Likewise, well-functioning represents a contrast to the dys-functioning feature of many mental disorders. Emotions, cognitions and behaviors can all be functional, and as such belong to the wellbeing domain. We need, however, to work towards clarifications of 'functional' for *whom*, in *what ways*, and criteria for *determining whether* a condition is functional.

16.2.2 Eudaimonic Wellbeing as Well-Moving

Although a clear-cut definition of eudaimonic wellbeing might be scientifically premature, we think it is useful to approach a definition by pointing to core characteristics (Huta & Waterman, 2014). Eudaimonic wellbeing includes phenomena such as growth, self-realization, pursuit of intrinsic goals, developing one's best self, and engagement (Huta & Waterman, 2014; Ryan & Deci, 2001; Vitterso, 2013). We will argue that these phenomena share some variant of development, process, change or movement. Therefore we propose the term *well-moving* as reflecting the core nature of eudaimonic phenomena, and as such an important part of wellbeing. Moving well is an integral aspect of self-actualization and growth, is central to the pursuit of intrinsic goals, and is often associated with experiences of engagement and interest. Being in a process of movement towards a desired goal, rather than being happy or satisfied from having reached the goal, is a core feature of many phenomena typically labelled eudaimonic wellbeing.

As we next move into the field of genetics and twin studies we will review recent findings on phenomena that are typically labelled eudaimonic in the literature. However, we will return to the notion of eudaimonia as well-moving and address the question of whether eudaimonia and hedonia should be seen as the Big Two of human wellbeing.

16.3 Genetically Informative Research

Since the draft sequences of the human genome were published in 2001, our understanding of genomic structure and function has progressed rapidly. Yet, for most psychological characteristics, deeper understanding of the complex relationship between genes and environmental influences has proved challenging and surprisingly little is still known about the specific pathways linking DNA variants to wellbeing (Boomsma et al., 2002; Plomin, 2013; Polderman et al., 2015). This is likely due to such characteristics being highly *complex*, *multi-factorial* (i.e., multiple genetic and environmental processes involved) and *polygenetic* (i.e., many genes with differing effects are involved in genetic variation) with risk and protective factors acting in a probabilistic fashion. Most of the genetic variants involved are also likely to be *pleiotropic*, meaning that they are involved in multiple functions throughout the brain (e.g., biochemical processes).

Broadly speaking, two main research paradigms investigate genetic and environmental sources of wellbeing, namely *molecular* and *behaviour genetics*. Molecular genetics seek to trace the causal pathways from specific DNA variants to given characteristics using a range of methods such as candidate-gene association studies which target pre-identified genetic markers (i.e., candidate genes) and genome wide association studies (GWAS) which practically scan the entire genome (exploratory) for associations between common gene variations (e.g., single-nucleotide polymorphisms, copy number variations) and given characteristics. Overall, most of the genetic variants identified through such methods seem to have small effects (<1 % of the variation), the findings have not replicated well, and to date very few have examined the molecular genetic underpinnings of "eudaimonic" characteristics (Bartels, 2015; De Neve, Christakis, Fowler, & Frey, 2012; Rietveld, Cesarini, Benjamin, Koellinger, & De Neve 2013).

In contrast to molecular genetic designs, behaviour genetic methods are fundamentally statistical and permit estimation of genetic and environmental influences on variation in wellbeing without specifying actual DNA sequences or specific environmental circumstances. Instead, overall effects of (unknown) genes and environmental factors are inferred, or modelled as latent variables, using statistical methods (Boomsma et al., 2002; Plomin, DeFries, Knopik, & Neiderhiser, 2013). To this end, behaviour genetics builds on the known genetic and environmental relationship between family members – most often monozygotic (MZ) and dizygotic (DZ) twins. Basic univariate twin designs explore *whether* and *to what extent* genetic factors are involved (i.e., estimate heritability), whilst more advanced multivariate designs explore *how* genetic and environmental influences are involved – for example whether the importance of genetic and environmental influences varies across males and females, are contingent on other variables, are specific to a given characteristic (e.g., social wellbeing), or shared with other traits (e.g., extraversion). Such specificity or commonality will be reflected in the genetic (r_g) and environmental (r_e) correlations between the given characteristics. These correlations can be quite different from the genetic and environmental contributions to the covariance. For example, the genetic contribution to two characteristics (e.g., optimism and pessimism) may be minor, implying low genetic covariance. Yet, the genetic correlation could be very strong, implying that the same genes are essentially affecting both traits although weakly. To some extent, such multivariate designs might inform the debate on the "jingle" and "jangle" fallacies – i.e. the discussion about whether characteristics labelled similarly actually are different, or whether constructs with different names might be essentially the same – at least from an etiological perspective.

Most behaviour genetic studies employ the classical twin design – comparing MZ and DZ reared-together twins (Boomsma et al., 2002). This design allows for estimation of *two* types of genetic effects (additive and non-additive) and *two* types of environmental effects (shared and non-shared). Additive genetic effects refer to the effects from individual genetic loci that combine in an additive fashion, whilst non-additive genetic effects refer to interaction between alleles at the same locus (dominance) or across loci (epistasis). The total genetic effect is termed *heritability* and is either estimated in a broad (i.e., include additive and non-additive influences) or narrow (i.e., only additive effects) sense. The *shared environment* comprises all non-genetic influences leading to family resemblance and might incorporate prenatal influences, nutrition, socioeconomic status, and illness – not just family socialization processes. The *non-shared environment* includes all non-genetic influences contributing to differences between family members plus measurement error and stochastic chance effects (Bouchard, 2004; Plomin et al., 2013).

The genetic and environmental effects are derived by specifying a mathematical model according to the differential degree to which pairs of MZ and DZ co-twins are correlated for genetic and environmental effects. Since MZ co-twins have identical DNA, genetic additivity and non-additivity are perfectly correlated in these pairs. By contrast, DZ co-twins share on average 50 % of their segregating genes (i.e. like other first-degree relatives) giving a genetic correlation of 0.5 (additivity) and 0.00–0.25 (non-additivity). As the shared environment includes all environmental influences causing similarity between co-twins regardless of zygosity, it is correlated 1.0 in all zygosity groups, whereas the non-shared environment is by definition uncorrelated. Figure 16.1 depicts the basic twin model with observed phenotypes, latent variables for the additive genetic (A), common/shared environement (C) and non-shared environment (E) factors, and constrained correlations according to the genetic relatedness of MZ and DZ twins (non-additive genetic factors, D, not shown in model). Structural equation modelling is used to test models against data to obtain parameter estimates and model fit.

Heritability represents the part of the total variation attributable to genetic variation – in a specific population at a specific point in time. As such, heritability is a *relative* estimate, and does not refer to genetic influences at the individual level. The relativity of the heritability estimate also implies that heritability indexes *what is* in a population at a specific time and not what *could be* (Plomin et al., 2013). Contrary to what many people believe, high heritability does not necessarily limit the potential of policy efforts and interventions aiming to improve wellbeing levels. To use body height as an example – height is highly heritable (80–90 %) in current western societies. However, height might have been less heritable a century ago, as the environmental variance (e.g. childhood nutrition) was greater and therefore the relative influence of the genetic factor was smaller. Also, despite the high heritability (i.e. genetic influence on variance within the current population) we have witnessed substantial increases in mean height during the last century (differences between cohorts that are not included in models of the living population). In a similar way we need to acknowledge that potential wellbeing interventions are not included in the equations estimating current heritabilities. That is, only the naturally occurring environmental influences are captured, and the addition of an effective intervention could possibly increase the environmental variance and thereby reduce the relative genetic effect.

Another important point is that the heritability estimate is based on the assumption that the genetic and environmental influences are independent. However, people are active agents in their lives, choosing and influencing their circumstances thus violating this basic assumption. Consequently, the heritability estimate might index the direct genetic effects as well as the effects of certain types of gene-environment interplay such as *gene environmental correlation* (CorGE) and *gene-environment interaction* (G × E) which might be highly relevant for wellbeing research. CorGE refers to the fact that an indi-

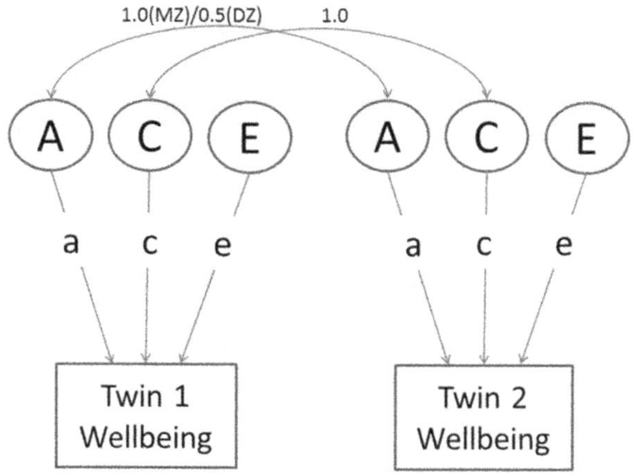

Fig. 16.1 A basic univariate twin model, including additive genetic factors (*A*), common/shared environment (*C*) and non-shared environment (*E*). *MZ* monozygotic, *DZ* dizygotic

vidual's genotype is likely to influence the probability of exposure to environmental risk and protective factors (i.e., we are not exposed to a random environment) which is known as *social selection* in the developmental literature and *reverse causation* or *confounding* in epidemiology. Individuals tend to be active agents in selecting and shaping their environments (active CorGE), and to trigger responses to their behaviour (evocative CorGE), which in turn strengthen their genetically based dispositions. Those who are sociable with high self-esteem are likely to seek contexts that match their partly genetic disposition (active CorGE) and tend to elicit more positive feedback from others than those who are angry or withdrawn (evocative CorGE). *Gene-environment interaction* (G × E) refers to interaction between specific DNA sequences and specific measured environments. There has been an explosion of interest in G × E in recent years, and G × E has been suggested to be the norm in relating specific polymorphisms to behaviour (Canli, 2004). Most studies have been conducted within the *diasthesis-stress* perspective (Monroe & Simons, 1991) and a number of studies have shown specific genetic variants (e.g., *5-HTTLPR* "short" allele) to increase risk of psychopathology given environmental adversity (Caspi, Sugden, Moffitt, Taylor, & Craig, 2003; Karg, Burmeister, Shedden, & Sen, 2011). As an alternative to the diasthesis-stress perspective, the *differential susceptibility* framework (Belsky, 1997; Belsky & Pluess, 2009a) predicts that specific genetic variants (e.g., *5-HTTLPR* "short" allele) are disproportionally susceptible to both negative *and* positive environmental stimuli (i.e., being particularly malleable). So, given a harsh environment such genetic variants might confer risk of pathology (e.g., anxiety), but given a warm and supportive environment the same genetic variant might contribute to a positive development (e.g., increase self-esteem). The concept of *vantage sensitivity* (Pluess & Belsky, 2013) has been used to refer to the "bright side" of differential susceptibility to indicate that some individuals – partly for genetic reasons, might benefit more than others from positive life experiences.

16.3.1 Results from Behaviour Genetic Studies

Behaviour genetic studies have investigated genetic and environmental sources of wellbeing characteristics since the 1980s, but mostly using hedonic indicators such as life satisfaction and positive affect (Bartels & Boomsma, 2009; Lykken & Tellegen, 1996; Nes, Røysamb, Tambs, Harris, & Reichborn-Kjennerud, 2006; Røysamb, Harris, Magnus, Vitterso, & Tambs, 2002; Røysamb, Tambs, Reichborn-Kjennerud, Neale, & Harris, 2003). As noted, two recent meta-analyses of wellbeing have shown average heritabilities in the range of 32–40 % (Bartels, 2015; Nes & Røysamb, 2015). Interestingly, but not surprisingly, heritability was found to vary across samples and/or constructs and 70 % of this variability was found to reflect true heterogeneity in heritability rather than random variation in estimates (Nes & Røysamb, 2015). That is, the heritability of wellbeing is not a fixed statistic but will depend on environmental variance and varies across populations and measures. These meta-analyses include data from a number of different countries and a total sample size of up to more than 55,000 individuals – providing solid evidence for the importance of both genetic and environmental effects.

Most behaviour genetic studies of eudaimonic wellbeing characteristics have been published over the past few years. These studies have been based on data from several different twin registers (e.g., the MIDUS,[1] the VETSA,[2] the Italian Twin Registry, the Swedish Twin Registry, the TWIN-E study) and have included a number of different indicators (e.g., the Ryff Psychological Wellbeing (PWB) Scales, the Rosenberg Self-Esteem Scale) with most studies employing the classical twin design. Quite consistently, variation in eudaimonic wellbeing has been found to be attributable to both genetic and environmental factors with these factors being partly common (i.e., genetic and environmental commonality), partly specific to the given indicators or dimensions (i.e., genetic and environmental specificity). The presence of partly distinct genetic and environmental sources indicates that more than one set of genetic and environmental factors are involved (i.e., multidimensionality at the genetic and environmental level). The environmental influences seem to be largely *non-shared* and commonly account for 40–70 % of the total variation. Influences from *shared* environmental factors appear to be minor, and mostly negligible – at least in adult samples, indicating that family similarity essentially is due to shared genes, and not to shared environments.

Altogether six different studies have utilized the Ryff Psychological Wellbeing (PWB) Scales (either 42 or 18 item versions) which include six correlated wellbeing components, including *personal growth*, *social relations*, *autonomy*, *environmental mastery*, *purpose in life* and *self-acceptance*. The heritability of the overall PWB scale has been estimated in the 47–52 % range (Keyes et al., 2010; Kubarych, Prom-Wormley, Franz, Panizzon, & Dale, 2012) and genetic influences are consistently reported for all six components, with heritabilities of 30–64 %. There seems to be a substantial etiological overlap across the six components – particularly for genetic influences. Such genetic commonality has also been shown between the PWB components and other eudaimonic characteristics such as self-esteem (Franz et al., 2012; Kubarych et al., 2012), hedonic wellbeing (e.g., life satisfaction), susceptibility to depression (Franz et al., 2012), and personality (Keyes et al., 2015). For example, exploring commonality and specificity underpinning wellbeing and illbeing using the 18-item PWB scale, a single item life satisfaction measure, the Rosenberg Self-Esteem Scale (Rosenberg, 1965), the Wellbeing subscale of the Multidimensional Personality Questionnaire (MPQWB), and the Center for Epidemiological Studies Depression Scale (CES-D; (Radloff, 1977)), Franz and colleagues (2012) reported two latent wellbeing factors – both influenced by genes and environmental factors. PWB and self-esteem loaded most strongly on the first factor, which was strongly heritable ($h^2 = 79\,\%$) and appeared to primarily reflect self-appraisal. LS loaded only on the second factor which was more influenced by environmental factors ($h^2 = 34\,\%$). The CES-D also loaded on both latent factors, and was thus associated with both wellbeing dimensions, albeit in different ways.

Another study employing the full 42-item PWB scale reported the six PWB components to reflect five distinct genetic effects (Archontaki et al., 2013). One genetic factor was associated with all six components, with *self-acceptance* showing the highest loading. This general factor was provisionally labelled *self-control* and suggested to reflect a top-down control mechanism impacting on multiple systems processing emotional, reward-incentive and motivational information related to PWB. The four additional genetic factors were termed *purpose* (loading on

[1]Midlife Development in the United States.

[2]Vietnam Era Twin Study of Aging.

purpose and personal growth), *social relations*, *growth* (loading on growth and autonomy) and *agency* (loading on autonomy and environmental mastery). No obvious meaningful theoretical structure was indicated for the environmental influences.

Keyes and colleagues (2010) estimated genetic and environmental influences on the higher-order construct of *mental wellbeing* as indicated by three facets including psychological (PWB scale, 18 items), emotional and social wellbeing. The heritability of the common factor (i.e., mental wellbeing) was substantial and estimated to be 72.3 %, whilst heritabilities for the three facets ranged between 45 % (social wellbeing) and 52 % (psychological wellbeing). Genetic influences on PWB were almost entirely shared (99 %) with the common factor, whereas the respective estimates for emotional and social wellbeing were 61 % and 65 %. Trait-specific genetic influences were thus more important to social and emotional rather than psychological wellbeing. The environmental commonality was likewise more substantial for psychological wellbeing (42 %) than for social (19 %) and emotional (24 %) wellbeing. In a more recent study, Keyes and colleagues (2015) examined associations between *flourishing* (termed mental wellbeing in the previous study) and personality, finding that a third of the genetic variance was distinctive from overall personality traits.

Another recent study (Gatt, Burton, Schofield, Bryant, & Williams, 2014) used a new, copyrighted, 26-item wellbeing scale (COMPAS-W) also consisting of moderately heritable dimensions, including total wellbeing (h^2=48 %) and sub-scales (composure, own-worth, mastery, positivity, achievement, and satisfaction) with heritabilities ranging from 32 % to 48 %. The genetic and environmental factors were correlated across most sub-dimensions but with the magnitude of the associations varying across sub-dimensions and across genetic and environmental factors. For example, Composure and Satisfaction were highly etiologically correlated (r_g=0.87; r_e=0.57), whilst Mastery and Positivity (r_g=0.31; r_e=0.00) were entirely unrelated in terms of the environment and very modestly genetically related. However, as the scales were constructed as a combination of items from different instruments the findings are somewhat unclear. Almost half the items were from the NEO Five-Factor Inventory (McCrae & Costa, 2004), which was developed to measure personality traits rather than wellbeing.

Using data from 444 adult Swedish twin pairs, Mosing and colleagues investigated genetic and environmental influences underpinning *flow proneness* in three central life domains including work, leisure, and maintenance (Mosing, Pedersen, Cesarini, Johannesson, & Magnusson, 2012). The heritability estimates were reported to range between 29 % and 35 %, and to be almost entirely shared, suggesting a general proneness to flow experiences across different life arenas that is moderately influenced by genes. Contrasting the findings for the genetic effects, influences from the non-shared environment were mostly specific to each of the three sub-scales.

Twin studies have also examined heritability for the 24 *strengths* and *virtues* (e.g., creativity, curiosity, hope, gratitude) included in the Values in Action (VIA) (Peterson & Seligman, 2004), with significant genetic and non-shared environmental effects estimated for 21 out of the 24 character strengths (Steger, Hicks, Kashdan, Krueger, & Bouchard, 2007). The VIA strengths correlated moderately with personality traits (MPQ) and genetic influences on personality accounted for most but not all of the heritable influences on character strengths. Steger and colleagues also investigated the heritability, commonality and specificity of *meaning in life*, *religiousness* and *spirituality*, finding substantial shared genetic and environmental factors.

Lastly, two studies have examined *trait resilience* and reported sex differences in heritability estimates. Boardman and colleagues reported genetic influences to account for 52 % and 38 % of the variation for males and females respectively (Boardman, Blalock, & Button, 2008). Waaktaar and Torgersen used a multi-informant twin-family design (i.e., information from adolescent twins and their parents) and reported the heritability estimates to range between 50 % and 75 % for boys, and 41 % and 66 % for girls

(Waaktaar & Torgersen, 2012). The heritability estimates in this latter study was also shown to vary across raters with the highest heritability estimated from maternal ratings.

The collective findings thus indicate that eudaimonic wellbeing and related characteristics are moderately heritable with differences in the magnitude of the estimates likely related to the specific constructs explored, the psychometric qualities and the given design, including the number and type of respondents. As such, the results fit well with findings for characteristics such as hedonic wellbeing, personality traits, liability to depression and distress, which quite consistently show moderate genetic influences and negligible influences from the shared environment, but moderate to substantial influences from the non-shared environment (McGue, 2010; Nes & Røysamb, 2015). Environmental influences are thus highly important but do not generally operate on a family-by-family basis (e.g., parenting style and shared family events do not have general effects), but rather on an individual-by-individual basis (affects siblings differently). Additionally, the eudaimonic indicators tend to share a genetic core, with environmental influences being somewhat more distinct. Etiological influences are also partly shared between eudaimonic and hedonic indicators (Caprara et al., 2009; Franz et al., 2012), and between eudaimonic indicators and personality traits (Keyes et al., 2010; Steger et al., 2007).

16.3.2 Results from Molecular Genetic Studies

Wellbeing-related characteristics are increasingly studied in molecular genetics and the first wellbeing GWAS just recently published (Bartels et al., 2015). Overall, molecular genetic studies of hedonic and eudaimonic wellbeing have shown mixed result and many studies have been limited by small sample sizes and short self-report scales with only moderate reliability. As noted, the most investigated genetic variant is perhaps the serotonin transporter-linked polymorphic region (*5-HTTLPR*) of the serotonin transporter gene (SLC6A4) which has been studied in psychiatric genetics for more than 20 years (e.g., De Neve et al., 2012; Stein, Campbell-Sills, & Gelernter, 2009). The "short" variant has been suggested to constitute a risk allele for neuroticism and anxiety-related traits (Munafo et al., 2003), to confer heightened sensitivity to negative environmental stimuli and to increase the risk of both anxiety (Lesch et al., 1996) and depression in response to adversity (Caspi et al., 2003; Karg et al., 2011). Recent studies also indicate that the *5-HTTLPR* is involved in wellbeing-related characteristics (i.e., eudaimonia) such as enhanced sensitivity to motivationally relevant stimuli. For example, individuals with the homozygous "long" variant have been shown to display significant bias towards processing of positive information and selectively avoiding negative information (Fox, Ridgewell, & Ashwin, 2009).

Although the "short" allele was initially regarded as a risk factor for negative emotion (e.g., sadness, depression) in response to adversity (e.g., abuse, trauma), whereas the "long" variant was assumed to constitute a protective factor, recent reports indicate that the "short" variant might confer particular benefits when exposed to a positive or adversity-free environment (Beevers et al., 2011; Belsky et al., 2015; Belsky & Pluess, 2009b; Fox, Zougkou, Ridgewell, & Garner, 2011). The "short" variant might therefore represent a plasticity factor rather than a risk factor, coding for a general sensitivity or heightened susceptibility to environmental conditions, and is recently suggested to function as an amplifier of both positive and negative emotion (Haase et al., 2015).

Eudaimonic wellbeing clearly consists of partly overlapping, partly independent components that are multi-factorial, polygenetic and influenced by several neurobiological systems. Neuroscientific research has indicated that two subcortical neurotransmitter systems seem to be particularly relevant for positive emotional states in the brain. Genetic variants impacting on these two systems are therefore likely to constitute important molecular foundations of hedonic and eudaimonic wellbeing experiences. The two systems are suggested to generate positive emotions by regulating core components of "liking" and "wanting" (Burgdorf & Panksepp, 2006). The opiate and GABA system appears to be involved in the "liking" system that is processing sensory pleasures (e.g. hedonic tastes, consummating behaviour), whereas the reward-seeking wanting system (appetitive behaviour) is associated, at least partly, with psycho-stimulants (e.g. dopamine, cocaine and amphetamine).

Recently another molecular genetic strategy has been used to study both hedonic and eudaimonic wellbeing, using RNA transcripts as outcomes (i.e., "expression profiling", "transcriptome profiling). The collection of genes which are expressed, or transcribed from genomic DNA (i.e., transcriptome) constitutes an important determinant of cellular function. Using such procedures, Fredrickson and colleagues (2013) have reported highly divergent transcriptional response to adversity (CTRA; pro-inflammatory, anitviral and antibody-related genes) for hedonic and eudaimonic wellbeing despite the two constructs being highly correlated, suggesting that the two types of wellbeing engage distinct gene regulatory programs despite similar effects on overall wellbeing (Fredrickson et al., 2013; Fredrickson, this volume). Hence, the authors speculated that the human genome might be more sensitive to qualitative variations in wellbeing than are our conscious affective experiences. Of note, these findings have been subject to heated debate. For example, Brown and colleagues (2014) claim important conceptual and methodological shortcomings (e.g., collinearity) and suggest that the results entirely reflect methodological artefacts (Brown, MacDonald, Samanta, Friedman, & Coyne, 2014). Fredrickson and colleagues have replicated their findings in a more recent and somewhat larger study (Fredrickson et al., 2015). Using the same transcriptome profiling technique, eudaimonic (purpose and meaning) wellbeing has also been indicated to have the potential to compensate for the adverse impact of loneliness on CTRA gene expression (Cole, Levine, Arevalo, Ma, & Weir, 2015).

The recent interest in the molecular genetic underpinnings of wellbeing testifies that wellbeing is put on the molecular genetic research agenda and represents an important topic for future research. However, there are very few studies, most findings have not (yet) been replicated and very little is still known about the putative molecular genetic pathways involved in wellbeing.

16.4 Implications

In the following we will focus on two main topics – one conceptual, another more practical, namely (i) how genetically informative studies may contribute to conceptual clarification in the eudaimonic research field, and (ii) how the notion of positive gene-environmental interplay might be relevant for wellbeing promotion in the eudaimonic field.

16.4.1 Eudaimoic and Hedonic Wellbeing. The Big Two of Human Wellbeing?

Do eudaimonia and hedonia represent two major types of wellbeing, or in other words, is the eudaimonic-hedonic distinction a major line of division (Proctor, Tweed, & Morris, 2015; Proctor & Tweed, this volume)? Findings from recent twin studies indicate that various wellbeing constructs – including both hedonic and eudaimonic types – *share common genetic factors*. These genetic factors tend to have larger effects than the genetic factors unique to the different constructs. For example, *social*, *psychological* (eudaimonic) and *emotional* (hedonic) wellbeing are influenced by a single underlying, and highly heritable (0.72), common factor (Keyes et al., 2010). The genetic correlation between *psychological wellbeing* (eudaimonic) and *life satisfaction* (hedonic) is also high (0.73) (Franz et al., 2012). Thus, most of the genetic influences on eudaimonic and hedonic wellbeing seem to be shared.

Although factor analyses support distinctions between eudaimonic and hedonic wellbeing (Keyes, Shmotkin, & Ryff, 2002; Ryan & Deci,

2001; Vitterso et al., 2010; Waterman, 2008), phenotypic correlations between the factors are also high. For example, correlations between *subjective* and *psychological wellbeing* have been estimated to 0.70 and 0.84 (models with and without cross-loadings, respectively) in a large and population based US sample (Keyes et al., 2002). Likewise, correlations between hedonia and eudaimonia have been estimated to 0.96 in a sample of 7,617 participants from 109 different countries (Disabato, Goodman, Kashdan, Short, & Jarden, 2015), and reported to range between 0.75 and 0.85 when eudaimonia and hedonia were experienced in connection with personally salient activities (Waterman, 2008).

If eudaimonia and hedonia represent the Big Two of wellbeing, we should expect correlations within each domain to exceed correlations across the domains. We therefore examined such correlations in two large studies; a MIDUS based study of *subjective wellbeing* (life satisfaction, positive and negative affect) and *psychological wellbeing* (the six subscales of Ryff's PWB scale) (Keyes et al., 2002), and a recent study of *hedonia* (life satisfaction, happiness and depression) and *eudaimonia* (the Ryff scales) based on the International Wellbeing Study (Disabato et al., 2015). These two studies might not be representative of all relevant studies, but both are based on large samples, are published in high ranking journals and involve highly respected wellbeing researchers. Figure 16.2 shows the magnitude of correlations within and across domains. The two studies converge on relatively high correlations among the hedonic constructs, more moderate correlations among the eudaimonic constructs, and importantly; equally high or higher correlations between the hedonic and eudaimonic variables. Although the eudaimonic constructs were limited to the Ryff scales, we believe the within-eudaimonia correlations might be further reduced if additional eudaimonic constructs (e.g., meaning, excellence, flow, engagement, authenticity, competence) were included.

Other studies seem to confirm this picture. For example, in a study of *emotional* (hedonic), *social* and *psychological* (both eudaimonic) wellbeing, Keyes et al. (2010) found support for a common factor (labelled mental well-being) underlying the three components. Based on the reported loadings, the cross-domain correlation between emotional and psychological wellbeing is estimated to 0.60, whilst the within-domain correlation between psychological and social wellbeing is estimated to 0.53.

In addition to the abovementioned correlational and etiological findings, common operationalizations and measures of wellbeing also illustrate the point. Consider the four following statements:

1. If I could live my life over, I would change almost nothing.
2. The past had its ups and downs, but in general I wouldn't want to change it.
3. When I look at the story of my life, I am pleased with how things have turned out.
4. So far I have gotten the important things I want in life.

These four statements seem relatively similar, mostly tapping into the same underlying phenomenon. If so, is this phenomenon hedonic or eudaimonic? Wellbeing researchers familiar with well-established measures might recognize the four items as belonging to two different instruments – one measuring hedonic wellbeing, the other one eudaimonic wellbeing. Items 1 and 4 belong to the Satisfaction With Life Scale (Diener, Emmons, Larsen, & Griffin, 1985), one of the most frequently used instruments in the hedonic wellbeing tradition. Items 2 and 3 belong to the Self-Acceptance sub-scale of the Ryff Psychological Wellbeing Scales (Ryff & Keyes, 1995), a commonly used measure of eudaimonic wellbeing.

Admitted, this is a selected set of items, and the items are not entirely identical. Yet, their obvious similarity (in particular when contrasted with other items intended to measure and operationalize either type of wellbeing) does not point in the direction of a Big Two of wellbeing. It is also noteworthy that self-acceptance is not a peripheral component of eudaimonia. Rather,

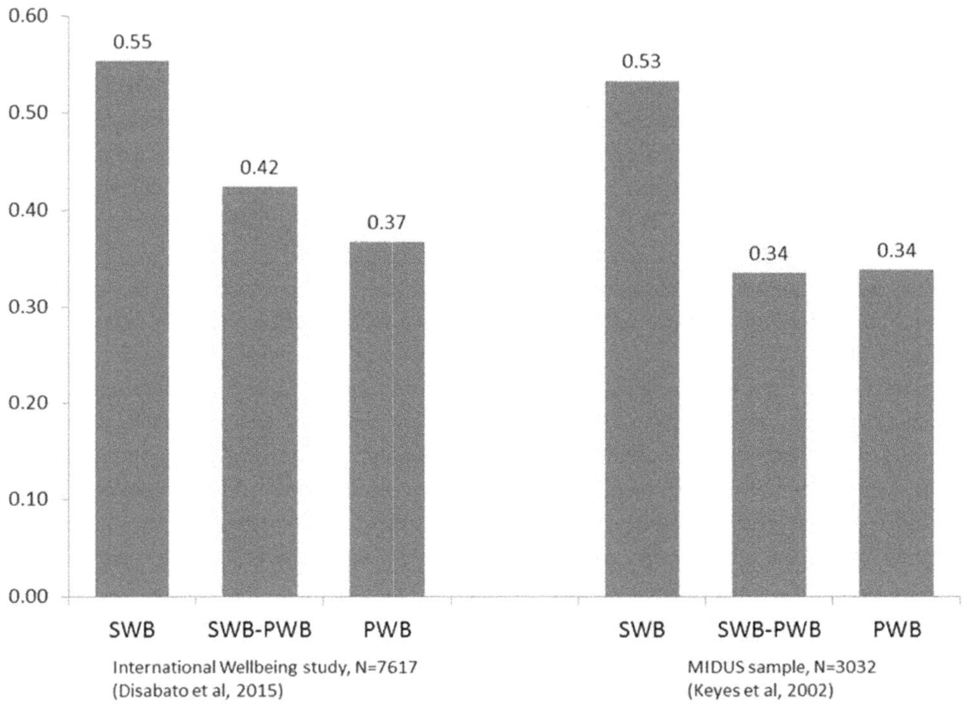

Fig. 16.2 *Bars* indicate mean correlation within domains (*SWB* and *PWB*) and across domains (*SWB-PWB*)

self-acceptance has been found to have the highest loading on a general factor of PWB (Archontaki et al., 2013).

High correlations within the eudaimonic domain are not a necessary requirement for continued demarcation of this domain. There might be shared features, common etiology, and theoretical reasons to retain a certain domain of constructs. Yet, inasmuch as the empirical evidence indicate that hedonic phenomena are as related to eudaimonic phenomena as the eudaimonic phenomena are interrelated, we believe it is time to question the hedonic-eudaimonic distinction as a major line of division in the wellbeing field.

Others have also questioned the use of eudaimonia and hedonia as two separate wellbeing domains. For example, Keyes and Annas (2009) regard hedonism as an aspect of eudaimonism: "*It is one of the options within eudaimonism. Eudaimonism presents us with an unspecific framework within which we get rival claims about what it is that constitutes eudaimonia, and pleasure is one* (p.198)" (Keyes & Annas, 2009).

In line with Waterman (2008), we discourage the use of the term hedonic wellbeing when referring to phenomena such as life satisfaction, positive and negative affect. The term is not very precise, has somewhat negative connotations, and captures neither the negative affect component nor the essence of life satisfaction – which theoretically involves an evaluation of life, potentially based on experiences of self-realization, growth, good social relations and meaning. Also in line with Waterman (2008), we find the term *subjective wellbeing* useful, well-established, and clearly defined (including life satisfaction and positive/negative affect). If there is a need for a Greek term denoting this class of phenomena we suggest *Eutychia* (ευτυχία). Eutychia is a Greek goddess of happiness, the etymological meaning of the word is *good* (eu) *luck* (tychia), and the term literally means happiness in modern Greek.

We see two alternative ways forward. First, the term eudaimonia refers to the good life, and could be seen as corresponding to *wellbeing* in general – including both *feeling good* and *functioning well*, comprising a number of components such as subjective, psychological and social wellbeing. If eudaimonic wellbeing is to encompass all the different terms previously suggested (e.g., environmental mastery, social coherence, flow, engagement, meaning), yet is partly indistinguishable from theoretically non-eudaimonic phenomena, then eudaimonia is basically a wide-ranging and heterogeneous conceptual landscape with vague borders.

Alternatively, the term eudaimonic wellbeing could be reserved for a more narrow class of phenomena, and would be operationalized through more pure indicators with high convergent and discriminant validity, thereby establishing clear distinctions from non-eudaimonic wellbeing. Within such an approach we suggest eudaimonia to be about *well-moving*. That is, a core feature of eudaimonic wellbeing is a process, development or movement towards a goal, a potential activation of the genetically based 'wanting' system, and feedback mechanisms that signal potential progress towards a goal. Constructs such as self-realization, growth, fulfilling of potentials and engagement fit into this taxonomy. Well-moving can be distinguished from *well-staying*, an aspect of wellbeing reflected in the satisfaction of having reached a goal and remaining there. Further, well-moving is also distinguishable from *ill-moving*, being in a process towards a threat or loss, typically involving experiences of fear, anxiety or anger.

In Fig. 16.3 we outline a tentative model of Well/Ill-Staying/Moving (WISM), with two underlying dimensions of *positive-negative* and *stability-change*. The upper right quadrant, well-moving, includes typical aspects of eudiamonic wellbeing, is characterized by movement, dynamics, progress towards desired goals and approach mechanisms. The lower right quadrant, well-staying, is characterized by satisfaction with things-as-they-are, happiness and contentment, focus on goals accomplished, gratitude and preservation of that which is good. Correspondingly, the left side quadrants represent ill-being, including ill-staying, which involves loss, continuation of negatives, little prospect for change, and hopelessness – and in the upper quadrant ill-moving, which involves threats, uncertainty about the

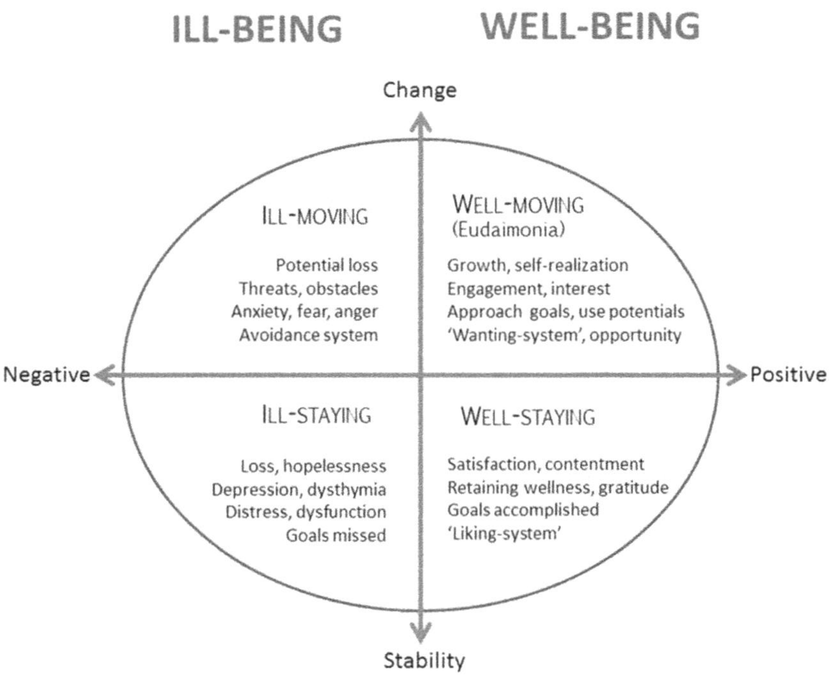

Fig. 16.3 A structural model of Well/Ill-Staying/Moving (WISM)

future, potential of loss, avoidance motives, anxiety and anger. So far this is a theoretical model in need for empirical validation, yet potentially useful as a way to structure well- and illbeing, and to define potential core features of eudaimonia.

The process of delineating the structure, dimensionality and taxonomy of wellbeing could benefit from using more genetically informative designs such as twin studies. In the field of mental disorders such studies have provided important knowledge of the genetic and environmental structures underlying various disorders (Kendler, Aggen, Czajkowski, Røysamb, & Tambs, 2008, Kendler, Aggen, Knudsen, Røysamb, & Neale, 2011), for example providing evidence for distinctions between internalizing and externalizing disorders, and between clinical and personality disorders. With genetically informative designs, such as twin studies, it is possible to extract genetic correlations (i.e. correlations between the genetic factors influencing a set of traits) as well as environmental correlations. These correlation matrices can subsequently be subjected to exploratory and confirmatory factor analyses to identify the underlying genetic and environmental structures, which might be highly informative of the most important dimensions and types of wellbeing.

16.4.2 Positive Gene-Environment Interplay

How to improve wellbeing constitutes a main topic in current wellbeing research and a number of interventions have been shown to be effective (Bolier, Haverman, Westerhof, Riper, & Smit, 2013). However, much still remains to be learned about how to prevent maladaptive and promote constructive development – in different individuals and subgroups of the population. The last decades of behavior and molecular genetic findings have contributed to change how we look upon causal mechanisms – one example being findings indicating that environmental influences do not confer the same risk – or protection – across individuals, suggesting that "genetically tailored interventions" might be particularly useful.

We have previously introduced *gene-environment matchmaking* as a general concept referring to positive interplay and collaboration between genes and environmental factors (Røysamb et al., 2014). Optimal matchmaking could include both amplifying and compensatory processes. By amplifying processes or interventions we refer to active seeking or creation of activities that provide opportunities to express (partly) genetic talents and potentials. Compensatory processes or interventions might include identification and acceptance of vulnerabilities and risk factors (e.g., anxieties, addictions, self-doubt), or less developed characteristics which constitute "wellbeing thieves", for example by limiting behavioral flexibility or impeding optimal development. Identification of such vulnerabilities could then be followed by activities for building experiences and competencies that balance these vulnerabilities or channel them into functional pathways. Compensatory strategies might therefore complement amplifying strategies and activities in important ways.

Gene-environment interplay occurs naturally, some variants of such interplay are highly beneficial, and intervention studies could benefit further from explicitly addressing gene-environmental matchmaking – building on findings from both behavior and molecular genetic research. The essential processes are implicitly present in the recent focus on personalized medicine (Gordon, 2007) and treatment-matching (Gastfriend & McLellan, 1997) and incorporated in several wellbeing promoting strategies. For example, "use of signature strengths in a new way" (Seligman, Steen, Park, & Peterson, 2005) involve identifying character strengths (which are genetically influenced) and exploring new and novel ways to use these strengths. Research has shown that such intrinsically motivating strengths are particularly useful in enhancing wellbeing. Recent studies also indicate that a balanced approach in which both the most and the least developed strengths are targeted (i.e., amplifying and compensatory interventions) might be the most effective route to create and sustain wellbeing (Young, Kashdan, & Macatee, 2015). Along with notions of *person-*

activity fit which has been proposed as the key moderator of the effects from positivity enhancing activities (Lyubomirsky & Layous, 2013; Sheldon & Lyubomirsky, 2007), such findings are congruent with a model of gene-environment matchmaking which incorporate both amplifying and compensatory processes.

Self-realization is seen as a key component in eudaimonic perspectives (Huta & Waterman, 2014; Ryan & Deci, 2001). We will argue that self-realization is an archetypal example of positive gene-environmental interplay. Environments might prevent or promote people's realization of potentials, and *match-making* between environments and genetic potentials might be a crucial factor in wellbeing promotion. For example, a person with a genetic potential for creativity – or musicality, sports or math – might realize this potential in many different directions, but mostly so when the environmental conditions allow for, and support, such realizations. Positive gene-environment interplay may be created through gene-environment correlations (CorGE) and interactions (G×E). The notions of vantage sensitivity (Pluess & Belsky, 2013), differential susceptibility (Belsky & Pluess, 2009a), and gene-environmental match-making (Røysamb et al., 2014) all point in a direction of increased attention to the potential of positive and fruitful interplay between genetic and environmental factors in promoting wellbeing for individuals and societies alike.

16.5 Conclusions

We have witnessed an exciting growth of research on eudaimonia during recent years. Our main focus in this chapter has been the genetic and environmental influences on eudaimonic wellbeing. Genetically informative studies provide strong evidence of the causal role of both genetic and environmental factors for most, if not all wellbeing conditions. They also indicate strong evidence for dynamic interplay between genes and environmental factors.

We have addressed the conceptual and taxonomic nature of wellbeing, and the potential of genetically informative studies for this work. We have argued that (a) there is a need for clarifying constructs and for moving towards a more stringent and consensual use of terms, (b) wellbeing research might benefit from lessons learned in the scientific process of establishing taxonomies of mental disorders, and that (c) despite supporting the focus on eudaimonia, we do not believe current evidence support the distinction between eudaimonia and hedonia as a major line of division in wellbeing research. One possible way forward would be to develop a more narrow and clear demarcation of eudaimonia, and we suggest *well-moving* to potentially represent a core feature. We also believe that findings from genetic and environmental studies might prove useful for establishing major dimensions of wellbeing and suggest that positive gene-environment interplay is a promising avenue for future research on interventions and human growth.

References

APA. (2013). *Diagnostic and statistical manual of mental disorders* (5th ed.). Washington, DC: American Psychiatric Association.

Archontaki, D., Lewis, G. J., & Bates, T. C. (2013). Genetic influences on psychological well-being: A nationally representative twin study. *Journal of Personality, 81*(2), 221–230.

Bartels, M. (2015). Genetics of wellbeing and its components satisfaction with life, happiness, and quality of life: A review and meta-analysis of heritability studies. *Behavior Genetics, 45*(2), 137–156.

Bartels, M., & Boomsma, D. I. (2009). Born to be happy? The etiology of subjective well-being. *Behavior Genetics, 39*(6), 605–615.

Bartels, M., Okbay, A., Derringer, J., Baselmans, B., De Neve, J. E., Rietveld, C., … Koellinger, P. (2015). Genome-wide association meta-analyses for happiness, satisfaction with life and wellbeing; the sequel. *Behavior Genetics, 45*(6), 642–642.

Beevers, C. G., Marti, C. N., Lee, H. J., Stote, D. L., Ferrell, R. E., Hariri, A. R., et al. (2011). Associations between serotonin transporter gene promoter region (5-HTTLPR) polymorphism and gaze bias for emotional information. *Journal of Abnormal Psychology, 120*(1), 187–197.

Belsky, J. (1997). Variation in susceptibility to environmental influence: An evolutionary argument. *Psychological Inquiry, 8*(3), 182–186.

Belsky, J., Newman, D. A., Widaman, K. F., Rodkin, P., Pluess, M., Fraley, R. C., … Roisman, G. I. (2015).

Differential susceptibility to effects of maternal sensitivity? A study of candidate plasticity genes. *Development and Psychopathology, 27*(3), 725–746.

Belsky, J., & Pluess, M. (2009a). Beyond diathesis stress: Differential susceptibility to environmental influences. *Psychological Bulletin, 135*(6), 885–908.

Belsky, J., & Pluess, M. (2009b). The nature (and nurture?) of plasticity in early human development. *Perspectives on Psychological Science, 4*(4), 345–351.

Bergeman, C., Plomin, R., Pedersen, N. L., & McClearn, G. (1991). Genetic mediation of the relationship between social support and psychological well-being. *Psychology and Aging, 6*(4), 640–646.

Boardman, J. D., Blalock, C. L., & Button, T. M. M. (2008). Sex differences in the heritability of resilience. *Twin Research and Human Genetics, 11*(1), 12–27.

Bolier, L., Haverman, M., Westerhof, G. J., Riper, H., Smit, F., & Bohlmeijer, E. (2013). Positive psychology interventions: A meta-analysis of randomized controlled studies. *BMC Public Health, 13*, 119.

Boomsma, D., Busjahn, A., & Peltonen, L. (2002). Classical twin studies and beyond. *Nature Reviews Genetics, 3*(11), 872–882.

Bouchard, T. J., Jr. (2004). Genetic influence on human psychological traits: A survey. *Current Directions in Psychological Science, 13*(4), 148–151.

Bradburn, N. M. (1969). *The structure of psychological well-being*. Oxford, UK: Aldine.

Brannan, D., Biswas-Diener, R., Mohr, C. D., Mortazavi, S., & Stein, N. (2013). Friends and family: A cross-cultural investigation of social support and subjective well-being among college students. *Journal of Positive Psychology, 8*(1), 65–75.

Brown, N. J. L., MacDonald, D. A., Samanta, M. P., Friedman, H. L., & Coyne, J. C. (2014). A critical reanalysis of the relationship between genomics and well-being. *Proceedings of the National Academy of Sciences of the United States of America, 111*(35), 12705–12709.

Burgdorf, J., & Panksepp, J. (2006). The neurobiology of positive emotions. *Neuroscience and Biobehavioral Reviews, 30*(2), 173–187.

Canli, T. (2004). Functional brain mapping of extraversion and neuroticism: Learning from individual differences in emotion processing. *Journal of Personality, 72*(6), 1105–1132.

Caprara, G. V., Fagnani, C., Alessandri, G., Steca, P., Gigantesco, A., Sforza, L. L. C., et al. (2009). Human optimal functioning: The genetics of positive orientation towards self, life, and the future. *Behavior Genetics, 39*(3), 277–284.

Caspi, A., Sugden, K., Moffitt, T. E., Taylor, A., Craig, I. W., Harrington, H., … Poulton, R. (2003). Influence of life stress on depression: Moderation by a polymorphism in the 5-HTT gene. *Science, 301*(5631), 386–389.

Christakopoulou, S., Dawson, J., & Gari, A. (2001). The community well-being questionnaire: Theoretical context and initial assessment of its reliability and validity. *Social Indicators Research, 56*(3), 321–351.

Cole, S. W., Levine, M. E., Arevalo, J. M., Ma, J., Weir, D. R., & Crimmins, E. M. (2015). Loneliness, eudaimonia, and the human conserved transcriptional response to adversity. *Psychoneuroendocrinology, 62*, 11–17.

Csikszentmihalyi, M. (2000). The contribution of flow to positive psychology. *Science of Optimism and Hope, 2*, 387–395.

De Neve, J.-E., Christakis, N. A., Fowler, J. H., & Frey, B. S. (2012). Genes, economics, and happiness. *Journal of Neuroscience, Psychology, and Economics, 5*(4), 193–211.

Deaton, A., & Stone, A. A. (2014). Evaluative and hedonic wellbeing among those with and without children at home. *Proceedings of the National Academy of Sciences of the United States of America, 111*(4), 1328–1333.

Diener, E., Emmons, R. A., Larsen, R. J., & Griffin, S. (1985). The satisfaction with life scale. *Journal of Personality Assessment, 49*(1), 71–75.

Diener, E., Oishi, S., & Lucas, R. E. (2009). *Subjective well-being: The science of happiness and life satisfaction Oxford handbook of positive psychology* (2nd ed., pp. 187–194). New York: Oxford University Press.

Diener, E., Suh, E. M., Lucas, R. E., & Smith, H. L. (1999). Subjective well-being: Three decades of progress. *Psychological Bulletin, 125*(2), 276–302.

Disabato, D. J., Goodman, F. R., Kashdan, T. B., Short, J. L., & Jarden, A. (2015). Different types of well-being? A cross-cultural examination of hedonic and eudaimonic well-being. *Psychological Assessment, 28*, 471–482.

Fave, A. D. (2013). *Chapter: Past, present, and future of flow the Oxford handbook of happiness* (pp. 60–72). New York: Oxford University Press.

Fox, E., Ridgewell, A., & Ashwin, C. (2009). Looking on the bright side: Biased attention and the human serotonin transporter gene. *Proceedings of the Royal Society B-Biological Sciences, 276*(1663), 1747–1751.

Fox, E., Zougkou, K., Ridgewell, A., & Garner, K. (2011). The serotonin transporter gene alters sensitivity to attention bias modification: Evidence for a plasticity gene. *Biological Psychiatry, 70*(11), 1049–1054.

Frankenburg, F. R. (2001). Perspectives on spiritual well-being and aging. *American Journal of Psychiatry, 158*(8), 1348–1349.

Franz, C. E., Panizzon, M. S., Eaves, L. J., Thompson, W., Lyons, M. J., Jacobson, K. C., … Kremen, W. S. (2012). Genetic and environmental multidimensionality of well- and ill-being in middle aged twin men. *Behavior Genetics, 42*(4), 579–591.

Fredrickson, B. L., Grewen, K. M., Algoe, S. B., Firestine, A. M., Arevalo, J. M. G., Ma, J., & Cole, S. W. (2015). Psychological Well-Being and the Human Conserved Transcriptional Response to Adversity. *PLoS One, 10*(3), e0121839.

Fredrickson, B. L., Grewen, K. M., Coffey, K. A., Algoe, S. B., Firestine, A. M., Arevalo, J. M. G., … Cole, S. W. (2013). A functional genomic perspective on human well-being. *Proceedings of the National Academy of Sciences of the United States of America, 110*(33), 13684–13689.

Gastfriend, D. R., & McLellan, A. T. (1997). Treatment matching – theoretic basis and practical implications. *Medical Clinics of North America, 81*(4), 945.

Gatt, J. M., Burton, K. L. O., Schofield, P. R., Bryant, R. A., & Williams, L. M. (2014). The heritability of mental health and wellbeing defined using COMPAS-W, a new composite measure of wellbeing. *Psychiatry Research, 219*(1), 204–213.

Gomez, R., & Fisher, J. W. (2003). Domains of spiritual well-being and development and validation of the Spiritual Well-Being Questionnaire. *Personality and Individual Differences, 35*(8), 1975–1991.

Gordon, E. (2007). Integrating genomics and neuromarkers for the era of brain-related personalized medicine. *Personalized Medicine, 4*(2), 201–215.

Haase, C. M., Beermann, U., Saslow, L. R., Shiota, M. N., Saturn, S. R., Lwi, S. J., … Levenson, R. W. (2015). Short alleles, bigger smiles? The effect of 5-HTTLPR on positive emotional expressions. *Emotion, 15*(4), 438–448.

Huppert, F. A., & So, T. T. C. (2013). Flourishing across Europe: Application of a new conceptual framework for defining well-being. *Social Indicators Research, 110*(3), 837–861.

Huta, V., & Waterman, A. S. (2014). Eudaimonia and its distinction from Hedonia: Developing a classification and terminology for understanding conceptual and operational definitions. *Journal of Happiness Studies, 15*(6), 1425–1456.

Karg, K., Burmeister, M., Shedden, K., & Sen, S. (2011). The serotonin transporter promoter variant (5-HTTLPR), stress, and depression meta-analysis revisited evidence of genetic moderation. *Archives of General Psychiatry, 68*(5), 444–454.

Kendler, K. S., Aggen, S. H., Czajkowski, N., Røysamb, E., Tambs, K., Torgersen, S., … Reichborn-Kjennerud, T. (2008). The structure of genetic and environmental risk factors for DSM-IV personality disorders a multivariate twin study. *Archives of General Psychiatry, 65*(12), 1438–1446.

Kendler, K. S., Aggen, S. H., Knudsen, G. P., Røysamb, E., Neale, M. C., & Reichborn-Kjennerud, T. (2011). The structure of genetic and environmental risk factors for syndromal and subsyndromal common DSM-IV axis I and all axis II disorders. *American Journal of Psychiatry, 168*(1), 29–39.

Keyes, C. L. M. (1998). Social well-being. *Social Psychology Quarterly, 61*(2), 121–140.

Keyes, C. L. M. (2000). Subjective change and its consequences for emotional well-being. *Motivation and Emotion, 24*(2), 67–84.

Keyes, C. L. M. (2007). Promoting and protecting mental health as flourishing – a complementary strategy for improving national mental health. *American Psychologist, 62*(2), 95–108.

Keyes, C. L. M. (2013). *Promotion and protection of positive mental health: Towards complete mental health in human development. The Oxford handbook of happiness* (pp. 915–925). New York: Oxford University Press.

Keyes, C. L. M., & Annas, J. (2009). Feeling good and functioning well: Distinctive concepts in ancient philosophy and contemporary science. *Journal of Positive Psychology, 4*(3), 197–201.

Keyes, C. L. M., Kendler, K. S., Myers, J. M., & Martin, C. C. (2015). The genetic overlap and distinctiveness of flourishing and the big five personality traits. *Journal of Happiness Studies, 16*(3), 655-668.

Keyes, C. L. M., Myers, J. M., & Kendler, K. S. (2010). The structure of the genetic and environmental influences on mental well-being. *American Journal of Public Health, 100*(12), 2379–2384.

Keyes, C. L. M., Shmotkin, D., & Ryff, C. D. (2002). Optimizing well-being: The empirical encounter of two traditions. *Journal of Personality and Social Psychology, 82*(6), 1007–1022.

Kubarych, T. S., Prom-Wormley, E. C., Franz, C. E., Panizzon, M. S., Dale, A. M., Fischl, B., … Kremen, W. S. (2012). A multivariate twin study of hippocampal volume, self-esteem and well-being in middle-aged men. *Genes Brain and Behavior, 11*(5), 539–544.

Lau, A. L. D., Cummins, R. A., & McPherson, W. (2005). An investigation into the cross-cultural equivalence of the Personal Wellbeing Index. *Social Indicators Research, 72*(3), 403–430.

Lesch, K. P., Bengel, D., Heils, A., Sabol, S. Z., Greenberg, B. D., Petri, S., … Murphy, D. L. (1996). Association of anxiety-related traits with a polymorphism in the serotonin transporter gene regulatory region. *Science, 274*(5292), 1527–1531.

Lucas, R. E., & Diener, E. (2008a). Personality and subjective well-being. In O. P. John, R. W. Robins, & L. A. Pervin (Eds.), *Handbook of personality: Theory and research* (3rd ed., pp. 795–814). New York: Guilford Press.

Lucas, R. E., & Diener, E. (2008b). Subjective well-being. In M. Lewis, J. M. Haviland-Jones, & L. F. Barrett (Eds.), *Handbook of emotions* (3rd ed., pp. 471–484). New York: Guilford Press.

Luhmann, M., Hawkley, L. C., Eid, M., & Cacioppo, J. T. (2012). Time frames and the distinction between affective and cognitive well-being. *Journal of Research in Personality, 46*(4), 431–441.

Lykken, D., & Tellegen, A. (1996). Happiness is a stochastic phenomenon. *Psychological Science, 7*(3), 186–189.

Lyubomirsky, S., & Layous, K. (2013). How do simple positive activities increase well-being? *Current Directions in Psychological Science, 22*(1), 57–62.

McCrae, R. R., & Costa, P. T. (2004). A contemplated revision of the NEO Five-Factor Inventory. *Personality and Individual Differences, 36*(3), 587–596.

McGue, M. (2010). The end of behavioral genetics? *Behavior Genetics, 40*(3), 284–296.

Monroe, S. M., & Simons, A. D. (1991). Diathesis stress theories in the context of life stress research – implications for the depressive-disorders. *Psychological Bulletin, 110*(3), 406–425.

Mosing, M. A., Pedersen, N. L., Cesarini, D., Johannesson, M., Magnusson, P. K., Nakamura, J., … Ullen, F. (2012). Genetic and environmental influences on the relationship between flow proneness, locus of control and behavioral inhibition. *PLoS One, 7*(11), e47958.

Muffels, R., & Headey, B. (2013). Capabilities and choices: Do they make sen'se for understanding objective and subjective well-being? An empirical test of Sen's capability framework on German and British panel data. *Social Indicators Research, 110*(3), 1159–1185.

Munafo, M. R., Clark, T. G., Moore, L. R., Payne, E., Walton, R., & Flint, J. (2003). Genetic polymorphisms and personality in healthy adults: A systematic review and meta-analysis. *Molecular Psychiatry, 8*(5), 471–484.

Nes, R. B. (2010). Happiness in behaviour genetics: Findings and implications. *Journal of Happiness Studies, 11*(3), 369–381.

Nes, R. B., & Røysamb, E. (2015). The heritability of subjective well-being: Review and meta-analysis. In M. Pluess (Ed.), *Genetics of psychological well-being* (pp. 75–96). Oxford, UK: Oxford University Press.

Nes, R. B., Røysamb, E., Tambs, K., Harris, J., & Reichborn-Kjennerud, T. (2006). Subjective well-being: Genetic and environmental contributions to stability and change. *Psychological Medicine, 36*(7), 1033–1042.

Novin, S., Tso, I. F., & Konrath, S. H. (2014). Self-related and other-related pathways to subjective well-being in Japan and the United States. *Journal of Happiness Studies, 15*(5), 995–1014.

Oswald, A. J., & Wu, S. (2010). Objective confirmation of subjective measures of human well-being: Evidence from the USA. *Science, 327*(5965), 576–579.

Pavot, W., & Diener, E. (1993). Review of the satisfaction with life scale. *Psychological Assessment, 5*(2), 164–172.

Peterson, C., & Seligman, M. E. P. (2004). *Character strengths and virtues: A handbook and classification*. Washington, DC: American Psychological Association/Oxford University Press.

Plomin, R. (2013). Commentary: Missing heritability, polygenic scores, and gene-environment correlation. *Journal of Child Psychology and Psychiatry, 54*(10), 1147–1149.

Plomin, R., DeFries, J. C., Knopik, V. S., & Neiderhiser, J. M. (2013). *Behavioral genetics* (6th ed.). New York: Worth Publishers.

Pluess, M., & Belsky, J. (2013). Vantage sensitivity: Individual differences in response to positive experiences. *Psychological Bulletin, 139*(4), 901–916.

Polderman, T. J. C., Benyamin, B., de Leeuw, C. A., Sullivan, P. F., van Bochoven, A., Visscher, P. M., et al. (2015). Meta-analysis of the heritability of human traits based on fifty years of twin studies. *Nature Genetics, 47*(7), 702.

Proctor, C., Tweed, R., & Morris, D. (2015). The naturally emerging structure of well-being among young adults: "Big Two" or other framework? *Journal of Happiness Studies, 16*(1), 257–275.

Radloff, L. S. (1977). The CES-D scale: A self-report depression scale for research in the general population. *Applied Psychological Measurement, 1*(3), 385–401.

Rietveld, C. A., Cesarini, D., Benjamin, D. J., Koellinger, P. D., De Neve, J.-E., Tiemeier, H., … Bartels, M. (2013). Molecular genetics and subjective well-being. *PNAS Proceedings of the National Academy of Sciences of the United States of America, 110*(24), 9692–9697.

Robinson, M. D. (2000). The reactive and prospective functions of mood: Its role in linking daily experiences and cognitive well-being. *Cognition & Emotion, 14*(2), 145–176.

Rosenberg, M. (1965). *Society and the adolescent self-image*. Princeton, NJ: Princeton University Press.

Røysamb, E., Harris, J. R., Magnus, P., Vitterso, J., & Tambs, K. (2002). Subjective well-being. Sex-specific effects of genetic and environmental factors. *Personality and Individual Differences, 32*(2), 211–223.

Røysamb, E., Kendler, K. S., Tambs, K., Orstavik, R. E., Neale, M. C., Aggen, S. H., … Reichborn-Kjennerud, T. (2011). The joint structure of DSM-IV axis I and axis II disorders. *Journal of Abnormal Psychology, 120*(1), 198–209.

Røysamb, E., Nes, R. B., & Vitterso, J. (2014). Well-being: Heritable and changeable. In K. Sheldon & R. E. Lucas (Eds.), *Stability of happiness*. New York: Elsevier.

Røysamb, E., Tambs, K., Reichborn-Kjennerud, T., Neale, M. C., & Harris, J. R. (2003). Happiness and health: Environmental and genetic contributions to the relationship between subjective well-being, perceived health, and somatic illness. *Journal of Personality and Social Psychology, 85*(6), 1136–1146.

Ryan, R. M., & Deci, E. L. (2001). On happiness and human potentials: A review of research on hedonic and eudaimonic well-being. *Annual Review of Psychology, 52*, 141–166.

Ryan, R. M., Huta, V., & Deci, E. L. (2008). Living well: A self-determination theory perspective on eudaimonia. *Journal of Happiness Studies, 9*(1), 139–170.

Ryff, C. D. (1989). Happiness is everything, or is it – explorations on the meaning of psychological well-being. *Journal of Personality and Social Psychology, 57*(6), 1069–1081.

Ryff, C. D., & Keyes, C. L. M. (1995). The structure of psychological well-being revisited. *Journal of Personality and Social Psychology, 69*(4), 719–727.

Ryff, C. D., & Singer, B. H. (2008). Know thyself and become what you are: A eudaimonic approach to psychological well-being. *Journal of Happiness Studies, 9*(1), 13–39.
Seligman, M. E. P. (2002). *Authentic happiness: Using the new positive psychology to realize your potential for lasting fulfillment. 2002*. New York: Free Press.
Seligman, M. E. P. (2011). *Flourish: A visionary new understanding of happiness and well-being*. New York: Free Press.
Seligman, M. E. P., & Csikszentmihalyi, M. (2000). Positive psychology: An introduction. *American Psychologist, 55*(1), 5–14.
Seligman, M. E. P., Steen, T. A., Park, N., & Peterson, C. (2005). Positive psychology progress: Empirical validation of interventions. *American Psychologist, 60*(5), 410–421.
Shapiro, A., & Keyes, C. L. M. (2008). Marital status and social well-being: Are the married always better off? *Social Indicators Research, 88*(2), 329–346.
Sheldon, K. M., & Lyubomirsky, S. (2007). Is it possible to become happier? (And if so, how?). *Social and Personality Psychology Compass, 1*(1), 129–145.
Simsek, O. F. (2009). Happiness revisited: Ontological well-being as a theory-based construct of subjective well-being. *Journal of Happiness Studies, 10*(5), 505–522.
Sirgy, M. J., Widgery, R. N., Lee, D. J., & Yu, G. B. (2010). Developing a measure of community well-being based on perceptions of impact in various life domains. *Social Indicators Research, 96*(2), 295–311.
Steger, M. F., Hicks, B. M., Kashdan, T. B., Krueger, R. F., & Bouchard, T. J., Jr. (2007). Genetic and environmental influences on the positive traits of the values in action classification, and biometric covariance with normal personality. *Journal of Research in Personality, 41*(3), 524–539.
Steger, M. F., Kashdan, T. B., & Oishi, S. (2008). Being good by doing good: Daily eudaimonic activity and well-being. *Journal of Research in Personality, 42*(1), 22–42.
Stein, M. B., Campbell-Sills, L., & Gelernter, J. (2009). Genetic variation in 5HTTLPR is associated with emotional resilience. *American Journal of Medical Genetics Part B-Neuropsychiatric Genetics, 150b*(7), 900–906.
Steptoe, A., Deaton, A., & Stone, A. A. (2015). Subjective wellbeing, health, and ageing. *Lancet, 385*(9968), 640–648.
Tomyn, A. J., Tyszkiewicz, M. D. F., & Cummins, R. A. (2013). The personal wellbeing index: Psychometric equivalence for adults and school children. *Social Indicators Research, 110*(3), 913–924.
Vitterso, J. (2013). Functional well-being: Happiness as feelings, evaluations, and functioning. In S. A. David, I. Boniwell, & A. Conley Ayers (Eds.), *The Oxford handbook of happiness* (pp. 227–244). New York: Oxford University Press.
Vitterso, J., Soholt, Y., Hetland, A., Thoresen, I. A., & Roysamb, E. (2010). Was Hercules happy? Some answers from a functional model of human well-being. *Social Indicators Research, 95*(1), 1–18.
Waaktaar, T., & Torgersen, S. (2012). Genetic and environmental causes of variation in trait resilience in young people. *Behavior Genetics, 42*(3), 366–377.
Wakefield, J. C. (1992). Disorder as harmful dysfunction – a conceptual critique of Dsm-Iii-Rs definition of mental disorder. *Psychological Review, 99*(2), 232–247.
Waterman, A. S. (2008). Reconsidering happiness: A eudaimonist's perspective. *The Journal of Positive Psychology, 3*(4), 234–252.
WHO. (1992). *The ICD-10 classification of mental and behavioural disorders: Clinical descriptions and diagnostic guidelines*. Geneva, Switzerland: World Health Organization.
Widiger, T. A., & Samuel, D. B. (2005). Diagnostic categories or dimensions? A question for the diagnostic and statistical manual of mental disorders – fifth edition. *Journal of Abnormal Psychology, 114*(4), 494–504.
Young, K. C., Kashdan, T. B., & Macatee, R. (2015). Strength balance and implicit strength measurement: New considerations for research on strengths of character. *Journal of Positive Psychology, 10*(1), 17–24.

The Feeling of Excellent Functioning: Hedonic and Eudaimonic Emotions

17

Joar Vittersø

17.1 Introduction

> The overarching aim in the study of well-being is to identify the ultimate human goodness
>
> (Crisp, 2005)

In *A Midsummer Night's Dream*, Shakespeare invites us, his audience, to imagine that if the juice of a little western flower is dripped into a sleeping person's eye, it will "cause the sleeper to fall in love with the first person he or she sees on waking" (Oatley, 2011, p. 14). When Shakespeare created this scene, he could have had Titania hit by Cupid's arrow rather than by a drop of juice. But Cupid's arrow was already a cliché when Shakespeare wrote the play. Thus, as Oatley points out, introducing an unknown juice rather than the familiar arrow makes the love scene strange. And strangeness attracts our attention in a way that sometimes generates intense positive feelings that are not experienced as pleasure or satisfaction; but rather as interest, awe, and engagement.

Scientific knowledge is in agreement with Shakespeare's insights into the psychology of strangeness and complexity. Evolution, it seems, has equipped us with a system of feelings that responds differently when confronted with something new, complex, or uncertain, as opposed to something familiar and simple. The function of the "strangeness" feeling is to prepare our minds to step out of its default mode of "lazy" and automatized thinking, also referred to as System 1 cognition (Kahneman, 2011). What we need when confronted with strangeness is the active kind of effortful and analytic thinking that is carried out by System 2 rationality.

What I am going to say in the present chapter, with an analogy to the two systems of information processing, is that human goodness also comes in two different forms. One is simple and the other is complex. They are related to, but certainly not identical with, System 1 and System 2 thinking. In terms of functionality, the simple kind of goodness is associated with a need for regulating stability—a need humans share with other biological organisms (Damasio, 2010; Denton, 2005; Panksepp & Biven, 2012; Watts & Donovan, 2010). The complex kind of goodness is related to a need equally important for us: the need to manage change (Law & Staudinger, Chap. 9, this volume; Magnusson & Mahoney, 2003; Piaget, 1952; Valsiner, 1998). These two major classes of functioning cover biological, psychological, and social aspects of our lives, or biopsychosocial functioning as Engel (1977) named it. The two classes of functioning are, I shall argue, related to the distinction between hedonic and eudaimonic well-being.

Hedonic well-being reflects a goodness that is familiar. It is a simple kind of goodness defined

J. Vittersø (✉)
UiT The Arctic University of Norway,
Tromsø, Norway
e-mail: joar.vitterso@uit.no

J. Vittersø (ed.), *Handbook of Eudaimonic Well-Being*, International Handbooks of Quality-of-Life,
DOI 10.1007/978-3-319-42445-3_17

by satisfaction and pleasant feelings. Eudaimonic well-being is more complex and much harder to conceptualize. Only a rough sketch of its constitution will be offered in this chapter, presented in the section on Functioning and Well-being. Thus, the idea of eudaimonic feelings is not proposed as a theory of eudaimonic well-being. Rather, these feelings only represent some of the ingredients needed in the ongoing struggle of articulating a common conceptual language on eudaimonia.

Eudaimonic well-being is strange. It contains a kind of complex goodness that is not necessarily associated with pleasure—and it may be valued only after a bit of reflection. Logically, the distinction between a simple and a complex form of goodness is not intuitively correct. By reason alone, it makes sense to say that if H is good and E is good, then both H and E are good. However, perception and other mental activities do not behave in accordance with the syllogistic logic proposed by Aristotle when he argued that if A is B, and B is C, then A is C. Thus, empirical observations suggest that the hedonic kind of goodness comes more easily to mind when we are asked to name or recall good elements in our lives. For reasons to be further discussed below, the hedonic kind of goodness is therefore overrepresented in empirical studies of well-being. There is also a tendency, the chapter argues, for the hedonic kind of goodness to be related to the class of functioning that helps maintain stability, and consequently with System 1 thinking. Eudaimonic goodness, in contrast, is associated with efforts and strivings that are not spontaneously associated with goodness. In this respect, it is related to System 2 thinking and other psychological mechanisms not identified with pleasure and satisfaction.

The best illustration of how these two kinds of goodness can be separate entities is given, I think, by Fiske, Cuddy, and Glick (2007). In a comprehensive review of research on social perception, Fiske and her co-authors identified two different ways in which goodness could be attributed to other people. The first dimension is recognized among people who are happy, popular, helpful, and honest, what Fiske et al. describe as being warm. The second kind of goodness involves traits such as skillful, persistent, imaginative, and serious, what the authors describe as competence. In explaining the functionality of the two dimensions these authors point out that during our evolutionary past, social contact involved judgments about friendliness and hostility in others, particularly in early stages of the interaction. At stake when initiating social encounters is the question of whether the other is a friend or foe. But the next important thing to establish is whether the other person is skillful enough to act on these intentions to help or harm, in other words if the person is sufficiently enabled for collaboration or competition. Thus, warmth and competence are the two kinds of goodness we look for in other people, and empirical studies show that the two factors account for about 80 % of the variance in perceptions of everyday social behaviors (Fiske et al., 2007).

Social functioning is characterized by a two-dimensional structure of goodness, and we should not be surprised to find a similar structure of goodness at the individual level as well. Indeed, it seems that people who observe themselves—and in particular when introspecting about their positive feelings—often make a distinction that approximately parallels the dimensions of warmth and competence. In the domain of subjective experiences, the two are referred to as pleasure and striving, respectively. If this analogy holds, it is tempting to suggest that the two categories of goodness described above have clear parallels to hedonic and eudaimonic well-being. The three arguments offered to back up this claim are as follows: The first, briefly stated below and more extensively debated elsewhere (Vittersø, forthcoming), is that a theory of well-being ought to be articulated within a framework of biopsychosocial functioning. Second, I shall argue that the function of hedonic well-being is associated with the maintenance of a homeostatic stability, which implies the sustainment of physical and psychological equilibrium. The third argument develops around the idea of eudaimonic well-being as reflecting a complex goodness of a non-homeostatic nature, directed towards developing one's capacity to master a constantly changing environment. These adjustments take place in our biology, in our psychology, and in our social relations. As a psychologist I will primarily focus on the changes that occur in cognitive structures and skills.

17.2 Functioning and Well-being

Functioning was central to ancient theories of the human good. Aristotle's "Function argument" stated, generally, that in order to establish goodness for a living being, its 'function' or characteristic activity needs to be identified (Casebeer, 2003; Crisp, 2005; Korsgaard, 2008; Megone, 1994; Ross, 2009; Thorsrud, 2015; Whiting, 1988). The essence of human goodness is therefore found in its proper and particular functioning, which according to Aristotle was "in the activity of the rational part of the soul performed well, which is to say, in accordance with virtue (NE 1.7 1098a15–17)" (cited in Korsgaard, 2008, p. 129). The function argument has admittedly generated some serious objections over the years, many of them summarized by Korsgaard. One objection is that even if something is part of our evolutionary heritage, it is not necessarily good for us (Besser, Chap. 5, this volume). As exemplified by Thin (Chap. 37, this volume), violence, greed, and social anxiety are all part of our nature, but that does not make them particularly good.

Despite the limitations of the "human nature" approach, several theories of well-being are concerned with the concept of functioning. Doyal and Gough (1991) theory of human needs is one example, and the capability approach is another. The latter, introduced by Sen in 1979 as a neo-Aristotelian and generic theory of human functioning, originates from a philosophical idea of human nature (e.g., Phillips, 2006). Sen's concept of functioning is rather vague, dealing roughly with 'doing' and 'being.' More important than the doing and being as such, though, is Sen's concept of capabilities, or the freedom to pursue valuable doings and beings. The literature offered to explain and analyze the capability approach, or Nussbaum's capabilities approach, is rich (see Alkire, 2010; Binder & Coad, 2011; Burchardt & Vizard, 2011; Dean, 2009; Jayawickreme & Pawelski, 2012; Muffels & Headey, 2013; Nussbaum, 2011; Skidelsky & Skidelsky, 2013) and will not be examined further in the current chapter. Let it suffice herein to say that a principal assumption for the function argument in the writing of Sen and Nussbaum hinges on the idea that human goodness can only be determined in light of knowledge about human nature and how to "fulfill" it.

But when it comes to human nature, science is probably ahead of philosophy. Further progress along these lines are more likely achieved within a scientific—and not a philosophical—framework. Hence, I will investigate the notion of functioning from a psychological perspective and in particular analyze the function of feelings, which I suggest have been overlooked in some theories of well-being.

17.3 Feelings and Functioning

Nothing about feelings makes sense except in the light of functioning, one could be tempted to say, freely paraphrasing Dobzhansky's renowned formulation about evolution.[1] Hence, the distinction some researchers have created between feelings as a marker of hedonic well-being and functioning as a marker of eudaimonic well-being (e. g., Keyes & Annas, 2009), is not very convincing. The function of pleasure (or displeasure), for example, is to inform us about goodness (or badness) in our immediate inner and outer environments. A pleasant feeling is a subjective comment about the favorability of the environment, as William James put it. He believed that without the ability to experience such feelings, nothing in the universe would have more importance than another (James, 1902, cited in Wessman & Ricks, 1966, p. 2).

The functions of pleasure span from the obvious to the sophisticated. Pleasant feelings serve

[1]Dobzhansky's formulation comes in different versions, the most cited being: "Nothing in biology makes sense except in the light of evolution" (Olson, 2015).

us, for instance, by helping to discriminate fresh from rotten food, regulating body temperature, or signaling that the intention of a social encounter is cooperative. Pleasure, or rather displeasure, reminds us to breathe, drink, rest, and put on a warm coat if we for some reason attempt to avoid these necessities—without requiring detailed knowledge about nutrition, the effect of sleep, or the biology of temperature regulation (e.g., Johnston, 1999).

Pleasure is also good for us in less obvious ways. As illustrated in the so-called Capgras syndrome, subtle feelings of pleasure help establish a conceptual understanding of familiar objects such as a dear friend. A person with Capgras syndrome has lost the ability to supply well-known objects with affective meaning. As a consequence, familiar faces no longer wake the emotional feelings used as a cue in identifying the object, and patients suffering from Capgras syndrome do not experience a sense of familiarity when seeing a friend or a family member, believing instead thatan imposter has replaced that individual (Duncan & Barret, 2007; Ramachandran, 2011).

Thus far I have focused the functional argument on feelings, with little mention of emotions. Feelings and emotions do have related functions, yet they are different concepts. Emotions comprise several subcomponents and feeling is only one of them. Other major components of emotions are physiological reactions and bodily expressions. Feelings on the other hand, are not always emotional, but they are always present in a conscious mind; being awake always feels like something, as Nagel (1974) famously told us. As for their overall function, Arnold (1960) proposed early on that feelings operate quite broadly to signal enhanced or impeded functioning in general. By contrast, the function of emotions is more action-specific. Emotion is felt action tendency, Arnold said (cited in Frijda, 1986, p. 244).

In detail, Oatley has explained that emotions are "part of a solution to problems of organizing knowledge and action in a world that is imperfectly known and in which we have limited resources" (Oatley, 1992, p. 3). Sadness, for example, which is one of the four basic emotions in Oatley and Johnson-Laird's (1987) taxonomy,[2] will typically occur when a major plan fails or an important goal (i.e., something valuable) is lost. Its function is to temporarily disengage the sad person from further involvement in these ill-fated goals. This function is achieved by a passive action tendency that restrains the sad person from building new plans for his or her life. Anger, another basic emotion, occurs when an active plan is frustrated and it prompts the angry person to work harder towards his or her goal, sometimes assisted with aggression. The overall function of this action tendency is to adjust social relations.

Summarizing the functions of positive emotions, Fredrickson (1998) maintains that happiness creates an urge to play, whereas contentment brings about thankfulness and the urge to savor current life circumstances. Interest, which according to Fredrickson shares conceptual space with intrinsic motivation and flow, serves to integrate information into new views of the self and of the world. Citing Izard (1977), Fredrickson writes that interest generates "a feeling of wanting to investigate, become involved, or extend or expand the self by incorporating new information and having new experiences with the person or object that has stimulated the interest" (Fredrickson, 1998, p. 305).

With a few exceptions—notably some so-called set-point theories that appear to have put the cart before the horse by arguing that our biology has evolved with the purpose of ensuring that a stable amount of pleasures is felt in our lives—scientific understanding has converged on the view that emotions and feelings are there to assist in the regulation of our biological, psychological, and social lives. The literature supporting this notion is gigantic (e.g., Averill & More, 2000; Barrett, 2012; Bonanno, Goorin, & Coifman, 2008; Bruce 2010; Cabanac, 2010; Cacioppo & Gardner, 1999; Damasio & Carvalho, 2013; De Dreu, Baas, & Nijstad, 2008; Forgas, Haselton, &

[2]These "big four" are happiness, sadness, anger, and fear. Disgust was included as a fifth basic emotion in an earlier version of the theory (Oatley & Johnson-Laird, 1996).

Von Hippel, 2007; Fredrickson, 2001; Frijda, 1994; Harmon-Jones, Gable, & Peterson, 2010; Hochschild, 1983; Izard, 2007, 2011; Johnston, 2003; Lang & Bradley, 2010; LeDoux, 2012; Mar & Oatley, 2008; Moors, Ellsworth, Scherer, & Frijda, 2013; Nesse, 1991; Oatley, 2011; Scherer, 2009; Schwarz & Clore, 1988; Shiota et al., 2014; Silvia, 2008; Yiend, 2010; Zajonc, 2001). To narrow down this ample research, what follows will reflect only a small sample of the knowledge attesting to the diverse roles played by feelings and emotions as facilitators of the important needs of stability and change.

17.4 Hedonic Feelings and Their Functions

The term hedonic has to do with pleasure (e.g., Vittersø, 2009), and pleasure has been defined as "the condition of consciousness or sensation induced by the enjoyment or anticipation of what is felt or viewed as good or desirable" (Simpson & Weiner, 1989). Although this definition captures something essential about pleasure and goodness, conceptualizing pleasure is a bit more problematic than the conceptualization suggests. Controversies about pleasure have, after all, been with us since the dawn of critical thinking. Thus, Epicurus objected to Aristippus's idea of pleasure as being restricted to one's own physical, positive, momentary feelings. To Epicurus, pleasure was a mental state; it was even a mental state that *had* to be just and moral to be called pleasant (McMahon, 2006).

Plato presented several views on pleasure. Michalos and Robinson (2012) identified at least five meanings to which Plato applied the concept: a desire satisfaction theory, a needs satisfaction theory, a harmony theory, a true pleasures theory, and a class theory of pleasure. The functional perspective in Plato's need satisfaction theory is actually quite consistent with how modern biologists think about pleasure as a principal player in the regulation of homeostatic processes. Plato's view belongs to a tradition referred to by Katz (2009) as the "Improvement indicator view," meaning that Plato saw pleasure as the satisfaction generated when a need is fulfilled. Such a need could stem from a biological disequilibrium (belonging to the body), or from imperfect knowledge (belonging to the soul). In Plato's ideal world, needs did not exist because it was a place without bodies and mental ignorance. This implies that no deficit mental states or biological imbalances could be set on such a scene, and further improvement from status quo was impossible. Thus, Plato reasoned that a perfect life was one without pleasure.

To Aristotle, pleasure did not regulate homeostatic balances. He held what Katz refers to as a "Perfection in functioning view," indicating that pleasure arises from being active, and different activities, or ways of performing them, produced different kinds of pleasure. To Aristotle then, pleasure could be an expression of the best life conceivable and Katz describes the role of pleasure in Aristotelian eudaimonics as "living a life that brings our biologically highest capacities to their complete development and then exercises them without impediment upon their naturally best and most suitable objects brings the most pleasant pleasure with it" (Katz, 2009, p. 28). Pleasure could, however, also signal less worthy activities, which is why pleasure in itself cannot be taken as an infallible indicator of a good life. Here is Aristotle's own words again: "Trivial or ignoble pleasures are sought instead by those who are stunted in their capacities or opportunities for higher activities, or else fail to develop the intellectual and moral virtues needed to use these well, and consequently fall short of the natural human goal" (Katz, 2009, p. 28).

After Darwin, scientists realized that "lower pleasures," or"bodily pleasures," are essential for survival and optimal functioning. At a general level this idea was grasped by many of the ancient thinkers as well, but modern knowledge allows for a more precise understanding of how pleasure is related to goodness. It is crucial, we now know, for biological organisms to have a representation of the current state of their living tissue, as well as a representation of what the desirable state of that tissue is. Damasio (2010) refers to such an optimal state as a homeostatic goal. In order for this set-up to be operative, the organism also needs an internal scale to compare its current state with the desirable goal. The solution evolution came up with for this challenging task was to invent feelings of pleasure and pain. In homeostatic processes, displeasure communicates to our minds that a state of deficit is building up whereas the message broadcasted by pleasure is that the return to a homeostatic set point is about to be, or has been, successful (Denton, 2005; Leyton, 2010; Panksepp, 1998).

From a phylogenetic perspective, a primitive form of pleasure may have had a role to play even before the homeostatic processes became governed by a central nervous system. Tracing the hedonic mechanisms back to their earliest origin, Humphrey (2002) finds that the rudiments of pleasure started when simple life forms, such as amoebas, began to monitor their body surface with an evaluative response. Even very primitive organisms must have developed an ability to classify their environments according to a simple category of goodness and badness, in order to cope with the essential question: "What is happening to me?" The information needed to deal with this critical issue is subjective, present-tense, transient, and qualitative. It is felt. It is felt by an organism as pleasure or displeasure and is interpreted by the experiencing organism as degrees of goodness and badness. Thus, the essence of a pleasant feeling is the evolutionary advantage of being able to "figure out" whether one's inner and outer environments are good or bad.

An informative description of the goodness function of pleasure was provided by a participant in a classic study investigating what a hedonic odor feels like: "When I say *pleasant* it doesn't stand for anything more than I would smell it more if I could. I am not able to discriminate anything beside that in most cases" (Young, 1927, p. 180). This verbal report goes to the heart of the functionality of pleasure—which is to make attractive to the experiencing subject whatever it is that appears as pleasant. Actually, such an account of pleasure has been maintained in scientific psychology since its very beginning. James (1890), for example, pointed out that feelings of pleasure facilitate life-enhancing activities and that we would not have such feelings if they had not served some useful purpose in our evolutionary history (cited in Denton, 2005, p. 8). In Germany, Wundt did not only consider pleasure as an irreducible mental element. He also understood it to be evaluative in the sense that pleasure implies acceptance of the stimulus or of the experience itself (cited in Frijda, 1986, p. 179). Wundt formulated the doctrine of "affective primacy" to describe how instant likes and dislikes prompt subjects to either approach or avoid a stimuli (see Haidt, 2012).

Consistent with these ideas, Cabanac (2010, 2014) reminds us about a fundamental task that dominates human lives: assessing our biological needs against the opportunities, or treats, presented by the environment. As a rule, Cabanac argues, the functional choice is that which takes us from an unfavorable state to a favorable one. "For this to happen, the required resource must first exhibit a gradient in the external environment. Otherwise, there will be nowhere better to move to" (Cabanac, 2009, p. 47). Needless to say, the resource in question is pleasure. Because of its amazing capacity to simplify a multitude of human experiences down to a one-dimensional preference scale,[3] which is what we need in order to prioritize among competing behaviors, Cabanac (1992) refers to pleasure as our "common currency."

To illustrate how pleasure transcends different sense modalities onto a single good-bad dimension, Cabanac (2009) had participants taste drinks of increasing sourness. For each sip, the participants reported how pleasant or unpleasant the drink was. Next, participants rated samples of increasingly sweet liquids. In the third and final phase of the experiment, participants were given samples of sour liquids, and could freely add as much sugar to the drink they preferred in order to make the best tasting drink. Based on each participant's preference for sourness and sweetness (provided by their previous pleasure ratings),

[3]The essence of this idea is adopted by thinkers and ideologists who model humans as rational agents. But the classic model of a rational agent assumes that preferences are stable, and this assumption is not included in the scientific models of momentary pleasures.

Cabanac could predict how much sugar each participant would add to their drinks by simply adding the two pleasure ratings. The study demonstrates that the displeasure of sourness is perfectly comparable to the pleasure of sweetness, and that behavior (at least in a laboratory) can be predicted by an algorithm that estimates the highest level of pleasure by calculating the sum of the sourness displeasure and the sweetness pleasure.

The hedonic dimension is not the only element of a feeling state, though. Besides varying in pleasantness, a feeling comprises a distinct quality, or "qualia" as philosophers often call it. Cabanac (2009) emphasizes that even if pleasure reflects the utility of a stimulus, it is the *quality* of a feeling state that describes its nature. The function of a feeling's quality, then, is discriminative in the sense that it enables us to categorize, or give meaning to, the stimulus at hand. Quantity is the third dimension of feeling states and its role is to describe the intensity of a stimulus. The fourth and final dimension of sensations is duration, which signals how long the stimulus is present (Cabanac, 2010).

Although all four elements of a feeling state have been mixed up in the literature on well-being, it is the difference between the pleasure element and the quality element that typically causes confusion. To some, pleasure is considered an umbrella term under which all positive emotions/feelings are grouped (e.g., Katz, 2009). Some psychologists follow a related practice, by defining pleasure as part of the quality dimension of an experience, on par with other qualities, such as feeling joy or fear (Schimmack & Crites, 2005; Schimmack, Oishi, Diener, & Suh, 2000). Other psychologists side with Cabanac and consider pleasure to be a hedonic element and not a feeling quality as such. According to this view, pleasure is like a "gloss of niceness" that comes on top of a feeling or an emotion, as Frijda described it. "Pleasure is not a feeling, not 'an experience of pleasure', not some felt inner state. (….) It is a niceness gloss to whatever the pleasure is about" (Frijda, 2007, pp. 66–67).

To illustrate the important difference between the quality component and the pleasure component of a feeling state, consider the taste of sweetness. Chocolate is typically both sweet (reflecting the quality dimension) and pleasant (reflecting the hedonic dimension). But it is only pleasant until one has eaten enough. Having too much chocolate is unpleasant even if the chocolate still tastes sweet, which shows that sweetness and pleasure are separable dimensions of a feeling state (Small, Zatorre, Dagher, Evans, & Jones-Gotman, 2001). Similarly, having a cold shower feels pleasant in a state of hyperthermia and unpleasant in a state of hypothermia (Cabanac, 2010), but in both cases we feel the quality of the water as cold.

The above examples are about sensational feelings, but the principle that separates the hedonic element from the quality element seems to apply for emotional and other mental feelings as well. Lazarus (1991) has pointed out that feeling drowsy can be either pleasant or unpleasant. "When one is lying in bed with nothing pressing to do, being drowsy is pleasant, but when one is sitting in a class or meeting at which one must pay attention, being drowsy is a distressing state that must be fought" (Lazarus, 1991, p. 824). Further empirical evidence for the distinction between qualias and hedonics comes from studies showing that feelings of interest can be be associated with stimuli that are either pleasant, neutral, or unpleasant (Lang, Bradley, & Cuthbert, 1990). More specifically, these researchers found that the images in the International Affective Picture System (IAPS) formed a unidimensional gradient from unpleasant to pleasant stimuli, whereas the relation between these pictures and interest was U-shaped. Hence, the emotional feeling quality of interestingness seems to be independent of its pleasantness.

Even feelings of happiness can presumably be disentangled from its hedonic component. Pleasure, satisfaction, and happiness are typically used synonymously, in ordinary language usage, so self-report research will normally not distinguish these terms from each other. Nevertheless, it seems reasonable to conceive of a dieter, say, having a feeling of both pleasantness and unhappiness when giving in to the temptation to consume an ice cream sundae. Similarly, the combination of extreme fatigue and a spectacular achievement could create feelings of both unpleasantness and happiness in a mountaineer who reaches the summit after a strenuous ascent. The important message from this line of reasoning is that something can be subjectively experienced as good without being felt as pleasant.

17.5 Hedonism: The Vulgar Version of Hedonics

The literature reviewed thus far illustrates how pleasure theorists consider hedonic feelings as indispensable and highly functional. Some refer to pleasure as a virtue, and Cabanac has gone so far as to put it on equal footing with the four forces in physics (i.e., gravity, electromagnetism, strong nuclear, and weak nuclear influences). Just as these forces act on masses and particles, pleasure acts on our brains. Hence, Cabanac (2009) proposes that pleasure is the "fifth element" of the forces of the universe.

But there is another idea about pleasure, widespread in some circles, that hedonia represents everything except virtues or importance. Rather, in this account pleasant feelings are signs of laziness, vulgarism, and bad morality. For instance, when Steger, Kashdan, and Oishi (2008) invited colleagues to propose phrases suitable for items intended to measure hedonic well-being, the suggestions they received included statements such as "Having sex purely to get pleasure," "Getting drunk," and "Masturbating." Likewise, when constructing the "Orientation to happiness scale" Peterson, Park, and Seligman (2005) created a pleasure dimension with items such as "Life is short—eat dessert first" setting the tone.

These approaches to hedonic well-being confuse the idea of hedonia (having to do with pleasure) with vulgar hedonism (having to do with rampant drinking, wantonness, gluttony, etc.). This unfortunate misconception is further illustrated by Wong (2011), who associates hedonic happiness with phrases such as "eat, drink, and be merry," and Steger and colleagues who refer to pleasure seeking as the doctrine of "doing whatever the hell I want to" (Steger, Shin, Shim, & Fitch-Martin, 2013, p. 164).

The idea of hedonics as something vulgar is much too crude to explain the complexities and functions of pleasure, a feeling that humans can not live without. As Kringelbach explains, "Pleasure can be defined as a way of fulfilling the evolutionary imperatives of survival and procreation. This leads to a classification of pleasure in fundamental (sensory, sexual, and social pleasures) and higher-order pleasures (for example monetary, artistic, musical, altruistic, and transcendent pleasures)" (Kringelbach, 2009, p. 10). If one, in contrast, equates pleasure with immoral behavior, then it cannot come as a big shock that Peterson et al.'s (2005) pleasure scale has turned out to be unrelated to both the experience of pleasant feelings (Vittersø, Dyrdal, & Røysamb, 2006) and to hedonic behavior (Henderson, Knight, & Richardson, 2014). Neither can it be very surprising to learn that Steger et al. (2008) find that people who often get drunk also report lower well-being than those who get drunk less often. By using items of vulgar hedonism, it is doubtful that researchers will discover anything essential about hedonic and eudaimonic well-being.

17.6 Satisfaction Is Hedonic

Life satisfaction is a cornerstone in the scientific study of well-being. It has traditionally been conceptualized as a rational comparison between what a person has with what that person thinks he or she deserves (Campbell, Converse, & Rodgers, 1976; Michalos, 1985; Shin & Johnson, 1978). More recently, however, life satisfaction has been conceived in less specific terms. Ed Diener, who is usually taken to be the doyen of subjective well-being, defines life satisfaction as "a report of how a respondent evaluates or appraises his or her life taken as a whole. It is intended to represent a broad, reflective appraisal that a person makes of his or her life" (Diener, 2006, p. 401). Another broad understanding of life satisfaction is offered by Wayne Sumner, a philosopher who claims that evaluating one's life favorably is the same as saying "that I am well off, or that I am flourishing" (Sumner, 1996, p. 20). Similarly,

Veenhoven (2003) insists that self-reports on overall happiness[4] provide reliable information about everything we need to know about participants' happiness. The prestigious "Stiglitz report" follows a similar line of thought, maintaining that measures of life satisfaction provide a convenient and reliable aggregate of people's various experiences and preferences. Snap-judgments about life satisfaction are even considered to "reflect the diversity of people's views about what is important in their lives" (Stiglitz, Sen, & Fitoussi, 2009, p. 145).

A little bit of reflection on our mental capacities brings to light some obvious troubles with this way of thinking. Humans are simply not equipped with the mental capacity to evaluate "everything important about their happiness." To put the amount of work needed for such systematic mental operations in context, consider the effort it takes to compare a series of very simple propositions against each other. According to Johnson-Laird, Girotto, and Legrenzi (2004), a set of 100 true/false propositions allows for 2^{100} possibilities, which would take over 40 thousand million million to examine (given that each possibility could be checked in a millionth of a second). Compare this, then, to the 2.2 s that people typically spend deciding how happy or satisfied they are with their entire lives (Robinson & Clore, 2002).

The discrepancy between what life satisfaction is supposed to be about, and what it possibly *can* be about—given the constraints of our mental capacities—is not only an unsolved puzzle in the research on subjective well-being. It is often ignored. For instance, in a thorough review, Diener, Inglehart, and Tay (2013) conclude that measures of life satisfaction "validly reflect the quality of respondents' lives." But if the term *valid* is taken to mean that life satisfaction scales are actually measuring what they are supposed to measure, i.e., a broad, reflective appraisal of everything important in a person's life, then Diener and his co-authors fall short of evidence. What it really would have taken to prove that "self-reported life satisfaction is a valid measure" is something showing that the variation captured with these scales are causally produced by changes in everything that is important in the participants' lives (Markus & Borsboom, 2013). In other words, for a life satisfaction measure to be considered valid, researchers must establish that the responses given to it are caused by "a broad, reflective appraisal made by a respondent regarding his or her entire life" (e.g., Diener, 2006, p. 401).

The validity claim about life satisfaction is further weakened by general knowledge about how responses to survey items are generated. After reviewing the relevant literature, Clore and Robinson (2012) concluded that, as a rule, self-reports are neither thoughtful nor reflective. To the contrary, they come from mental processes that are quick and easily produced. This is important, because fast/rapid information processing is biased towards that which is familiar and pleasant and away from events that are unfamiliar and complex (Gilovich & Griffin, 2010; Kahneman, 2011; Schwarz, 2004; Winkielman, Halberstadt, Fazendeiro, & Catty, 2006; Winkielman, Schwarz, Fazendeiro, & Reber, 2003). According to Tetlock (1992), it takes unusually powerful incentives to force people to make deeper analyses of self-report items (cited in Gilovich, Epley, & Hanko, 2005, p. 68). The typical self-assessment is therefore done relatively spontaneously and automatically. Moreover, rapid self-reports seem to be governed by an optimism bias, which leads the statements in a favorable direction (e.g., Baumeister, Vohs, Aaker, & Garbinsky, 2013; Newman, De Freitas, & Knobe, 2015; Schlegel, Hicks & Christy, Chap. 14, this volume). These insights have been further elaborated by Gilovich and colleagues, who argue that self-evaluations are biased towards favorable verdicts because of illusions most of us hold about our personal worth. "Because we try our best to structure our lives to produce positive experiences, the associations that are most accessible are likely to be positive" (Gilovich et al., 2005, p. 72).

[4]As many others (e.g., Adler, 2013; Christoffersen, Beyeler, Eichenberger, Nannestad, & Paldam, 2014; Easterlin, 2004; Helliwell, Huang, Grover, & Wang, 2014) I use life satisfaction and overall happiness interchangeably in this chapter, even if the overlap between them is not complete (e.g., Kahneman & Deaton, 2010).

Hence, when participants search for the information they need to answer questions about life satisfaction, it is a favorable self-view that most readily comes to their minds. And on the rare occasions that our optimism bias is corrected, responses are then modified through a conscious and effortful process of adjustment (Gilovich et al., 2005). What goes on mentally when self-reports on life satisfaction are produced is therefore strongly influenced by hedonic processes.

The hedonic element involved in survey responses to life satisfaction items is not necessarily pleasure in the sense of an intense feeling. Subjective judgments of goodness and badness need not be experienced intensely in order to be categorized as hedonic (Pratto, 1994). Because of their functional similarity, both pleasant feelings and rapid good-bad evaluations of low experiential intensity are plausibly referred to as hedonic (Roskos-Ewoldsen & Fazio, 1992). The purpose of both is to quickly inform the organism about the goodness and badness of their environments. Consider for instance the following observations by Zajonc: "When we meet a stranger, we know within a fraction of a second whether we like the person or not. The reaction is instantaneous and automatic. Perhaps the feeling is not always precise, perhaps we are not always aware of it, but the feeling is always there. If our later experience with the stranger conflicts with the first impression, we are terribly surprised. We consider it an exception" (Zajonc, 1980, p. 157).

If life satisfaction reports comprise a clear hedonic element, one could expect them to be unstable and to vary as a consequence of brief changes in temporary feelings and mood. Some argue that this is exactly what is going on. For instance, the mood-as-information paradigm, spearheaded by Norbert Schwarz (Messner & Wänke, 2011; Schwarz & Clore, 2003; Schwarz, Strack, Kommer, & Wagner, 1987), presents data to show that feelings and moods influence life satisfaction judgments. A classic example is the Schwarz and Clore (1983) study that documents how participants reported higher satisfaction with their lives as a whole on a sunny day than on a rainy day. More recently, Deaton (2012) showed how merely reminding survey participants about politicians, and by this presumably lowering their moods(!), reduced the estimated level of life satisfaction among US-citizens more than the 2008 economic crisis did. Despite these somewhat spectacular demonstrations of the influence of temporary feelings on overall life satisfaction, it turns out that mood and other ad hoc phenomena do not account for much of the variation observed in life satisfaction measures. For instance, both Eid and Diener (2004) and Schimmack and Oishi (2005) found that stable, or "chronically accessible information," accounts for over 70 % of the life satisfaction variance, whereas the influence from temporary sources account for less than 20 % of the variance.

Diener and colleagues think that this "chronically accessible" information about one's well-being reflects "facets of people's lives that they think are important and relevant to evaluations of their life, and are areas for which they often have a ready appraisal, such as marriage, health, and work" (Diener et al., 2013, p. 509). Similarly, Oishi (2012) argues that even if life satisfaction responses are quick, they need not be simple or hedonic. Fast self-report responses can reflect complex content, given that the answer has been well-practiced. After all, people often think about their happiness, most of us at least once a day according to Lyubomirsky and Lepper (1999). Given the assumption that people regularly and systematically analyze all the important elements of their lives, snap-judgments of life satisfaction can be well-informed, and provide valid clues as to how well the life of a respondent is going. When asked to evaluate their lives, the argument goes, people's idiosyncratic preferences do come to mind, even if they are of a complex nature. "Hedonists might judge their lives based on how much pleasure they feel each day, while moralists might judge their lives based on how virtuous their lives have been" (Oishi, 2012, p. 12).

Some of my own research casts doubt on this argument. For instance, in a demonstration of how evaluation of goodness and badness are hedonically biased, Lucie Glede Collet and I asked participants from a convenience sample in Norway ($N = 108$) to look at a set of photos, and for each image report how good or bad they

Table 17.1 Means and Standard Deviations (SD) for images rated either very good or very interesting

					Difficult		Difficult	
	Goodness		Interesting		Goodness		Interesting	
Type of image	Mean	SD	Mean	SD	Mean	SD	Mean	SD
Basically good	6.55	0.62	4.43	1.54	1.71	1.09	2.37	1.24
Basically interesting	3.54	1.17	5.28	1.22	3.30	1.68	2.65	1.30

N=108

evaluated it to be. We also asked how interesting the images were. Finally, the participants reported how easy or difficult it was to rank the images along the good-bad dimension, and along the interesting-uninteresting dimension (Collett, 2015). The results from the study showed that a picture of flowers and a picture of a palm beach got very high scores on the goodness scale and very low scores on the interesting scale. A picture of Mother Teresa and an image used in a campaign by Amnesty International[5] got very high scores on the interest scale and very low scores on the goodness scale. The next thing Collett and I did was to combine the flower image and beach image into a "basically good" variable, and the Mother Teresa and Amnesty images into a "basically interesting" variable. As shown in Table 17.1, the good images were significantly easier to evaluate than the interesting images. A within-participants *t*-test of the goodness scores gave a t-value (with df=107) of 9.31, $p<0.001$. Even the responses to the interesting scale were easier to produce for the good images, $t(107)=2.21$, $p=0.029$. What is most important, however, is that the participants had a hard time rating the extent to which the interesting images were good.

In addition to rating the goodness and interestingness of a total of 12 images, the participants in the Collet study also reported their level of life satisfaction, using the Satisfaction With Life Scale (SWLS; Diener, Emmons, Larsen, & Griffin, 1985), and their level of personal growth, using the Personal Growth Composite (PGC; Vittersø, Oelmann, & Wang, 2009). A multilevel path analysis showed that the SWLS predicted the tendency to rate images as good, but not as interesting. On the other hand, personal growth predicted participants' tendency to rate images as interesting, but not as good. Moreover, the within-participant correlation between ratings of interest and goodness was only $r=0.13$ ($p=0.003$). Hence, for the average participant, goodness ratings were only weakly associated with interestingness ratings. At the between-participant level on the other hand, the correlation between goodness and interestingness was much higher, $r=0.91$ ($p<0.001$). These numbers suggest that individuals tend to be disposed to give either high or low ratings of both goodness and interestingness, but that within their own range of responses, participants clearly differentiate between the two dimensions (Fig. 17.1).

In a different study I used a priming technique to illustrate how life satisfaction is biased towards hedonia, in the sense of being oriented towards pleasure and effortless activities. By random assignment, half of the participants were handed a questionnaire that started out with the five life satisfaction items (the SWLS) and then proceeded to an anagram puzzle. The other half started out with the personal growth items (the PGC) before the anagrams were presented. The hypothesis was that a mere exposure to the notion of life satisfaction would prime participants to put less effort into the problem solving task, as compared with participants exposed to the notion of personal growth. To measure the motivation to work hard on the problem, participants were able to choose how difficult the task would be. The choice was between four levels of difficulty, defined by the number of letters per anagram: four, five, six, or seven letters. As expected, participants in the "personal growth items first" condition preferred to work with more difficult problems, on average 6.4 letters as compared to 5.9 letters in the "life satisfaction items first"

[5]The image illustrated a barbed wire against a blue sky. The barbs at the end of the wire turned into birds that flew away into the sky.

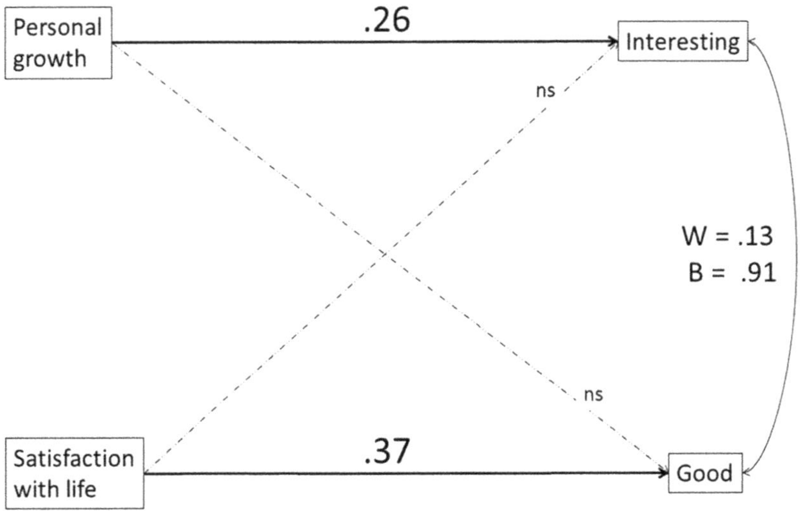

Fig. 17.1 A multilevel path model showing how life satisfaction predicts good-bad responses on a series of images, whereas personal growth predicts responses of interestingness. The numbers along the paths are standardized regression weights (betas) and W is the within-participant correlation coefficient and B is the between-participant correlation (all significant at $p < 0.05$)

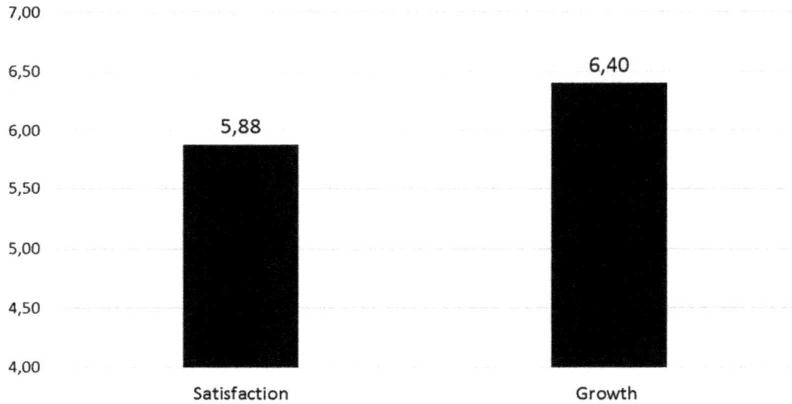

Fig. 17.2 Preferred level of difficulty for groups primed by either the Satisfaction With Life Scale (Mean = 5.88 letters) or the Personal Growth Composite (Mean = 6.40 letters). The difference is significant at $p = 0.018$

condition. The size of the difference between them, expressed as Cohen's d, was 0.63. The difference was significant, $t(62) = 2.43$, $p = 0.018$. See Fig. 17.2.

The two studies reported above provide support for the notion that ratings of life satisfaction reflect hedonic judgments in several ways. First, stimuli that are judged to be good are easier to rate than stimuli that are judged to be interesting. If this tendency generalizes across stimuli and events, the results suggest that areas in our lives that are interesting may be ignored when people self-report their life satisfaction. This follows from the tendency for easy elements to dominate the content of survey items. Second, individuals with high scores on life satisfaction also give high ratings to images that are judged to be good, but not to images that are judged to be interesting. For people with high scores on a personal growth scale, this trend was reversed. Third, compared with participants who had been exposed to a measure of personal growth, those who had been exposed to a measure of life satisfaction became motivated to perform easier tasks.

In general, an abundance of research shows that hedonic feelings tend to stimulate superficial information processing and prevent engagement in effortful activity (e.g., Forgas, 2014). The studies presented above extend these finding by illustrating that a similar tendency seems to operate for life satisfaction as well.

17.7 Eudaimonic Feelings and Their Functions

When Seligman and Csikszentmihalyi (2000) introduced the positive psychology movement in the "millennium issue" of American Psychologist, they did not use the term eudaimonia or eudaimonic well-being. They could have done so, however, because the two authors immediately warned against the limits of hedonic well-being. Just as neuroscientists try to tell us that "pleasure is only half of the happiness story" (Kringelbach & Berridge, 2009), Seligman and Csikszentmihalyi wrote about the difference between pleasure and enjoyment, as they called it. "Pleasure is the good feeling that comes from satisfying homeostatic needs such as hunger, sex, and bodily comfort. Enjoyment, on the other hand, refers to the good feelings people experience when they break through the limits of homeostasis—when they do something that stretches them beyond what they were—in an athletic event, an artistic performance, a good deed, a stimulating conversation. Enjoyment, rather than pleasure, is what leads to personal growth and long-term happiness" (Seligman & Csikszentmihalyi, 2000, p. 12).

Seligman and Csikszentmihalyi's note on pleasure and the regulation of homeostasis is certainly in line with common knowledge. Their use of the term enjoyment is more controversial. Enjoyment is sometimes used in the sense of being fully engaged in what one is doing, but more typically, its meaning comes closer to that of joy and pleasure (Ainley & Hidi, 2014; Renninger & Hidi, 2016). The similarities between pleasure and enjoyment was articulated already by Dewey (1913), who proposed that the paradigmatic experience associated with intellectual growth is interest, not enjoyment. Following up on this distinction, Tomkins (1962) pointed out that enjoyment (or "Enjoyment-Joy" in his terminology) is different from the emotions that serve a growth function, which he referred to as "Interest-Excitement." The difference between enjoyment and interest has also been elaborated in detail by Izard (1977). In an empirical test of their differentiation, Reeve (1989) found that it is interest, and not enjoyment, that characterized the kind of situations described by Seligman and Csikszentmihalyi as those that "break through the limits of homeostasis" (p. 12).

Seligman and Csikszentmihalyi are not the only scholars to ignore the concept of interest when looking for an experiential and functional contrast to pleasure. The long-lasting tradition of separating lower from higher pleasures has touched on this issue, as noted in the above review of Plato and Aristotle. In the twentieth century, still obeying the somewhat archaic terminology, Fromm (1947) proposed that lower pleasures follow from the satisfaction of needs, whereas higher pleasures are associated with the growth of insight (cited in Maslow, 1962). Writing in approximately the same period, Gordon Allport was an eager spokesman for separating the two different kinds of psychological functioning. He reasoned that humans must have evolved needs for both stability and variety, and the feeling of interest was among the regulating mechanisms for the latter. About the emotional regulation of stability and variety, Allport noted that "Along with striving, we may mention interest, tendency, disposition, expectation, planning, problem solving, and intention (…) While we want dependable modes of reduction tension we also abandon old habits and take risks in searching our new courses of conduct. It is only through risk-taking and variation that growth can occur. But risk-taking and variation are fraught with new and often avoidable tensions, which however we scorn to avoid" (Allport, 1955, p. 66). Other leading figures in the first wave of humanistic psychology were also concerned with the distinction between stability and change. Maslow (e.g., 1970) wrote extensively about the difference between deficit motivation and being motivation, and Carl Rogers admitted, after a long life as a psychotherapist, that the good life is not a state of contentment, happiness, or homeostasis. Rather, the fully functioning person strives in Rogers's opinion to gain an increasingly deeper understanding of his or her inner life (Rogers, 1961).

The concept of a fully functioning person is often taken to reflect eudaimonia, at least implicitly (e.g., Ryff, 1989; Waterman, 2013). According to Rogers (1963), the core characteristic of a fully functioning person is openness to experience. The prototypical feeling of openness is interest (e.g., Silvia & Kashdan, 2009; Vittersø & Søholt, 2011) and in more rare instances, awe (e.g., Keltner & Haidt, 2003; Danvers, O'Neil & Shiota, Chap. 21, this volume; Shiota, Keltner, & Mossman, 2007). Thus, in debating which subjective experiences are relevant to eudaimonia, I have chosen to use interest as a paradigmatic example for the feeling of personal growth. Awe is thought to be a good example of the kind of feelings associated with rare and dramatic moments of insight. They often have a social component, which fits with the idea of developing civic virtues. Employing interest and awe as examples of feelings that can be associated with eudaimonia is not to say that these feelings constitute eudaimonic well-being. Rather, they are but a few of several key features of eudaimonia. Neither am I arguing that interest and awe are the only feelings that accompany eudaimonia. Rather, my intention in the sections below is to illustrate that indicators of hedonic well-being (i.e., pleasure and self-reported life satisfaction) poorly reflect optimal functioning in areas that have to do with change and development. Interest and awe describe more precisely what personal growth and the development of virtues feels like. They are, for this reason, better indicators than pleasure and satisfaction when it comes to the experiential dimension of eudaimonic well-being.

A somewhat extensive review might be necessary to demonstrate the fundamental difference between the concepts of pleasure and interest. When it comes to awe, a review is provided by Danvers, O'Neil, and Shiota (Chap. 21, this volume) and it will therefore not be offered below. The in-depth investigation counters a widespread impression about hedonic and eudaimonic feelings as being almost identical. True, some frequently used measures of eudaimonia do overlap with measures of hedonic well-being (e.g., Disabato, Goodman, Kashdan, Short, & Jarden, 2016; Ward & King, Chap. 35, this volume; Proctor & Tweed, Chap. 18, this volume). However, the self-report measures in question tap in to only a fragment of the many elements that make hedonic and eudaimonic well-being different. For example, even if a self-report measure uses words and phrases that point in the direction of eudaimonic well-being, such a wording is not by itself sufficient to eliminate the hedonic biases inherent in these kinds of assessments. This point was articulated in section 17.6 about the hedonic nature of self-reported life satisfaction. Hence, in order to erect a fruitful debate, discussants of hedonic and eudaimonic well-being must avoid falling back on procedures of operationalism. For a long time now, operationalism in science has been considered flawed, since it is hard to see how a concept can be constituted by its 'operational definition' (e.g., Koch, 1992; Michell, 1999). Consequently, the concept of eudaimonic well-being cannot be eliminated because some self-report measures of it correlate highly with measures of hedonic well-being (see also Fredrickson et al., 2015; Fredrickson, Chap. 12, this volume; Smith, Tong, & Ellsworth, 2014).

17.8 Interest and Pleasure

The systematic investigation of the distinction between interest and pleasure began empirically with Berlyne and theoretically with Tomkins. Berlyne (1960) realized the importance of developing a fine-graded conceptualization of positive emotions, and his extensive studies of them suggested that the function of pleasure was related to satiation and stability, whereas interest prompts us to actively seek out "new sensations, new experiences and new knowledge" (Berlyne, 1949, p. 192).

The scientific understanding of the distinction between pleasure and interest also benefitted from Tomkins's (1962) amazingly clear understanding of the functional elements of feelings and affect. What Tomkins realized early on was that pleasure (or enjoyment) cannot sustain the kind of focused attention needed to handle a complex task or to motivate long term and effortful endeavors. When it comes to perception, for instance, a new and unfamiliar stimulus needs to be analyzed by a cognitive step-by-step process in order for us to understand its meaning. An unfamiliar object must be perceived both in detail and as a whole, Tomkins maintained, and complex surroundings must therefore be approached with a focused and sustained attention. Pleasure is simply not the right experiential mode when concentration is needed in order to analyze a complex stimulus. As illustrated by Fredrickson in her Broaden-and-build theory (Fredrickson, Chap. 12, this volume), pleasant feelings have the opposite effect on our attention. This is one reason why pleasure is not optimally functional in the face of challenges, complexities, and novel situations. Greenfield (2009) claims it is rather the opposite. Building on neuropsychological knowledge about how episodes of intense pleasure tend to temporarily shut down the parts of the brain involved in understanding difficult stimuli, she argues that pleasant feelings thwart the complicated analysis of the "what" part of meaning making. Pleasure reduces the capacity to do the step-by-step information processing sequences needed in order to understand and incorporate the nuts and bolts of a complex world into a meaningful whole.

In a dramatic and beautifully narrated introspection of an extremely blissful moment, Taylor (2008) has animated some of these mechanisms. As a neurologist hit by a stroke, Taylor could observe how a euphoric feeling of a joy "finer than the finest of pleasures" contributed to shutting down parts of her prefrontal cortex. "I had spent a lifetime of 37 years being enthusiastically committed to 'do-do-doing' lots of stuff at a very fast pace. On this special day, I learned the meaning of simply 'being.' When I lost my left hemisphere and its language centers, I also lost the clock that would break my moments into consecutive brief instances. Instead of having my moments prematurely stunted, they became open-ended, and I felt no rush to do anything. Like walking along the beach or just hanging out in the beauty of nature, I shifted from the going-consciousness of my left brain to the being-consciousness of my right brain. (…) I was not capable of deliberating about past or future-related ideas because those cells were incapacitated. All I could perceive was right here, right now, and it was beautiful" (Taylor, 2008, p. 74).

Taylor's description of her exceptional "stroke of insight" is anecdotal. It occurred during an instance of acute brain damage and is hard to generalize or replicate. Nevertheless, from a variety of sources, evidence now accumulates to suggest that pleasure impedes rather than stimulates the psychological processes needed for a thorough understanding of ourselves and our environments. Although this literature is not restricted to debating only pleasure and interest, a brief review of the studies on this particular distinction may be valuable in the effort to understand the differences between hedonic and eudaimonic elements of well-being.

17.9 Perception and Problem Solving

The distinction between pleasure and interest has been extensively researched within a paradigm of perception and problem solving. Quite often geometric figures such as polygons have been used as study stimuli. Day (1967) for example, asked participants to rank polygons of varying complexity and observed that as complexity increased, feelings of pleasure decreased and feelings of interest rose. Other studies have replicated this pattern (Aitken, 1974; Eisenman, 1966; Reeve, 1989). Silvia (2005) reported that participants who were asked to pick the most interesting polygon out of a sample that varied in complexity selected more complex polygons than participants who were instructed to pick the most enjoyable polygon.

In another context, Crozier (1974) factor analyzed subjective responses to music and sound sequences. He found that descriptions such as pleasant, good, and nice were accounted for by a different factor than descriptions like active, varied, and complex. Crozier referred to this structure as the "evaluative, activity model" of music perception. Elaborating on these principles, Gaver and Mandler (1987) fitted the findings on interest into the more general principles of cognition. Equipped with the concept of a schema and Piaget's analysis of cognitive development, Gaver and Mandler found that simple assimilation requires virtually no mental effort, whereas massive accommodation may demand extensive processing. Using music to illustrate their line of reasoning, the authors claimed that we find music that fits an existing schema pleasant, although such music is not interesting. In contrast, great works of music may emerge as interesting, even if they are not considered pleasant. The reason is that the complexity of great music cannot be easily assimilated, and this is exactly why it is interesting. Empirical data reported in Gaver and Mandler's article suggest that interestingness operates as an index of deviation from typicality.

My own research corroborates and extends the presented knowledge on how pleasure and interest differ. For instance, in one study conducted at a Folk High School in Lofoten, Norway, I invited the students to work on a small mathematical puzzle that could either be solved by System 1 thinking or System 2 thinking (Kahneman, 2011). A person activates his or her System 1 for easy and routinized information processing, like reporting the result of 2+2. It requires more effort and a different mentality to figure out the result of 17 times 24. The 17×24 puzzle can, for most of us, only be solved with logical reasoning and some computational efforts, i.e., System 2 thinking.

There are fascinating tests available to reveal whether people are allocating their attention to System 1 or System 2 reasoning. One such measure is Frederick's Cognitive Reflection Test (Frederick, 2005), which asks participants to solve the following mathematical problem: "A bat and a ball cost $1.10. The bat costs $1.00 more than the ball. How much does the ball cost?"

This was the puzzle presented to the students in Lofoten (using Norwegian currency), and 44 of them (53 %) answered 10 cents, and 38 students provided the 5 cent answer. The 10 cent answer is intuitive, but wrong, and it is attributed to System 1 thinking. The 5 cent answer is correct and requires the activation of System 2 thinking. Immediately after completing the bat and ball problem, the students were asked how happy and interested they felt when they labored on solving the problem. The 10 cent group and the 5 cent group were equally happy; the size of the difference between them, expressed as Cohen's d, was $d=0.12$, $t(80)=0.55$, $p=0.581$. For interest, on the other hand, the difference was substantial, with $d=0.82$, $t(80)=3.67$, $p<0.001$. The results graphically illustrated in Fig. 17.3 show how interest—but not happiness—discriminates between simple and complex reasoning.

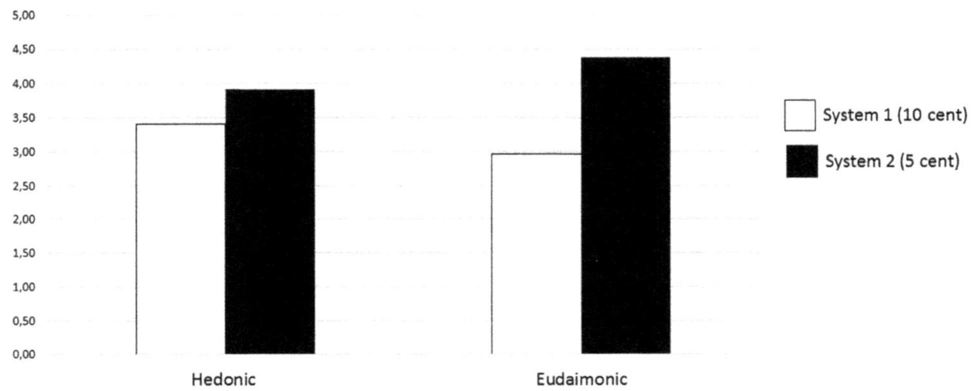

Fig. 17.3 Hedonic feelings (happiness) and eudaimonic feelings (interestingess) during System 1 and System 2 thinking

17.10 The Neuroscience of Eudaimonic Feelings

In his early review, Arnold (1906) proposed that interest's function is to broadcast a message about a possible pleasure that lies ahead. The feeling of interest itself, he said, is not pleasant. This idea was further developed by one of the most celebrated studies of the early days of neuroscience. The research took place in a primitive laboratory that James Olds had borrowed from Donald Hebb at McGill University. While looking for learning structures in the central nervous system, Olds and graduate student Peter Milner erroneously administered an electrical shock to the wrong part of a rat's brain, and thus stumbled upon one of the most fascinating phenomena ever discovered in biopsychology. What Olds and Milner (1954) found was that if rats, when wired to a self-administered device that gave electrical stimulation to a particular area of the brain, were given the choice to stimulate themselves, they would do so almost all the time. Rather than eating, drinking, or having sex, rats would press the lever to self-stimulate thousands of times in a row. The brain-area stimulated in these studies became known as the "pleasure center".

One thing, however, seems to have escaped the attention of most observers of this so-called intra-cranial self-stimulation (ICSS). It is that the behavior displayed by the rats in these states does not at all resemble anything akin to pleasant or hedonic behavior. Rather than the rewarding and consuming activities that typically accompany pleasant feelings, the self-stimulating animals look excessively excited, even crazed, when they work for this kind of stimulation. Thus, Panksepp (1998) suggests that terms such as intense interest and engaged curiosity better reflect the feeling systems involved in the ICSS behavior.

Berridge has suggested that the state elicited in Olds and Milner's rats is better described as "wanting" than as pleasure (Berridge, 1996). Wanting is a kind of incentive motivation that can be differentiated from pleasure, or "liking" in Berridge's terminology. A long series of studies documents how the two concepts differ, anatomically, physiologically, and phenomenologically (e.g., Kringelbach & Berridge, 2010b). According to Kringelbach and Berridge, it is *liking* that corresponds to the hedonic component of well-being: "'liking' without 'wanting' would be akin to what has been described by some world religions as bliss or "true" happiness" (Kringelbach & Berridge, 2010a, p. 11). A literature on the neurology of liking and wanting and how these states are associated with hedonic and eudaimonic well-being, respectively, is now growing fast (Berridge & Kringelbach, 2011, 2013; Kringelbach & Berridge, 2009; Lewis, Kanai, Rees, & Bates, 2014; Naor, Ben-Ze'ev, & Okon-Singer, 2014).

17.11 Other Differences Between Pleasure and Interest

The differences found between pleasure and interest when it comes to perception, problem solving, and neurological structures tell a convincing story about why all positive feelings should not be classified in the same category. Research from other areas adds to this view. For instance, Ekman (2003), p. 204 noted that all positive emotions, except interest and awe, share smiles as their facial signal. This finding has been corroborated in a recent cross-cultural study, reporting that interest, surprise, and awe were the only positive emotions not associated with a genuine smile, the so-called "Duchenne" smile (Cordaro & Keltner, 2015). From a review of the function of positive emotions, Campos and coauthors conclude that contentment and satisfaction are generally evoked by an appreciation for present circumstances and are associated with feeling satisfied and secure. Interest on the other hand, is typically evoked by environmental novelty and is associated with exploration (Campos & Keltner, 2014, p. 57). This group of researchers also found that among eight positive emotions, interest was the only feeling state that promoted exploration of novel stimuli (Campos, Shiota, Keltner, Gonzaga, & Goetz, 2012).

Smith et al. (2014) have proposed a taxonomy for positive emotions in which "benefit-related" emotions are separated from "opportunity-related" emotions. The former category covers emotions such as pleasure and happiness, whereas interest, challenge, and engagement exemplify the "opportunity-related" emotions. In the Functional well-being approach (FWA; Vittersø, 2013), a comparable separation between two categories of positive emotions and feelings has been made, although the labels are different. The FWA sorts positive emotions according to their role in sustaining the basic needs of stability and change. The argument offered by the FWA for choosing these labels follows from the central role played by these concepts, as reviewed above and testified in past work (Denton, 2005; Magnusson & Mahoney, 2003; Panksepp & Biven, 2012; Piaget, 1952; Staudinger & Glück, 2011; Valsiner, 1998).

In the FWA, and in the present chapter, the study of well-being is attached to the concepts of stability and change. Such a move, I hope, is a step towards grounding the concept of well-being onto a general scientific body of knowledge. After all, the idea that human functioning develops arounds stability and change is perhaps the most fundamental insight generated in the sciences of humans and other biological organisms. The needs for stability and change reflect, in the words of Bless and Fiedler (2006), the common theoretical denominator that connects all aspects of behavior regulation and adaptive functions.

17.12 Conclusion

William Shakespeare created strangeness in his plays to open up our minds. Strangeness in a dream-world may help us to look behind the immediate appearance of things, because sometimes the immediate appearance clutters the understanding we hold about ourselves and the world around us (Oatley, 2011). Human functioning also operates in a dynamic between dimensions that are immediately familiar to us and those that are yet to be discovered. No one appreciated this like Piaget, who also wrote wisely about dreams and fantasies (e.g., Piaget, 1962). During phases of assimilation, when reality is taken in without constraints, life events are easily processed and accompanied by feelings of pleasure (Eckblad, 1981). Conversely, a novelty that does not fit the existing schemas will challenge the conceptual status quo, and to understand it, the old schema must be revised according to the principles of accommodation. As realized by Piaget (along with Shakespeare and many others), the confrontation of a mental equilibrium is emotionally arousing, and not seldom experienced as unpleasant and thus avoided if possible. Hence, optimal human functioning works, as elaborated by Block (1982), by the following imperative: "Assimilate if you can; accommodate if you must!"

What these insights suggest is that human functioning operates at different levels and with different complexities and depths. If goodness is defined in relation to optimal functioning, it seems tenable to assume that it, too, should be categorized at different levels. It is good to be able to regulate homeostatic principles and to feel rewarded when important goals have been successfully achieved. Pleasure and satisfaction are the experiential instruments evolution developed to help maintain this kind of goodness. But sometimes it is good to stretch beyond the homeostatic balance and the "mental celebration" provided by hedonic feelings. Our biology uses a different and non-hedonic set of feelings to help manage this kind of goodness, and interest and awe are among these experiences.

The empirical literature on well-being is biased towards the first form of goodness, which is the simpler one. The reason is partly due to the extensive use of self-report data in the study of hedonic and eudaimonic well-being. While such measures work reasonably well for hedonic well-being, they fall short when it comes to eudaimonic well-being. Eudaimonia reflects a deeper kind of goodness, and a wider scope of more sophisticated methods are needed in order to grasp its complexities. Although the urge to gather numbers is strong in science, statistics will not rescue us from the premature state of knowledge that currently characterizes the study of eudaimonia. We cannot measure something unless we know what it is we want to measure.

Until more solid knowledge is available, we would be wise to heed the advice of Nussbaum (1992): "It is better to be vaguely right than precisely wrong."

References

Adler, M. (2013). Happiness surveys and public policy: What's the use? *Duke Law Journal, 62*, 1509–1601.

Ainley, M., & Hidi, S. (2014). Interest and enjoyment. In R. Pekrun & L. Linnenbrink-Garcia (Eds.), *International handbook of emotions in education* (pp. 205–227). New York: Routledge.

Aitken, P. P. (1974). Judgments of pleasingness and interestingness as functions of visual complexity. *Journal of Experimental Psychology, 103*, 240–244. doi:10.1037/h0036787.

Alkire, S. (2010). *Human development: Definitions, critiques, and related concepts*. Retrieved from OPHI Working Paper No. 36: http://ssrn.com/abstract=1815263.

Allport, G. W. (1955). *Becoming: Basic considerations for a psychology of personality*. New Haven, Connecticut: Yale University Press.

Arnold, F. (1906). The psychology of interest (I). *Psychological Review, 13*, 221–238. doi:10.1037/h0075836.

Arnold, M. (1960). *Emotion and personality*. New York: Columbia University Press.

Averill, J. R., & More, T. A. (2000). Happiness. In M. Lewis & J. Haviland-Jones (Eds.), *Handbook of emotions* (2nd ed., pp. 663–676). New York: Guilford.

Barrett, L. F. (2012). Emotions are real. *Emotion, 12*, 413–429. doi:10.1037/a0027555.

Baumeister, R. F., Vohs, K. D., Aaker, J. L., & Garbinsky, E. N. (2013). Some key differences between a happy life and a meaningful life. *The Journal of Positive Psychology, 8*, 505–516. doi:10.1080/17439760.2013.830764.

Berlyne, D. E. (1949). 'Interest' as a psychological concept. *British Journal of Psychology. General Section, 39*, 184–195. doi:10.1111/j.2044-8295.1949.tb00219.x.

Berlyne, D. E. (1960). *Conflict, arousal, and curiosity*. London: McGraw-Hill.

Berridge, K. C. (1996). Food reward: Brain substrates of wanting and liking. *Neuroscience & Biobehavioral Reviews, 20*, 1–25. doi:10.1016/0149-7634(95)00033-B.

Berridge, K. C., & Kringelbach, M. L. (2011). Building a neuroscience of pleasure and well-being. *Psychology of Well-Being, 1*, 1–26. doi:10.1186/2211-1522-1-3.

Berridge, K. C., & Kringelbach, M. L. (2013). Towards a neuroscience of well-being: Implications of insights from pleasure research. In H. Brockmann & J. Delhey (Eds.), *Human happiness and the pursuit of maximization* (pp. 81–100). Dordrecht, The Netherlands: Springer.

Binder, M., & Coad, A. (2011). Disentangling the circularity in Sen's capability approach: An analysis of the co-evolution of functioning achievement and resources. *Social Indicators Research, 103*, 327–355. doi:10.1007/s11205-010-9714-4.

Bless, H., & Fiedler, K. (2006). Mood and the regulation of information processing and behavior. In J. P. Forgas (Ed.), *Affect in social thinking and behavior* (pp. 65–84). New York: Psychology Press.

Block, J. (1982). Assimilation, accomodation, and the dynamics of personality development. *Child Development, 53*, 281–295.

Bonanno, G. A., Goorin, L., & Coifman, K. G. (2008). Sadness and grief. In M. Lewis, J. M. Haviland-Jones, & L. F. Barrett (Eds.), *Handbook of emotions* (3rd ed., pp. 797–810). London: The Guilford Press.

Bruce, H. F. (2010). Feelings and the body: The Jamesian perspective on autonomic specificity of emotion. *Biological Psychology, 84*, 383–393. doi:10.1016/j.biopsycho.2009.10.006.

Burchardt, T., & Vizard, P. (2011). 'Operationalizing' the capability approach as a basis for equality and human rights monitoring in twenty - first - century Britain. *Journal of Human Development and Capabilities, 12*, 91–119. doi:10.1080/19452829.2011.541790.

Cabanac, M. (1992). Pleasure. The common currency. *Journal of Theoretical Biology, 155*, 173–200.

Cabanac, M. (2009). *The fifth influence. The dialectics of pleasure*. Bloomington, IN: iUniverse.

Cabanac, M. (2010). The dialectics of pleasure. In M. L. Kringelbach & K. C. Berridge (Eds.), *Pleasures of the brain* (pp. 113–124). Oxford, UK: Oxford University Press.

Cacioppo, J. T., & Gardner, W. L. (1999). Emotion. *Annual Review of Psychology, 50*, 191–214.

Campbell, A., Converse, P. E., & Rodgers, W. L. (1976). *The quality of American life*. New York: Sage.

Campos, B., & Keltner, D. (2014). Shared and differentiating features of the positive emotion domain. In J. Gruber & J. T. Moskowitz (Eds.), *Positive emotion: Integrating the light sides and dark sides* (pp. 52–71). Oxford, UK: Oxford University Press.

Campos, B., Shiota, M. N., Keltner, D., Gonzaga, G. C., & Goetz, J. L. (2012). What is shared, what is different? Core relational themes and expressive displays of eight positive emotions. *Cognition and Emotion, 27*, 37–52. doi:10.1080/02699931.2012.683852.

Casebeer, W. D. (2003). *Natural ethical facts: Evolution, connectionism, and moral cognition*. New York: Cambridge University Press.

Christoffersen, H., Beyeler, M., Eichenberger, R., Nannestad, P., & Paldam, M. (2014). *The good society. A comparative study of Denmark and Switzerland*. New York: Springer.

Clore, G. C., & Robinson, M. D. (2012). Knowing our emotions: How do we know what we feel? In S. Vazire & T. D. Wilson (Eds.), *Handbook of self-knowledge* (pp. 194–209). New York: The Guilford Press.

Collett, L. G. (2015). *Images of a good life: Distinctions between pleasant and interesting elements in wellbeing.* (Unpublished Bachelor Thesis), UiT The Arctic University of Norway.

Cordaro, D. T., & Keltner, D. (2015). Universals and cultural variations in 22 emotional expressions across five cultures. *Manuscript in preparation.*

Crisp, R. (2005). Well-being. In E. N. Zalta (Ed.), *The Stanford encyclopedia of philosophy.* Stanford, Connecticut: Stanford University.

Crozier, J. B. (1974). Verbal and exploratory responses to sound sequences varying in uncertainty level. In D. E. Berlyne (Ed.), *Studies in the new experimental aesthetics: Steps toward and objective psychology of aesthetic appreciation* (pp. 27–90). New York: Wiley.

Damasio, A. (2010). *Self comes to mind: Constructing the conscious brain.* New York: Pantheon Books.

Damasio, A., & Carvalho, G. B. (2013). The nature of feelings: Evolutionary and neurobiological origins. *Nature Review Neuroscience, 14*, 143–152.

Day, H. (1967). Evaluations of subjective complexity, pleasingness and interestingness for a series of random polygons varying in complexity. *Perception and Psychophysics, 2*, 281–286.

De Dreu, C. K., Baas, M., & Nijstad, B. A. (2008). Hedonic tone and activation level in the mood-creativity link: Toward a dual pathway to creativty model. *Journal of Personality and Social Psychology, 94*, 739–756.

Dean, H. (2009). Critiquing capabilities: The distractions of a beguiling concept. *Critical Social Policy, 29*, 261–278. doi:10.1177/0261018308101629.

Deaton, A. (2012). The financial crisis and the well-being of Americans. *Oxford Economic Papers, 64*, 1–26. doi:10.1093/oep/gpr051.

Denton, D. (2005). *The primordial emotions: The dawning of consciousness.* Oxford, UK: Oxford University Press.

Dewey, J. (1913). *Interest and effort in education.* Boston: Riverside.

Diener, E. (2006). Guidelines for national indicators of subjective well-being and ill-being. *Journal of Happiness Studies, 7*, 397–404. doi:10.1007/s10902-006-9000-y.

Diener, E., Emmons, R. A., Larsen, R. J., & Griffin, S. (1985). The Satisfaction With Life Scale. *Journal of Personality Assessment, 49*, 71–75. doi:10.1207/s15327752jpa4901_13.

Diener, E., Inglehart, R., & Tay, L. (2013). Theory and validity of life satisfaction scales. *Social Indicators Research, 112*, 497–527. doi:10.1007/s11205-012-0076-y.

Disabato, D. J., Goodman, F. R., Kashdan, T. B., Short, J. L., & Jarden, A. (2016). Different types of well-being? A cross-cultural examination of hedonic and eudaimonic well-being. *Psychological Assessment, 28*, 471–482. doi:10.1037/pas0000209.

Doyal, L., & Gough, I. (1991). *A theory of human needs.* London: Macmillan.

Duncan, S. C., & Barret, L. F. (2007). Affect is a form of cognition: A neurobiological analysis. *Cognition and Emotion, 21*, 1184–1211.

Easterlin, R. A. (2004). The economics of happiness. *Daedalus, 133*, 26–33.

Eckblad, G. (1981). *Scheme theory. A conceptual framework for cognitive-motivational processes.* London: Academic.

Eid, M., & Diener, E. (2004). Global judgments of subjective well-being: Situational variability and long-term stability. *Social Indicators Research, 65*, 245–277. doi:10.1023/B:SOCI.0000003801.89195.bc.

Eisenman, R. (1966). Pleasing and interesting visual complexity: Support for Berlyne. *Perceptual and Motor Skills, 23*, 1167–1170.

Ekman, P. (2003). *Emotions revealed: Recognizing faces and feelings to improve communication and emotional life.* New York: Henry Holt.

Engel, G. (1977). The need for a new medical model: A challenge for biomedicine. *Science, 196*, 129–136. doi:10.1126/science.847460.

Fiske, S. T., Cuddy, A. J. C., & Glick, P. (2007). Universal dimensions of social cognition: Warmth and competence. *Trends in Cognitive Science, 11*, 77–83.

Forgas, J. P. (2014). On the downside of feeling good. In J. Gruber & J. T. Moskowitz (Eds.), *Positive emotion: Integrating the light sides and dark sides* (pp. 301–322). Oxford, UK: Oxford University Press.

Forgas, J. P., Haselton, M. G., & Von Hippel, W. (2007). *Evolution and the social mind: Evolutionary psychology and social cognition.* New York: Psychology Press.

Frederick, S. (2005). Cognitive reflection test. *Journal of Economic Perspectives, 19*, 25–42.

Fredrickson, B. L. (1998). What good are positive emotions? *Review of General Psychology, 2*, 300–319.

Fredrickson, B. L. (2001). The role of positive emotions in positive psychology. The Broaden-and-build theory of positive emotions. *American Psychologist, 56*, 218–226.

Fredrickson, B. L., Grewen, K. M., Algoe, S. B., Firestine, A. M., Arevalo, J. M. G., Ma, J., et al. (2015). Psychological well-being and the human conserved transcriptional response to adversity. *PloS One, 10*, e0121839. doi:10.1371/journal.pone.0121839.

Frijda, N. H. (1986). *The emotions.* Cambridge, UK: Cambridge University Press.

Frijda, N. H. (1994). Emotions are functional, most of the time. In P. Ekman & R. J. Davidson (Eds.), *The nature of emotion. Fundamental questions* (pp. 112–122). New York: Oxford University Press.

Frijda, N. H. (2007). *The laws of emotions.* Mahwah, NJ: Lawrende Erlbaum Associates.

Fromm, E. (1947). *Man for himself.* New York: Holt, Rinehart and Winston.

Gaver, W. W., & Mandler, G. (1987). Play it again Sam: On liking music. *Cognition and Emotion, 1*, 259–282.

Gilovich, T. D., Epley, N., & Hanko, K. (2005). Shallow thoughts about the self: The automatic components of self-assessment. In M. D. Alicke, D. Dunning, & J. Krueger (Eds.), *The self in social judgment* (5th ed., pp. 67–84). New York: Psychology Press.

Gilovich, T. D., & Griffin, D. W. (2010). Judgment and decision making. In S. T. Fiske, D. T. Gilbert, & G. Lindzey (Eds.), *Handbook of social psychology* (5th ed., pp. 542–588). Hoboken, NJ: Wiley.

Greenfield, S. (2009). *ID. The quest for meaning in the 21st century*. London: Sceptre.

Haidt, J. (2012). *The righteous mind: Why good people are divided by politics and religion*. London: Penguin.

Harmon-Jones, E., Gable, P. A., & Peterson, C. K. (2010). The role of asymmetric frontal cortical activity in emotion-related phenomena: A review and update. *Biological Psychology, 84*, 451–462. doi:10.1016/j.biopsycho.2009.08.010.

Helliwell, J. F., Huang, H., Grover, S., & Wang, S. (2014). *Good governance and national well-being: What are the linkages?* Paris: OECD Publishing.

Henderson, L. W., Knight, T., & Richardson, B. (2014). The hedonic and eudaimonic validity of the orientations to happiness scale. *Social Indicators Research, 115*, 1087–1099. doi:10.1007/s11205-013-0264-4.

Hochschild, A. R. (1983). *The managed heart: Commercialization of human feeling*. Berkeley, CA: University of California Press.

Humphrey, N. (2002). *The mind made flesh. Essays from the frontiers of psychology and evolution*. Oxford, UK: Oxford University Press.

Izard, C. E. (1977). *Human emotions*. New York: Plenum Press.

Izard, C. E. (2007). Basic emotions, natural kinds, emotion schemas, and a new paradigm. *Perspectives on Psychological Science, 2*, 260–280. doi:10.1111/j.1745-6916.2007.00044.x.

Izard, C. E. (2011). Forms and functions of emotions: Matters of emotion–cognition interactions. *Emotion Review, 3*, 371–378. doi:10.1177/1754073911410737.

James, W. (1890). *Principles of psychology*. New York: Henry.

Jayawickreme, E., & Pawelski, J. O. (2012). Positivity and the capabilities approach. *Philosophical Psychology, 26*, 383–400. doi:10.1080/09515089.2012.660687.

Johnson-Laird, P. N., Girotto, V., & Legrenzi, P. (2004). Reasoning from inconsistency to consistency. *Psychological Review, 111*, 640–661.

Johnston, V. S. (1999). *Why we feel: The science of human emotions*. Reading, MA: Perseus Books.

Johnston, V. S. (2003). The origin and function of pleasure. *Cognition and Emotion, 17*, 169–179.

Kahneman, D. (2011). *Thinking, fast and slow*. New York: Penguin.

Kahneman, D., & Deaton, A. (2010). High income improves evaluation of life but not emotional well-being. *Proceedings of the National Academy of Sciences, 107*, 16489–16493.

Katz, L. (2009). Pleasure. In E. N. Zalta (Ed.), *The Stanford encyclopedia of philosophy* (Fall 2009 ed.): Available from: http://plato.stanford.edu/archives/fall2009/entries/pleasure

Keltner, D., & Haidt, J. (2003). Approaching awe, a moral, spiritual, and aesthetic emotion. *Cognition and Emotion, 17*, 297–314. doi:10.1080/02699930302297.

Keyes, C. L. M., & Annas, J. (2009). Feeling good and functioning well: Distinctive concepts in ancient philosophy and contemporary science. *Journal of Positive Psychology, 4*, 197–201.

Koch, S. (1992). Psychology's Bridgman vs Bridgman's Bridgman. *Theory & Psychology, 2*, 261–290.

Korsgaard, C. M. (2008). *The constitution of agency: Essays on practical reason and moral psychology*. New York: Oxford University Press.

Kringelbach, M. L. (2009). *The pleasure center. Trust your animal instincts*. New York: Oxford University Press.

Kringelbach, M. L., & Berridge, K. C. (2009). Towards a functional neuroanatomy of pleasure and happiness. *Trends in Cognitive Sciences, 13*, 479–487. doi:10.1016/j.tics.2009.08.006.

Kringelbach, M. L., & Berridge, K. C. (2010a). Fundamental pleasure questions. In M. L. Kringelbach & K. C. Berridge (Eds.), *Pleasures of the brain* (pp. 7–23). Oxford, UK: Oxford University Press.

Kringelbach, M. L., & Berridge, K. C. (Eds.). (2010b). *Pleasures of the brain*. Oxford, UK: Oxford University Press.

Lang, P. J., & Bradley, M. M. (2010). Emotion and the motivational brain. *Biological Psychology, 84*, 437–450. doi:10.1016/j.biopsycho.2009.10.007.

Lang, P. J., Bradley, M. M., & Cuthbert, B. N. (1990). Emotion, attention, and the startle reflex. *Psychological Review, 97*, 377–395.

Lazarus, R. S. (1991). Progress on a cognitive-motivational-relational theory of emotion. *American Psychologist, 46*, 819–834.

LeDoux, J. (2012). Rethinking the emotional brain. *Neuron, 73*, 653–676. doi:10.1016/j.neuron.2012.02.004.

Lewis, G. J., Kanai, R., Rees, G., & Bates, T. C. (2014). Neural correlates of the 'good life': Eudaimonic well-being is associated with insular cortex volume. *Social Cognitive and Affective Neuroscience, 9*, 615–618. doi:10.1093/scan/nst032.

Leyton, M. (2010). The neurobiology of desire: Dopamine and the regulation of mood and motivational states in humans. In M. L. Kringelbach & K. C. Berridge (Eds.), *Pleasures of the brain* (pp. 222–243). Oxford, UK: Oxford University Press.

Lyubomirsky, S., & Lepper, H. S. (1999). A measure of subjective happiness: Preliminary reliability and construct validation. *Social Indicators Research, 46*, 137–155. doi:10.1023/A:1006824100041.

Magnusson, D., & Mahoney, J. L. (2003). A holistic person approach for research on positive development. In L. G. Aspinwall & U. M. Staudinger (Eds.), *A psychology of human strengths. Fundamental questions and directions for a positive psychology* (pp. 227–243). Washington, DC: American Psychologcal Association.

Mar, R. A., & Oatley, K. (2008). The function of fictionis the abstraction and simulation of social experience. *Perspectives on Psychological Science, 3*, 173–193.
Markus, K. A., & Borsboom, D. (2013). *Frontiers of test validity theory: Measurement, causation, and meaning [Kindle]*. New York: Routledge.
Maslow, A. (1962). *Toward a psychology of being*. New York: Van Nostrand.
Maslow, A. (1970). *Motivation and personality* (2nd ed.). New York: Harper and Row.
McMahon, D. (2006). *The pursuit of happiness. A history from the Greeks to the present*. London: Allen Lane.
Megone, C. (1994). Quality of life: Starting from Aristotle. In S. Baldwin, C. Godfrey, & C. Propper (Eds.), *Quality of life: Perspectives and policies* (pp. 28–41). London: Routledge.
Messner, C., & Wänke, M. (2011). Good weather for Schwarz and Clore. *Emotion, 11*, 436–437.
Michalos, A. C. (1985). Multiple discrepancies theory (MDT). *Social Indicators Research, 16*, 347–413.
Michalos, A. C., & Robinson, S. R. (2012). The good life: Eighth century to third century BCE. In K. C. Land, A. C. Michalos, & M. J. Sirgy (Eds.), *Handbook of social indicators and quality of life research* (pp. 23–61). Dordrecht, The Netherlands: Springer.
Michell, J. (1999). *Measurement in psychology: Critical history of a methodological concept*. New York: Cambridge University Press.
Moors, A., Ellsworth, P. C., Scherer, K. R., & Frijda, N. H. (2013). Appraisal theories of emotion: State of the art and future development. *Emotion Review, 5*, 119–124. doi:10.1177/1754073912468165.
Muffels, R., & Headey, B. (2013). Capabilities and choices: Do they make Sen'se for understanding objective and subjective well-being? An empirical test of sen's capability framework on German and British panel data. *Social Indicators Research, 110*, 1159–1186.
Nagel, T. (1974). What is it like to be a bat? *Philosophical Review, 83*, 435–450.
Naor, N., Ben-Ze'ev, A., & Okon-Singer, H. (2014). The modern search for the Holy Grail: Is neuroscience a solution? *Frontiers in Human Neuroscience, 8*, 505–516. doi:10.3389/fnhum.2014.00388.
Nesse, R. M. (1991). What good is feeling bad? *The Sciences, 31*, 30–37.
Newman, G. E., De Freitas, J., & Knobe, J. (2015). Beliefs about the true self explain asymmetries based on moral judgment. *Cognitive Science, 39*, 96–125. doi:10.1111/cogs.12134.
Nussbaum, M. C. (1992). Human functioning and social justice: In defense of Aristotelan essentialism. *Political Theory, 20*, 202–246.
Nussbaum, M. C. (2011). *Creating capabilities. The human development approach*. Cambridge, MA: The Belknap Press.
Oatley, K. (1992). *Best laid schemes. The psychology of emotions*. Cambridge, UK: Cambridge University Press.
Oatley, K. (2011). *Such stuff as dreams. The psychology of fiction*. Sussex, UK: Wiley-Blackwell.
Oatley, K., & Johnson-Laird, P. N. (1987). Towards a cognitive theory of emotions. *Cognition and Emotion, 1*, 29–50.
Oatley, K., & Johnson-Laird, P. N. (1996). The communicative theory of emotions: Empirical tests, mental models, and implications for social interaction. In L. L. Martin & A. Tesser (Eds.), *Striving and feeling. Interactions among goals, affect, and self-regulation* (pp. 363–394). Mahwah, NJ: Lawrence Erlbaum.
Oishi, S. (2012). *The psychological wealth of nations. Do happy people make a happy society?* Sussex, UK: Wiley-Blackwell.
Olds, J., & Milner, P. (1954). Positive reinforcement produced by electrical stimulation of septal area and other regions of rat brain. *The Journal of Comparative Physiological Psychology, 47*, 419–427.
Olson, R. (2015). *Houston, we have a narrative: Why science needs story [Kindle]*. Chicago: University of Chicago Press.
Panksepp, J. (1998). *Affective neuroscience. The foundations of human and animal emotions*. New York: Oxford University Press.
Panksepp, J., & Biven, I. (2012). *The archaeology of mind. Neuroevolutionary origins of human emotions*. New York: Norton.
Peterson, C., Park, N., & Seligman, M. E. P. (2005). Orientations to happiness and life satisfaction: The full life versus the empty life. *Journal of Happiness Studies, 6*, 25–41.
Phillips, D. (2006). *Quality of life: Concept, policy and practice*. London: Routledge.
Piaget, J. (1952). *The origins of intelligence in children*. New York: International Universities Press.
Piaget, J. (1962). *Play, dreams and imitation in childhood*. London: Routledge & Kegan Paul.
Pratto, F. (1994). Consciousness and automatic evaluation. In P. M. Niedenthal & S. Kitayama (Eds.), *The heart's eye. Emotional influences in perception and attention* (pp. 115–143). London: Academic.
Ramachandran, V. S. (2011). *The tell-tale brain. Unlocking the mystery of human nature*. London: Wiliam Heinemann.
Reeve, J. (1989). The interest-enjoyment distinction in intrinsic motivation. *Motivation and Emotion, 13*, 83–103.
Renninger, K. A., & Hidi, S. (2016). *The power of interest for motivation and engagement [Kindle]*. London: Routledge.
Robinson, M. D., & Clore, G. L. (2002). Belief and feeling: Evidence for an accessibility model of emotional self report. *Psychological Bulletin, 128*, 934–960.
Rogers, C. R. (1961). *On becoming a person*. Boston: Houghton Mifflin.
Rogers, C. R. (1963). The concept of the fully functioning person. *Psychotherapy: Theory, Research & Practice, 1*, 17–26. doi:10.1037/h0088567.

Roskos-Ewoldsen, D. R., & Fazio, R. H. (1992). On the orienting value of attitudes: Attitude accessibility as a determinant of an object's attraction of visual attention. *Journal of Personality and Social Psychology, 63*, 198–211. doi:10.1037/0022-3514.63.2.198.

Ross, W. D. (2009). *Aristotle: The Nicomachean ethics*. New York: Oxford University Press.

Ryff, C. D. (1989). Happiness is everything, or is it? Explorations on the meaning of psychological well-being. *Journal of Personality and Social Psychology, 57*, 1069–1081. doi:10.1037/0022-3514.57.6.1069.

Scherer, K. (2009). The dynamic architecture of emotion: Evidence for the component process model. *Cognition and Emotion, 23*, 1307–1351.

Schimmack, U., & Crites, S. L. (2005). The structure of affect. In D. Albarracín, B. T. Johnson, & M. P. Zanna (Eds.), *The handbook of attitudes* (pp. 397–435). Mahwah, NJ: Lawrence Erlbaum.

Schimmack, U., & Oishi, S. (2005). The influence of chronically and temporarily accessible information on life satisfaction judgments. *Journal of Personality and Social Psychology, 89*, 395–406.

Schimmack, U., Oishi, S., Diener, E., & Suh, E. (2000). Facets of affective experiences: A framework for investigations of trait affect. *Personality and Social Psychology Bulletin, 26*, 655–668.

Schwarz, N. (2004). Meta-cognitive experiences in consumer judgment and decision making. *Journal of Consumer Psychology, 14*, 332–348.

Schwarz, N., & Clore, G. L. (1983). Mood, misattribution and judgments of well-being: Information and directive functions of affective states. *Journal of Personality and Social Psychology, 45*, 513–523.

Schwarz, N., & Clore, G. L. (1988). How do I feel abuot it? The informative function of affective states. In K. Fiedler & J. P. Forgas (Eds.), *Affect, cognition and social behavior* (pp. 44–62). Toronto, Canada: C.J. Hogrefe.

Schwarz, N., & Clore, G. L. (2003). Moods as information: 20 years later. *Psychological Inquiry, 14*, 296–303.

Schwarz, N., Strack, F., Kommer, D., & Wagner, D. (1987). Soccer, rooms, and the quality of your life: Mood effects on judgments of satisfaction with life in general and with specific domains. *European Journal of Social Psychology, 17*, 69–79. doi:10.1002/ejsp.2420170107.

Seligman, M., & Csikszentmihalyi, M. (2000). Positive psychology: An introduction. *American Psychologist, 55*, 5–14. doi:10.1037/0003-066X.55.1.5.

Shin, D. C., & Johnson, D. M. (1978). Avowed happiness as an overall assessment of the quality of life. *Social Indicators Research, 5*, 475–492.

Shiota, M. N., Keltner, D., & Mossman, A. (2007). The nature of awe: Elicitors, appraisals, and effects on self-concept. *Cognition and Emotion, 21*, 944–963. doi:10.1080/02699930600923668.

Shiota, M. N., Neufeld, S. L., Danvers, A. F., Osborne, E. A., Sng, O., & Yee, C. I. (2014). Positive emotion differentiation: A functional approach. *Social and Personality Psychology Compass, 8*, 104–117. doi:10.1111/spc3.12092.

Silvia, P. J. (2005). What is interesting? Exploring the appraisal structure of interest. *Emotion, 5*, 89–102.

Silvia, P. J. (2008). Interest—the curious emotion. *Current Directions in Psychological Science, 17*, 57–60. doi:10.1111/j.1467-8721.2008.00548.x.

Silvia, P. J., & Kashdan, T. B. (2009). Intersting things and curious people: Exploration and engagement as transient states and enduring strengths. *Social and Personality Compass, 3*, 785–797.

Simpson, J. A., & Weiner, E. (1989). *The Oxford English dictionary* (2nd ed.). Oxford, UK: Oxford University Press.

Skidelsky, R., & Skidelsky, E. (2013). *How much is enough: The love of money and the case for the good life [Kindle]* (2nd ed.). New York: Penguin.

Small, D. M., Zatorre, R. J., Dagher, A., Evans, A. C., & Jones-Gotman, M. (2001). Changes in brain activity related to eating chocolate. From pleasure to aversion. *Brain, 124*, 1720–1733.

Smith, C. A., Tong, E. M. W., & Ellsworth, P. C. (2014). The differentiation of positive emotional experience as viewed through the lens of appraisal theory. In M. M. Tugade, M. N. Shiota, & K. N. Kirby (Eds.), *Handbook of positive emotions* (pp. 11–27). New York: Guilford.

Staudinger, U. M., & Glück, J. (2011). Psychological wisdom research: Commonalities and dofferences in a growing field. *Annual Review of Psychology, 62*, 215–241.

Steger, M. F., Kashdan, T. B., & Oishi, S. (2008). Being good by doing good: Daily eudaimonic activity and well-being. *Journal of Research in Personality, 42*, 22–42. doi:10.1016/j.jrp.2007.03.004.

Steger, M. F., Shin, J. Y., Shim, Y., & Fitch-Martin, A. (2013). Is meaning in life a flagship indicator of well-being? In A. Waterman (Ed.), *The best witin us: Positive psychology perspectives on eudaimonia* (pp. 159–182). Washington, DC: American Psychological Association.

Stiglitz, J. E., Sen, A., & Fitoussi, J.-P. (2009). *Report by the Commission on the measurement of economic performance and social progress*. Retrieved from Paris, France: http://www.stiglitz-sen-fitoussi.fr/en/index.htm.

Sumner, L. W. (1996). *Welfare, happiness, and ethics*. Oxford, UK: Clarendon.

Taylor, J. B. (2008). *My stroke of insight [Kindle]*. London: Hodder & Stoughton.

Tetlock, P. E. (1992). The impact of accountability on judgment and choice: Toward a social contingency model. In *Advances in experimental social psychology* (Vol. 25, pp. 331–376). San Diego, CA: Academic.

Thorsrud, H. (2015). Aristotle's dichotomous anthropology: What is most human in the Nicomachean ethics? *Apeiron, 48*, 346–367.

Tomkins, S. S. (1962). *Affect, imagery, consciousness. Vol 1. The positive affects*. New York: Springer.

Valsiner, J. (1998). The development of the concept of development: Historical and epistemological perspectives. In W. Damon & R. M. Lerner (Eds.), *Handbook of child psychology* (pp. 189–231). New York: Wiley.

Veenhoven, R. (2003). Happiness. *The Psychologist, 16*, 128–129.

Vittersø, J. (2009). Hedonics. In S. J. Lopez (Ed.), *The encyclopedia of positive psychology* (Vol. I, pp. 473–478). Malden, MA: Wiley-Blackwell.

Vittersø, J. (2013). Functional well-being: Happiness as feelings, evaluations and functioning. In S. David, I. Boniwell, & A. C. Ayers (Eds.), *The Oxford handbook of happiness* (pp. 227–244). Oxford, UK: Oxford University Press.

Vittersø, J. (forthcoming). *Oh, my goodness. Scientific approaches to a good life*. New York: Springer.

Vittersø, J., Dyrdal, G. M., & Røysamb, E. (2006). *Why we can't measure engagement with life satisfaction scales: Some theoretical and empirical arguments about their distinctiveness*. Paper presented at the 3th European Conference on Positive Psychology, Braga, Portugal, 3–6 July 2006, Brage, Portugal.

Vittersø, J., Oelmann, H., & Wang, A. L. (2009). Life satisfaction is not a balanced estimator of the good life. Evidence from reaction time measures and self-reported emotions. *Journal of Happiness Studies, 10*, 1–17. doi:10.1007/s10902-007-9058-1.

Vittersø, J., & Søholt, Y. (2011). Life satisfaction goes with pleasure and personal growth goes with interest: Further arguments for separating hedonic and eudaimonic well-being. *Journal of Positive Psychology, 6*, 326–335. doi:10.1080/17439760.2011.584548.

Waterman, A. (2013). Introduction: Considering the nature of a life well lived-intersections of positive psycholgy and eudaimonist philosophy. In A. Waterman (Ed.), *The best witin us: Positive psychology perspectives on eudaimonia* (pp. 3–17). Washington, DC: American Psychological Association.

Watts, A. G., & Donovan, C. M. (2010). Sweet talk in the brain: Glucosensing, neural networks, and hypoglycemic counterregulation. *Frontiers in Neuroendocrinology, 31*, 32–43. doi:10.1016/j.yfrne.2009.10.006.

Wessman, A. E., & Ricks, D. F. (1966). *Mood and personality*. New York: Holt, Reinehart & Winston.

Whiting, J. (1988). Aristotle's function argument: A defense. *Ancient Philosophy, 8*, 33–48.

Winkielman, P., Halberstadt, J., Fazendeiro, T., & Catty, S. (2006). Prototypes are attractive because they are easy on the mind. *Psychological Science, 17*, 799–806. doi:10.1111/j.1467-9280.2006.01785.x.

Winkielman, P., Schwarz, N., Fazendeiro, T. A., & Reber, R. (2003). The hedonic marking of processing fluency: Implications for evaluative judgment. In J. Musch & K. C. Klauer (Eds.), *The psychology of evaluation. Affective processes in cognition and emotion* (pp. 189–217). Mahwah, NJ: Lawrence Erlbaum.

Wong, P. T. P. (2011). Positive psychology 2.0: Towards a balanced interactive model of the good life. *Canadian Psychology/Psychologie canadienne, 52*, 69–81. doi:10.1037/a0022511.

Yiend, J. (2010). The effects of emotion on attention: A review of attentional processing of emotional information. *Cognition & Emotion, 24*, 3–47.

Young, P. T. (1927). Studies of affective psychology. *The American Journal of Psychology, 38*, 157–193.

Zajonc, R. B. (1980). Feelings and thinking: Preferences need no inferences. *American Psychologist, 35*, 151–175.

Zajonc, R. B. (2001). Feeling and thinking. Closing the debate over the independence of affect. In J. P. Forgas (Ed.), *Feeling and thinking. The role of affect in social cognition* (pp. 31–58). Cambridge, UK: Cambridge University Press.

18 Measuring Eudaimonic Well-Being

Carmel Proctor and Roger Tweed

18.1 Introduction

The concept of eudaimonia is not widely understood outside of the positive psychology and philosophy fields and not consistently defined within them. As noted by Huta and Waterman (2014), eudaimonia is often loosely or vaguely defined, "without clear identification of the concepts believed to be a core part of the definition and concepts believed to be correlates" (p. 1426). Perhaps, what is understood by most is the idea of individual progress and development towards the "good life" (e.g., Maslow, 1999; Rogers, 1961). This idea of progress on a path to the good life makes intuitive sense based on theories of human development and plays on our understanding of ourselves as teleological beings in process towards an end goal. For example, Rogers' view of the meaning of the good life was based on his conception of the "fully functioning" person – that is, a person-in-process, a person continually changing in growth oriented ways. Similarly, Maslow (1954) suggested that once our basic needs are met, human beings have an innate tendency towards constant betterment – "metamotivation" towards satisfaction of higher needs and self-actualization.

Philosophers, most notably Aristotle (c. 330 BCE/1925), argued that there needs to be more to living than just being; that is, that there must be some ultimate function of human beings, and that exercising this function is what gives meaning to our being. The exact nature of Aristotle's meaning regarding this ultimate function is less clear. In particular, the meaning of living well or exercising the eudaimon life (i.e., human flourishing) as presented by Aristotle remains in dispute (e.g., Huta & Waterman, 2014).

Even though details of Aristotle's meaning remain in dispute, some elements of his intention seem clear from his writings. In particular, Aristotle wished to convey that eudaimonia is achieved through the pursuit and exercising of virtue or excellence. Eudaimonia is good moral activity (moral excellence) or good intellectual activity (intellectual excellence). Activities that produce excellence are virtuous – that is, avoid excess and deficit. According to Aristotle (c. 330 BCE/1925), what must be sought is the mean or intermediate relative to us – acts must be done "at the right times, with reference to the right objects, towards the right people, with the right motive, and in the right way" (p. 38). Indeed, Aristotle suggests that in doing virtuous acts we become

C. Proctor (✉)
PPRC, PO Box 544, St. Peter Port,
Guernsey GY1 6HL, UK
e-mail: carmel@pprc.gg

R. Tweed
Kwantlen Polytechnic University,
12666 – 72nd Avenue, Surrey, BC V3W 2M8,
Canada
e-mail: roger.tweed@kpu.ca

J. Vittersø (ed.), *Handbook of Eudaimonic Well-Being*, International Handbooks of Quality-of-Life,
DOI 10.1007/978-3-319-42445-3_18

virtuous, but this is hinged on doing such acts with the knowledge and desire to do them *because* they are virtuous and to carry them out *as* a virtuous person of good character would do them (see Aristotle, c. 330 BCE/1925, p. 35). That is, Aristotle acknowledges that it is possible to do acts that appear to be virtuous, but are carried out without being "good". He also makes clear that one cannot carry out immoral or "bad" acts "at the right time, and in the right way" because "to do any of them is to go wrong" – "there is no mean nor any excess and deficiency, but however they are done they are wrong" (Aristotle, c. 330 BCE/1925, p. 39).

According to Aristotle (c. 330 BCE/1925), virtue also has an essential connection with pleasure and pain. Indeed, Aristotle notes that "virtuous actions must be in themselves pleasant" (p. 17). He said this because he believed that doing apparently virtuous actions out of painful duty indicates that the underlying virtue has not yet been attained: "the man who does not rejoice in noble actions is not even good; since no one would call a man just who did not enjoy acting justly, nor any man liberal who did not enjoy liberal actions" (p. 16). Initially, therefore, actions that appear virtuous may require the type of self-control or willpower that Baumeister and Tierney (2011) have argued is the greatest human strength. According to Aristotle, once virtue has been attained, the behavioral manifestations will not be difficult or painful. He believed that virtue, in contrast, is pained by vice, so we can "measure even our actions, some of us more and others less, by the rule of pleasure and pain. For this reason then, our whole inquiry must be about these; for to feel delight and pain rightly or wrongly has no small effect on our actions" (p. 33). This ideal outcome of taking pleasure in the right cannot be attained quickly. In fact, he defined eudaimonia as the ultimate end, but noted that it is a process that requires habituation. Much like Rogers (1961) concept of "becoming" a fully functioning person, Aristotle espoused habituating into virtue (i.e., becoming virtuous) as a means of working towards the objectively desirable life – to know and experience oneself as living well. Similarly, Maslow's (1999) concept of the hierarchy of needs that describe human growth towards "self-actualization" – is another concept or construct that involves striving towards an ultimate end, but also involves a progressive enhancement of our being. Similarly, eudaimonia is an ongoing process during one's life – a process of pleasures and pains associated with the actions and passions of life (Aristotle, c. 330 BCE/1925).

In contrast, pleasure or hedonia, according to Aristotle, is not a transition or process (Aristotle, c. 330 BCE/1925). Therefore, pleasure is not an ultimate function of human beings or an end in itself, because it is complete in the time that it occurs. However, pleasure is a *good*, which differs in kind according to different activities, and may even be the *summum bonum* or essential element of eudaimonia.

Even though eudaimonia and hedonia are distinct – eudaimonia is a process and hedonia is not – the two are related. Indeed, Aristotle believed that the eudaimonic process will enhance pleasure and transform other activities to make them pleasurable. In particular, Aristotle particularly argued that for someone who has not made steps toward a eudaimonic character, it will be difficult to exert self-control (or willpower) when engaging in particular acts of good; for example, abstaining from unhealthy bodily pleasures to become temperate. For this person, restraining unhealthy bodily desires will be frustrating – such a person is, in accordance with Plato, being pained by virtue instead of being "pained by the things that we ought [i.e., vice]" (Aristotle, c. 330 BCE/1925, p. 32). In contrast, the person who has made steps toward eudaimonia will find pleasure in acts of good; for example, when we have abstained from unhealthy bodily pleasures and become temperate, we are more easily able to abstain and take pleasure in doing so. Thus, both pleasure and pain result from eudaimonia – indeed "[n]ow for most men their pleasures are in conflict with one another…but the lovers of what is noble find pleasant the things that are by nature pleasant; and virtuous actions are such, so that these are pleasant for such men…Their life, therefore, has no further need of pleasure as a sort of adventitious charm, but has its pleasure in itself" (Aristotle, c. 330 BCE/1925, p. 16).

In this chapter we define eudaimonia based on Aristotle's definition and philosophical conceptualization. Aristotle was concerned with what the ultimate good was for humans – what the most enviable life was. According to Aristotle, life consists of the pursuit of ends. Ends are goods that can be aimed at, activities themselves, or products of activities. However, for Aristotle there is one end that is most desirable – an end in itself – eudaimonia. He believed that this end must be chosen for itself, for its own sake, and be satisfying with no need for supplementation. By Aristotle's definition, eudaimonia is:

> [A]ctivity of soul [(i.e., virtuous or intellectual activity)] exhibiting excellence, and if there are more than one excellence [(or virtue)], in accordance with the best and most complete. But we must add 'in a complete life'. For one swallow does not make a summer, nor does one day; and so too one day, or a short time, does not make a man blessed and happy. (Aristotle, c. 330 BCE/1925, p. 14)

The purpose of this chapter is to provide a brief review of the concept of eudaimonia, explore the challenges associated with its measurement, and offer suggestions for researchers currently choosing measures of eudaimonia. In terms of measurement challenges, we consider the extent to which the heterogeneous conceptualizations of eudaimonia as the "ultimate good" might inherently make it difficult to measure. Also, even if we achieve consensus on a concept of eudaimonia, the concept may be difficult to measure because of issues related to measuring virtue. We posit that a defining factor in the measurement of eudaimonia that makes it different from the assessment of other related constructs, is the inclusion of the assessment of virtue. The lack of virtue measurement in a number of common assessments of eudaimonic well-being given Aristotle's definition is presented.

18.2 Measurement Challenges

Measuring eudaimonia appears to be inherently challenging, this is due in part to the majority of research and discussions of eudaimonia placing minimal emphasis on the heart of Aristotle's original intended meaning. Admittedly, language and definitions change over time; therefore, if modern researchers and philosophers were to replace Aristotle's definition with a widely agreed upon definition that facilitated research and communication, then departing from Aristotle's definition might make sense. However, departing into a variety of distinct definitions and assumptions is problematic because these distinct definitions become barriers to communication and research. At times, it seems that the main consensus regarding eudaimonia, is what eudaimonia does not mean. Indeed, among modern users of this term, "eudaimonia" would possibly be defined with most consensus when defined negatively. In particular, eudaimonia is well-being that is not mere pleasure. Other definitions have been offered, but the varieties of definitions are hard to reconcile, therefore eudaimonia is often defined most simply by saying what it is not. This negative definition alone lacks satisfactory value however because a negative definition like this could allow the concept of eudaimonia to grow to encompass almost all positively valued human variables, thus losing its distinctive value.

Historical precedent exists for using negative definitions for complex concepts. For example, ancient writers, such as Dionysius the Pseudo-Areopagite, proposed that negative definitions have value when something is too difficult to describe. Dionysius reasoned that the divine was too difficult to understand, and therefore it was best described by saying what it was not. This type of approach, despite re-appearing occasionally throughout history (e.g., *The Cloud of Unknowing*), has proved problematic and failed to solve problems of scholarly debate. Thus, possibly there is value in departing from negative definitions of eudaimonia and seeking a return to a greater emphasis on Aristotle's ideas concerning virtue and excellence. Within our discussion, we hope to demonstrate, not a rejection of modern definitions, but a proposition that modern definitions are more firmly rooted when related to virtue and excellence.

18.2.1 The Lack of Attention to the Virtue Hypothesis

Admittedly, Aristotle's emphasis on virtue as central to well-being is echoed in some modern work discussing well-being. For example, as noted by Robbins (2008), "the virtue hypothesis predicts that happiness is derived from the cultivation of virtue" (p. 103).

One of the most surprising characteristics of measures of eudaimonia, however, is the glaring absence or at least minimal representation of virtue-related constructs. Admittedly, some scholars have expanded the definition of eudaimonia to encompass more than the pursuit of virtue and excellence, and therefore, it may make sense from their perspective, to include additional elements in their operationalization of eudaimonia. For example, Huta and Waterman (2014) argue that the modern concept of eudaimonia should not be limited to the original concept from Aristotle, but be expanded to include both ways of functioning and subjective states that result from the pursuit of virtue and excellence (see also Huta, Chap. 15, this volume).

Nonetheless, the pursuit of virtue and excellence are central to the original definition of eudaimonia, so one would expect virtue to at least have a strong representation within measures of eudaimonia. Yet, virtue is minimally present or even absent in most measures currently used to assess eudaimonia.

This tendency suggests that currently used measures of eudaimonia are incomplete because of their minimal representation of virtue. The construct of personal meaning illustrates this tendency. Measures of personal meaning have been suggested as indicators of eudaimonia (Huta & Waterman, 2014) with reasonable justification (Huta & Ryan, 2010; Wong, 2011). The most common self-report measure of meaning is perhaps the Meaning in Life Questionnaire (MLQ) created by Steger and Shin (2010). This scale has many desirable aspects, including good internal consistency and evidence of convergent and discriminant validity (Steger & Shin, 2010) – its use by various scholars also suggests its value in testing other hypotheses. The MLQ assesses whether one is experiencing a sense of meaning and whether one is searching for meaning. However, as the scale does not assess virtue, there is no means of determining from what ends meaning is being derived. We do not mean to demean the utility of Steger and Shin's excellent measure, nor the reasonable suggestion that personal meaning can have a role in assessing eudaimonia (Huta & Waterman, 2014), but instead intend to point out that a complete measure of eudaimonia would need to also assess whether meaning is being derived from virtuous ends. Similarly, one could consider the Flourishing Scale (FS; Diener et al., 2009). The measurement of flourishing was proposed as a measure of well-being distinct from assessment of positive and negative emotions (hedonia), and it is often used an indicator of eudaimonic well-being. However, only two of the items assess whether the experience of flourishing is derived from virtuous ends, those being: "I actively contribute to the happiness and well-being of others" and "I am a good person and live a good life" (Diener et al., 2009). Our conclusion about the Flourishing Scale is similar to that about the meaning items of the MLQ: The measure seems to serve its intended purpose fairly well, but would not be complete as solitary indicator of eudaimonia.

Indeed, in order to be in keeping with Aristotle's notion of virtue, scales would need to not only consider virtue, but also to distinguish it from vice:

> For instance, both fear and confidence and appetite and anger and pity and in general pleasure and pain maybe felt both too much and too little, and in both cases not well; but to feel them at the right times, with reference to the right objects, towards the right people, with the right motive, and in the right way, is what is both intermediate and best, and this is characteristic of virtue...Virtue, then, is a state of character concerned with choice, lying in a mean, i.e., the mean relative to us, | this being determined by rational principle, and by that principle by which the man of practical wisdom would determine it. Now it is a mean between two vices, that which depends on excess and that which depends on defect; and again it is a mean because the vices respectively fall short of or exceed what is right in both passions and actions, while virtue both finds and chooses that which is intermediate. (Aristotle, c. 330 BCE/1925, p. 38–39)

The minimal presence of virtue or vice in most operationalizations of eudaimonia is surprising given the fact that moral rectitude is at the very root of the concept of eudaimonia. As discussed earlier, the term eudaimonia is inextricably linked to virtue. Nevertheless, as noted by Robbins (2008), "positive psychology engages in the activity of normative ethics to the extent that it aspires to a eudaimonic concept of ethics, which identifies the state of happiness with the acquisition of virtue", but does not admit to being "engaged in the activity of *prescriptive* valuation" (p. 103).

One might question why the virtue aspect is largely absent from the measures of eudaimonia. Possibly, researchers are swayed by the view of science as value-free, and therefore avoid discussion of virtue. Perhaps researchers are uncomfortable discussing virtue because they know they fall short of their own virtue ideal. Perhaps virtue is difficult to assess because respondents, in our experience, even those engaged in behavior that society judges as immoral, often perceive themselves as relatively virtuous (e.g., criminal offenders who seem to devote significant attention to thinking about their own virtue compared to others who commit worse crimes, or compared to others who fail to adhere to particular standards for social interaction). Nevertheless, as suggested by Robbins (2008), the "value neutral position is not a realistic aspiration for a researcher or therapist" (p. 104).

We too know that it can be difficult to write about virtue when we know we are not exemplars of complete virtuous achievement. Aristotle, likewise, believed complete virtue is a target that is never completely achieved. Nonetheless, unless one proposes a radically different definition of eudaimonia, discussion of eudaimonia requires discussion of virtue.

One of the few exceptions to this principle is the work of Wong (2011). Wong has defined eudaimonia as meaning plus virtue. "A meaning orientation with a focus on virtues becomes a eudaimonic orientation" (Wong, 2011, p. 75). Wong has refused to give up his strong convictions in order to follow the prevailing trends in research. He has highlighted an important element that deserves more inclusion in measures of eudaimonia. According to Wong, "[w]hat is good, depends on the purpose it serves. *Good* must mean good for *something*...[t]he good life demands the presence of virtue" (p. 73). Some others have agreed. For example, Sandstrom and Dunn (2011) have spoken of a blind spot of psychology being the relative absence of a focus on virtue.

Because efforts toward virtue can become misguided, Aristotle also suggested a role for practical wisdom. In fact, a genuinely Aristotelian perspective of eudaimonia demands the use of virtues in everyday life with the guidance of practical wisdom, or *phronesis* – having the knowledge of the rules of morality, as well as "an intelligent understanding of the reason for them" (Aristotle, c. 330 BCE/1925, p. xvi; Robbins, 2008). In keeping with Aristotle, Schwartz and Sharpe (2006) define practical wisdom as the "master virtue", "essential for orchestrating the other virtues into an effective and happy life" (p. 383). Indeed, according to Aristotle, the essential nature of practical wisdom in living a eudaimon life is self-evident (Schwartz & Sharpe, 2006).

Huta and Waterman (2014) suggest an expansion of the modern concept of eudaimonia. Accordingly, we argue for researchers to include virtue as an essential element. To that end, measures of eudaimonia could treat eudaimonia as a conjunctive construct – Wong's (2011) ideas illustrate this point. He argued that virtue must be present for eudaimonia to be genuine. If a person has some elements of eudaimonia, but not virtue, the person does not have 50 % of eudaimonia; instead one is completely lacking eudaimonic well-being.

Perhaps an analogy of a well-functioning vehicle will further help illustrate the concept of a conjunctive construct. Imagine a person renting a car to drive from Beijing to Shanghai. Imagine if the renter asks the owner whether the car works well, and the owner says, "Oh yes, the car works pretty well". But then the passenger finds out that the transmission has seized up and won't operate. Even though almost all parts of the car work well, the driver would be wrong to say the car works pretty well. No, a well-functioning car is a conjunctive construct that requires all the essential elements to be operating. The absence of any essential element means the car is not functioning. Similarly, eudaimonia, according to traditional definitions, would require one's behavior to be virtuous. Virtue is not merely a desirable element that makes eudaimonia even better: Virtue is essential for eudaimonia to be present.

This does not mean that existing measures are lacking utility; instead, to be complete, they would need to be supplemented by an implementation that treats virtue as an essential element of virtue. In other words, the researcher would need to treat eudaimonia as conjunctive.

18.3 Measurement of Eudaimonia

In light of the prior discussion, it is worth considering some current measures that can be used to assess eudaimonia. The organization of this brief review of measures of eudaimonia is designed to quickly help researchers find a measure that may match their research needs. There are many possible measures of eudaimonia, and this review is not intended to be comprehensive. Our method of organizing this review of measures relies heavily on Huta and Waterman's (2014) insightful classification for organizing the concept of eudaimonia. They differentiate definitions of eudaimonia into four types, those focused on: (1) orientations or motives, (2) behaviors, (3) experiences, and (4) functioning. For the purposes of this review, the last two categories are combined, so the review examines measures of eudaimonic motives, behaviors, and outcomes. Additionally, because most measures of eudaimonia put less emphasis on virtue than Aristotle in his original discussion, virtue receives little emphasis in this section. Thus, possible strategies for assessing this element are discussed separately.

18.3.1 Measuring Eudaimonic Motivation

One fascinating aspect of eudaimonia is that some behaviors could be lacking eudaimonia for one person, but be eudaimonic for another person. For example, consider a person playing a cello, perhaps playing a Bach solo on their cello. The playing may be purely hedonic and lacking eudaimonia; for example, the person may be playing the song early in the morning to gain amusement by annoying a neighbor (hedonic, not eudaimonic). But another person may play the song while seeking self-improvement, or while seeking to bring joy to someone else, or simply as part of habit of daily practice. Any one of these could be considered eudaimonic as long as the playing is being done at the right time for a right purpose. For a third person, the behavior may be both eudaimonic and hedonic. In particular, the person could be playing at an appropriate time, place, and purpose while also gaining pleasure by doing so. The person may simply enjoy playing, or could be playing in an effort to forget the emotional tribulation of a painful relationship. Within the Aristotelian framework, seeking pleasure is not antithetical to virtue; therefore, eudaimonia and hedonia often co-occur.

The cello example illustrates that motivation can be one factor determining whether a behavior is eudaimonic (i.e., has a virtuous motive) and/or hedonic (motivated by pursuit of positive emotions or avoidance of painful emotions). Some researchers have put great emphasis on this motivational aspect in their theory and measurement (e.g., Huta, 2013). Researchers seeking to assess this motivational aspect of eudaimonia (i.e., eudaimonic orientation) will want to select a related measure, such as the Hedonic and Eudaimonic Motives for Activities (Huta & Ryan, 2010).

Hedonic and Eudaimonic Motives for Activities (HEMA; Huta & Ryan, 2010)

The HEMA, as its name implies, was designed to assess eudaimonic and hedonic motives. In the short history of this scale, research of impressive quality has helped to explore the structure of the scale and the relation of these constructs to other variables. The items assess eudaimonic orientation and also two types of hedonic orientation (seeking pleasure and seeking comfort, i.e., avoidance of pain) (Huta, Pelletier, Baxter, & Thompson, 2012). The eudaimonic items assess an orientation toward authenticity, excellence, or growth, which seems to capture the excellence component of Aristotle's ideal. All the items can be reworded to assess short-term *state* motivations or long-term *trait* motivations. The items have also been used to have a third person rate the participant (Huta et al., 2012). People scoring high on the eudaimonic subscale tend to have high sense of personal meaning, more frequent experiences of awe, and a feeling of connection with something larger than themselves. In a fascinating intervention study, people nudged toward a eudaimonic orientation had elevated well-being 3 months later, as opposed to a shorter term benefit for those nudged toward a hedonic orientation (Huta & Ryan, 2010). The intervention was conducted by asking participants to add one activity to each day for 10 days. They were assigned to add either all eudaimonic activities or all hedonic activities, but were required to vary the specific activity (eudaimonic or hedonic) across the 10 days. One advantage of the HEMA is that it uses the same format to provide scores for eudaimonia and hedonia, so the two orientations can be directly compared as predictors and outcomes in larger studies. The items are currently available at http://veronikahuta.weebly.com/.

18.3.2 Measuring Eudaimonic Behavior

The prior section focused on eudaimonic motives, but as Huta and Ryan (2010) suggest, a researcher could instead choose to focus on assessing the presence of eudaimonic behavior. Admittedly, defining whether behavior is eudaimonic can be challenging. As suggested above, eudaimonic behavior is focused on pursuit of excellence and virtue, but that definition can include many possible behaviors. Pursuit of excellence and virtue could include behavior that is personally expressive or altruistic, but then again, choosing to relax and be content is a reasonable part of a virtuous life, so even that could be considered eudaimonic if done at the right time. In spite of these challenges, some measures have been designed to assess eudaimonic behavior.

Personally Expressive Activities Questionnaire (PEAQ; Waterman, 1993)

The PEAQ asks respondents to identify five of their own behaviors that demonstrate what they are like. The respondents then rate each behavior on 12 items assessing the extent to which the behavior is engaging or expresses their true self (eudaimonia) and is pleasurable (hedonia). The PEAQ, thus, allows any behavior to be considered eudaimonic, as long as the participant rates it to be such.

Daily Behaviors Scale (DBS; Steger, Kashdan, & Oishi, 2008)

The DBS was designed to assess the frequency of behaviors that are particularly associated with eudaimonia. The behaviors were selected in part by five experts who had published on eudaimonia and hedonia. The scale was originally used to serve the purposes of a larger study, and therefore the authors may not have expected any more widespread use. The scale is interesting however, and has potential for broader use as long as users are aware of the limitations in labeling only a small subset of behaviors as eudaimonic. The DBS asks participants how often they engage in each of seven eudaimonic behaviors, such as giving money, volunteering, writing out goals, persevering, and building relationships. The internal consistency was not high in the original study (e.g., Cronbach's Alpha = 0.62), but one could debate whether internal consistency is an appropriate expectation for this type of behavior frequency rating. In particular, engaging in one type of eudaimonic behavior does not necessarily predispose a person to engage in other types of eudaimonic behaviors (as opposed to attitudinal surveys for which researchers usually expect internal consistency within each construct), unless one believes that virtue is a truly unified construct, such that all virtues will be developed simultaneously (see Annas, 2011 for a discussion). The complete DBS also includes items to assess frequency of hedonic behaviors, providing a basis for comparing eudaimonic and hedonic behavior. In the original study, eudaimonic behaviors were associated with scores on other measures of hedonic and eudaimonic well-being concurrently, but similar effects for hedonic behaviors were largely absent or smaller. The eudaimonic behaviors also predicted an increased sense of meaning (sometimes treated as an outcome of eudaimonia) on the subsequent day. As stated above, any precise identification of certain behaviors as eudaimonic will be problematic because of the large influence of context. Nonetheless, the DBS was carefully constructed to be consistent with expert opinions, and also underwent further refinement through empirical testing. Also, the findings of that original study were consistent with theoretical expectations. These factors suggest that the DBS may be a useful measure of eudaimonic and hedonic behavior. The items on the DBS are reported in the original article (Steger et al., 2008).

18.3.3 Measuring Eudaimonic Outcome

Living eudaimonically could be expected to create particular outcomes. Thus, one way of assessing eudaimonic living would be to assess whether the participant has achieved outcomes that one would expect to emerge from eudaimonic living.

Personal Growth Composite (PGC; Vitterso, Oelmann, & Wang, 2009)

Perhaps the most intuitively obvious outcome of pursuing excellence and virtue (i.e., living eudaimonically) is an experience of personal growth. In other words, a person who seeks excellence and virtue could be expected to experience positive personal change and the subjective experiences that accompany this. Some research justifies this emphasis on personal growth as distinct from hedonia (Compton, Smith, Cornish, & Qualls, 1996; Ryff, Chap. 6, this volume; Schmutte & Ryff, 1997). Theoretical roots for this personal growth construct can be found in Maslow's (1943) work.

Vitterso, Oelmann, et al. (2009) have called this emphasis on experiences that accompany growth, a subjective approach to eudaimonia. They have argued that personal growth will be accompanied by three experiences: (1) interest, (2) engagement, and (3) curiosity. If they are correct, then one could use measures of these as indicators of eudaimonia. They systematized this approach by using four distinct psychological measures as indicators of growth: A measure of (1) curiosity (Amabile, Hill, Hennessey, & Tighe, 1994), (2) flow (Kashdan, 2004), (3) complexity (using the IPIP (2002) items for Cattel's 16 Personality Factor Questionnaire (16PF; Cattell, Eber, & Tatsuoka, 1970 construct of "openness to change"), and (4) competence (using the IPIP (2002) items for Cloninger's Temperament and Character Inventory (TCI; Cloninger, 1994)). They also provided evidence that the resulting composite has reasonable internal consistency and seems to be quite distinct from life satisfaction (Vitterso, Oelmann, et al., 2009). A recent incarnation of the scale includes three items per subscale (Vitterso & Soholt, 2011). We have included the PGC in this section on outcomes of eudaimonia, but one could reasonably debate whether this measure instead deserves a different categorization because of the constituent subscales – it could be argued, that emphasis is placed on traits rather than outcomes.

One concern with this growth-focused approach to eudaimonic outcome is that self-evaluations of personal growth may often be strongly related to the personality trait of openness (Compton et al., 1996; Schmutte & Ryff, 1997). In fact, one element of the PGC scale is called "complexity", but is derived from a construct originally called "openness to change" (IPIP, 2002). This close relation to personality is potentially problematic because many researchers assessing eudaimonia will be more interested in measuring an outcome (well-being), even if that outcome becomes stable and trait-like, rather than a cause (personality). Conceptually, this emphasis on growth as an indicator of eudaimonia makes sense, and admittedly other measures of eudaimonia will also have relationships with personality. Nonetheless, future researchers using growth-oriented measures could consider statistically controlling for the personality trait of openness to assess the role of personal growth experiences beyond those predictable from the personality trait of openness.

Basic Emotions State Test: Interestingness (BEST-I; Vitterso, Overwien, & Martinsen, 2009)

The BEST, like the PGC, builds on a personal growth oriented understanding of eudaimonia, but is focused on short-term state emotions during a particular activity and is very brief (three-items). The BEST uses three emotion-related terms (engagement, inspiration, interest) to assess short-term emotional states theorized to result from experiences of eudaimonia. Participants report the extent to which a particular activity produced each of these emotions. This scale has good internal consistency and produces correlations that make sense (e.g., associated with personal growth, but not life satisfaction (Vitterso, Oelmann, et al., 2009); may also predict personal growth (Vitterso & Soholt, 2011); associated with analyzing, but not replaying happy moments (Vitterso, Overwien, et al., 2009)). The full scale not only includes a eudaimonia-related subscale called the interestingness subscale, but also subscales assessing pleasantness and negative emotions. A related trait-oriented measure is also available that assesses the related constructs of engagement, pleasure, and negative emotions (Vitterso, Oelmann, et al., 2009).

Meaning in Life Questionnaire: Presence (MLQ-P; Steger, Frazier, Oishi, & Kaler, 2006)

If a researcher is seeking to assess a eudaimonic outcome, and minimize confounding with hedonia, a measure of personal meaning or purpose might be appropriate. Theoretically, this link between eudaimonia and meaning makes sense because seeking to live a life consistent with one's own values could be expected to create a sense that one is living a meaningful life (Huta & Ryan, 2010; Wong, 2011). Also, empirically, there is evidence that a sense of meaning clearly fits the negative definition of eudaimonia addressed above: Having a sense of meaning is minimally related to mere pleasure. In particular, in a recent analysis of well-being measures, presence of meaning showed the greatest independence from hedonic elements, such as short-term affect and happiness (Proctor, Tweed, & Morris, 2015a). Further, evidence also suggests that even though meaning is distinct from hedonia, it is central to well-being. For example, in a measure of flourishing (Diener et al., 2009), the meaning item had the highest item-total correlation.

The presence subscale of the MLQ provides the advantage of having good internal consistency, reliability, widespread use, and clear face validity. Alongside the good face validity comes transparency. Thus, the questionnaire has value in research contexts, but probably less so in environments in which participants are motivated to bias their own responding (e.g., personnel selection contexts). The search subscale of the same scale assesses a distinct construct that represents not merely an absence of meaning, but instead something that may often be representative of dysphoria (e.g., Proctor et al., 2015a). Steger et al. (2008) have also developed a much shorter, two-item meaning presence indicator that may be useful for daily diary studies for which extreme brevity is essential. The many advantages of the MLQ explain its widespread use.

One disadvantage of the MLQ questionnaire is that it allows participants to use their own definition of meaning. Thus, each participant may be scoring himself or herself on a different concept of what it is to have meaning in one's life, though a similar criticism could be made of many psychological scales. The items are currently available at http://www.michaelfsteger.com/?page_id=13.

The Brief Personal Meaning Profile (PMP-B; McDonald, Wong, & Gingras, 2012)

If one instead desires a more consistent and theoretically-based construct to be used among all participants, one could select one of Paul Wong's measures. Wong has written voluminously on meaning, and provided a helpful review of measures of meaning including his own *Personal Meaning Profile* which has now been reduced to 21 items (see McDonald et al., 2012).

This questionnaire assesses meaning in the domains of achievement, relationships, religion, self-transcendence, self-acceptance, intimacy, and fair treatment. One further advantage of the PMP-B (Wong, 1998) is that virtue has a central role. In particular, according to Wong's conceptualization, meaning is not real unless it is integrated with responsible action (see McDonald et al., 2012). However, once one defines the nature of meaning as extensively and precisely as Wong has, room for disagreement sets in; thus researches will need to examine the specific items and his justifications to see whether they agree with Wong's conceptualization of meaning. The items are available in the original chapter (see McDonald et al., 2012).

Sources of Meaning and Meaning in Life Questionnaire (SoMe; Schnell, 2009)

Another interesting scale is the SoMe. The SoMe is quite long at 151 items, and thus may not be appropriate unless meaning is a central part of any given study. However, the SoMe provides an interesting combination of the advantages of the Steger scale (Steger et al., 2006, 2008) and the Wong scale (Wong, 1998). Like the Steger scale (Steger et al., 2006), the SoMe provides an assessment of whether life as a whole is meaningful. The SoMe also provides a fine-grained analysis of the extent to which the person's meaning is derived from each of 26 different possible sources of meaning, thus reflecting some of the advantages of the PMP-B. Because the number of subscales is so large, it would take significant research efforts to validate each subscale, but there is some support for validity of the major subscales (Schnell, 2009). For a study with a major focus on eudaimonia, as manifested in a sense of meaning, the SoMe may be appropriate.

Basic Psychological Needs Scale (BPNS; Gagne, 2003; Kasser, Davey, & Ryan, 1992)

Based on prior theory, one would expect eudaimonic living to produce more than growth and personal meaning. In particular, a sense of autonomy may result from eudaimonic living because eudaimonic living may require rejection of cultural norms and instead a conscious choice of an alternate lifestyle. Similarly, eudaimonic living may produce a sense of relatedness because the allocentrism of eudaimonic living may tend to improve relationships. Also, one could expect eudaimonic living to produce a sense of competence, because pursuit of excellence is central to eudaimonia, and this pursuit would increase one's competence, admittedly however, the growth construct of the PGC already includes elements of self-perceived competence (Vitterso & Soholt, 2011). These three hypothesized outcomes (autonomy, relatedness, competence) would fulfill the needs that self-determination theory suggests are central to human well-being (Deci & Ryan, 2000, 2008). The BPNS assesses the extent to which one has fulfilled these needs for autonomy, competence, and relatedness, and thus may have relevance as a measure of eudaimonic outcome. A qualification deserves mention, because a recent analysis suggests that a sense of personal meaning may provide a more pure measure of eudaimonic outcome than would fulfillment of the needs for autonomy, relatedness, and competence (Proctor et al., 2015a). In particular, there may be more overlap between hedonic measures and fulfillment of the relatedness and autonomy needs, than there is between hedonia and meaning. Nonetheless, the 21-item BPNS assesses the extent to which one has met the need for autonomy, competence, and relatedness and, when combined with a measure of personal meaning, may provide a more complete picture of eudaimonic outcome than would a measure of meaning alone.

18.3.4 A Qualification Regarding Life Satisfaction

Life satisfaction deserves brief mention here. A eudaimonic life might produce life satisfaction or a positive assessment of a person's quality of life (Shin & Johnson, 1978). Therefore, the life satisfaction construct might deserve a place in studies of eudaimonia. However, the relation between eudaimonia and life satisfaction is complex. For example, life satisfaction should not be viewed solely as an outcome – that is, it is not only a related outcome of eudaimonia and hedonia, but also an important predictor of psychological states (Proctor et al., 2015a; Proctor, Linley, & Maltby, 2007). Thus, even though life satisfaction may result from eudaimonia, it is not in itself a pure measure of it. Indeed, Aristotle is clear in indicating that eudaimonic living may lead us to judge our lives positively, however he prescribed virtue as the normative standard against which this judgment is made (Diener, 1984). As a further indicator of the complexity, recent research has demonstrated that life satisfaction is associated with presence of meaning, positive affect (Proctor et al., 2015a), and pleasant experiences, but not personal growth (Vitterso, Oelmann, et al., 2009). Nonetheless, in keeping with Aristotelian theory, life satisfaction appears to be an outcome of the Rogerian personal growth orientation of the fully functioning person (Proctor, Tweed, & Morris, 2015b). Thus, the link between life satisfaction and eudaimonia is not a simple one.

18.3.5 Measures Combining More Than One Level (Orientation, Behavior, Outcome)

Some measures do not fit neatly into the Huta and Waterman (2014) categories we have discussed. These assess more than one of the different aspects of eudaimonia.

Psychological Well-Being (PWB; Ryff, 1989)

The Ryff scales of PWB have had value in efforts to highlight the importance of well-being that is not merely subjective well-being (SWB). We discuss the scale because of its wide usage and historical value, but other measures might be better for future researchers. The items, it has been argued, assess one's ability to successfully face the more existential demands of being (Keyes, Shmotkin, & Ryff, 2002). Subscales assess self-acceptance, positive relations, autonomy, environmental mastery, purpose in life, and personal growth.

There may be problems with the theorized structure of the scale. The scale was intended to assess PWB distinct from SWB, and three subscales (purpose in life, personal growth, and positive relations) are distinct from SWB as intended (Keyes et al., 2002). Two subscales (environmental mastery and self-acceptance), however, overlap with SWB, and one (autonomy) has only a weak relation to both SWB and the three internally consistent PWB scales (purpose in life, personal growth, positive relations). One report (Disabato, Goodman, Kashdan, Short, & Jarden, in press) suggests that the Ryff scales are almost completely confounded with hedonia. However, that analysis could deserve qualification because the statistical analysis treated depression as the opposite of hedonia, but not the opposite of eudaimonia (a theoretically debatable assumption), and treated the Ryff scales as unitary, in spite of evidence that they may not be (Keyes et al., 2002). The PWB scale does have stronger relations to some outcomes, such as finances and health, than do SWB measures (Ryff, 1989), suggesting it does have some value.

The original form of the inventory is quite long (120 items), and the briefest version (18 items) has problems with internal consistency possibly because the items for the shorter scales were selected to maximize conceptual breadth of each construct rather than internal consistency (Ryff & Keyes, 1995). Thus, the PWB has had an important role in the study of well-being, but problems with the scale suggest it would need refinement to justify continued widespread usage.

Comprehensive Inventory of Thriving (CIT; Su, Tay, & Diener, 2014)

One of the more comprehensive measures of well-being to emerge in recent years is the CIT. It includes subscales representing elements of eudaimonic motivation (community subscale), eudaimonic outcomes of personal growth (engagement, self-efficacy, skills, and accomplishment subscales), meaning, hedonia (positive and negative emotion subscales), life satisfaction, and trust. The scale is interesting and has potential because of its breadth and relative brevity. A structural analysis is supportive of the theoretical framework, and correlational analyses suggest the scale is associated with a variety of measures of well-being including health-related outcomes (Su et al., 2014). The scale does not include simple summary scores of eudaimonia and hedonia that can be compared; therefore, the structure would hinder studies focused on simple comparisons of eudaimonia and hedonia. Furthermore, greater understanding of the validity and distinctiveness of its subscales is needed and could be derived in part by explorations of relations between them and some of the eudaimonia scales reviewed in this chapter. Nonetheless, the scale deserves further attention and possibly widespread use because of its comprehensiveness, brevity, and preliminary evidence of utility (Su et al., 2014). The items are currently available at http://internal.psychology.illinois.edu/~ediener/CIT_BIT.html.

18.3.6 Measures of Virtue Component of Eudaimonia

The measures of eudaimonia reviewed to this point, still leave virtue underemphasized. Measuring virtue is challenging for a variety of reasons, and currently a number of these challenges cannot be completely resolved. As a result, some challenges in the measurement of virtue are worth mentioning before describing potential measures.

Measurement challenges related to virtue include, but are not limited to: (1) bias introduced by socially desirable responding, (2) cultural variability in standards for virtue, (3) individual variability in level of habituation towards virtuous ends (e.g., as virtuous acts become habitual, they may require less conscious effort and possibly become less amenable to self-report), (4) standards for determining the degree of habituation attained and individual awareness of progress, (5) determining frequency, meaning, and utility of acts as they relate to virtuous ends, (6) assessing traits/behaviors as they relate to being in excess or deficit rather than simply assuming that more of a particular desired trait is always better, and (7) development of a strategy for combining a virtue indicator with other indicators of eudaimonia: Psychological researchers often assume that combining multiple measures of a trait leads to a more valid score than using a single indicator. One strategy would be to simply create a composite score for eudaimonia that strongly weights a measure of virtue. That composite score approach may be the best strategy for empirical research. However, as we have argued, virtue is essential to eudaimonia; therefore, conceptually it would be best for any score to reflect the essential nature of virtue. Perhaps, each other indicator (e.g., personal growth or meaning) could be multiplied by a virtue score in order that the score is moderated by the extent to which it is being experienced in a virtuous direction. However, before committing to any such strategy, it would be important to conduct empirical research assessing any proposed strategy for combining virtue with other indicators of eudaimonia. It is premature to prescribe exactly how to combine a virtue score with other indicators of eudaimonia to create an overall score.

Several possible measures of virtue will be described and evaluated, however further work is needed to improve measures of virtue and determine how to integrate them into studies of eudaimonia.

VIA Survey (VIA; Peterson & Park, 2009; Peterson & Seligman, 2004)

The VIA Survey was designed to assess 24 character strengths, each of which was thought to be an expression of one of six virtues: wisdom, courage, humanity, justice, temperance, and transcendence (Peterson & Seligman, 2004). The original title of this survey, the *Values in Action Inventory of Strengths* (Peterson & Park, 2009; Peterson & Seligman, 2004) shows the creators' assumption that character requires a combination of right values and active behavioral expression. The items are largely focused on behavior. The name of this survey was later changed to its acronym: VIA.

A structural analysis with over a million cases (McGrath, 2015b) found three higher order virtues explaining relations between the 24 strengths. The three categories were caring (e.g., kindness, teamwork, love, and gratitude), self-control (e.g., prudence, self-regulation, perseverance, and honesty), and inquisitiveness (e.g., creativity, curiosity, bravery, and love of learning). The analysis also suggested that the caring and self-control factors were more strongly related, but the inquisitiveness component somewhat distinct. This finding suggests that inquisitiveness items are prominent in this inventory. Inquisitiveness does fit with Aristotle's value placed on intellectual excellence and therefore may be appropriate, but does not tend to typically appear this prominently or even at all in other traditional lists of virtues. Thus, one could wonder whether inquisitiveness has such a prominent role in the VIA Survey because the designers, being academics, overrepresented intellectual strengths in this group of virtues. McGrath's evidence that the VIA Survey assesses mainly care, self-control, and inquisitiveness contrasts somewhat with the six originally intended overarching virtues (i.e., wisdom and knowledge, courage, humanity, justice, temperance, transcendence) thought to link these 24 character strengths (Peterson & Seligman, 2004).

Some evidence of convergent validity exists which means that there is evidence that VIA constructs have theoretically sensible relations with other indicators, such as vocational interests, that may be manifestations of the same underlying constructs (e.g., Proyer, Sidler, Weber, & Ruch, 2012). Also evidence of test-retest reliability exists (e.g., Ruch et al., 2010), and versions of the VIA Survey have been developed for youth (Park & Peterson, 2006) and children (Toner, Haslam, Robinson, & Williams, 2012).

The creators of the VIA Survey sought to overcome the problem of cultural specificity by including only character strengths that were valued across cultures, and they make a good case for a least partial success on that criterion (see Peterson & Park, 2004, 2009). The questionnaire has received use in a number of cultural contexts and has produced similar mean responses for the various constructs across nations (McGrath, 2015a).

One disadvantage is that the questionnaire is transparent; the intended purpose of the questions is often somewhat obvious (e.g., in the youth version, gratitude is assessed in part with a question asking whether the participant is a grateful person); therefore a person wishing to fake good could easily do so. Thus, the questionnaire might have less value in a personnel selection task or other context in which participants might seek to create a particular impression and fool the tester. For instance, high scores across multiple scales on the VIA Survey could indicate a high level of virtue, faking good, or even very high self-esteem. Therefore, users of the survey often look, not at raw scores, but instead at the tops five (signature) strengths associated with a person's scores. Possibly, researchers could control for social desirability or self-esteem by simultaneously administering measures of these constructs (e.g., Crowne & Marlowe, 1964; Rosenberg, 1965), and then statistically control for them during analyses. Further, the VIA approach has also been criticized because it treats virtue as a collection of different traits, rather than as a single construct (cf. Annas, 2011). The scale can be used for personal development. Common practice in positive psychology tends to focus on developing existing strengths. In other words, people who are grateful would be told that they can work to use their gratitude strength more often (cf. Rust, Diessner, & Reade, 2009). A virtue approach, however, might focus on developing all virtues.

The possibility of using the VIA Survey as a measure of virtue deserves exploration. This approach admittedly deviates from Aristotle because his ideas about the mean suggest that more of a strength is not always better (see Schwartz & Sharpe 2006; Schwartz & Wrzesniewski, Chap. 8, this volume for a discussion).

Nonetheless, for psychometric purposes, this strategy of adding together virtue scores may have value. For example, there is a limit above which higher scores for self-esteem are probably are not desirable in terms of living successfully. Nonetheless, for research purposes, using a simple linear analysis, assuming that more is better, can have utility, in analysis of self-esteem, and possibly also in analyses of virtue scales.

Character Strength Rating Form (CSRF; Ruch, Martinez-Marti, Proyer, & Harzer, 2014)

This 24-item scale is a brief measure of these same strengths. The CSFR is available in English and German, and has acceptable correlations on many of its dimensions with the VIA Survey, at least for research purposes. For individual testing and assessment, the longer VIA Survey might be more appropriate because longer questionnaires can be more accurate. The CSRF items are available through a link within the original article (Ruch et al., 2014) that provides access to supplementary materials.

Even greater brevity in terms of a measure of virtue may be provided by selecting a subset of items from the previously mentioned DBS (Steger et al., 2008), which includes seven eudaimonic items, several of which assess virtue. It has the added advantage of not being correlated with socially desirable responding (Steger et al., 2008), however, a researcher would have to select a focused subset of virtue items. For example, the giving money and volunteering time items map well onto virtue, but the confiding in another person items possibly less so.

Measure of Vice: Short Dark Triad (SD3; Jones & Paulhus, 2014)

Because virtue is so difficult to measure well, researchers could choose to measure part of the virtue construct by instead assessing vice, the opposite of virtue – fitting with Aristotle's ideas discussed above. They could then mathematically reverse the vice score and use it as an indicator of virtue. As previously stated, one of the three major VIA classification components (McGrath, 2015b) is care. The care component of virtue (McGrath, 2015b) could possibly be assessed with reversed scores from the SD3 (Jones & Paulhus, 2014) scale. The items are currently available at http://www2.psych.ubc.ca/~dpaulhus/Paulhus_measures/. The SD3 provides an assessment of the dark triad of Machiavellianism, narcissism, and psychopathy (Jones & Paulhus, 2014), and therefore could potentially work well as a measure of what might be its opposite, care for others. The self-control component of the VIA Survey might not need this type of reverse approach, but if one were to try nonetheless, a scale such as the Barratt Impulsiveness Scale 11 (Patton & Stanford, 1995) might be appropriate, though admittedly that scale contains some items worded in the impulsive direction and some in the opposite direction. Giving prominence to impulsivity when measuring vice would fit well with Baumeister and Tierney's (2011) proposition that its opposite, willpower, is the greatest human strength. Whereas, the inquisitiveness component of virtue could be assessed with a scale that would not need to be reversed, such as a curiosity scale (e.g., PGC; Amabile et al., 1994; Vitterso, Oelmann, et al., 2009).

Another way to assess virtue would be to ask participants to rate the virtue of their own behavior. Participants could be asked to select a subset of behaviors important to them and rate those in terms of their adherence to their own virtue ideals and a prescribed list of virtues. However, effect sizes from this type of approach might be small due to the measurement difficulties associated with rating only a small subset of behavior. Nonetheless, the idea of having people rate virtue using their own values and a prescribed standard list of values might deserve further attention – and is more in keeping with subjective approaches. Alternatively, rather than rating their own behavior, the participants could rate the extent to which goals related to virtue are central to their daily lives. This could be done retrospectively, with daily diaries, or with smartphone-based experience sampling.

Berlin Wisdom Paradigm (Law & Staudinger, 2016)

The focus here has been on measures that can be fairly easily added to an existing study. Thus, measures that require more extensive preparation or coding practice have not been included. Nonetheless, the Berlin Wisdom Paradigm (Law & Staudinger, 2016) is worth briefly mentioning.

Within this paradigm, wisdom is measured by coding participant responses to standardized stories of life dilemmas. The paradigm is interesting because the concept of wisdom requires not pure selflessness, but a practical wisdom that is able to balance the goals of others with one's own personal goals. In that sense, this paradigm closely matches the Aristotelian concept of virtue because it requires a balanced rather than extreme response and an ability to know the right response in the right situation. This view of wisdom also fits with other thinkers, such as Annas (2011), that decry simple lists of distinct virtues and argue that virtue requires not only extensive practice, but also deep personal transformation, rather than merely acting out a set of behaviors prescribed as virtuous. However, using the Berlin Wisdom Paradigm requires careful coding, and thus could not be as easily implemented as other measures mentioned here. For those willing to devote the time to implementing this measure in their research, the benefits might be significant.

Finally, if one wanted to assess eudaimonia at an organizational level, there also exists a measure of organizational virtue (Cameron, Bright, & Caza, 2004). In the earliest years of positive psychology, some of the leaders (e.g., Seligman, Steen, Park, & Peterson, 2005) aspired for this new discipline to study institutions that promote well-being and character strengths. Perhaps that focus on the positive psychology of institutions could be facilitated by efforts to assess the virtue of organizations. At an even higher level of measurement, efforts have also been attempted in regard to assessing the virtue of nations (www.goodcountry.org).

18.4 Conclusion

Various measures associated with the concept of eudaimonia have been presented and reviewed according to three categories of definitions: motives, behaviors, and outcomes. Reflections of commonalities and differences between the measures presented have been considered along with some of the conceptual challenges associated with measuring eudaimonia and the potential benefits of different individual measures. The chapter presents Aristotle's conceptualization of eudaimonia and considers this based on modern conceptualizations and measurement.

We propose that what emerges from a review of this ancient concept is the embedded foundation of virtue in any conceptualization. Indeed, unless a new/modern definition of eudaimonia is proposed, it appears that positive psychological measures of eudaimonia require measurement of virtue. Moreover, measurement of virtue includes distinguishing it from vice – albeit, often a point of confusion, hedonia (or pleasure) can co-occur with and even result from eudaimonia, and yet pain will not be eradicated. Awareness of an injustice or other vice may produce pain for a person living eudaimonically. Finally, in keeping with Wong (2011), Aristotle suggests that the exercising of virtue provides meaning to being and thus is our ultimate function.

Overall, this review highlights that, not only is there lack of consensus with regards to the definition and measurement of eudaimonia, but also there is lack of understanding of Aristotle's original meaning. As noted by Diener (1984):

> Aristotle wrote that eudaemonia is gained mainly by leading a virtuous life, he did not mean [merely] that virtue leads to feelings of joy. Rather, Aristotle was prescribing virtue as the normative standard against which people's live can be judged. Therefore, eudaemonia is not happiness in the modern senses of the word, but a desirable state judged from a particular value framework.

Indeed, it is this value framework that appears to be missing in modern conceptualizations and measurements of eudaimonia. In fact, it appears that we are missing the heart of the matter. Aristotle's philosophy suggests, what we might call today, making a "lifestyle" choice. That is to say, adoption of a way of being, such that we become our choices. Said another way, Aristotle suggests that by choosing to practice virtue, we will become by nature the very thing for which we strive. For Aristotle, we must practice virtue to become virtuous – making virtuous characteristics our own. Doing so will involve both pleasure and pain, however neither will matter if we do not understand the rules of morality and choose ourselves and our actions based on an intelligent understanding of the reason for them – that is, exercise practical wisdom. Modern research into the measurement of eudaimonia provides tools that enable us to further explore these ideas and larger questions about the causes, nature, and outcomes of well-being.

References

Amabile, T. M., Hill, K. G., Hennessey, B. A., & Tighe, E. M. (1994). The work preferences inventory: Assessing intrinsic and extrinsic motivational orientation. *Journal of Personality and Social Psychology, 66*, 950–967.

Annas, J. (2011). *Intelligent virtue*. Oxford, UK: Oxford University Press.

Aristotle. (c. 330 BCE/1925). *The Nicomachean ethics* (trans: Ross, D.). New York: Oxford.

Baumeister, R. F., & Tierney, J. (2011). *Willpower: Rediscovering the greatest human strength*. New York: Penguin Press.

Cameron, K. S., Bright, D., & Caza, A. (2004). Exploring the relationship between organizational virtuousness and performance. *American Behavioral Scientist, 47*(6), 766–790.

Cattell, R. B., Eber, H. W., & Tatsuoka, M. M. (1970). *Handbook for the Sixteen Personality Factor questionnaire (16PF)*. Champaign, IL: Institute for Personality and Ability Testing.

Cloninger, C. R. (1994). *The Temperament and Character Inventory (TCI): A guide to its development and use*. St. Louis, MO: Center for Psychobiology of Personality, Washington University.

Compton, W. C., Smith, M. L., Cornish, K. A., & Qualls, D. L. (1996). Factor structure of mental health measures. *Journal of Personality and Social Psychology, 71*(2), 406–413. doi:10.1037/0022-3514.71.2.406.

Crowne, D., & Marlowe, D. (1964). *The approval motive*. New York: Wiley.

Deci, E. L., & Ryan, R. M. (2000). The 'what' and 'why' of goal pursuits: Human needs and the self-determination of behavior. *Psychological Inquiry, 11*(4), 227–268.

Deci, E. L., & Ryan, R. M. (2008). Self-determination theory: A macrotheory of human motivation, development, and health. *Canadian Psychology, 49*(3), 182–185.

Diener, E. (1984). Subjective well-being. *Psychological Bulletin, 95*(3), 542–575.

Diener, E., Wirtz, D., Tov, W., Kim-Prieto, C., Choi, D., Oishi, S., et al. (2009). New measure of well-being: Flourishing and positive and negative feelings. *Social Indicators Research, 39*, 247–266.

Disabato, D. J., Goodman, F. R., Kashdan, T. B., Short, J. L., & Jarden, A. (in press). Different types of well-being? A cross-cultural examination of hedonic and eudaimonic well-being. *Psychological Assessment*.

Gagne, M. (2003). The role of autonomy support and autonomy orientation in prosocial engagement. *Motivation and Emotion, 27*(3), 199–223.

Huta, V. (2013). Pursuing eudaimonia versus hedonia: Distinctions, similarities, and relationships. In A. Waterman (Ed.), *The best within us: Positive psychology perspectives on eudaimonic functioning* (pp. 139–158). Washington, DC: APA Books.

Huta, V., Pelletier, L. G., Baxter, D., & Thompson, A. (2012). How eudaimonic and hedonic motives relate to the well-being of close others. *The Journal of Positive Psychology, 7*(5), 399–404.

Huta, V., & Ryan, R. M. (2010). Pursuing pleasure or virtue: The differential and overlapping well-being benefits of hedonic and eudaimonic motives. *Journal of Happiness Studies, 11*, 735–762. doi:10.1007/s10902-009-9171-4.

Huta, V., & Waterman, A. S. (2014). Eudaimonia and its distinction from hedonia; Developing a classification and terminology for understanding conceptual and operational definitions. *Journal of Happiness Studies, 15*, 1425–1456. doi:10.1007/s10902-013-9485-0.

IPIP. (2002). *International personality item pool: A scientific collaboration for the development of advanced measurement of personality traits and other individual differences*. Retrieved from http://ipip.ori.org

Jones, D. N., & Paulhus, D. L. (2014). Introducing the short dark triad (SD3): A brief measure of dark personality traits. *Assessment, 21*(1), 28–41.

Kashdan, T. B. (2004). The assessment of subjective well-being (issues raised by the Oxford happiness questionnaire). *Personality and Individual Differences, 36*, 1225–1232.

Kasser, T., Davey, J., & Ryan, R. M. (1992). Motivation and employee-supervisor discrepancies in a psychiatric vocational rehabilitation setting. *Rehabilitation Psychology, 37*(3), 175–187.

Keyes, C. L. M., Shmotkin, D., & Ryff, C. D. (2002). Optimizing well-being: The empirical encounter of two traditions. *Journal of Personality and Social Psychology, 82*(6), 1007–1022.

Law, A., & Staudinger, U. M. (2016). Eudaimonia and wisdom. In J. Vitterso (Ed.), *Handbook of eudaimonic wellbeing*. New York: Springer.

Maslow, A. H. (1943). A theory of human motivation. *Psychological Review, 50*(4), 370–396. doi:10.1037/h0054346.

Maslow, A. H. (1954). *Motivation and personality*. New York: Harper.

Maslow, A. H. (1999). *Toward a psychology of being*. New York: Wiley.

McDonald, M. J., Wong, P. T. P., & Gingras, D. T. (2012). Meaning in life measures and development of a brief version of the personal meaning profile. In P. T.

P. Wong (Ed.), *The human quest for meaning* (2nd ed., pp. 237–382). New York: Routledge.
McGrath, R. E. (2015a). Character strengths in 75 nations: An update. *The Journal of Positive Psychology, 10*(1), 41–52. doi:10.1080/17439760.2014.888580.
McGrath, R. E. (2015b). Integrating psychological and cultural perspectives on virtue: The hierarchical structure of character strengths. *Journal of Positive Psychology, 10*(5), 407–424. doi:10.1080/17439760.2014.994222.
Park, N., & Peterson, C. (2006). Moral competence and character strengths among adolescents: The development and validation of the values in action inventory of strengths for youth. *Journal of Adolescence, 29*(6), 891–909.
Patton, J. H., & Stanford, M. S. (1995). Factor structure of the Barratt impulsiveness scale. *Journal of Clinical Psychology, 51*(6), 768–774.
Peterson, C., & Park, N. (2004). Classification and measurement of character strengths: Implications for practice. In P. A. Linley & S. Joseph (Eds.), *Positive psychology in practice* (pp. 433–446). Hoboken, NJ: Wiley.
Peterson, C., & Park, N. (2009). Classifying and measuring strengths of character. In S. J. Lopez & C. R. Snyder (Eds.), *Oxford handbook of positive psychology* (2nd ed., pp. 25–33). New York: Oxford University Press.
Peterson, C., & Seligman, M. E. P. (2004). *Character strengths and virtues: A classification and handbook.* Washington, DC: American Psychological Association.
Proctor, C. L., Linley, P. A., & Maltby, J. (2007). *Youth life satisfaction: A review of the literature.* Paper presented at the Centre for Applied Positive Psychology: 1st Applied Positive Psychology Conference – People at their best in work, education and health, Warwick University, Warwick, Warwick University.
Proctor, C., Tweed, R., & Morris, D. (2015a). The naturally emerging structure of well-being among young adults: "Big Two" or other framework? *Journal of Happiness Studies, 16*(1), 257–275. doi:10.1007/s10902-014-9507-6.
Proctor, C., Tweed, R., & Morris, D. (2015b). The Rogerian fully functioning person: A positive psychology perspective. *Journal of Humanistic Psychology.* doi:10.1177/0022167815605936. Advanced online publication.
Proyer, R. T., Sidler, N., Weber, M., & Ruch, W. (2012). A multi-method approach to studying the relationship between character strengths and vocational interests in adolescents. *International Journal for Educational and Vocational Guidance, 12*(2), 141–157.
Robbins, B. D. (2008). What is the good life? Positive psychology and the renaissance of humanistic psychology. *The Humanistic Psychologist, 36*, 96–112. doi:10.1080/08873260802110988.
Rogers, C. R. (1961). *On becoming a person: A therapist's view of psychotherapy.* London: Constable.
Rosenberg, M. (1965). *Society and the adolescent self-image.* Princeton, NJ: Princeton University Press.
Ruch, W., Martinez-Marti, M. L., Proyer, R. T., & Harzer, C. (2014). The Character Strengths Rating Form (CSRF): Developmental and initial assessment of a 24-item rating scale to assess character strengths. *Personality and Individual Differences, 68*, 53–58.
Ruch, W., Proyer, R. T., Harzer, C., Park, N., Peterson, C., & Seligman, M. E. P. (2010). Values in Action Inventory of Strengths (VIA-IS): Adaptation and validation of the German version and the development of a peer-rating form. *Journal of Individual Differences, 31*(3), 138–149.
Rust, T., Diessner, R., & Reade, L. (2009). Strengths only or strengths and relative weaknesses? A preliminary study. *The Journal of Psychology, 143*(5), 465–476.
Ryff, C. D. (1989). Happiness is everything, or is it? Explorations on the meaning of psychological well-being. *Journal of Personality and Social Psychology, 57*(6), 1069–1081. doi:10.1037/0022-3514.57.6.1069.
Ryff, C. D., & Keyes, C. L. M. (1995). The structure of psychological well-being revisited. *Journal of Personality and Social Psychology, 69*(4), 719–727. doi:10.1037/0022-3514.69.4.719.
Sandstrom, G. M., & Dunn, E. W. (2011). The virtue blind spot: Do affective forecasting errors undermine virtuous behavior? *Social and Personality Psychology Compass, 5*(10), 720–733. doi:10.1111/j.1751-9004-2011-00384.x.
Schmutte, P. S., & Ryff, C. D. (1997). Personality and well-being: Reexamining methods and meanings. *Journal of Personality and Social Psychology, 73*(3), 549–559. doi:10.1037/0022-3514.73.3.549.
Schnell, T. (2009). The sources of meaning and meaning in life questionnaire (SoMe): Relations to demographics and well-being. *The Journal of Positive Psychology, 4*(6), 483–499.
Schwartz, B., & Sharpe, K. E. (2006). Practical wisdom: Aristotle meets positive psychology. *Journal of Happiness Studies, 7*(3), 377–395.
Seligman, M. E. P., Steen, T. A., Park, N., & Peterson, C. (2005). Positive psychology progress: Empirical validation of interventions. *American Psychologist, 60*(5), 410–421. doi:10.1037/0003-066X.60.5.410.
Shin, D., & Johnson, D. M. (1978). Avowed happiness as an overall assessment of the quality of life. *Social Indicators Research, 5*, 475–492.
Steger, M. F., Frazier, P., Oishi, S., & Kaler, M. (2006). The meaning in life questionnaire: Assessing the presence of and search for meaning in life. *Journal of Counseling Psychology, 53*(1), 80–93.
Steger, M. F., Kashdan, T. B., & Oishi, S. (2008). Being good by doing good: Daily eudaimonic activity and well-being. *Journal of Research in Personality, 42*, 22–42.
Steger, M. F., & Shin, J. Y. (2010). The relevance of the meaning in life questionnaire to therapeutic practice: A look at the initial evidence. *The International Forum for Logotherapy, 33*, 95–104.

Su, R., Tay, L., & Diener, E. (2014). The development and validation of the Comprehensive Inventory of Thriving (CIT) and the Brief Inventory of Thriving (BIT). *Applied Psychology: Health and Well-Being, 6*(3), 251–279. doi:10.1111/aphw.12027.

Toner, E., Haslam, N., Robinson, J., & Williams, P. (2012). Character strengths and wellbeing in adolescence: Structure and correlates of the values in action inventory of strengths for children. *Personality and Individual Differences, 52*(5), 637–642.

Vitterso, J., Oelmann, H. I., & Wang, A. L. (2009). Life satisfaction is not a balanced estimator of the good life: Evidence from reaction time measures and self-report emotions. *Journal of Happiness Studies, 10*(1), 1–17. doi:10.1007/s10902-007-9058-1.

Vitterso, J., Overwien, P., & Martinsen, E. (2009). Pleasure and interest are differentially affected by replaying versus analyzing a happy life moment. *Journal of Positive Psychology, 4*, 14–20. doi:10.1080/174397/60802060602.

Vitterso, J., & Soholt, Y. (2011). Life satisfaction goes with pleasure and personal growth goes with interest: Further arguments for separating hedonic and eudaimonic well-being. *The Journal of Positive Psychology, 6*(4), 326–335. doi:10.1080/17439760.2011.584548.

Waterman, A. S. (1993). Two conceptions of happiness: Contrasts of personal expressiveness (eudaimonia) and hedonic enjoyment. *Journal of Personality and Social Psychology, 64*, 678–691.

Wong, P. T. P. (1998). Implicit theories of meaningful life and the development of the personal meaning profile. In *The human quest for meaning* (pp. 111–140). Mahwah, NJ: Erlbaum.

Wong, P. T. P. (2011). Positive psychology 2.0: Towards a balanced interactive model of the good life. *Canadian Psychology, 52*(2), 69–81.

Part III

Living Eudaimonically

19 Well-Doing: Personal Projects and the Social Ecology of Flourishing

Brian R. Little

Philosophers have explored the nature of human flourishing for over two millennia and in recent decades psychologists have joined in the quest. But have incursions by psychologists truly advanced our understanding of the quality of lives? Not all philosophers are convinced they have. Indeed, Nussbaum (2008) claims that some influential research in positive psychology ignores or obscures features of human lives that are constitutive of flourishing. My goal here is to engage with this debate.

I will present the elements of a research program on personality and well-being in which the personal projects of daily lives play a vital role. I propose that flourishing comprises felicitous action or "well-doing" and is achieved through the *sustainable pursuit of core personal projects* (Little, 2014a, b). This perspective is intended to advance both psychological and philosophical inquiry on the quality of lives.

The chapter proceeds as follows: First, I present a social ecological framework in which personal projects are the pivotal units of analysis. Second, I review how analyzing the content, appraisal and impact of personal projects provides a granular analysis of diverse aspects of well-being. Third, I propose a research agenda in which psychologists and philosophers continue to join forces to illuminate and enhance the quality of lives.

19.1 Personal Projects and the Social Ecology of Flourishing

Personal projects are extended sets of personally salient activity in context. They can range from the mundane tasks of Monday mornings (e.g. "change my print cartridge yet again") to the defining aspirations of a lifetime (e.g. "be a better social justice warrior") (Little, 1983, 1989).[1] Personal projects may be solitary, selfish pursuits but they may also be capacious and wholly altruistic. Each project may facilitate or frustrate other projects, both within the individual and between people. As sources of fun, pleasure and delight personal projects can promote hedonic well-being; as sources of value, meaning and self-expression they can promote eudaimonic well-being.

Personal projects research has been developed within a social ecological framework (Little, 2000; Little & Ryan, 1979; Little, Salmela-Aro &

B.R. Little (✉)
University of Cambridge, Cambridge, UK
e-mail: bl321@cam.ac.uk

[1] Like most psychological research our samples are largely WEIRD (i.e. white, educated, industrialized, rich, and democratic) (see Henrich, Heine and Norenzayan (2010) although that is gradually changing in our own research program.

J. Vittersø (ed.), *Handbook of Eudaimonic Well-Being*, International Handbooks of Quality-of-Life,
DOI 10.1007/978-3-319-42445-3_19

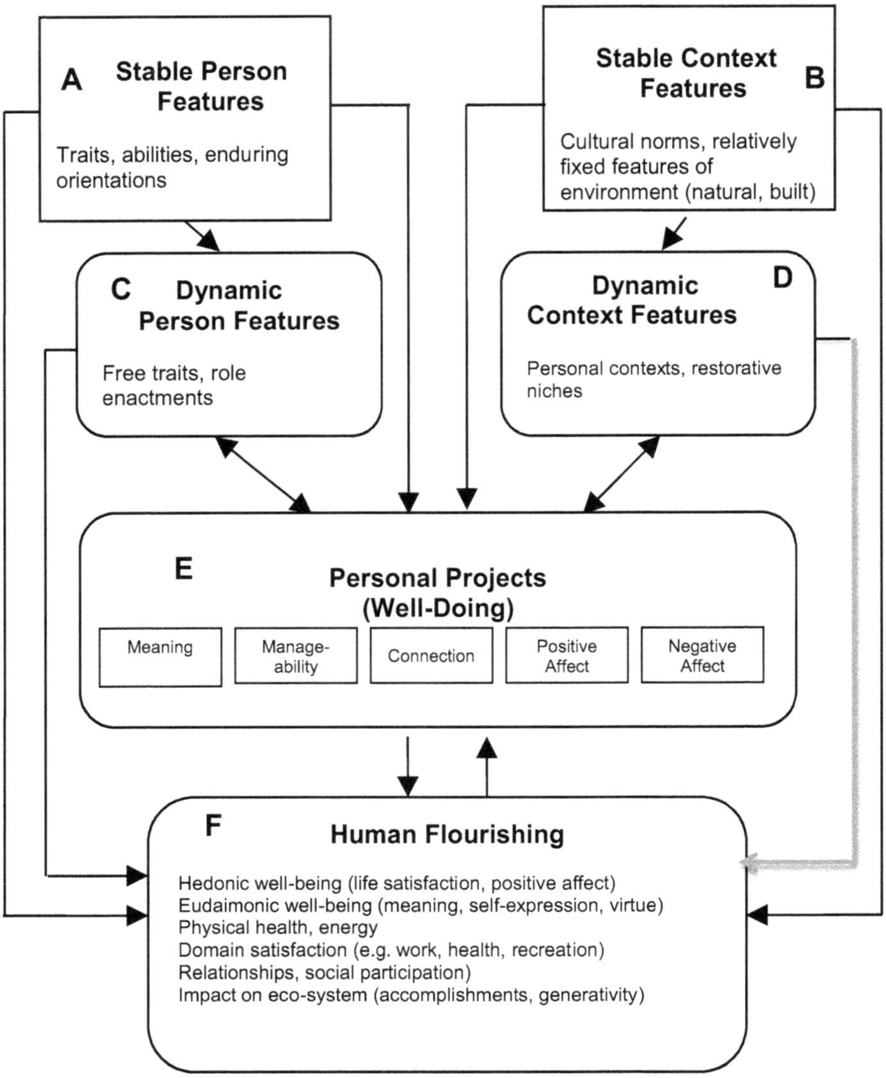

Fig. 19.1 A social ecological model of human flourishing (Adapted from Little, 1999a, 2000)

Phillips, 2007).[2] Figure 19.1 presents the six elements of the framework (Little, 1999a; Little and Coulombe, 2015). Human flourishing (Box F) is influenced by five factors: relatively stable features of a person such as enduring traits, interests and orientations (Box A); relatively stable or slow moving features of the environment such as the cultural, historical and material features of a person's life (Box B); dynamic features of persons such as their personal constructs and "free traits" (to be explained below) (Box C); more dynamic and singular features of their environments such as their intimate relationships (Box D) and, most pivotally and consequentially, the point of convergence of these different sources of influence, the individual's personal projects (Box E).

The six blocks of the framework can be briefly sketched.

Block F comprises diverse features of hedonic and eudaimonic well-being, accomplishments

[2]Social ecological models examine the systems of influences that are conducive to human well-being broadly conceived. Those influences involve physical, social, economic and historical factors that help shape lives. See also Bronfenbrenner (1979), Oishi and Graham (2010).

and the impact people have on their social ecology. Methodologically, Block F comprises a multivariate set of quasi-dependent or outcome measures with Blocks A-E serving as sets of predictor variables with direct, indirect, bidirectional and interactive effects on human flourishing. The diversity of measures contained in Box F acknowledges the complex and potentially contestable nature of living well whether by personal or objective standards.

Block A comprises relatively stable and enduring temperamental and personality traits such as the Big Five traits of openness, conscientiousness, extraversion, agreeableness and neuroticism. The traits of extraversion and neuroticism, for example, are strongly linked to consequential outcomes relating to subjective well-being, happiness, life satisfaction, health and accomplishments (Ozer and Benet-Martínez (2006). Hedonic happiness, for example, is reliably associated with stable extraversion (Costa & McCrae, 1980; DeNeve & Cooper, 1998; Steel, Schmidt and Shultz (2008). These linkages may be due to shared neurobiological mechanisms underlying traits and well-being (DeYoung, 2010, 2015; Depue & Collins, 1999).

Block B consists of the relatively stable and slow moving features of contexts such as cultural norms and eco-system influences. Cultures differ, for example, in their average levels of happiness (Helliwell, Layard, & Sachs, 2012). But they also differ in the criteria they invoke when appraising well-being. Individualist cultures favour more agentic and hedonic forms of well-being while collectivist cultures favour more eudaimonic forms (Diener & Suh, 2000). Cultural influences also include material features that may be conducive to flourishing and we include in Block B the natural and built environments that shape daily lives (Little, 2010).

Box C comprises the more dynamic features of personality that are shaped strategically by individuals to meet their needs, aspirations and role demands. A key concept here is what we call "free traits " that contrast with the more stable traits in Box A. Free traits are *strategic enactments of social scripts to advance a personal project*, such as when an introverted person acts in an extraverted fashion in order to fulfill a valued task or role (Little, 2000; Little & Joseph, 2007).

Box D, similarly, refers to the dynamic features of environments, the *personal contexts* that derive from a person's idiosyncratic ways of construing the environment. One central feature of Box D is the presence of other people. When we ask individuals to list and describe images of their lived day those images are dominated by relationships and interactions with intimate others (Little, 1996). The dynamic nature of contexts is also apparent when individuals have been engaging in free traits. They avail themselves of different features of their objective environment to discover personally relevant "restorative niches" that provide respite from having acted out of character (Little & Joseph, 2007).

Box E focuses on our key analytic concept, personal projects. They have direct effects on flourishing and also serve as the conduit for the indirect effects arising from person and context influences. Personal projects are assessed by a methodology, Personal Projects Analysis (PPA), a modular assessment technique for assessing the content, appraisal, dynamics and impact of personal projects. PPA is based on a set of explicit criteria about the level and type of measurement required for the study of personality and well-being (see Little, 2006; Little & Gee, 2007).

19.2 Personal Projects: What's Up? How's It Going?

Research on the content, appraisal and social ecology of project pursuit explores how individuals think and feel about the doings of their daily lives. In the following section I will selectively review this research and illustrate how the way in which individuals pursue their personal projects is conducive to living well, or not so well.

19.2.1 What's Up? The Content of Personal Projects

The content of everyday personal projects provides an answer to the everyday question "What's up?" or "What are you doing?" We assess this with an open Elicitation Module that prompts participants to list the personal projects that they are currently pursuing or thinking about pursuing. Typically participants list about 15 projects. The most frequent types of projects listed are work (or, for students, academic), interpersonal, health, and recreational projects. Less frequently listed but consequential for well-being are intrapersonal projects—those that focus on the self and "estate" projects involving home repairs and maintenance.

The social ecological framework specifies that both personal and contextual factors will influence the content of personal projects (Little, 1999b; McGregor & Little, 1998; McGregor, McAdams & Little, 2006; Salmela-Aro & Little, 2007).

The content of personal projects also has a genetic source that is shared with big five trait dimensions. For example, in a major study of personality and personal projects in identical and non-identical twins openness to experience shared a common genetic link with being engaged in educational projects Salmela-Aro et al. (2012). More curiously, the study also showed that people low on both openness and agreeableness engage in the more concrete deeds of daily life, such as home maintenance projects. It is not yet known if such projects are carried out zealously, spitefully, or in mere resignation to the eternal tedium of Sisyphean tasks.

Cultural factors also influence the kinds of personal projects people pursue. Normative, age-graded expectations of society are particular influential in shaping the types of projects engaged in across the life course (Cantor, 1990; Little, 1999a). Well-being is enhanced if personal projects align with these social and cultural expectations during development such as the transition from university to work, having a family, and retirement (Salmela-Aro, 2009).

Intrapersonal projects, such as "try to be more outgoing," deal with aspects of one's self or identity. they are consequential for well-being. Although not among the more frequently elicited project categories, *intrapersonal* projects are associated with depressive affect and vulnerability (Little, 1989; Salmela-Aro, 1992). But they also serve as sources of self-expression for highly creative individuals (Melia-Gordon, 1994).[3]

By invoking issues of the origin and self-expressiveness of projects we enter into consideration of the appraisal dimensions that form the bulk of our research. Knowing "what's up" is an essential starting point for understanding a person's daily life and how it is going. Knowing "*how* it's going" takes us even farther.

19.2.2 How's It Going? Meaning, Manageability, Connection and Affect in Project Pursuit

The Appraisal Module of PPA asks individuals to rate each of their elicited personal projects on dimensions that we posit as having theoretical importance and relevance for applied interventions to improve the quality of lives. Early versions of PPA asked individuals to rate (on 0–10 scales) each elicited project on seventeen appraisal dimensions that formed five factors of project meaning structure community, efficacy and stress (Little, 1983, 1989).[4] Generally, those scoring high on subjective well-being were engaged in projects that were meaningful, well structured, efficacious, supported by others, and not stressful. Those whose lives were not going well were engaged in personal projects that were meaningless, chaotic, hopeless and stressful. And nobody else really cared (Little, 1989).

These early studies were examined meta-analytically to determine which of the appraisal factors were the most robust predictors of well-

[3]Consider the personal project " try to be more outgoing. " Why might this be depressing for some and salutary for others? Who initiated the project seems pivotal. If it is pursued because one's socially gregarious spouse insists on it, the course of that project may be demanding, and potentially depressogenic. If it originates with the project pursuer herself it is more likely to be construed as a self-exploratory adventure.

[4]Examples of dimensions defining these factors are: Meaning (value congruency, self-identity,), Structure (control, time-adequacy), Community (e.g. visibility, others' support), Efficacy (progress, outcome likelihood) and Stress (difficulty, stress).

being. Project efficacy (likelihood of successful completion of the project) and stress (inversely) were consistently found to be the best predictors. What was surprising was the relatively unimportant role played by project meaning in predicting life satisfaction relative to the other dimensions (Little, 1998). Subsequent research provided a compelling explanation. Sheldon and Kasser (1998) showed that mere efficacy in project pursuit was insufficient to predict well-being. Rather, one's pursuits needed to be personally meaningful in order to enhance satisfaction with one's life.[5]

Here is where PPA meets one of the enduring questions of moral philosophy. What is to count as meaningful pursuit? Can objective criteria be invoked that gather consensual reflective agreement that a project is deservingly called meaningful? Or is this primarily a matter of subjective judgement? If the project pursuer regards a project as enjoyable, congruent with her values, important and self-expressive, is this either necessary or sufficient to count as a truly meaningful pursuit? This is, I believe, a question for philosophical adjudication. But I do believe that psychologists can play an essential role in informing such adjudication (Little, 2015); see also Kristjánsson (2013).

Here's an example. Consider the current debate about whether hedonic and eudaimonic well-being are linked or independent aspects of flourishing (Kashdan, Biswas-Diener, & King, 2008; Ward & King, Chap. 35, this volume; Vittersø & Søholt, 2011; Vittersø, Chap. 17, this volume). In our early version of PPA the affective dimensions were restricted to enjoyment and stress. More recently, we have used the modular flexibility of PPA to add more dimensions tapping into a broader array of positive and negative emotions associated with each project. How might this change the factor structure of personal projects appraisal? Do the meaning dimensions and the positive affect dimensions merge or separate?

As listed in Box E of Table 19.1, this new structure comprised five factors: meaning, manageability (a blend of structure and efficacy dimensions), connection (primarily social support) and two independent affect factors – positive and negative.[6] In other words, when we look at the personal projects that individuals pursue, we confirm the view that hedonic and eudaimonic meaning are independent, not merged, features of the well-lived life.

But research with PPA does more than sharpen theoretical debate. It allows us to drill down to the specific projects that generate feelings of enjoyment and satisfaction as well as value congruency and self-identity and hence inform at a granular level issues related to hedonic and eudaimonic well-being (Little & Coulombe, 2015). Moreover, this level of analysis is relevant to social policy. We can pose inquiries such as: what are the joyful pursuits of adolescents in rural areas? What are the most challenging but self-expressive projects of older people in residential centers? Are the intimate projects of LBGT individuals more stressful than their work projects? (Little 2014a, b; Little & Frost, 2013).

19.3 Well-Doing: The Sustainable Pursuit of Core Projects

I want to summarize the argument so far. I have presented the case that the study of people's personal projects opens up a perspective on human flourishing that is granular and consequential. I want to move now to what may be a more conten-

[5]Take a famous example proposed by John Rawls. He asks if the project of "counting blades of grass" outside the Widener Library at Harvard can be regarded as meaningful or worthwhile. Although the example is meant to underscore that some life pursuits are not intrinsically meaningful, from a psychological perspective this might be approached rather differently. There is a big difference in the merit of the grass project if it is being pursued by a despondent, addicted and suicidal street kid or if by an eccentric professor emeritus who wants to experience an example made famous by John Rawls. I must confess that I spent 14 min of my life doing exactly this and I was neither despondent, addicted, suicidal nor a kid at that time. I may have been eccentric, however.

[6]Interestingly, the dimension of ambivalence loaded on the negative affect factor but not on positive. Also, at the dimension level, challenge is linked to both meaning and stress, suggesting that challenging projects are more aligned with the kind of effortful pursuit associated with some views of eudaimonic well-being.

Table 19.1 Methodological criteria for PPA

Reflexive	The constructs invoked apply equally to researchers and agents
Evocative	Gives agent an opportunity for self-reflection and new insights about themselves
Ecologically representative	Samples the daily experiences of agents
Temporally sensitive	Documents the dynamic nature of personal projects through their stages of progression.
Social Indicator potential	Provides policy-relevant data on the quality of the social ecological settings where the subjects evolve.
Systemic	Studies the interrelations between the multiple projects pursued concomitantly by the agent, and which, aggregated, form the personal project system.
Middle-level	Provides access to both lower order (i.e. acts) and higher order (values and aspirations) aspects of human experience.
Modular	Provides modules that can be selected, adapted and supplemented to offer the best answer to the study question, in the specific research setting.
Conjointly idiographic and normative	Facilitates measurement of relations between projects dimensions at the individual level (across each agent's different projects) and the sample level (across all agents' project systems).
Integrative	Provides a single instrument to document cognitive, behavioral, affective and ecological aspects of the agent's experience, integrated around their personal projects.
Direct applicability	Focuses on a tractable unit of analysis that can be targeted in individual and social interventions to promote well-being.

Adapted from Little, 1999b

tious claim. What if we think of indices based on an individual's personal projects not as predictors of outcome measures of flourishing or well-being but as the outcome measures themselves? What if we thought of human flourishing as well-doing? A shift away from the various states of happiness and well-being to the activity that creates such states would be a concession not only to Aristotelian conceptions of human flourishing but also to other philosophical traditions in which action and its consequences are pivotal to understand the human good.

From such a perspective, human flourishing comprises *the sustainable pursuit of core projects in one's life*. Core projects are those that are central to the project system as a whole and without which a life may be seen as aimless and empty. They are highly resistant to change, in part because changing them would entail a major shift in the rest of a person's project system (Little, 2014). Indeed, Williams (1982) suggests that without such ground projects people may wonder whether it is possible to go on at all. How might these core projects, these vital sources of direction in a person's life, be sustained? There are two broad strategies: internal motivational strategies and external, social ecological strategies.

Internally, personal projects are more sustainable if they are congruent with one's basic dispositions than if they require action that runs counter to them. For example, extraverted individuals experience greater efficacy in their interpersonal projects than in academic pursuits while neurotic individuals feel their projects are ineffectual in both academic and social domains (Little, Lecci & Watkinson, 1992).

But people are frequently called upon to engage in counter-dispositional behaviour, to engage in what we call "free traits". An introverted academic might be called upon to host a major social event that is vitally important to the university's international stature. For the duration of this event the academic acts as a pseudo-extravert. While this promotes his well-being by advancing the core project of "securing the next international congress at my university," it may deplete his physiological coping resources and lead to burnout (Little, 2011). But there may be unanticipated eudaimonic effects of engaging in free traits as well. Free traits can help us grow and flourish in domains that we had previously thought were beyond the bounds of our competency.

The sustainable pursuit of core projects also requires successful management of the external or social ecological environment by the project pursuer. A person's projects may be personally meaningful and prudentially managed. But beyond the questions of "what's up?" and "how's it going?" there is another crucial question to ask of individuals about their project pursuit: Who cares?" As depicted in Table A one of the key factors of project appraisal is the extent to which it involves connection with others. Projects may be isolated and isolating ventures or they may be animated and intertwined by the pursuits of other people. The social ecological framework sees such connections as hierarchically organized, from the micro level support of an intimate partner to the meso-level organizational climate of one's work place to the macro-level political orthodoxies of one's country. At each of these levels other people may facilitate or frustrate, promote or proscribe the pursuit of one's projects with consequences for both individual and collective quality of life. And there is a crucial question about a core project that is callous or criminal or simply evil. Such projects supply the limiting case of how sustainable pursuit constitutes human flourishing. From a value perspective such pursuits ought not to be regarded as aspects of a flourishing life. From a pragmatic perspective "bad projects" will likely be met with push-back, ostracism, or attack and their sustainability, one hopes, will be compromised.

Each of these levels of connection has been studied in research with personal projects. The emotional support of one's partner is highly significant as a factor in pregnancy, including subjective and objective aspects of delivery (McKeen, 1984) as well as in entrepreneurial success (Dowden, 2004). The number of personal projects shared with one's romantic partner predicts relationship satisfaction (Hwang, 2004). The organizational climate of work places is critical to sustainable project pursuit, with males preferring a climate that facilitates autonomy in pursuits and women preferring a climate that builds connection with others (Phillips, Little & Goodine, 1997).[7] And at the macro level, the pursuit of intimacy projects amongst LGBT individuals has been shown to be frustrated by macro-system variables such as political institutions (Little & Frost, 2013).

19.4 Collaborative Inquiry: Personal Projects and the Quality of Lives

By looking at human flourishing as the sustainable pursuit of core projects can we meet any of the concerns that Nussbaum (2008) raised about poverty of psychological approaches to well-being? Certainly moral philosophy has invoked personal projects as important analytic units for guidance on how agents ought to make choices about their pursuits. Williams (1982) makes a forceful argument that respect for an individual's ground projects with which the agent identifies and hold dear should outweigh the claims of either Utilitarian or Kantian claims about life choices. Similarly, Lomasky (1984, 1987) treats respect for personal project pursuit as the very core of his theory of human rights. In short, there is already a space within philosophical discourse and moral philosophy in particular in which personal projects are given a central role.

More recently, two philosophers have incorporated aspects of psychological insights about project pursuit into their philosophical treatments of morality and life choices. Betzler (2013) provides a nuanced analysis of the normative importance of personal projects in moral choice and anticipates and answers alternative views from utilitarian philosophers. Finally,

[7] It should be noted, however, that many of the women in these organizations were in the job for a shorter period of time than their male counterparts. It is possible that the gender effect may actually be more a "newcomer" effect, where forming social connections is part of the process of learning the ropes in a new institutional setting (Phillips, Little & Goodine, 1997).

Tiberius (2015) presents a compelling case for viewing personal projects as the instantiation of values driving reflective life choices (see also Tiberius (2008) and Tiberius, Chap. 38, this volume). I see considerable value in facilitating collaborative inquiry between psychologists and philosophers on personal project pursuit and well-being. The analytic tools of personality psychology can provide specific granular instances of how individuals plan for, engage with and occasionally complete projects. We can provide information on how projects become meaningful, whether they are manageable, what emotional consequences they entail and who else, if anyone, cares for our pursuits. We can specify how projects are embodied in our daily action and embedded within temporal, spatial, social and value contexts. Philosophers can bring their own distinctive strengths of conceptual clarity and rigour to the shared enterprise and can enrich the exploration of these consequential issues. That, at least, is my vision and my nascent project.

References

Betzler, M. (2013). The normative significance of personal projects. In M. Kühler & N. Jelinek (Eds.), *Autonomy and the self.* New York: Springer. (forthcoming).

Bronfonbrenner, U. (1979). *The ecology of human development: Experiments by nature and design.* Cambridge, UK: Harvard University Press.

Cantor, N. (1990). From thought to behavior: "having" and "doing" in the study of personality and cognition. *American Psychologist, 45*, 735–750.

Costa, P. T., & McCrae, R. R. (1980). Influence of extraversion and neuroticism on subjective well-being: Happy and unhappy people. *Journal of Personality and Social Psychology, 38*(4), 668–678.

DeNeve, K. M., & Cooper, H. (1998). The happy personality: A meta-analysis of 137 personality traits and subjective well-being. *Psychological Bulletin, 124*, 197–229.

Depue, R. A., & Collins, P. F. (1999). Neurobiology of the structure of personality: Dopamine, facilitation of incentive motivation, and extraversion. *Behavioral and Brain Sciences, 22*, 491–569.

DeYoung, C. G. (2010). Personality neuroscience and the biology of traits. *Social and Personality Psychology Compass, 4*(12), 1165–1180.

DeYoung, C. G. (2015). Cybernetic big five theory. *Journal of Research in Personality, 56*, 33–58.

Diener, E., & Suh, E. M. (Eds.). (2000). *Culture and subjective well being*. Cambridge, MA: MIT Press.

Dowden, C. (2004). *Managing to be free: Personality, personal projects and well-being in entrepreneurs.* Unpublished Doctoral dissertation, Carleton University, Ottawa, Canada.

Helliwell, J. R., Layard, R., & Sachs, J. (2012). *World happiness report*. New York: United Nations.

Henrich, J., Heine, S. J., & Norenzyan, A. (2010). The weirdest people in the world? *Behavioural and Brain Sciences, 33*, 61–83.

Hwang, A. A. (2004). *Yours, mine, ours: The role of joint personal projects in close relationships*. Unpublished Doctoral dissertation, Harvard University, Cambridge, MA.

Kashdan, T. B., Biswas-Diener, R., & King, L. A. (2008). Reconsidering happiness: The costs of distinguishing between hedonics and eudaimonia. *Journal of Positive Psychology, 3*, 219–233.

Kristjánsson. (2013). *Virtues and vices in positive psychology: A philosophical critique*. Cambridge, UK: Cambridge University Press.

Little, B. R. (1983). Personal projects: A rationale and method for investigation. *Environment and Behavior, 15*, 273–309. (205–244). New York: Wiley.

Little, B. R. (1989). Personal projects analysis: Trivial pursuits, magnificent obsessions, and the search for coherence. In D. Buss & N. Cantor (Eds.), *Personality psychology: Recent trends and emerging directions* (pp. 15–31). New York: Springer-Verlag.

Little, B. R. (1996). Free traits, personal projects and idiotapes: Three tiers for personality psychology. *Psychological Inquiry, 7*(4), 340–344.

Little, B. R. (1998). Personal project pursuit: Dimensions and dynamics of personal meaning. In P. T. P. Wong & P. S. Fry (Eds.), *The human question for meaning: A handbook of psychological research and clinical applications* (pp. 197–221). Thousand Oaks, CA: Sage.

Little, B. R. (1999a). Personal projects and social ecology: Themes and variation across the life span. In J. Brandtstadter & R. M. Lerner (Eds.), *Action and self-development: Theory and research through the life span* (pp. 197–221). Thousand Oaks, CA: Sage.

Little, B. R. (1999b). Personality and motivation: Personal action and the conative evolution. In L. A. Pervin & O. P. John (Eds.), *Handbook of personality theory and research* (2nd ed., pp. 501–524). New York: Guilford.

Little, B. R. (2000). Free traits and personal contexts: Expanding a social ecological model of well-being. In W. B. Walsh, K. H. Craik, & R. H. Price (Eds.), *Person environment psychology: New directions and perspectives* (2nd ed., pp. 87–116). Mahwah, NJ: Lawrence Erlbaum.

Little, B. R. (2006). Personality science and self-regulation: Personal projects as integrative units. *Applied Psychology: An International Review, 55*(3), 419–427.

Little, B. R. (2010). Opening space for project pursuit: Affordance, restoration and chills. In C. W. Thompson, P. Aspinall, & S. Bell (Eds.), *Innovative approaches to researching landscape and health* (Open space: People space 2, pp. 163–178). New York: Routledge.
Little, B. R. (2011). Personality science and the northern tilt: As positive as possible under the circumstances. In K. M. Sheldon, T. B. Kashdan, & M. F. Steger (Eds.), *Designing positive psychology: Taking stock and moving forward* (pp. 228–247). New York: Oxford University Press.
Little, B. R. (2014a). *Me, myself and us: The science of personality and the art of well-being*. New York: Public Affairs Books.
Little, B. R. (2014b). Well-doing: Personal projects and the quality of lives. *Theory and Research in Education, 12*, 329–346.
Little, B. R., & Coulombe, S. (2015). Personal projects analysis. In *International encyclopedia of social and behavioral sciences* (2nd ed., pp. 757–765). Oxford, UK: Elsevier.
Little, B. R., & Frost, D. (2013). Aspects of love: Connecting, romancing and caring. In M. Hojjat & D. Cramer (Eds.), *Positive psychology of love* (pp. 162–176). New York: Oxford University Press.
Little, B. R., & Gee, T. L. (2007). The methodology of personal projects analysis: Four modules and a funnel. In B. R. Little, K. Salmela-Aro, & S. D. Phillips (Eds.), *Personal project pursuit: Goals, action, and human flourishing* (pp. 51–94). Mahwah, NJ: Lawrence Erlbaum.
Little, B. R., & Joseph, M. F. (2007). Personal projects and free traits: Mutable selves and well beings. In B. R. Little, K. Salmela-Aro, & S. D. Phillips (Eds.), *Personal project pursuit: Goals, action, and human flourishing* (pp. 375–400). Mahwah, NJ: Lawrence Erlbaum.
Little, B. R., Lecci, L., & Watkinson, B. (1992). Personality and personal projects: Linking big five and PAC units of analysis. *Journal of Personality, 1992*(60), 501–525.
Little, B. R., & Ryan, T. J. (1979). A social ecological model of development. In K. Ishwaran (Ed.), *Childhood and adolescence in Canada* (pp. 273–301). Toronto, Canada: McGraw-Hill Ryerson.
Little, B. R., Salmela-Aro, K., & Phillips, S. D. (Eds.). (2007). *Personal project pursuit: Goals, action and human flourishing*. Mahwah, NJ: Lawrence Erlbaum.
Lomasky, L. E. (1984). Personal projects as the foundation for basic rights. *Social Philosophy and Policy, 1*, 35–55.
Lomasky, L. E. (1987). *Persons, rights, and the moral community*. New York: Oxford University Press.
McGregor, I., & Little, B. R. (1998). Personal projects, happiness and meaning: On doing well and being yourself. *Journal of Personality and Social Psychology, 74*, 494–512.
McKeen, N. A. (1984). *The personal projects of pregnant women*. Unpublished Bachelor thesis, Carleton University, Ottawa, Canada.
Melia-Gordon, M. (1994). *The measurement and meaning of personal projects creativity*. Unpublished Master's thesis, Carleton University, Ottawa, Canada.
Nussbaum, M. (2008). Who is the happy warrior? Philosophy poses questions to psychologists. *Journal of Legal Studies, 37*(52), S81–S113.
Oishi, S., & Graham, J. (2010). Social ecology: Lost and found in psychological science. *Perspectives on Psychological Science, 5*, 356–377.
Ozer, D. J., & Benet-Martínez. (2006). Personality and the prediction of consequential outcomes. *Annual Review of Psychology, 57*, 401–421.
Phillips, S. D., Little, B. R., & Goodine, L. A. (1997). Reconsidering gender and public administration: Five steps beyond conventional research. *Canadian Public Administration, 40*, 563–581.
Salmela-Aro, K. (1992). Struggling with self: The personal projects of students seeking psychological counselling. *Scandinavian Journal of Psychology, 33*(4), 330–338.
Salmela-Aro, K. (2009). Personal goals and well-being during critical life transitions: The four C's—channelling, choice, co- agency and compensation. *Advances in Life Span Research, 14*, 63–73.
Salmela-Aro, K., & Little, B. R. (2007). Relational aspects of project pursuit. In B. R. Little, K. Salmela-Aro, & S. D. Phillips (Eds.), *Personal project pursuit: Goals, action, and human flourishing* (pp. 199–219). Mahwah, NJ: Lawrence Erlbaum.
Salmela-Aro, K., Read, S., Nurmi, J.-E., Vuoksimaa, E., Siltala, M., Dick, D. M., et al. (2012). Personal goals and personality traits among young adults: Genetic and environmental effects. *Journal of Research in Personality, 46*(3), 248–257. ISSN 0092-6566.
Sheldon, K. M., & Kasser, T. (1998). Pursuing personal goals: Skills enable progress, but not all progress is beneficial. *Personality and Social Psychology Bulletin, 24*(12), 1319–1331.
Steel, P., Schmidt, J., & Shultz, J. (2008). Refining the relationship between personality and subjective well-being. *Psychological Bulletin, 134*(1), 138–161.
Tiberius, V. (2008). *The reflective life: Living wisely with our limits*. New York: Oxford University Press.
Tiberius, V. (2015). *Well-being, virtue and personal projects: A normative framework for virtue ethics and public policy*. Unpublished ms., Department of Philosophy, Minneapolis: University of Minnesota.
Vittersø, J., & Søholt, Y. (2011). Life satisfaction goes with pleasure and personal growth goes with interest: Further arguments for separating hedonic and eudaimonic well-being. *Journal of Positive Psychology, 6*, 326–335.
Williams, B. (1982). *Moral luck*. Cambridge, UK: Cambridge University Press.

20 The Eudaimonics of Human Strengths: The Relations Between Character Strengths and Well-Being

Claudia Harzer

20.1 Introduction

Research within the area of positive psychology is focused on the investigation of what makes individuals' lives most worth living; Seligman & Csikszentmihalyi, 2000). This focus facilitates research on conditions and processes that enable human flourishing and optimal functioning (Gable & Haidt, 2005). Three topics are at the center of positive psychology: (a) positive subjective experiences like positive emotions and well-being; (b) positive individual traits like character strengths; and (c) positive institutions (e.g., families or workplaces) (Peterson, 2006; Seligman & Csikszentmihalyi, 2000). A core proposition regarding the interplay between these three topic states that positive institutions enable the development and/or display of positive traits like character strengths, which in turn foster positive experiences (Peterson, 2006) and lead people to positive behaviors (Peterson & Park, 2006). The chapter at hand is focused on the relations between character strengths as positive traits and positive experiences with a special emphasis on well-being considering two different approaches (i.e., hedonic well-being and eudaimonic well-being).

20.1.1 Character Strengths

Clinical psychologists, psychiatrists, and social workers use classification schemes like the *Diagnostic Statistic Manual of Mental Disorders* (DSM) or the *International Classification of Diseases* (ICD) for classifying and diagnosing patients. However, the positive psychologists' desk reference is the so-called *Manual of the Sanities* by Peterson and Seligman (2004) describing human strengths as positive traits rather than weaknesses and pathologies. The good character is seen as an important instance of optimal functioning (Park & Peterson, 2007; Peterson & Seligman, 2004). Peterson and Seligman introduced the Values in Action classification of strengths (VIA classification) as an extensive framework for the investigation of individuals' character strengths.

The character strengths are defined as positively valued trait-like individual differences with demonstrable generality across different situations and stability across time (Peterson & Seligman, 2004). Character strengths manifest in the range of individuals' thoughts (e.g., looking positively ahead), feelings (e.g., being grateful for getting help), and behaviors (e.g., working well in a team). They are widely recognized and

C. Harzer (✉)
Section on Psychological Assessment, Department of Psychology, University of Kassel,
Holländische Str. 36-38, 34127 Kassel, Germany
e-mail: harzer.c@gmail.com

J. Vittersø (ed.), *Handbook of Eudaimonic Well-Being*, International Handbooks of Quality-of-Life,
DOI 10.1007/978-3-319-42445-3_20

desired across cultures (Peterson & Seligman, 2004). Accordingly, researchers have found empirical support indicating that character strengths can be observed in individuals of, and are valued by the members of various cultures (cf. Biswas-Diener, 2006; Park, Peterson, & Seligman, 2006).

The VIA classification includes a list of 24 character strengths that were derived from an extensive review of various sources describing positive personality traits (e.g., literature on good character from different disciplines like psychiatry, philosophy, youth development, and psychology; brainstorming in core groups of scholars; see Peterson & Seligman, 2004, for more a detailed overview). To reduce the initially derived list of positive personality traits, ten criteria were used to identify character strengths among those traits (cf. Peterson & Seligman, 2004). For example, traits not valued across cultures (e.g., cleanliness, frugality, and silence) were excluded and redundancies were combined. Furthermore, other criteria defined character strengths as contributing to individual fulfillment, satisfaction, and happiness broadly construed (i.e., optimal functioning), and as being valued in their own right and not for tangible outcomes they may produce (although character strengths can and do produce desirable outcomes). Table 20.1 shows the 24 character strengths included in the VIA classification and short definitions describing their core meaning.

The current gold standard measure for the assessment of the 24 character strengths presented in Table 20.1 in adults is the *Values in Action Inventory of Strengths* (*VIA-IS*; Peterson, Park, & Seligman, 2005a). The VIA-IS is a questionnaire consisting of 240 items with a 5-point answer format (from 1 = *very much unlike me* to 5 = *very much like me*) measuring the 24 character strengths of the VIA classification (10 items for each strength). The responses are averaged across the ten items per character strength with higher scores indicating a stronger and more frequent manifestation of this character strength in an individual's thoughts, feelings, and behaviors. A sample item is "I am always coming up with new ways to do things" (creativity). The 24 scales have shown satisfactory psychometric characteristics (e.g., with respect to reliability and validity). The VIA-IS has been used in numerous studies and is available in various language versions in addition to the original English language version (e.g., German, Hebrew, Japanese, and Spanish; cf. Azañedo, Fernández-Abascal, & Barraca, 2014; Littman-Ovadia & Lavy, 2012; Otake et al., 2005; Ruch, Proyer et al., 2010).

Previous research showed that character strengths are meaningfully related to optimal functioning as postulated in this set of criteria. For example, various studies showed that character strengths are linked to dealing successfully with adversities in life like illnesses or stress at work (e.g., Harzer & Ruch, 2015; Park, Peterson, & Seligman, 2004b; Peterson, Park, & Seligman, 2006). Furthermore, character strengths are positively related to positive outcomes like stable interpersonal relationships or performance at work (e.g., Harzer & Ruch, 2014; Peterson & Park, 2007).

On the other hand, in order to study the relations between character strengths and optimal functioning on a more general level, it may be of interest to examine the role of character strengths for individual well-being. Two large research traditions with very different philosophical roots, the hedonic and the eudaimonic approach, form major perspectives in current research on well-being (Ryan & Deci, 2001). These will be described in more detail in the following subsections of this chapter. Subsequently, an overview about research on the relations between character strengths and well-being – with respect to each of the two approaches to well-being – will be presented.

20.1.2 Hedonic and Eudaimonic Well-Being

Well-being is a concept that deals with optimal psychological functioning and experience (Ryan & Deci, 2001). Early on in intellectual history, philosophers discussed what makes life a good one (i.e., a life which is full of optimal experience; cf. Ryan & Deci, 2001; Ryff, 1989; Chap. 6, this volume; 2014; Ryff & Singer, 2008). Depending on the approach (i.e., hedonism vs.

Table 20.1 The 24 character strengths included in the values in action classification of strengths (Peterson & Seligman, 2004) and short descriptions defining the strengths

1. Cognitive strengths that entail the acquisition and use of knowledge – strengths of wisdom and knowledge
Creativity [*originality, ingenuity*]: thinking of novel and productive ways to conceptualize and do things; includes artistic achievement but is not limited to it
Curiosity [*interest, novelty-seeking, openness to experience*]: taking an interest in ongoing experience for its own sake; finding subjects and topics fascinating; exploring and discovering
Judgment [*open-mindedness, critical thinking*]: thinking things through and examining them from all sides; not jumping to conclusions; being able to change one's mind in light of evidence; weighing all evidence fairly
Love of learning: mastering new skills, topics, and bodies of knowledge, whether on one's own or formally; obviously related to the strength of curiosity but goes beyond it to describe the tendency to add systematically to what one knows
Perspective [*wisdom*]: being able to provide wise counsel to others; having ways of looking at the world that make sense to oneself and to other people
2. Emotional strengths that involve the exercise of will to accomplish goals in the face of opposition, external or internal – strengths of courage
Bravery [*valor*]: *not* shrinking from threat, challenge, difficulty, or pain; speaking up for what is right even if there is opposition; acting on convictions even if unpopular; includes physical bravery but is not limited to it
Perseverance [*persistence, industriousness*]: finishing what one starts; persisting in a course of action in spite of obstacles; "getting it out the door"; taking pleasure in completing tasks
Honesty [*authenticity, integrity*]: speaking the truth but more broadly and presenting oneself in a genuine way and acting in a sincere way; being without pretense; taking responsibility for one's feelings and actions
Zest [*vitality, enthusiasm, vigor, energy*]: approaching life with excitement and energy; not doing things halfway or halfheartedly; living life as an adventure; feeling alive and activated
3. Interpersonal strengths that involve "tending and befriending" others – strengths of humanity
Love [*capacity to love and be loved*]: valuing close relations with others, in particular those in which sharing and caring are reciprocated; being close to people
Kindness [*generosity, nurturance, care, compassion, altruistic love, "niceness"*]: doing favors and good deeds for others; helping them; taking care of them
Social intelligence [*emotional intelligence, personal intelligence*]: Being aware of the motives and feelings of other people and oneself; knowing what to do to fit into different social situations; knowing what makes other people tick
4. Civic strengths that underlie healthy community life – strengths of justice
Teamwork [*citizenship, social responsibility, loyalty*]: working well as a member of a group or team; being loyal to the group; doing one's share
Fairness: treating all people the same according to notions of fairness and justice; not letting personal feelings bias decisions about others; giving everyone a fair chance
Leadership: encouraging a group of which one is a member to get things done and at the time maintain time good relations within the group; organizing group activities and seeing that they happen
5. Strengths that protect against excess – strengths of temperance
Forgiveness [*mercy*]: forgiving those who have done wrong; accepting others' shortcomings; giving people a second chance; not being vengeful
Modesty [*humility*]: letting one's accomplishments speak for themselves; not regarding oneself as more special than one is
Prudence: being careful about one's choices; not taking undue risks; *not* saying or doing things that might later be regretted
Self-regulation [*self-control*]: regulating what one feels and does; being disciplined; controlling one's appetites and emotions
6. Strengths that forge connections to the larger universe and provide meaning – transcendence/theological strengths
Appreciation of beauty and excellence [*awe, wonder, elevation; short name: appreciation*]: noticing and appreciating beauty, excellence, and/or skilled performance in various domains of life, from nature to art to mathematics to science to everyday experience

(continued)

Table 20.1 (continued)

Gratitude: being aware of and thankful for the good things that happen; taking time to express thanks
Hope [*optimism, future-mindedness, future orientation*]: expecting the best in the future and working to achieve it; believing that a good future is something that can be brought about
Humor [*playfulness*]: liking to laugh and tease; bringing smiles to other people; seeing the light side; making (not necessarily telling) jokes
Spirituality [*religiousness, faith, purpose*]: having coherent beliefs about the higher purpose and meaning of the universe; knowing where one fits within the larger scheme; having beliefs about the meaning of life that shape conduct and provide comfort

Note. The character strengths are grouped together content-wise on a theoretical basis. Labels of character strengths and expressions in brackets emphasize family resemblance to acknowledge heterogeneity of strengths and to minimize subtle (political or otherwise) connotations (Peterson & Seligman, 2004)

eudaimonism), the views differ with respect to what is considered as a good life. Although they do overlap in some aspects (e.g., considering emotions), they take different perspectives. For example, the hedonic approach would consider mourning about a dead loved one as detrimental for well-being. Contrary, the eudaimonic approach would consider mourning to be more fully functioning (i.e., greater well-being) than avoiding the feeling of sadness (cf. Ryan & Deci, 2001, Ryan & Martela, Chap. 7, this volume). In the following both approaches will be described in more detail.

Hedonic Well-Being

Well-being – with respect to the hedonic view – is defined by pleasures and happiness. Aristippus, a Greek philosopher living from 435 to 356 BC, was one of the very first highlighting that a good life is a life that is aimed at maximizing the amount of pleasurable experiences and minimizing displeasure in life (cf. Ryan & Deci, 2001; Seligman, Steen, Park, & Peterson, 2005). In psychological research mostly *subjective well-being* (Diener, Suh, Lucas, & Smith, 1999) is used as an indicator for the degree to which hedonic well-being is represented in individuals' lives (Ryan & Deci, 2001). Subjective well-being is defined as frequent positive affect, infrequent negative affect, and high life satisfaction[1] (e.g., Diener et al., 1999; Diener, Lucas, & Oishi, 2005). Positive and negative affect are the emotional aspects of subjective well-being, and life satisfaction is the cognitive component of subjective well-being.

Positive affect and negative affect are defined as being closely related to the dispositions to experience certain sets of feelings and moods (e.g., Watson, Clark, & Tellegen, 1988). Higher levels of positive affect go along with high energy, full concentration, and pleasurable engagement, whereas lower levels of positive affect go along with sadness and lethargy (Watson et al., 1988). Higher levels of negative affect are linked to negative moods like anger, guilt, and fear; lower levels of negative affect relate to calmness and serenity (Watson et al., 1988). Life satisfaction is typically defined as a cognitive (vs. emotional) evaluation of the positivity of one's life as a whole (Diener, 1994). The constructs of life satisfaction and affect are related to some degree, but are distinct from each other (i.e., show considerable discriminant validity), indicating the need to consider all of them in studies on subjective well-being in order to comprehensively capture it (e.g., Diener et al., 1999).

Widely utilized measures to assess the three indicators of subjective well-being (i.e., positive affect, negative affect, global life satisfaction) are the *Positive and Negative Affect Schedule* (*PANAS*; Watson et al., 1988) and the *Satisfaction with Life Scale* (*SWLS*; Diener, Emmons, Larsen, & Griffin, 1985). Both measures showed satisfactory psychometric characteristics (e.g., with respect to reliability and validity).

[1]On a more nuanced level, domain specific satisfactions (e.g., with work, family or self) can be distinguished as well (cf. Diener et al., 1999). However, this will not be of interest in the present chapter.

The *Positive and Negative Affect Schedule* (*PANAS*; Watson et al., 1988) is a 20-item measure of the frequency of positive affect (PA) and negative affect (NA) of adults. The PA scale entails ten items reflecting moods like interested, active, and proud. The NA scale has ten items reflecting moods like hostile, guilty, and nervous. The PANAS uses a 5-point answer format (from 1 = *little or not at all* to 5 = *all of the time*), which participants use to indicate the extent they have felt the moods, for example, in the past month. Other instructions are available referring to other time frames (e.g., at the moment, in the past weeks, generally). Responses are averaged across the ten items per scale to compute a total score for positive affect and negative affect; higher scores indicate more frequent experiences of positive affect and negative affect. The PANAS is available in various language versions in addition to the original English language version (e.g., German, French, Hebrew, and Spanish; cf. Anaby, Jarus, & Zumbo, 2010; Gaudreau, Sanchez, & Blondin, 2006; Krohne, Egloff, Kohlmann, & Tausch, 1996; Sandín et al., 1999).

The *Satisfaction with Life Scale* (*SWLS*; Diener et al., 1985) is a five-item measure for the assessment of global life satisfaction, which utilizes a 7-point answer format (from 1 = *strongly disagree* to 7 = *strongly agree*). Responses are added up or averaged across the five items to compute a total score for global life satisfaction; higher scores indicated a higher life satisfaction. A sample item is "The conditions of my life are excellent". The SWLS is available in various language versions in addition to the original English language version (e.g., German, French, Hebrew, and Spanish; cf. Anaby et al., 2010; Atienza, Balaguer, & García-Merita, 2003; Blais, Vallerand, Pelletier, & Brière, 1989; Glaesmer, Grande, Braehler, & Roth, 2011; Ruch, Harzer, Proyer, Park, & Peterson, 2010; Ruch, Proyer et al., 2010; Ruch, Proyer, & Weber, 2010).

An overall subjective well-being score is often computed by summing the z-standardized scores of positive affect and life satisfaction, and subtracting negative affect (cf. Diener, 1994; Sheldon & Elliot, 1999; Sheldon & Niemiec, 2006; Sheldon, Chap. 36, this volume). Hence, higher scores indicate higher overall subjective well-being.

Eudaimonic Well-Being

Well-being – with respect to the eudaimonic view – is defined by knowing one's unique talents and strengths, and nurturing them to bring them to reality (e.g., Ryan & Deci, 2001; Ryff, 2014). Hence, a central part of eudaimonic well-being is personal growth and self-actualization (cf. Ryan & Deci, 2001; Ryff, 2014; Ryff & Singer, 2008). From the eudaimonic perspective, a hedonic life is a vulgar way of life, because aiming for momentary pleasures can be detrimental for personal growth on the long run (cf. Peterson, Park, & Seligman, 2005b; Ryan & Deci, 2001; Ryff, 2014; Ryff & Singer, 2008). The eudaimonic approach to well-being dates back to Aristotle, a Greek philosopher living from 384 to 322 BC. In psychological research often *psychological well-being* (Ryff, 1989) is used as an indicator for the degree to which eudaimonic well-being is represented in individuals' lives.

Ryff (1989) identified six recurring, defining themes of optimal psychological functioning in philosophical as well as humanistic, existential, developmental, and clinical psychological literature about human growth and development. Table 20.2 presents an overview about the six dimension including short definitions to describe their core meaning.

Table 20.2 shows that an individual with pronounced psychological well-being (a) manages life situations well (i.e., environmental mastery), (b) makes use of personal talents and potential (i.e., personal growth), (c) feels that life has meaning and direction (i.e., purpose in life), (d) lives in line with personal convictions (i.e., autonomy), (e) knows and accepts own strengths and limitations (i.e., self-acceptance), and (f) has deep connections with significant others (i.e., positive relationships) (cf. Ryff, 1989, 2014; Ryff & Singer, 2008). Research showed, that these six dimensions form related, yet distinct dimensions of psychological well-being (cf. Ryff, 1989, 2014) indicating the need to consider all of them in studies on psychological well-being in order to comprehensively capture it.

Table 20.2 The six key dimensions of psychological well-being and short descriptions defining the dimensions (Ryff, 1989)

Environmental mastery
High scorer: has a sense of mastery and competence in managing the environment; controls complex array of external activities; makes effective use of surrounding opportunities; able to choose or create contexts suitable to personal needs and values
Low scorer: has difficulty managing everyday affairs; feels unable to change or improve surrounding context; is unaware of surrounding opportunities; lacks sense of control over external world
Personal growth
High scorer: has a feeling of continued development; sees self as growing and expanding; is open to new experiences; has sense of realizing his or her potential; sees improvement in self and behavior over time; is changing in ways that reflect more self-knowledge and effectiveness
Low scorer: has a sense of personal stagnation; lacks sense of improvement or expansion over time; feels bored and uninterested with life; feels unable to develop new attitudes or behaviors
Purpose in life
High scorer: has goals in life and a sense of directedness; feels there is meaning to present and past life; holds beliefs that give life purpose; has aims and objectives for living
Low scorer: lacks a sense of meaning in life; has few goals or aims, lacks sense of direction; does not see purpose in past life; has no outlooks or beliefs that give life meaning
Autonomy
High scorer: is self-determining and independent; able to resist social pressures to think and act in certain ways; regulates behavior from within; evaluates self by personal standards
Low scorer: is concerned about the expectations and evaluations of others; relies on judgments of others to make important decisions; conforms to social pressures to think and act in certain ways
Self-acceptance
High scorer: possesses a positive attitude toward the self; acknowledges and accepts multiple aspects of self, including good and bad qualities; feels positive about past life
Low scorer: feels dissatisfied with self; is disappointed with what has occurred in past life; is troubled about certain personal qualities; wishes to be different than what he or she is
Positive relationships (also labeled as positive relations with others)
High scorer: has warm, satisfying, trusting relationships with others; is concerned about the welfare of others; capable of strong empathy, affection and intimacy; understands give and take of human relationships
Low scorer: has few close, trusting relationships with others; finds it difficult to be warm, open, concerned about others; is isolated and frustrated in interpersonal relationships; not willing to make compromises to sustain important ties with others

The *Psychological Well-Being Scales* (*PWBS*; Ryff, 1989; Ryff & Essex, 1992) are widely utilized to measure the six core dimensions of psychological well-being (i.e., environmental mastery, personal growth, purpose in life, autonomy, self-acceptance, and positive relationships; Ryff & Keyes, 1995) as well as overall psychological well-being. Example items are "I have confidence in my opinions, even if they are contrary to the general consensus" (autonomy) and "I like most parts of my personality" (self-acceptance). Participants are asked to rate the degree to which they (dis)agree with each of the statements presented in the items by utilizing a 6-point answer format (from 1 = *completely disagree* to 6 = *completely agree*). The responses are averaged across the respective items per scale with higher scores indicating higher psychological well-being. There are different versions of the PWBS, which differ with respect to scale length. Research indicated that the scales should not be shorter than 7 items to insure the quality of the measurement, and that the 14-item version is to be preferred (cf. Ryff, 2014). Taking this into account, the PWBS can be described as a measure that demonstrated satisfactory psychometric properties (e.g., with respect to reliability and validity). The PWBS are available in various language versions in addition to the original English language version (e.g., German, French, and Japanese; cf. Kishida et al., 2004; Risch, 2008; Risch, Strohmayer, & Stangier, 2005; Salama-Younes, Ismaïl, Montazeri, & Roncin, 2011; Van Dierendonck, 2005).

20.2 The Role of Character Strengths for Hedonic and Eudaimonic Well-Being

Most research studying character strengths in adult samples examined their relations to subjective well-being (with a special emphasis on life satisfaction). Little is known about the relations between character strengths and psychological well-being. In the remainder of this section a brief overview about existing research is given.

20.2.1 Character Strengths and Subjective Well-Being

Character strengths and overall *subjective well-being* share almost 50% of variance (Harzer, 2016). Especially the emotional and interpersonal strengths were related to overall subjective well-being, followed by the civic (except fairness) and theological strengths (except appreciation). Appreciation, prudence, and judgment showed the numerically weakest associations (Harzer, 2016).

Across different methods (self- vs. peer-ratings, paper-pencil vs. web-based testing, college students vs. community samples) and across samples from various nations, character strengths showed positive correlations with measures of *life satisfaction*. Hope, zest, curiosity, gratitude, and love were consistently among the character strengths with the strongest relations to life satisfaction (e.g., Gradišek, 2012; Littman-Ovadia & Lavy, 2012; Miljković & Rijavec, 2008; Park, Peterson, & Seligman, 2004a; Ruch, Proyer et al., 2010; Shimai, Otake, Park, Peterson, & Seligman, 2006). Character strengths like modesty, appreciation, creativity, judgment, and love of learning were less related to life satisfaction. However, none of the 24 character strengths showed statistically significant negative correlations with life satisfaction. This generally supports the idea that character strengths contribute to a satisfied life (Peterson & Seligman, 2004). Moreover, an intervention study supported the causal relation between character strengths and life satisfaction (see Proyer, Ruch, & Buschor, 2013). In line with these results for adults, the strongest predictors of adolescents' life satisfaction were the character strengths of hope, gratitude, love, and zest (e.g., Park & Peterson, 2006; Ruch, Weber, Park, & Peterson, 2014; Weber, Ruch, Littman-Ovadia, Lavy, & Gai, 2013).

With respect to *positive affect*, zest, hope, and curiosity were among those character strengths that correlated numerically highest with positive affect across studies utilizing different measures of positive affect, and samples stemming from different nations. Modesty, spirituality, prudence, and forgiveness were among those character strengths that showed the weakest associations with positive affect (e.g., Brdar & Kashdan, 2010; Güsewell & Ruch, 2012; Littman-Ovadia & Lavy, 2012; Martínez Martí & Ruch, 2014).

At the moment, few studies examined the relations between character strengths and *negative affect*. However, results are mixed across utilized samples and measurements of negative affect. Overall, results suggest that character strengths are negatively related to negative affect, but effect sizes are smaller than those reported for positive affect and life satisfaction. Hope, zest, humor, and curiosity were among the strongest correlates of negative affect, whereas appreciation and spirituality were among the weakest (e.g., Khumalo, Wissing, & Temane, 2008; Littman-Ovadia & Lavy, 2012; Martínez Martí & Ruch, 2014). Overall, especially the strengths of temperance (except prudence) and the emotional strengths (except bravery) correlated with negative affect (Harzer, 2016).

20.2.2 Character Strengths and Psychological Well-Being

Research on the relations between character strengths and psychological well-being (Ryff, 1989) is scarce. To the knowledge of the author there are (a) two studies examining the correlations between character strengths and psychological well-being on an aggregated level of character strengths (e.g., average scores for the groups of strengths as presented in Table 20.1 or on a higher-order factorial level) (cf. Leontopoulou & Triliva, 2012; Yanez, 2007); and (b) one study reporting the relations between character strengths and psychological well-being on scale level (i.e., 24 character strengths and 6 dimensions of psychological well-being plus overall psychological well-being) (cf. Harzer, 2016).

Across the two studies examining the relations on the level of aggregated character strengths, emotional strengths were especially related to environmental mastery, purpose in life, autonomy, and self-acceptance (Leontopoulou & Triliva, 2012; Yanez, 2007). Self-acceptance also went along with theological strengths. Cognitive strengths were substantially associated with personal growth. Interpersonal strengths showed the strongest correlations with positive relationships. Comparable results were reported in studies utilizing similar concepts like the ones defined by Ryff (1989) (e.g., autonomy and meaning; cf. Brdar & Kashdan, 2010; Huta & Hawley, 2010, Huta, Chap. 15, this volume).

Harzer (2016) reported results on the relations between the 24 character strengths and the six dimensions of psychological well-being. Overall, character strengths and psychological well-being shared 56 % of variance (Harzer, 2016). Environmental mastery was especially related to the emotional strengths bravery, perseverance, honesty, and zest as well as to the interpersonal strengths love, kindness, and social intelligence. Furthermore, it went along with hope, self-regulation, and curiosity. Personal growth showed consistent relations with the cognitive strengths creativity, curiosity, judgment, love of leaning, and perspective, but also with bravery, zest, and hope. The emotional and cognitive strengths were also consistently related to purpose in life (except judgment) as well as autonomy. The strongest relations to purpose in life exhibited the specific character strengths of hope, zest, and curiosity. Autonomy showed the strongest relations with bravery followed by curiosity, zest, honesty, and perspective. Self-acceptance went especially along with interpersonal strengths followed by teamwork, leadership, gratitude, hope, and humor. Its strongest relations were with zest and hope followed by curiosity, love, and forgiveness. All of the interpersonal and civic strengths were consistently associated with positive relationships. The numerically strongest relations exhibited love, zest, hope, social intelligence, and humor. Across all indicators of psychological well-being, the specific character strengths of prudence, modesty, appreciation, and spirituality exhibited the weakest associations.

20.3 Discussion

Positive psychology is aimed at studying what makes individuals' lives most worth living; Seligman & Csikszentmihalyi, 2000). This focus facilitates research on what enables human flourishing and optimal functioning (Gable & Haidt, 2005). Depending on the approach (i.e., hedonism vs. eudaimonism), the views differ with respect to what is considered as optimal experience. In psychological research mostly *subjective well-being* (i.e., positive affect, negative affect, global life satisfaction; e.g., Diener et al., 1999, 2005; Ryan & Deci, 2001) is used as an indicator for the degree to which hedonic well-being is represented in individuals' lives (Ryan & Deci, 2001). *Psychological well-being* (i.e., environmental mastery, personal growth, purpose in life, autonomy, self-acceptance, and positive relationships; Ryff, 1989) is often used as an indicator for the degree to which eudaimonic well-being is represented in individuals' lives.

Summarizing the existing research, it can be said that none of the character strengths systematically showed a correlation coefficient that indicated a detrimental relation between a strength and (indicators of) subjective and psychological well-being. On the contrary and as expected, character strengths seem to be important individual factors facilitating optimal functioning. Table 20.3 provides an overview about the numerically strongest relations between the 24 character strengths and the indicators of subjective well-being as well as psychological well-being that could be observed across the different studies summarized in the present chapter.

Table 20.3 Overview about the strongest relations between the 24 character strengths of the VIA classification and the indicators of subjective and psychological well-being across the different studies summarized in this chapter

	Subjective well-being			Psychological well-being					
Character strengths	PA	NA	LS	EM	PG	PL	A	SA	PR
Cognitive strengths									
Creativity					✓	✓	✓		
Curiosity	✓✓		✓	✓	✓✓	✓✓	✓✓	✓	✓
Judgment					✓		✓		
Love of learning					✓✓	✓	✓		
Perspective					✓	✓	✓✓		
Emotional strengths									
Bravery				✓	✓	✓	✓✓	✓	
Perseverance		✓		✓		✓✓	✓		
Honesty		✓		✓		✓	✓✓	✓	
Zest	✓✓	✓	✓✓	✓✓	✓	✓✓	✓✓	✓✓	✓✓
Interpersonal strengths									
Love	✓		✓	✓		✓		✓	✓✓
Kindness				✓				✓	✓
Social intelligence				✓				✓	✓✓
Civic strengths									
Teamwork								✓	✓
Fairness									✓
Leadership								✓	✓
Strengths of temperance									
Forgiveness		✓							
Modesty		✓							
Prudence									
Self-regulation		✓		✓		✓✓		✓	
Theological strengths									
Appreciation	✓								
Gratitude			✓					✓	
Hope	✓✓	✓	✓✓	✓✓	✓	✓✓	✓	✓✓	✓✓
Humor								✓	
Spirituality									

Note: Indicators of subjective well-being: *PA* Positive affect, *NA* Negative affect, *LS* Life satisfaction. Indicators of psychological well-being: *EM* Environmental mastery, *PG* Personal growth, *PL* Purpose in life, *A* Autonomy, *SA* Self-acceptance, *PR* Positive relationships. ✓ = Among the strongest correlations across the different studies summarized in this chapter, but correlations coefficient <0.40 in Harzer (2016); ✓✓ = Among the strongest correlations across the different studies summarized in this chapter, and correlations coefficient ≥0.40 in Harzer (2016)

Table 20.3 shows, that across all indicators of well-being (i.e., subjective well-being and psychological well-being) zest, hope, and curiosity were the most substantial correlates among the character strengths; the least often relevant character strengths were modesty, prudence, appreciation, and spirituality. Moreover, in addition to zest, hope, and curiosity, further character strengths were relevant for specific indicators of subjective well-being and psycho-

logical well-being as well. For example, forgiveness and modesty were among the strongest correlates of negative affect. Self-regulation, honesty, and perspective were among the strongest correlates of environmental mastery. Love of learning, bravery, and creativity were especially related to personal growth. Furthermore, bravery, honesty, and perspective were of specific relevance for autonomy. Love and forgiveness were among the strongest correlates of self-acceptance. Moreover, love, social intelligence, and humor were among the most substantial correlates of positive relationships. In the following these results are interpreted and discussed in more detail with a special emphasis on the eudaimonic approach of well-being (i.e., psychological well-being).

Why would the character strengths zest, hope, and curiosity be relevant for such a broad range of well-being indicators? These character strengths go along with behaviors and cognitions (cf. Peterson & Seligman, 2004) that by definition foster optimal functioning and a positive way to approach life (cf. Harzer, 2016). Feeling full of energy and activated (zest), believing that a good future is something that can be brought about (hope) as well as taking an interest in and exploring all of ongoing experience (curiosity), lead people to approach the tasks and challenges of everyday life in a proactive and self-efficacious way (cf. Cangiano & Parker, 2016). According to Parker, Bindl, and Strauss's (2010) model of proactive motivation there are three key motivational aspects that initiate and maintain proactivity. These are "energized to", "can do", and "reason to". These three aspects can be directly linked to the behaviors and cognitions related to zest, hope, and curiosity, respectively.

Forgiveness and modesty were among the relevant character strengths for negative affect in addition to the three character strengths noted above. According to Peterson and Seligman (2004), a forgiving person is able to accept the shortcomings of others, and a humble and modest person has an accurate awareness of own limitations or deficiencies without being overly sensitive to ego threats (see also Chancellor & Lyubomirsky, 2013; Tangey, 2000). Therefore, when expectations regarding oneself or with respect to others are violated, these two character strengths may buffer the negative effects of such a violation on an individual's mood. Consequently, lower levels of negative affect are likely in forgiving and modest individuals.

20.3.1 Character Strengths and Psychological Well-Being

Self-regulation, honesty, and perspective were specifically related to *environmental mastery*. Why would individuals with high levels in these character strengths possess high levels of environmental mastery? Behaviors, thoughts, and feelings linked to those character strengths may support the development of environmental mastery (cf. Harzer, 2016). For example, self-regulation helps individuals to control their behaviors, honesty leads people to behave in a sincere way and to take responsibility for their own behaviors, and perspective fosters integrating the information into a meaningful big picture (Peterson & Seligman, 2004). As environmental mastery is characterized by having a sense of competence in managing the environment, being able to control complex array of external activities, and making effective use of surrounding opportunities suitable to personal needs and values (Ryff, 1989, 2014; Ryff & Singer, 2008) these character strengths may specifically foster this dimension of psychological well-being (cf. Harzer, 2016).

Personal growth was most strongly related to love of learning, bravery, and creativity. It seems obvious that love of learning (e.g., mastering new skills) goes hand in hand with a feeling of continued development, which is a defining aspect of personal growth according to Ryff (1989, 2014; Ryff & Singer, 2008; cf. Harzer, 2016). Furthermore, the character strength creativity, defined as thinking of novel and productive ways to conceptualize and do things (Peterson & Seligman, 2004), might foster improvement in behavior over time and an increase in effectiveness (cf. Harzer, 2016). Both are core aspects of personal growth (Ryff, 1989, 2014; Ryff &

Singer, 2008). Learning and development – as relevant aspects of personal growth – are not always easy but include tackling challenges and difficulties, and bravery assists in not shrinking back from it (Peterson & Seligman, 2004).

Autonomy was especially related to bravery, honesty, and perspective. This makes sense, as an autonomous person is characterized by being self-determining and independent, and able to resist social pressures to think and act in certain ways (cf. Ryff, 1989, 2014; Ryff & Singer, 2008), all of which are characteristics of a brave individual (cf. Peterson & Seligman, 2004). Therefore, bravery appears to be a very central personality characteristic that enables autonomy (cf. Harzer, 2016). Furthermore, an autonomous person regulates behavior from within, which means that this person takes responsibility for own feelings and actions (cf. Ryff, 1989, 2014; Ryff & Singer, 2008). As this is a major element of the character strength honesty, the strong linkage between honesty and autonomy seems plausible (cf. Harzer, 2016). Finally, autonomy includes the evaluation of the self by personal standards (cf. Ryff, 1989, 2014; Ryff & Singer, 2008). Perspective is a characteristic that enables individuals to do so (cf. Peterson & Seligman, 2004); therefore, it appears to be a meaningful and obvious contributor to autonomy as well (cf. Harzer, 2016).

The dimension of *positive relationships* was substantially associated with the character strengths love, social intelligence, and humor. A person who scores high in in this dimension of psychological well-being has warm, satisfying, and trusting relationships with others, is capable of strong empathy, affection, and intimacy as well as understands give and take of human relationships (cf. Ryff, 1989, 2014; Ryff & Singer, 2008). People high in love value trusting, close relationships in which sharing and caring are reciprocated (Peterson & Seligman, 2004). This fosters positive relationships as defined by Ryff (1989) (cf. Harzer, 2016). Furthermore, one important aspect of social intelligence is the awareness of the motives and feelings of other people as well as to know what makes other people tick (Peterson & Seligman, 2004). Additionally, humor includes behaviors like bringing smiles to other people when they do not feel well (Peterson & Seligman, 2004). Both social intelligence and humor foster empathy, warmth, and affection, which are important in positive relationships as defined by (Ryff, 1989; cf. Harzer, 2016).

Finally, love and forgiveness were substantial correlates of *self-acceptance*. Also this linkage appears meaningful as both character strengths represent aspects of acceptance of others but also of the self (cf. Harzer, 2016). For example, the character strength love includes (beside the ability to love others) the acceptance of being loved by others (i.e., feeling worth of being loved) (cf. Peterson & Seligman, 2004). On the other hand, forgiveness is also closely related to acceptance, because forgiving individuals are able to accept the shortcomings of others (Peterson & Seligman, 2004), and might therefore more likely accept their own shortcomings as well. This means, individuals who can accept being loved by others, and can accept their own shortcomings more likely develop high levels of self-acceptance (cf. Harzer, 2016).

Contrary to this interpretation, where love and forgiveness foster self-acceptance, one might assume another causal direction here as well (i.e., self-acceptance enhances love and forgiveness). Self-acceptance includes a positive attitude toward the self as well as the acknowledgment and acceptance of multiple aspects of the self (i.e., including good and bad qualities) (Ryff, 1989, 2014; Ryff & Singer, 2008). These attitudes and cognitions might foster the capability of a person to value and accept being loved by significant others as well as to forgive the shortcomings others might have, because the own ones are known and accepted (cf. Harzer, 2016).

20.3.2 Outlook and Future Research

Study Designs and Their Consequences

Most of the studies summarized in the present chapter share several characteristics with respect to the study designs. Firstly, the cross-sectional designs do not allow for any conclusions about causal relations between the variables. Although causal directions and potential mechanisms were formulated in the chapter in order to describe the assumed role of character strengths for subjective and psychological well-being, more studies utilizing longitudinal and intervention designs are needed to address research questions regarding causality (cf. Harzer, 2016).

Relating to this, it is important to consider that well-being is not a static characteristic. For example, subjective well-being is defined as both affective and cognitive-evaluative processes that are based on individuals everyday experiences and circumstances (e.g., Diener et al., 1999). Furthermore, with respect to the eudaimonic approach, personal growth is considered as a central part of psychological well-being (e.g., Ryff, 1989). The role of character strengths regarding such processes may be studied within the scope of diary and/or longitudinal studies to get in-depth insights on causal and reciprocal effects. The *engine model of well-being* (Jayawickreme, Forgeard, & Seligman, 2012; Jayawickreme & Dahill-Brown, Chap. 31, this volume) and the *broaden-and-build theory* (Fredrickson, 2001; Chap. 12, this volume) might be useful theoretical frameworks for such endeavors (cf. Harzer, 2016).

Additionally, because data are predominantly self-reported, common method variance may have inflated correlations (cf. Doty & Glick, 1998). However, correlation pattern between character strengths and well-being varied across the different indicators of well-being. Therefore, it was concluded that the results were not overly affected by this bias. Self-ratings have often been the chosen source of data in the present study, because the experiences related to well-being have been considered to be in large parts intra-individual, and self-ratings were considered the most valid judgments for such variables. Nevertheless, studies are needed that utilize multiple data sources to eliminate the effects associated with common method variance.

Moreover, future studies might specifically recruit samples with low or medium education as data predominantly stemmed from a highly educated sample. Therefore, generalizability of results to less educated groups can be questioned and needs to be addressed in future research.

Further Thoughts on the Eudaimonics of Character Strengths

This chapter presented how specific (groups of) character strengths relate to specific aspects of psychological well-being. However, one important aspect of character strengths could not be acknowledged within the present chapter. That is, each person has an individual set of up to seven top or core strengths among the set of 24 that he/she especially owns (Peterson & Seligman, 2004). These strengths are labeled as 'signature' strengths (Peterson & Seligman, 2004). Activities (like one's work tasks, hobbies) that allow the application of the individual signature strengths are postulated to be fulfilling and most valued (e.g., Harzer & Ruch, 2012, 2013; Park & Peterson, 2007; Peterson & Seligman, 2004; Seligman, 2002, 2011). Several studies highlighted the relations between the application of individual signature strengths and various positive outcomes. For example, the application of individual signature strengths is related to positive experiences in life (e.g., life satisfaction, positive affect, and meaning in life) as well as to positive work-related outcomes (e.g., job satisfaction, pleasure at work, calling, and job performance (e.g., Harzer & Ruch, 2012, 2013, 2014, in press; Littman-Ovadia & Steger, 2010; Proctor, Maltby, & Linley, 2011; Proctor & Tweed, Chap. 18, this volume; Wood, Linley, Maltby, Kashdan, & Hurling, 2011). Well-being – with respect to the eudaimonic view – is defined by knowing one's unique talents and strengths, and bringing them to reality. This is exactly what is done when individual signature strengths are applied in everyday activities. Therefore, the application of individual signature strengths should show strong relations with the dimensions of psychological well-being. This needs to be addressed in future research.

20.4 Conclusion

Character strengths are systematically related to different aspects of well-being. Therefore, they can be considered as important resources for both hedonic and eudaimonic well-being. As character strengths are seen as being malleable and trainable (Peterson & Seligman, 2004), they seem to be valuable target variables to focus on when aiming at fostering individuals' well-being. Studies have already shown that character strengths can be fostered by systematic interventions (e.g., Gander, Proyer, Ruch, & Wyss, 2013; Proyer et al., 2013), and that this leads to an increase in life satisfaction and decrease in depression (e.g., Forest et al., 2012; Gander et al., 2013; Mitchell, Stanimirovic, Klein, & Vella-Brodrick, 2009; Quinlan, Swain, & Vella-Brodrick, 2012). Therefore, further intervention programs that foster character strengths or the use of individual signature strengths in order to increase specific aspects of hedonic or eudaimonic well-being need to be developed and evaluated. So far, research on strengths interventions primarily focused on life satisfaction and depression as outcomes. In the light of the present chapter there are many more indicators of well-being available that should be considered in future research.

References

Anaby, D., Jarus, T., & Zumbo, B. D. (2010). Psychometric evaluation of the Hebrew language version of the Satisfaction with Life Scale. *Social Indicators Research, 96*, 267–274. doi:10.1007/s11205-009-9476-z.

Atienza, F. L., Balaguer, I., & García-Merita, M. L. (2003). Satisfaction with life scale: Analysis of factorial invariance across sexes. *Personality and Individual Differences, 35*, 1255–1260. doi:10.1016/S0191-8869(02)00332-X.

Azañedo, C. M., Fernández-Abascal, E. G., & Barraca, J. (2014). Character strengths in Spain: Validation of the Values in Action Inventory of Strengths (VIA-IS) in a Spanish sample. *Clínica y Salud, 25*, 123–130. doi:10.1016/j.clysa.2014.06.002.

Biswas-Diener, R. (2006). From the equator to the North Pole: A study of character strengths. *Journal of Happiness Studies, 7*, 293–310. doi:10.1007/s10902-005-3646-8.

Blais, M. R., Vallerand, R. J., Pelletier, L. G., & Brière, N. M. (1989). L'Echelle de Satisfaction de vie: Validation canadienne-française du "Satisfaction With Life Scale" [The satisfaction scale: Canadian-French validation of the Satisfaction with Life Scale.]. *Canadian Journal of Behavioural Science, 21*, 210–223. doi:10.1037/h0079854.

Brdar, I., & Kashdan, T. B. (2010). Character strengths and well-being in Croatia: An empirical investigation of structure and correlates. *Journal of Research in Personality, 44*, 151–154. doi:10.1016/j.jrp.2009.12.001.

Cangiano, F., & Parker, S. K. (2016). Proactivity for mental health and well-being. In S. Clarke, T. M. Probst, F. W. Guldenmund, & J. Passmore (Eds.), *The Wiley Blackwell handbook of the psychology of occupational safety and workplace health* (pp. 228–250). Malden, MA: Wiley.

Chancellor, J., & Lyubomirsky, S. (2013). Humble beginnings: Current trends, state perspectives, and hallmarks of humility. *Social and Personality Psychology Compass, 7*, 819–833. doi:10.1111/spc3.12069.

Diener, E. (1994). Assessing subjective well-being. Progress and opportunities. *Social Indicators Research, 31*, 103–157. doi:10.1007/BF01207052.

Diener, E., Emmons, R. A., Larsen, R. J., & Griffin, S. (1985). The satisfaction with life scale. *Journal of Personality Assessment, 49*, 71–75. doi:10.1207/s15327752jpa4901_13.

Diener, E., Lucas, R. E., & Oishi, S. (2005). Subjective well-being: The science of happiness and life satisfaction. In C. R. Snyder & S. J. Lopez (Eds.), *Handbook of positive psychology* (pp. 63–73). New York: Oxford University Press.

Diener, E., Suh, E. M., Lucas, R. E., & Smith, H. L. (1999). Subjective well-being: Three decades of progress. *Psychological Bulletin, 125*, 276–302. doi:10.1037//0033-2909.125.2.276.

Doty, D. H., & Glick, W. H. (1998). Common method bias: Does common methods variance really bias results? *Organizational Research Methods, 1*, 374–406. doi:10.1177/109442819814002.

Forest, J., Mageau, G. V. A., Crevier-Braud, L., Bergeron, L., Dubreuil, P., & Lavigne, G. V. L. (2012). Harmonious passion as an explanation of the relation between signature strengths' use and well-being at work: Test of an intervention program. *Human Relations, 65*, 1233–1252. doi:10.1177/0018726711433134.

Fredrickson, B. (2001). The role of positive emotions in positive psychology. *American Psychologist, 56*, 218–226. doi:10.1037//0003-066X.56.3.218.

Gable, S. L., & Haidt, J. (2005). What (and why) is positive psychology? *Review of General Psychology, 9*, 103–110. doi:10.1037/1089-2680.9.2.103.

Gander, F., Proyer, R. T., Ruch, W., & Wyss, T. (2013). Strength-based positive interventions: Further evidence on their potential for enhancing well-being and alleviating depression. *Journal of Happiness Studies, 14*, 1241–1259. doi:10.1007%2Fs10902-012-9380-0.

Gaudreau, P., Sanchez, X., & Blondin, J.-P. (2006). Positive and negative affective states in a performance-related setting: Testing the factorial structure of the PANAS across two samples of French-Canadian participants. *European Journal of Psychological Assessment, 22*, 240–249. doi:10.1027/1015-5759.22.4.240.

Glaesmer, H., Grande, G., Braehler, E., & Roth, M. (2011). The German version of the Satisfaction with Life Scale (SWLS): Psychometric properties, validity, and population-based norms. *European Journal of Psychological Assessment, 27*, 127–132. doi:10.1027/1015-5759/a000058.

Gradišek, P. (2012). Character strengths and life satisfaction of Slovenian in-service and pre-service teachers. *Center for Educational Policies Studies Journal, 2*, 167–180.

Güsewell, A., & Ruch, W. (2012). Are only emotional strengths emotional? Character strengths and disposition to positive emotions. *Applied Psychology: Health and Well-Being, 4*, 218–239. doi:10.1111/j.1758-0854.2012.01070.x.

Harzer, C. (2016). *The relations of character strengths with subjective and psychological well-being.* Manuscript submitted for publication.

Harzer, C., & Ruch, W. (2012). When the job is a calling: The role of applying one's signature strengths at work. *The Journal of Positive Psychology, 7*, 362–371. doi:10.1080/17439760.2012.702784.

Harzer, C., & Ruch, W. (2013). The application of signature character strengths and positive experiences at work. *Journal of Happiness Studies, 14*, 965–983. doi:10.1007/s10902-012-9364-0.

Harzer, C., & Ruch, W. (2014). The role of character strengths for task performance, job dedication, interpersonal facilitation, and organizational support. *Human Performance, 27*, 183–205. doi:10.1080/08959285.2014.913592.

Harzer, C., & Ruch, W. (2015). The relationships of character strengths with coping, work-related stress, and job satisfaction. *Frontiers in Psychology, 6*, 165. doi:10.3389/fpsyg.2015.00165.

Harzer, C., & Ruch, W. (in press). Your strengths are calling: Preliminary results of a strengths-based online-intervention to increase calling. *Journal of Happiness Studies*. doi:10.1007/s10902-015-9692-y.

Huta, V., & Hawley, L. (2010). Psychological strengths and cognitive vulnerabilities: Are they two ends of the same continuum or do they have independent relationships with well-being and ill-being? *Journal of Happiness Studies, 11*, 71–93. doi:10.1007/s10902-008-9123-4.

Jayawickreme, E., Forgeard, M. J. C., & Seligman, M. E. P. (2012). The engine of well-being. *Review of General Psychology, 16*, 327–342. doi:10.1037/a0027990.

Khumalo, I. P., Wissing, M. P., & Temane, Q. (2008). Exploring the validity of the Values-In-Action Inventory of Strengths (VIA-IS) in an African context. *Journal of Psychology in Africa, 18*, 133–142.

Kishida, Y., Kitamura, T., Gatayama, R., Matsuoka, T., Miura, S., & Yamabe, K. (2004). Ryff's psychological well-being inventory: Factorial structure and life history correlates among Japanese university students. *Psychological Reports, 94*, 83–103. doi:10.2466/PR0.94.1.83-103.

Krohne, H. W., Egloff, B., Kohlmann, C. W., & Tausch, A. (1996). Untersuchungen mit einer deutschen Version der Positive and Negative Affect Schedule (PANAS) [Investigations with a German version of the Positive and Negative Affect Schedule (PANAS)]. *Diagnostica, 42*, 139–156.

Leontopoulou, S., & Triliva, S. (2012). Explorations of subjective wellbeing and character strengths among a Greek University student sample. *International Journal of Wellbeing, 2*, 251–270. doi:10.5502/ijw.v2.i3.6.

Littman-Ovadia, H., & Lavy, S. (2012). Character strengths in Israel: Hebrew adaptation of the VIA inventory of strengths. *European Journal of Psychological Assessment, 28*, 41–50. doi:10.1027/1015-5759/a000089.

Littman-Ovadia, H., & Steger, M. F. (2010). Character strengths and well-being among volunteers and employees: Toward an integrative model. *The Journal of Positive Psychology, 5*, 419–430. doi:10.1080/17439760.2010.516765.

Martínez Martí, M. L., & Ruch, W. (2014). Character strengths and well-being across the life span: Data from a representative sample of German-speaking adults living in Switzerland. *Frontiers in Psychology, 5*, 1253. doi:10.3389/fpsyg.2014.01253.

Miljković, D., & Rijavec, M. (2008). What makes us happy: Strengths of mind, strengths of heart or self-control? In M. Cindrić, V. Domović, & M. Matijevic (Eds.), *Collected papers of 2nd scientific research symposium: Pedagogy and the knowledge society* (Vol. 1, pp. 241–250). Zagreb, Croatia: Učiteljski fakulte.

Mitchell, J., Stanimirovic, R., Klein, B., & Vella-Brodrick, D. A. (2009). A randomised controlled trial of a self-guided internet intervention promoting well-being. *Computers in Human Behavior, 25*, 749–760. doi:10.1016/j.chb.2009.02.003.

Otake, K., Shimai, S., Ikemi, A., Utsuki, N., Peterson, C., & Seligman, M. E. P. (2005). Development of the Japanese version of the Values in Action Inventory of Strengths (VIA-IS). *Japanese Journal of Psychology, 76*, 461–467. doi:10.4992/jjpsy.76.461.

Park, N., & Peterson, C. (2006). Moral competence and character strengths among adolescents: The development and validation of the values in action inventory of strengths for youth. *Journal of Adolescence, 29*, 891–909. doi:10.1016/j.adolescence.2006.04.011.

Park, N., & Peterson, C. (2007). Methodological issues in positive psychology and the assessment of character strengths. In A. D. Ong & M. H. M. van Dulmen (Eds.), *Handbook of methods in positive psychology* (pp. 292–305). New York: Oxford University Press.

Park, N., Peterson, C., & Seligman, M. E. P. (2004a). Strengths of character and well-being. *Journal of Social and Clinical Psychology, 23*, 603–619. doi:10.1521/jscp.23.5.603.50748.

Park, N., Peterson, C., & Seligman, M. E. P. (2004b). Reply: Strengths of character and well-being: A closer look at hope and modesty. *Journal of Social and Clinical Psychology, 23*, 628–634. doi:10.1521/jscp.23.5.628.50749.

Park, N., Peterson, C., & Seligman, M. E. P. (2006). Character strengths in fifty-four nations and the fifty

US states. *Journal of Positive Psychology, 1*, 118–129. doi:10.1080/17439760600619567.

Parker, S. K., Bindl, U. K., & Strauss, K. (2010). Making things happen: A model of proactive motivation. *Journal of Management, 36*, 827–856. doi:10.1177/0149206310363732.

Peterson, C. (2006). *A primer in positive psychology*. Oxford, UK: Oxford University Press.

Peterson, C., & Park, N. (2006). Character strengths in organizations. *Journal of Organizational Behavior, 27*, 1149–1154. doi:10.1002/job.398.

Peterson, C., & Park, N. (2007). Attachment security and its benefits in context. *Psychological Inquiry, 18*, 172–176. doi:10.1080/10478400701512752.

Peterson, C., Park, N., & Seligman, M. E. P. (2005a). Assessment of character strengths. In G. P. Koocher, J. C. Norcross, & S. S. Hill III (Eds.), *Psychologists' desk reference* (2nd ed., pp. 93–98). New York: Oxford University Press.

Peterson, C., Park, N., & Seligman, M. E. P. (2005b). Orientations to happiness and life satisfaction: The full versus the empty life. *Journal of Happiness Studies, 6*, 25–41. doi:10.1007/s10902-004-1278-z.

Peterson, C., Park, N., & Seligman, M. E. P. (2006). Greater strengths of character and recovery from illness. *Journal of Positive Psychology, 1*, 17–26. doi:10.1080/17439760500372739.

Peterson, C., & Seligman, M. E. P. (2004). *Character strengths and virtues: A handbook and classification*. New York: Oxford University Press.

Proctor, C., Maltby, J., & Linley, P. A. (2011). Strengths use as a predictor of wellbeing and health-related quality of life. *Journal of Happiness Studies, 12*, 153–169. doi:10.1007/s10902-009-9181-2.

Proyer, R. T., Ruch, W., & Buschor, C. (2013). Testing strengths-based interventions: A preliminary study on the effectiveness of a program targeting curiosity, gratitude, hope, humor, and zest for enhancing life satisfaction. *Journal of Happiness Studies, 14*, 275–292. doi:10.1007/s10902-012-9331-9.

Quinlan, D., Swain, N., & Vella-Brodrick, D. A. (2012). Character strengths interventions: Building on what we know for improved outcomes. *Journal of Happiness Studies, 13*, 1145–1163. doi:10.1007/s10902-011-9311-5.

Risch, A. K. (2008). *Rezidivierende Depression: Psychologische Risikofaktoren und Prädiktoren des Störungsverlaufs* [Recurrent depression: Psychological risk factors and predictors of the progress of disease] (Doctoral dissertation, Friedrich Schiller Universitay Jena). Retrieved from http://www.db-thueringen.de/servlets/DerivateServlet/Derivate-17179/Risch/Dissertation.pdf

Risch, A. K., Strohmayer, C., Stangier, U. (2005). *Fragebogen zum Psychologischen Wohlbefinden – PWB* [Psychological Well-Being Scales – PWB]. Unpublished manuscript, Department of Psychology, Friedrich Schiller University Jena, Jena, Germany.

Ruch, W., Harzer, C., Proyer, R. T., Park, N., & Peterson, C. (2010). Ways to happiness in German-speaking countries: The adaptation of the German version of the orientations to happiness questionnaire in paper-pencil and internet samples. *European Journal of Psychological Assessment, 26*, 224–231. doi:10.1027/1015-5759/a000030.

Ruch, W., Proyer, R. T., Harzer, C., Park, N., Peterson, C., & Seligman, M. E. P. (2010). Values in Action Inventory of Strengths (VIA-IS): Adaptation and validation of the German version and the development of a peer-rating form. *Journal of Individual Differences, 31*, 138–149. doi:10.1027/1614-0001/a000022.

Ruch, W., Proyer, R. T., & Weber, M. (2010). Humor as character strength among the elderly: Empirical findings on age-related changes and its contribution to satisfaction with life. *Zeitschrift für Gerontologie und Geriatrie, 43*, 13–18. doi:10.1007/s00391-009-0090-0.

Ruch, W., Weber, M., Park, N., & Peterson, C. (2014). Character strengths in children and adolescents: Reliability and initial validity of the German Values in Action Inventory of Strengths for Youth (German VIA-Youth). *European Journal of Psychological Assessment, 30*, 57–64. doi:10.1027/1015-5759/a000169.

Ryan, R. M., & Deci, E. L. (2001). On happiness and human potentials: A review of research on hedonic and eudaimonic well-being. *Annual Review of Psychology, 52*, 141–166. doi:10.1146/annurev.psych.52.1.141.

Ryff, C. D. (1989). Happiness is everything, or is it? Explorations on the meaning of psychological well-being. *Journal of Personality and Social Psychology, 57*, 1069–1081. doi:10.1037/0022-3514.57.6.1069.

Ryff, C. D. (2014). Psychological well-being revisited: Advances in the science and practice of eudaimonia. *Psychotherapy and Psychosomatics, 83*, 10–28. doi:10.1159/000353263.

Ryff, C. D., & Essex, M. J. (1992). The interpretation of life experiences and well-being: The sample case of relocation. *Psychology and Aging, 7*, 507–517. doi:10.1037/0882-7974.7.4.507.

Ryff, C. D., & Keyes, C. L. M. (1995). The structure of psychological well-being revisited. *Journal of Personality and Social Psychology, 69*, 719–727. doi:10.1037/0022-3514.69.4.719.

Ryff, C. D., & Singer, B. H. (2008). Know thyself and become what you are: A eudaimonic approach to psychological wellbeing. *Journal of Happiness Studies, 9*, 13–39. doi:10.1007/s10902-006-9019-0.

Salama-Younes, M., Ismaïl, A., Montazeri, A., & Roncin, C. (2011). Factor structure of the French Ryff's psychological well-being scales for active older adults. In I. Brdar (Ed.), *The human pursuit of well-being: A cultural approach* (pp. 203–2012). New York: Springer Science+Business Media. doi:10.1007/978-94-007-1375-8_17.

Sandín, B., Chorot, P., Lostao, L., Joiner, T. E., Santed, M. A., & Valiente, R. M. (1999). Escala PANAS de afecto positivo y negativo: validación factorial y convergencia transcultural [The PANAS Scales of positive and negative affect: Factor analytic validation and cross-cultural convergence]. *Psicothema, 11*, 37–51.

Seligman, M. E. P. (2002). *Authentic happiness: Using the new positive psychology to realize your potential for lasting fulfillment*. New York: The Free Press.

Seligman, M. E. P. (2011). *Flourish: A visionary new understanding of happiness and well-being*. New York: The Free Press.

Seligman, M. E. P., & Csikszentmihalyi, M. (2000). Positive psychology: An introduction. *American Psychologist, 55*, 5–14. doi:10.1037//0003-066X.55.1.5.

Seligman, M. E. P., Steen, T. A., Park, N., & Peterson, C. (2005). Positive psychology progress: Empirical validation of interventions. *American Psychologist, 60*, 410–421. doi:10.1037/0003-066X.60.5.410.

Sheldon, K. M., & Elliot, A. J. (1999). Goal striving, need satisfaction, and longitudinal well-being: The self-concordance model. *Journal of Personality and Social Psychology, 76*, 482–497. doi:10.1037/0022-3514.76.3.482.

Sheldon, K. M., & Niemiec, C. P. (2006). It's not just the amount that counts: Balanced need satisfaction also affects well-being. *Journal of Personality and Social Psychology, 91*, 331–341. doi:10.1037/0022-3514.91.2.331.

Shimai, S., Otake, K., Park, N., Peterson, C., & Seligman, M. E. P. (2006). Convergence of character strengths in American and Japanese young adults. *Journal of Happiness Studies, 7*, 311–322. doi:10.1007/s10902-005-3647-7.

Tangey, J. P. (2000). Humility: Theoretical perspectives, empirical findings and directions for future research. *Journal of Social and Clinical Psychology, 19*, 70–82. doi:10.1521/jscp.2000.19.1.70.

Van Dierendonck, D. (2005). The construct validity of Ryff's scales of psychological well-being and its extension with spiritual well-being. *Personality and Individual Differences, 36*, 629–643. doi:10.1016/S0191-8869(03)00122-3.

Watson, D., Clark, L. A., & Tellegen, A. (1988). Development and validation of brief measures of positive and negative affect: The PANAS scales. *Journal of Personality and Social Psychology, 54*, 1063–1070. doi:10.1037/0022-3514.54.6.1063.

Weber, M., Ruch, W., LittmanOvadia, H., Lavy, S., & Gai, O. (2013). Relationships among higher-order strengths-factors, subjective well-being, and general self-efficacy – The case of Israeli adolescents. *Personality and Individual Differences, 55*, 322–327. doi:10.1016/j.paid.2013.03.006.

Wood, A. M., Linley, A. P., Maltby, J., Kashdan, T. B., & Hurling, R. (2011). Using personal and psychological strengths leads to increases in well-being over time: A longitudinal study and the development of the strengths use questionnaire. *Personality and Individual Differences, 50*, 15–19. doi:10.1016/j.paid.2010.08.004.

Yanez, A. P. (2007). *Character strengths and psychological well-being as predictors of life satisfaction among multicultural populations* (Doctoral dissertation). Retrieved from ProQuest Dissertations and Theses database. (UMI No. 3244003).

The Mind of the "Happy Warrior": Eudaimonia, Awe, and the Search for Meaning in Life

21

Alexander F. Danvers, Makenzie J. O'Neil, and Michelle N. Shiota

What makes a life good? This question has deep philosophical roots, but has only recently become a focus of experimental psychology (Seligman, 2002). On one hand, a good life might be one with a great deal of pleasure, and little if any pain; this definition is implicit in the most commonly used measure of subjective well-being (e.g., Diener & Diener, 1996). In her critique of positive psychology, however, Martha Nussbaum (2008) challenges this definition, using Wordsworth's "Character of the Happy Warrior" to illustrate what an authentically happy life might include. The happy warrior is not happy in the sense of feeling copious pleasure. Rather, his happiness is the consequence of a life well-lived, filled with meaningful activity, performed with excellence—a valuable life judged as a whole.

Nussbaum's account emphasizes two key insights we build upon in this chapter. First, authentic happiness occurs through the active pursuit of meaningful goals. We may fail to achieve these goals, thereby experiencing distress, but we must define and pursue them in order to achieve a good life. Second, positive emotions do not, in and of themselves, define a good life; they are instead the frequent result of pursuing meaningful goals. Our research suggests that positive emotions are not just subjectively pleasant—they evolved to serve distinct adaptive functions that map to major life tasks, and they facilitate accomplishing those tasks (Shiota et al., 2014). From this perspective, positive emotions may therefore promote living a good life in distinct ways.

In this chapter we explore the contrast between hedonic well-being, which emphasizes the experience of pleasure, and eudaimonic well-being, which emphasizes deeper meaning in our life and actions. Our analysis of eudaimonia highlights one aspect that has received relatively little emphasis, but is consistent with Nussbaum's account—the importance of having a coherent framework that defines the meaning of one's life. We then consider the ways that positive emotions might actually promote eudaimonic well-being, as well as serving as markers of a good life. In particular, we emphasize a role the emotion awe might play in eudaimonia, facilitating development of a personal sense of meaning in life.

21.1 Defining Eudaimonia

Aristotle's concept of eudaimonia—and its contrast with hedonia—sets the framework for studying what a good life is. Broadly, eudaimonia is thought of as living a deep, satisfying life, whereas hedonia is living a life focused on maximizing pleasure (Deci & Ryan, 2008). The

A.F. Danvers • M.J. O'Neil • M.N. Shiota (✉)
Department of Psychology, Arizona State University, 871104, Tempe, AZ 85287-1104, USA
e-mail: Lani.Shiota@asu.edu

J. Vittersø (ed.), *Handbook of Eudaimonic Well-Being*, International Handbooks of Quality-of-Life,
DOI 10.1007/978-3-319-42445-3_21

hedonic approach, which Nussbaum argued against, suggests that the good life can be measured along a single important dimension related roughly to utility. The concept of utility comes out of the philosophy of Bentham, who suggested that overall good can be calculated by adding up all an individual's pleasures and subtracting out all suffering (Bentham, 1789/1948). In psychology research, the hedonic approach is associated with early research by Kahneman and Diener (Deci & Ryan, 2008; Diener, 1994; Kahneman, Diener, & Schwarz, 1999). Because hedonic well-being is a summation of subjective experience over individual moments in time, it can be measured through regular assessment of how much positive affect is felt, and subtracting out the amount of negative affect.

Measuring eudaimonia is trickier, because it is presumed to be a function of many different aspects of a life beyond subjective pleasure, including the goals one pursues, the way one pursues them, and how one reflects upon life as a whole. Following Aristotle, a number of theorists have emphasized the role of excellence in eudaimonia. Thomas Nagel (1972) identifies two forms of eudaimonia in Aristotle's *Nichomachean Ethics*: an intellectualist eudaimonia, which involves excellence in the exercise of reason; and a comprehensive eudaimonia, which involves virtuous action across life's full domain. Nagel suggests that the distinction is related to a deeper ambiguity about human nature and what its "proper excellence" is. The intellectualist account suggests that the true purpose of all people is to reason, and therefore we will best fulfill our purpose by reasoning excellently. The comprehensive account, which Nussbaum endorses, suggests that eudaimonia can arise from excellence in a variety of domains—in friendship, in politics, in ethics, or in intellect. This comprehensive account opens the door to a plurality of good lives—all individuals have their own "good life" to lead, based on the particular domain in which they excel.

Seligman (2002) agrees with this, describing the "good/engaged" life as one in which individuals excel at applying their *signature strengths*—virtuous qualities, such as creativity, leadership, or humor—to their life tasks. He further describes the "meaningful" life as one where these personal signature strengths are used in the service of something larger than the self. This emphasis on signature strengths was also seen in Peterson's research and the Values-In-Action project, which was an attempt to create a taxonomy of positive qualities that would serve as a counterpoint to the *Diagnostic and Statistical Manual of Mental Disorders* (APA, 1994; Peterson & Park, 2009; Peterson & Seligman, 2004). Research on character strengths implies that we must each find a good life based on what we are good at.

Like Nussbaum, theorists have suggested that beyond excelling in some particular domain, there are multiple dimensions along which a good life can be measured. Carol Ryff's (1989, 1995, Chap. 6, this volume) Psychological Well-Being (PWB) scale explicitly reflects this, measuring six distinct constructs: self-acceptance, purpose in life, environmental mastery, positive relationships, autonomy, and personal growth. Ryff's approach specifically attempts to remedy shortcomings in hedonically-oriented approaches to well-being, and is based on a broad theoretical review that includes Aristotelian, existential, and humanist philosophies. Similarly, Deci and Ryan's self-determination theory posits that humans have three basic needs: autonomy, relatedness, and competence, and that eudaimonia is achieved by acting in ways that fulfill these needs (Deci & Ryan, 2008; Ryan, Huta, & Deci, 2008; Ryan & Martela, Chap. 7, this volume; Huta, Chap. 15, this volume). These important, pioneering theoretical frameworks help us measure aspects of a good life that are not readily captured by hedonically-oriented scales.

21.2 Meaning as a Core Aspect of Eudaimonia

Another important aspect of eudaimonic well-being, and the main focus in this chapter, is the sense that one's life is meaningful (Halusic & King, 2013; Ryff, 1989; Ryff & Singer, 1998; Steger, 2012, Chap. 11, this volume; Ward & King, Chap. 35, this volume). Rather than being studied as a facet of eudaimonia, however, meaning in life has largely been studied as a construct in its own right, and is the subject of a distinct, rich body of research. Meaning has been central to the ideas of many existential theorists (Debats, 1996; Frankl, 1984; Maddi, 2004), social psychologists (Baumeister, 1991; Emmons, 2003; Steger, 2012), evolutionary theorists (Klinger, 1998), developmentalists (Erikson, 1959/1974), clinicians (Wong & Fry, 1998; Yalom, 1980), and health psychologists (Antonovsky, 1984). Empirical studies find meaning in life to be related to a host of positive outcomes, such as higher self-reported happiness and lower levels of depression (Reker & Wong, 1988; Wong & Fry, 1998), more positive responses to psychotherapy (Debats, 1996), and better coping with negative life events (Farran, Miller, Kaufman, & Davis, 1997).

Drawing from conceptualizations across the literature cited above, we define a sense of meaning as having a deep, coherent, organizing conceptual framework for one's life, one that helps define who we are as individuals and what is most important to each of us. A sense of meaning provides a sense of purpose. Meaning is found in the aims we create for ourselves that extend beyond the present moment, across our lives. This definition of meaning does not require a single, universal set of values that each person must exemplify or achieve in order to have a meaningful life. Rather, each person defines his or her own framework of meaning, and associated values and/or goals. Because these frameworks extend forward into time, as well as back, they create a standard by which we can judge and direct our lives. Are we progressing on the goals we have set for ourselves? Are we living according to the principles we value most, whatever those may be? Having meaning in life involves both creating a meaning framework through which a life is understood, and fulfilling that framework through living (Debats, 1996).

Theories of meaning in life have proposed that humans have a deep-seated *need* to make meaning, and that this need is in some way homeostatic—people attempt to keep themselves above a certain meaning threshold through compensatory behaviors (Baumeister & Vohs, 2002; Heine, Proulx, & Vohs, 2006). Baumeister and Vohs emphasize the "framework" aspect of meaning, defining meaning as something that connects things that would be otherwise unconnected, and stressing that such connections are not inherent—they exist solely within the human mind, and must be identified by each individual. This connects their theory with existential philosophy, which similarly assumes that meaning is something people must create.

This perspective also assumes that meaning exists along a continuum. As Baumeister and Vohs (2002) argue, and as further developed in the Meaning Maintenance Model (MMM; Heine et al., 2006), feeling a loss of meaning can come from something as small as getting negative feedback on a personality test (Baumeister & Jones, 1978), failing a trivia test (Cialdini et al., 1976), or just being given time pressure and a stressful environment in which to make a decision (Kruglanski & Webster, 1991). Compensatory actions, which are meant to increase meaning (often in a separate domain) after an insult to it, include things like: valuing certain aspects of your personality more, affiliating yourself with your college football team after wins, and rejecting people who have a different opinions. At this end of the meaning continuum, insults to meaning and the recovery efforts are only loosely associated with conscious feelings of purpose, coherence, and sense of fulfillment.

Although the MMM is not explicitly part of Terror Management Theory (TMT; Greenberg & Arndt, 2011), the latter makes similar assumptions about our deep-seated need to defend a sense of meaning against threats. TMT explicitly hypothesizes that experiences reminding us of our own mortality—which can be experimentally induced—lead to compensatory actions that help people achieve symbolic immortality through the continued survival of their in-group or worldview. For example, in one set of studies, mortality primes led people to evaluate in-group members and people who praised their worldview more favorably, and out-group members and those who criticized their worldview less favorably (Greenberg et al., 1990). This highlights the extent to which one's sense of meaning may be implicit, and its maintenance need not necessarily reflect conscious choice. This is in contrast to many existential theories, which emphasize conscious self-reflection as a fundamental source of meaning (Camus, 1955; Kierkegaard, 1843/1997; Sartre, 1956). The distinction between the two perspectives may reflect the difference between *developing* a personal framework for one's meaning in life, which may be a conscious activity, and *defending* that framework against threats, which may at times be automatic and reflexive.

The frameworks laid out by Baumeister and Vohs, Heine and colleagues, and Greenberg and colleagues are broad attempts to unify a diverse array of findings from experimental psychology, but they highlight a discrepancy between the conceptualizations of meaning used by experimental social psychologists versus philosophers. First, it's not clear that the way meaning is measured and manipulated in the MMM and TMT paradigms corresponds to meaning in the conscious, self-reflective sense. This is related to the distinction made between global and local meaning made by Park and Folkman (1997) in the coping literature. Second, it's not clear that the meaning-bolstering actions measured in the MMM and TMT studies would make people feel that their lives were more coherent, purposeful, or fulfilling—nor that meaning-bolstering actions would be universally effective.

Another research tradition, inspired by the existential psychology of Victor Frankl (1984), more strongly emphasizes the conscious, reflective sense of coherence, purpose, and fulfillment. Drawing on his experiences in Nazi concentration camps, Frankl identified having a sense of meaning as an important part of successful psychological functioning. In his logotherapy, patients were specifically treated for lacking a feeling of meaning. In order to measure whether individuals felt like their lives had meaning, self-report scales were developed. These explicit measures would be preferred to implicit measures based on the importance of self-examination and conscious choice in existential philosophy. For individuals suffering from a lack of meaning, what is important is not the implicit defense of meaning, but a conscious, global reflection on meaning in life.

Common self-report measures of meaning use Likert scale items or coding of written responses to open-ended questions (Auhagen, 2000; Chamberlain & Zika, 1988; Debats, 1999). Research with open-ended questions has identified several common sources of meaning—for example, having a commitment to family, friends, or romantic partners; being engaged in one's job, schooling, or other life occupation; striving for physical and mental health; or volunteering and helping others (Debats, 1999). Like Peterson and Seligman's research on signature strengths, this research suggests that there are a variety of ways to find meaning in life—no single approach captures a majority of responses.

Beyond open-ended responses, four Likert-type scales are commonly used to assess meaning, with each capturing a slightly different theoretical construct. The Purpose in Life Scale (PIL; Crumbaugh & Maholick, 1964) was designed to measure "noogenic neurosis"—Frankl's term for frustration by a lack of meaning. The scale was thus originally a clinical inventory, and low PIL scores have been related to negative outcomes such as drug use, imprisonment, and depression (Chamberlain & Zika, 1988). The Life Regard Index (LRI; Battista & Almond, 1973) was developed after the PIL, and includes two components, framework and fulfillment. Framework relates to having a coherent set of goals in life, whereas the fulfillment subscale relates to achieving these goals. This approach highlights the distinction between *creating* a meaning framework and *fulfilling* one's meaning, once a framework is in place. Separating these aspects of meaning led to the important empirical finding that many of the positive outcomes associated with meaning in life only occur when an individual reports fulfillment of meaning—not just having a framework (Debats, 1996; Shek, 1991).

The Sense of Coherence scale (SOC; Antonovsky, 1993) was developed to assess coherence among life's activities, which was regarded as a particularly important aspect of coping with stress. It has subscales assessing comprehensibility, or whether the world is predictable and well-ordered; manageability, or whether individuals thinks their life challenges can be met; and meaningfulness, or whether individuals thinks their current life challenges are worthy of being met. This scale foregrounds the idea that a meaningful life is one in which all the pieces fit together—meaning as coherence in perception, action, and cognition.

Most recently, Steger and colleagues have developed the Meaning in Life Questionnaire (MLQ; Steger, Frazier, Oishi, & Kaler, 2006). This questionnaire has subscales assessing the search for meaning and the feeling of having meaning in life. As expected, these are negatively related, suggesting that people who already have meaning need to seek it out less (Steger et al., 2006; Steger & Kashdan, 2007). Interestingly, however, Steger finds that seeking and having meaning are non-linearly related. He identified a threshold model where very low levels of meaning-having lead to very high meaning-seeking, and high levels of meaning-having lead to low levels of meaning-seeking, but there is a broad swath in the middle where increases in having don't strongly affect seeking (Steger, 2012). Most people settle on a moderate level of meaning-seeking, and don't significantly change that level unless they feel completely lost—or completely fulfilled.

These approaches to studying meaning in life have helped clarify several theoretical distinctions, such as the distinction between having a meaning framework vs. fulfilling that framework, and the distinction between seeking vs. having meaning in life. They also attempt to measure meaning in a psychometrically rigorous way that is consistent with the theoretical position that meaning is something people define through conscious reflection. However, this approach still does not explore deeply the question of *how* people find meaning. We believe that one answer to this question can be found in positive emotions.

21.3 Positive Emotions and Eudaimonia

As noted earlier, eudaimonia is not defined in terms of how much subjective pleasure is felt; positive affect is not the criterion for eudaimonic happiness, nor is the explicit pursuit of positive emotion a reliable strategy for achieving it (Mauss, Tamir, Anderson, & Savino, 2011). Nonetheless, we propose that positive emotions can be important *antecedents to*, as well as *consequences of*, eudaimonic well-being. This is because, in our view, positive emotions are not just subjectively gratifying experiences; they are specific, adaptive, complex responses to opportunities presented by the environment to fulfill important human motivations (Shiota et al., 2014). In this we follow a tradition of theorists who conceive of emotions as coordinated, functional responses to prototypical threats and opportunities (Darwin, 1872/1965; Ekman, 1992; Frijda, 1986; Izard, 1977; Lazarus, 1991; Plutchik, 1980; Tooby & Cosmides, 2008). Emotions are inherently multi-faceted, integrating a variety of physiological, perceptual, cognitive, and behavioral responses in order to promote an adaptive (on average) response to the eliciting situation (Ekman, 1992; Levenson, 1999; Tooby & Cosmides, 2008). From this perspective, positive emotions may facilitate achievement of the very goals that, for many people, define a good life: excellence in one's chosen work; investment in close relationships; successfully raising a family; making a positive impact on one's community and on the world.

Moreover, our account suggests that specific positive emotions may promote and/or reflect different aspects of eudaimonia. For example, pride might be particularly relevant for three of Ryff's (1989) dimensions of Psychological Well-Being: self-acceptance, personal growth, and positive relations with others. Pride is elicited by achievement in domains that are important to the individual and the individual's social group, and theorists have proposed that the function of pride is to enhance and display one's social status within that group (Tracy & Robins, 2007a; Williams & DeSteno, 2009). While personal achievement presents an opportunity to increase one's status through social behaviors, another likely consequence of pride is recalibration of our own sense of self-worth. Research shows that authentic pride—pride experienced in response to one's effortful achievement—is related to authentic self-esteem, feeling genuinely positive about oneself without narcissism or self-protection (Herrald & Tomaka, 2002; Tracy, Cheng, Robins, & Trzesniewski, 2009). Such feelings are closely related to Ryff's dimension of self-acceptance, which involves holding positive opinions about one's self while acknowledging both good and bad qualities, and making peace with the latter.

Pride can also prospectively promote eudaimonic well-being as individuals capitalize on prior successes by pursuing further achievement (Carver & Johnson, 2010; Higgins et al., 2001; Weiner, 1985). Pride can be empowering, and this can lead to individuals pushing themselves to try new things, or working harder toward the goals about which they care most. For example, one study found that salespeople imagining being in pride-eliciting situations tended to try harder and feel more effective (Verbeke, Belschak, & Bagozzi, 2004). Another set of studies found that people feeling experimentally induced, achievement-related pride persevered for longer at a subsequent difficult task (Williams & DeSteno, 2008). Feeling pride can therefore create a feedback loop between achievement and motivation that facilitates continued growth. Beyond reflecting excellence, pride can actually promote it. This aspect of eudaimonia is linked to Ryff's (1989) personal growth dimension of well-being, the feeling that one is constantly developing and improving.

Pride should also help to recalibrate others' opinions of you, with implications for relationships. In particular, authentic pride, in which one's achievement is attributed to effort (as distinct from hubristic pride or narcissism, where achievement is attributed to natural superiority)—is associated with better social relations (Tracy & Robins, 2007b). Attributing authentic pride to an individual makes people believe that individual is more prosocial (Wubben, De Cremer, & van Dijk, 2012). Authentic pride also predicts prestige-based social status—status based on merit rather than dominance—in self and peer reports (Cheng, Tracy, & Henrich, 2010). Those high on authentic pride tend to show more secure attachment styles, less rejection sensitivity, and greater feelings of support from others than people lower on pride (Tracy et al., 2009). These implications of pride all suggest that it facilitates concern for others and warm, secure relationships. In this way, pride appears to promote the "positive relations with others" dimension in Ryff's (1989) conceptualization of psychological well-being.

Pride is a particularly well-studied positive emotion, making it relatively easy to extrapolate from demonstrated empirical effects to implications for dimensions of human flourishing. Its relation to PWB also exemplifies many of the readily apparent ways positive emotions should help create a good life: by motivating people to feel good about themselves, to achieve more, and to have closer relationships. But positive emotions can also be profound. Although reflection is often depicted as a depressive, brooding activity, we propose that deep reflection can also be driven by positive emotion.

21.4 Positive Emotion and Meaning

How might positive emotions affect the development and fulfillment of a personal framework for life's meaning? Laura King's research has linked meaning-making with positive affect in general (Halusic & King, 2013; King, Hicks, Krull, & Del Gaiso, Krull, & Del Gaiso, 2006). King has found not only that having meaning makes people feel good, but that feeling good leads people to feel they have more meaningful lives—her team has found that experimentally inducing positive mood leads to greater self-reported meaning, suggesting a direct causal relationship (Hicks & King, 2008; Hicks, Trent, Davis, & King, 2012; King et al.King et al., 2006). King proposed that positive affect makes people receptive to meaning by freeing them from immediate concerns and shifting focus to more global issues, allowing them to perceive the underlying meaning across their experiences. One limitation of this approach is that it does not make fine-grained distinctions among positive emotions—which our lab group has found can be important in predicting the effects of emotion manipulations (e.g., Griskevicius, Shiota, & Neufeld, 2010; Shiota et al., 2014). Do all varieties of positive emotion have this effect, or only some? Shortly we will propose that a specific positive emotion is particularly likely to open this door to meaning-making.

Researchers have also connected meaning to hope (Feldman & Snyder, 2005). Hope involves two components: pathways, perceived ability to develop plans that will lead to goal fulfillment; and agency, the perceived ability to carry out those plans (Snyder et al., 1991). Having hope, then, is about developing and following through with one's chosen goals, and the road to achieving those goals. The pathways-agency distinction in the hope research closely mirrors the distinction between developing a meaning framework and fulfilling that framework, discussed earlier. Like pride, hope has been linked to a variety of positive outcomes, such as better academic performance, better physical and mental health, and better therapy outcomes (Barnum, Snyder, Rapoff, Mani, & Thompson, 1998, Snyder et al., 2000; 2002). In fact, psychometric studies have found that the Hope Scale (Snyder et al., 1991), the LRI, the SOC, and the PIL all load together on a single factor, suggesting that they tap into a common, underlying construct (Feldman & Snyder, 2005).

21.5 Awe and the Meaning Making Process

A number of positive emotions may play important roles in people's sense of meaning. Pride, hope, and love all facilitate behaviors that promote aspects of the good life, in the sense exemplified by the happy warrior. We propose, however, that the emotion of awe, and awe-evoking experiences, have the potential to play a distinct role in meaning-making—developing a coherent, personal "big picture" that integrates one's experience across situations and time, and links the self to something greater. In fact, the most commonly used theoretical definition of awe, supported by a growing body of empirical evidence, suggests that the function of awe itself may be closely related to meaning-making as we have defined it here.

21.5.1 What Is Awe?

Although awe has long been a subject of interest in disciplines such as sociology, anthropology, philosophy, and religious studies (e.g., Durkheim, 1887/1972; Otto, 1923; Weber, 1978), it was largely ignored by the psychology of emotion until recently. In his *Varieties of Religious Experience*, the early psychologist William James (1902/1985) discussed awe and wonder as aspects of mystical phenomenology. Decades later, Paul Ekman (1992) speculated that awe might someday be found to meet his strict criteria for a "basic" emotion, including universal eliciting events or stimuli; automatic appraisal; a distinct, universal facial or vocal expressive signal; and emotion-specific physiology. Between these two publications, however, awe received no empirical attention. No clear conceptual definition of awe been proposed on which to build a firm foundation for operational measures and hypotheses about awe's empirical effects.

This gap was filled by Keltner and Haidt (2003) in an article that set the stage for a new burst of theory and research on awe. Based upon a rich review of writings on awe across the social sciences, Keltner and Haidt proposed that awe is an emotional response to stimuli with two core characteristics. First, awe-eliciting stimuli are *vast*—they profoundly challenge the scale at which we usually experience the world. Prototypical awe stimuli, such as the Grand Canyon in Arizona, the Great Wall of China, and brilliant sunsets are literally, physically vast. However, stimuli can also be vast in abstract or conceptual ways. Einstein's theory of special relativity has vast implications for our understanding of the physical universe. Similarly, great works of art and literature can transform our understanding of the human experience. Historical events, such as the demolition of the Berlin Wall in 1989–1890, have vast social implications. Music and abstract art can be vast in terms of sensory complexity and detail. Even very small things, such as a snowflake, can be experienced as vast when examined at microscopic scale. In each of these cases, it is not just the sheer volume of information that provides the sense of vastness, but rather the perception of a single, integrated whole across that information. From a purely sensory standpoint, the Great Wall of China might not be that impressive without thinking of it as a single architectural structure constructed over centuries with a single purpose—but consideration of its historical as well as geographic scope promotes perception of its vastness.

The second proposed feature of awe stimuli is *need for accommodation*. In Piagetian cognitive theory, people flow back and forth between experiencing the world in two modes (Piaget, 1973). In *assimilation*, one perceives the current environment through the filters of prior conceptual knowledge, or "schemas" for people, things, and events. For example, if you are introduced at a party to a woman wearing a tie-dye dress with several beaded necklaces and tinted sunglasses and smelling of patchouli, you might reasonably apply the label "hippie" to her, and this label would come with a host of implicit assumptions about her personality and background. In *accommodation*, one instead takes in novel or unexpected information from the environment, and uses that information to reshape one's schemas or develop new ones. For example, if you were to learn that the woman above was a heart surgeon, this (presumably) unexpected information might grab your attention and provoke recalibration of your mental images. These two modes of cognition are complementary, and both are necessary for functioning in a complex environment. It is highly efficient to store conceptual information for future use, and to rely on that information whenever possible; however, it is also crucial to recognize when one's conceptual knowledge is inadequate to account for the current situation, and acquire new information from the environment.

Taken together, these elements suggest that the function of awe might be to promote intense cognitive accommodation when faced with a vast, novel stimulus that is not accounted for by one's current understanding of the world (Shiota, Keltner, & Mossman, 2007). This proposal is guiding, and supported by, a growing body of research. When asked to describe a time when they felt intense awe, participants in the United States report a variety of situations consistent with the definition above, including panoramic views, great works of art and music, remarkable human accomplishments, and major life transitions (marriage, death), all experienced for the first time (Shiota et al., 2007). Such stimuli challenge the frame of reference through which we normally perceive the world, and can provide a rich opportunity to expand our knowledge (Shiota, Thrash, Danvers, & Dombrowski, 2014). Studies have found that experimentally induced awe produces a variety of cognitive effects consistent with accommodation, such as increased reliance on careful, systematic analysis rather than heuristic, rule-of-thumb processing of persuasive messages (Griskevicius, Shiota & Neufeld, 2010), reduced reliance on event "scripts" when encoding the details of a novel story about a familiar kind of event (Danvers & Shiota, 2014), and enhanced memory for peripheral details of complex photographs (Osborne & Shiota, 2014).

21.5.2 Awe and Meaning-Making

Meaning-making is the development of a personal framework for understanding one's life as a coherent whole. Awe may provide an opportunity to shape and elaborate on our life frameworks as a byproduct of the perception of vastness, and general tendency toward accommodation, that awe entails. Awe encourages us to disengage from our mundane, day-to-day concerns and look at the big picture, not only out there in the world, but also as we fit into that world.

This proposal is supported by a growing body of empirical evidence. Compared with those in a positive emotion control condition (pride), participants reliving a personal experience of awe in one study reported stronger feelings of being small and insignificant, and aware of the presence of something greater than the self, yet connected to the surrounding world (Shiota et al.,

2007). Other studies have found that awe facilitates a sense of oneness not only with close friends, but also with people in general (Van Cappellen & Saroglou, 2011). Indeed, when asked to freely list completions of the stem "I am..." (the 20 Statements Test; Kuhn & McPartland, 1954), participants in an awe condition were found in one study to show increased use of "universal" self-descriptors such as "a living being" and "a human," relative to a control condition (Shiota et al., 2007). Researchers have pointed out that this integration of the self into something far greater lies at the heart of spirituality, a "tendency to orient oneself toward a larger transcendent reality," and found that awe promotes increased spirituality in this general sense (Saroglou, Buxant, & Tilquin, 2008).

For many people, religion is a powerful source of meaning in life. Studies examining the effects of awe on formal religiosity, or identification with a particular religion, have produced somewhat inconsistent and ambiguous results (Saroglou et al., 2008). However, a series of several recent studies has found that experimentally induced awe tends to increase "agency detection," the belief that events are caused by the efforts of intentional forces or beings (Valdesolo & Graham, 2014). While awe increased the perception that random number strings were actually generated by humans in one study, other studies found that awe also increased belief in supernatural forces such as God and karma. In an important twist, each of these effects appeared to be accounted for by the same mediator—an uncomfortable sense of uncertainty evoked by the awe manipulation.

This suggests an important aspect of the process by which awe might support development of a personal framework of meaning. Valdesolo and Graham (2014) argue that in broadening the scope of our awareness beyond comprehension, awe induces an aversive sense of randomness, prompting a search for a pattern or explanation. In their research, an explanation was sought for things out in the world. If this search for an explanation is applied to the personal problem of living, however, people may be spurred to find meaning—a sense of coherence among the various strands of one's life, and an explanation of who one truly is.

The process might begin with a momentary glimpse of the sublime, something that transcends the bounds of day-to-day living, generating a powerful feeling of awe. The discomfort with randomness documented by Valdesolo and Graham (2014) would prompt an effort to identify a theme in the chaos of personal history, perhaps even a commitment to what inspired the awe. This commitment, undergirded by a powerful emotional inspiration, could become an important source of meaning—both in the present and in guiding future action. In this way, we predict that awe might promote the perception of a coherent pattern across the many individual threads of one's life.

Notably, many conversion stories follow this narrative. In the Catholic tradition, the Apostle Paul was a persecutor of Christians until he was struck blind by a vision of God. The experience changed completely his framework for understanding his own life, and he emerged with a new way of making meaning for himself: devotion to promoting this new religion through writing and missionary work. Scientists may similarly find inspiration in confronting life's mysteries. As Einstein put it, "The most beautiful thing we can experience is the mysterious. It is the source of all true art and science" (Calaprice, 2000). The motivation for the overarching structure that gave his life meaning was not a rational deliberation, but an experience of awe. It is awe, he suggests, that inspires us to choose a life of art or of science.

21.6 Conclusion

The eudaimonic approach to well-being, particularly in Aristotle's comprehensive account, suggests that attempts to measure flourishing must account for the many ways in which people can live good, meaningful lives (Deci & Ryan, 2008; Nussbaum, 2008; Ryff, 1989). The eudaimonic approach also suggests that we will find authentic happiness not by seeking to maximize pleasure and minimize pain, but by developing a personal framework for what makes life meaningful, and engaging in life's important tasks with virtue and excellence. In this account, positive emotions are not goals in and of themselves, but they can be natural sequelae of goal pursuit.

We have expanded on this account, proposing that positive emotions can also *promote* eudaimonia indirectly by facilitating the accomplishment of important life goals. For example, pride in one's past accomplishments may empower us to reach for still greater heights in the future, and make us appealing partners for a variety of social connections. Our proposal resonates with a modern understanding of positive emotions as serving distinct functions (Shiota, et al., 2014). To the extent that specific emotions promote accomplishment of different kinds of goals (e.g., achievements, relationships, learning), they may facilitate different aspects of flourishing.

The connection of positive emotions with action-oriented outcomes such as achievement, proactive goal pursuit, and social connectedness is readily apparent, but we have argued that they can also underlie more contemplative aspects of eudaimonic well-being. The cognitive and motivational state inherent in awe, in particular, may facilitate meaning making—the development of a personal, coherent framework that conceptually organizes one's life, projects goals into the future, and sets standards against which to measure success. Since there are many ways to live the eudaimonic "good life," a meaning framework must be discovered and committed to by each individual. Provided that attention is directed toward one's own life while in an awe state, awe should help in this process by opening the mind to the "big picture" of that life and its place in the greater world (Shiota et al., 2007), while at the same time inducing discomfort with randomness and incoherence (Valdesolo & Graham, 2014), motivating a search for an organizing theme.

This account is based on a close reading of the empirical, theoretical, and philosophical literatures on awe and meaning, but it is also somewhat speculative, and thus suggests several new avenues for research. Can experiencing awe help individuals who have difficulty finding meaning in their lives? Does an awe experience automatically increase feelings of meaning, or are there important pre-conditions related to the context or the domain of the awe experience that help determine its effect on meaning making? Do continual re-infusions of awe in a life help to reinforce a meaning framework, or might too much awe destabilize otherwise useful meaning structures? There is still much to be learned about how to live a good life, and we believe awe will be an important part of the story going forward.

References

American Psychiatric Association. (1994). *Diagnostic and statistical manual of mental disorders*. Washington, DC: APA.

Antonovsky, A. (1984). A call for a new question—salutogenesis—and a proposed answer—the sense of coherence. *Journal of Preventive Psychiatry, 2*, 1–13.

Antonovsky, A. (1993). The structure and properties of the sense of coherence scale. *Social Science & Medicine, 36*(6), 725–733.

Auhagen, A. E. (2000). On the psychology of meaning of life. *Swiss Journal of Psychology/Schweizerische Zeitschrift für Psychologie/Revue Suisse de Psychologie, 59*(1), 34.

Barnum, D. D., Snyder, C. R., Rapoff, M. A., Mani, M. M., & Thompson, R. (1998). Hope and social support in psychological adjustment of children who have survived burn injuries and their matched controls. *Children's Health Care, 27*(1), 15–30.

Battista, J., & Almond, R. (1973). The development of meaning in life. *Psychiatry, 36*(4), 409–427.

Baumeister, R. F. (1991). *Meanings of life*. New York: Guilford Press.

Baumeister, R. F., & Jones, E. E. (1978). When self-presentation is constrained by the target's knowledge: Consistency and compensation. *Journal of Personality and Social Psychology, 36*(6), 608.

Baumeister, R. F., & Vohs, K. D. (2002). The pursuit of meaningfulness in life. In C. R. Snyder & S. J. Lopez (Eds.), *Handbook of positive psychology* (pp. 608–618). New York, NY: Oxford University Press.

Bentham, J. (1789). *An introduction to the principle of morals and legislations*. reprinted (Oxford, UK: Blackwell, 1948).

Calaprice, A. (2000). *The expanded quotable Einstein*. Princeton, NJ: Princeton University.

Camus, A. (1955). *The myth of Sisyphus and other essays*. New York: Knopf.

Carver, C. S., & Johnson, S. L. (2010). Authentic and hubristic pride: Differential relations to aspects of goal regulation, affect, and self-control. *Journal of Research in Personality, 44*(6), 698–703.

Chamberlain, K., & Zika, S. (1988). Measuring meaning in life: An examination of three scales. *Personality and Individual Differences, 9*(3), 589–596.

Cheng, J. T., Tracy, J. L., & Henrich, J. (2010). Pride, personality, and the evolutionary foundations of human social status. *Evolution and Human Behavior, 31*(5), 334–347.

Cialdini, R. B., Borden, R. J., Thorne, A., Walker, M. R., Freeman, S., & Sloan, L. R. (1976). Basking in reflected glory: Three (football) field studies. *Journal of Personality and Social Psychology, 34*(3), 366.

Crumbaugh, J. C., & Maholick, L. T. (1964). An experimental study in existentialism: The psychometric approach to Frankl's concept of noogenic neurosis. *Journal of Clinical Psychology, 20*(2), 200–207.

Danvers, A. F., & Shiota, M. N. (2014). *Effects of awe on schema-driven memory*. Poster at the 2014 inaugural meeting of the Society for Affective Science, Bethesda, MD.

Darwin, C. (1872/1965). *The expression of the emotions in man and animals* (Vol. 526). University of Chicago Press.

Debats, D. L. (1996). Meaning in life: Clinical relevance and predictive power. *British Journal of Clinical Psychology, 35*(4), 503–516.

Debats, D. L. (1999). Sources of meaning: An investigation of significant commitments in life. *Journal of Humanistic Psychology, 39*(4), 30–57.

Deci, E. L., & Ryan, R. M. (2008). Hedonia, eudaimonia, and well-being: An introduction. *Journal of Happiness Studies, 9*(1), 1–11.

Diener, E. (1994). Assessing subjective well-being: Progress and opportunities. *Social Indicators Research, 31*(2), 103–157.

Diener, E., & Diener, C. (1996). Most people are happy. *Psychological Science, 7*(3), 181–185.

Durkheim, E. (1887). Review of Guyau: L'irreÂligion de l'avenir. In *Revue Philosophique*, 23, 1887. Reprinted in A. Giddens (Ed.), *Emile Durkheim, Selected Writings* (1972). Cambridge: Cambridge University Press.

Ekman, P. (1992). An argument for basic emotions. *Cognition & Emotion, 6*(3–4), 169–200.

Emmons, R. A. (2003). Personal goals, life meaning, and virtue: Wellsprings of a positive life. In C. L. M. Keyes & J. Haidt (Eds.), *Flourishing: Positive psychology and the life well-lived* (pp. 105–128). Washington DC: American Psychological Association.

Erikson, E. H. (1959). Identity and the life cycle: Selected papers. *Psychological Issues, 1*, 1–171.

Farran, C. J., Miller, B. H., Kaufman, J. E., & Davis, L. (1997). Race, finding meaning, and caregiver distress. *Journal of Aging and Health, 9*(3), 316–333.

Feldman, D. B., & Snyder, C. R. (2005). Hope and the meaningful life: Theoretical and empirical associations between goal–directed thinking and life meaning. *Journal of Social and Clinical Psychology, 24*(3), 401–421.

Frankl, V. E. (1984). *Man's search for meaning: An introduction to logotherapy*. New York: Pocket Books.

Frijda, N. H. (1986). *The emotions*. Cambridge: Cambridge University Press.

Greenberg, J., & Arndt, J. (2011). Terror management theory. *Handbook of Theories of Social Psychology, 1*, 398–415.

Greenberg, J., Pyszczynski, T., Solomon, S., Rosenblatt, A., Veeder, M., Kirkland, S., et al. (1990). Evidence for terror management theory II: The effects of mortality salience on reactions to those who threaten or bolster the cultural worldview. *Journal of Personality and Social Psychology, 58*(2), 308.

Griskevicius, V., Shiota, M. N., & Neufeld, S. L. (2010). Influence of different positive emotions on persuasion processing: A functional evolutionary approach. *Emotion, 10*, 190–206.

Halusic, M., & King, L. A. (2013). What makes life meaningful: Positive mood works in a pinch. Washington DC: American Psychological Association.

Heine, S. J., Proulx, T., & Vohs, K. D. (2006). The meaning maintenance model: On the coherence of social motivations. *Personality and Social Psychology Review, 10*(2), 88–110.

Herrald, M. M., & Tomaka, J. (2002). Patterns of emotion-specific appraisal, coping, and cardiovascular reactivity during an ongoing emotional episode. *Journal of Personality and Social Psychology, 83*(2), 434.

Hicks, J. A., & King, L. A. (2008). Religious commitment and positive mood as information about meaning in life. *Journal of Research in Personality, 42*(1), 43–57.

Hicks, J. A., Trent, J., Davis, W. E., & King, L. A. (2012). Positive affect, meaning in life, and future time perspective: An application of socioemotional selectivity theory. *Psychology and Aging, 27*(1), 181.

Higgins, E. T., Friedman, R. S., Harlow, R. E., Idson, L. C., Ayduk, O. N., & Taylor, A. (2001). Achievement orientations from subjective histories of success: Promotion pride versus prevention pride. *European Journal of Social Psychology, 31*(1), 3–23.

Izard, C. E. (1977). *Human emotions*. New York: Plenum Press.

James, W. (1902/1985). *The varieties of religious experience: A study in human nature*. Cambridge, MA: Harvard University Press.

Kahneman, D., Diener, E., & Schwarz, N. (Eds.). (1999). *Well-being: Foundations of hedonic psychology*. New York: Russell Sage.

Keltner, D., & Haidt, J. (2003). Approaching awe, a moral, spiritual, and aesthetic emotion. *Cognition and Emotion, 17*(2), 297–314.

Kierkegaard, S. (1997). The sickness unto death. In H. Hong & E. Hong (Eds.), *The essential Kierkegaard* (pp. 350–372). Princeton, NJ: Princeton University Press. (Original work published 1848).

King, L. A., Hicks, J. A., Krull, J. L., & Del Gaiso, A. K. (2006). Positive affect and the experience of meaning in life. *Journal of Personality and Social Psychology, 90*(1), 179.

Klinger, E. (1998). The search for meaning in evolutionary perspective and its clinical implications. In P. T. P. Wong & P. S. Fry (Eds.), *The human quest for meaning. A handbook of psychological research and clinical applications* (pp. 27–50). Mahwah, NJ: Erlbaum.

Kruglanski, A. W., & Webster, D. M. (1991). Group members' reactions to opinion deviates and conformists at varying degrees of proximity to decision deadline and of environmental noise. *Journal of Personality and Social Psychology, 61*(2), 212.

Kuhn, M. H., & McPartland, T. S. (1954). An empirical investigation of self-attitudes. *American Sociological Review, 19*, 68–76.

Lazarus, R. S. (1991). *Emotion and adaptation*. New York: Oxford University Press.

Levenson, R. W. (1999). The intrapersonal functions of emotion. *Cognition & Emotion, 13*, 481–504.

Maddi, S. R. (2004). Hardiness: An operationalization of existential courage. *Journal of Humanistic Psychology, 44*(3), 279–298.

Mauss, I. B., Tamir, M., Anderson, C. L., & Savino, N. S. (2011). Can seeking happiness make people unhappy? Paradoxical effects of valuing happiness. *Emotion, 11*, 807–815.

Nagel, T. (1972). Aristotle on eudaimonia. *Phronesis, 17*, 252–259.

Nussbaum, M. C. (2008). Who is the happy warrior? Philosophy poses questions to psychology. *The Journal of Legal Studies, 37*(S2), S81–S113.

Osborne, E. A., & Shiota, M. N. (2014). *Motivated memory: Memory for gist and detail in complex positive images*. Poster at the 2014 inaugural meeting of the Society for Affective Science, Bethesda, MD.

Otto, R. (1923). *The idea of the holy*. London: Oxford University Press.

Park, C. L., & Folkman, S. (1997). Meaning in the context of stress and coping. *Review of General Psychology, 1*(2), 115.

Peterson, C., & Park, N. (2009). Classifying and measuring strengths of character. In S. J. Lopez & C. R. Snyder (Eds.), *Oxford handbook of positive psychology* (pp. 25-33). New York, NY: Oxford University Press.

Peterson, C., & Seligman, M. E. (2004). *Character strengths and virtues: A handbook and classification*. New York: Oxford University Press.

Piaget, J. (1973). *The child and reality* (A. Rosin, Trans.). New York: Grossman Publishers.

Plutchik, R. (1980). *Emotion: A psychoevolutionary synthesis*. New York: Harper & Row.

Reker, G. T., & Wong, P. P. (1988). Aging as an individual process: Toward a theory of personal meaning. In J. E. Birren & V. L. Bengtson (Eds.), *Emergent theories of aging* (pp. 214–246). New York, NY: Springer Publishing.

Ryan, R. M., Huta, V., & Deci, E. L. (2008). Living well: A self-determination theory perspective on eudaimonia. *Journal of Happiness Studies, 9*(1), 139–170.

Ryff, C. D. (1989). Happiness is everything, or is it? Explorations on the meaning of psychological well-being. *Journal of Personality and Social Psychology, 57*(6), 1069.

Ryff, C. D. (1995). Psychological well-being in adult life. *Current Directions in Psychological Science, 4*, 99–104.

Ryff, C. D., & Singer, B. (1998). The contours of positive human health. *Psychological Inquiry, 9*(1), 1–28.

Saroglou, V., Buxant, C., & Tilquin, J. (2008). Positive emotions as leading to religion and spirituality. *The Journal of Positive Psychology, 3*(3), 165–173.

Sartre, J. P. (1956). *Being and nothingness: A phenomenological essay on ontology* (H. E. Barnes, Trans.). New York: Washington Square (Original work published 1943).

Seligman, M. E. P. (2002). *Authentic happiness: Using the new positive psychology to realize your potential for lasting fulfillment*. New York: Free Press.

Shek, D. T. (1991). Meaning in life and psychological well-being: An empirical study using the Chinese version of the purpose in life questionnaire. *Journal of Genetic Psychology, 153*, 185–200.

Shiota, M. N., Keltner, D., & Mossman, A. (2007). The nature of awe: Elicitors, appraisals, and effects on self-concept. *Cognition and Emotion, 21*(5), 944–963.

Shiota, M. N., Neufeld, S. L., Danvers, A. F., Osborne, E. A., Sng, O., & Yee, C. I. (2014). Positive emotion differentiation: A functional approach. *Social and Personality Psychology Compass, 8*(3), 104–117.

Shiota, M. N., Thrash, T., Danvers, A. F., & Dombrowski, J. T. (2014). Transcending the self: Awe, elevation, and inspiration. In M. Tugade, M. N. Shiota, & L. Kirby (Eds.), *Handbook of positive emotion* (pp. 362–395). New York: Guilford Press.

Snyder, C. R., Harris, C., Anderson, J. R., Holleran, S. A., Irving, L. M., Sigmon, S. T., … & Harney, P. (1991). The will and the ways: development and validation of an individual-differences measure of hope. *Journal of personality and social psychology, 60*(4), 570.

Snyder, C. R., Ilardi, S. S., Cheavens, J., Michael, S. T., Yamhure, L., & Sympson, S. (2000). The role of hope in cognitive-behavior therapies. *Cognitive Therapy and Research, 24*(6), 747–762.

Snyder, C. R., Shorey, H. S., Cheavens, J., Pulvers, K. M., Adams, V. H., III, & Wiklund, C. (2002). Hope and academic success in college. *Journal of Educational Psychology, 94*(4), 820.

Steger, M. F. (2012). Experiencing meaning in life. In P. T. P. Wong (Ed.), *The human quest for meaning: Theories, research, and applications* (pp. 165–184). New York, NY: Routledge.

Steger, M. F., Frazier, P., Oishi, S., & Kaler, M. (2006). The meaning in life questionnaire: Assessing the presence of and search for meaning in life. *Journal of Counseling Psychology, 53*(1), 80.

Steger, M. F., & Kashdan, T. B. (2007). Stability and specificity of meaning in life and life satisfaction over one year. *Journal of Happiness Studies, 8*(2), 161–179.

Tooby, J., & Cosmides, L. (2008). The evolutionary psychology of the emotions and their relationship to internal regulatory variables. In L. Michael, J. M. Haviland-Jones, & L. F. Barrett (Eds.), *Handbook of emotions* (3rd ed.). New York: Guilford Press.

Tracy, J. L., Cheng, J. T., Robins, R. W., & Trzesniewski, K. H. (2009). Authentic and hubristic pride: The affective core of self-esteem and narcissism. *Self and Identity, 8*(2–3), 196–213.

Tracy, J. L., & Robins, R. W. (2007a). Emerging insights into the nature and function of pride. *Current Directions in Psychological Science, 16*(3), 147–150.

Tracy, J. L., & Robins, R. W. (2007b). The psychological structure of pride: A tale of two facets. *Journal of Personality and Social Psychology, 92*(3), 506.

Valdesolo, P., & Graham, J. (2014). Awe, uncertainty, and agency detection. *Psychological Science, 25*(1), 170–178.

Van Cappellen, P., & Saroglou, V. (2011). Awe activates religious and spiritual feelings and behavioral intentions. *Psychology of Religion and Spirituality, 4*(3), 223–236.

Verbeke, W., Belschak, F., & Bagozzi, R. P. (2004). The adaptive consequences of pride in personal selling. *Journal of the Academy of Marketing Science, 32*(4), 386–402.

Williams, L. A., & DeSteno, D. (2008). Pride and perseverance: The motivational role of pride. *Journal of Personality and Social Psychology, 94*(6), 1007–1017.

Williams, L. A., & DeSteno, D. (2009). Pride: Adaptive social emotion or seventh sin? *Psychological Science, 20*(3), 284–288.

Weber, M. (1978). Economy and society: An outline of interpretive sociology. In N. W. Biggart (Ed.), *Readings in economic sociology*. Malden, MA: Wiley-Blackwell.

Weiner, B. (1985). An attributional theory of achievement motivation and emotion. *Psychological Review, 92*(4), 548.

Wong, P. T., & Fry, P. S. (1998). The human quest for meaning. *Journal of Adult Development, 7*, 187–188.

Wubben, M. J., De Cremer, D., & van Dijk, E. (2012). Is pride a prosocial emotion? Interpersonal effects of authentic and hubristic pride. *Cognition & Emotion, 26*(6), 1084–1097.

Yalom, I. D. (1980). *Existential psychotherapy*. New York: Basic Books.

Heroism and Eudaimonia: Sublime Actualization Through the Embodiment of Virtue

22

Zeno E. Franco, Olivia Efthimiou, and Philip G. Zimbardo

22.1 Introduction

The notion of heroism as a virtuous existence endures in contemporary empirical studies of the phenomenon; "Heroism represents the ideal of citizens transforming civic virtue into the highest form of civic action, accepting either physical peril or social sacrifice" (Franco, Blau, and Zimbardo, 2011, p. 99). Anderson (1986, p. 592) observed that popular definitions of heroism centre around the notion of ideals such as "great bravery, daring, boldness, valor", including "virtue". Building on prior extensive work on moral exemplars Walker and Frimer (2008) explores "transcendence in the lives of moral heroes". Staats, Hupp, and Hugley (2008, p. 370) argue: "Heroism is a virtue in search of empirical measurement, not only with regard to persons and situations but also with regard to enabling and inhibiting factors (Peterson & Seligman, 2004)". The stories of heroism and heroic virtue that surmount national and world-wide crises are telling of the enduring relevance of these ancient ideals in our contemporary society.

The study of well-being and optimal human functioning has been a growing central preoccupation of research on human behaviour since the mid twentieth century. The past decade especially has witnessed a surge in research on heroism and heroic leadership. The reinstatement and recognition of the importance of heroism in the twenty first century is significant in terms of redefining our concept of well-being in contemporary culture. Introducing the concept of the "banality of heroism" (Franco & Zimbardo, 2006) escalates its centrality in everyday life, suggesting a transition toward a system of thought in which everyone is a *potential* hero. For example, a recent study conducted by Igou, Ritchie, and Kinsella (2012) highlighted "the importance of heroism in everyday life". This study acknowledges the wide-reaching effects of the phenomenon across the spectrum of human experience: "The term hero is universal and understood to provide important physical, psychological, and social benefits to people" (Kinsella, 2013, p. 1).

We argue here that the grounding of heroic action in the everyday and the universal should drive the phenomenological conceptualisation of heroic eudaimonia as *timeless phronetic wisdom*

Z.E. Franco (✉)
Department of Family and Community Medicine, Clinical and Translational Science Institute, Medical College of Wisconsin, 8701 Watertown Plank Road, 26509, Milwaukee, Wisconsin, USA
e-mail: zfranco@mcw.edu

O. Efthimiou
Murdoch University, Perth, Western Australia, Australia
e-mail: oliviaefi@gmail.com

P.G. Zimbardo
Stanford University, Stanford, CA, USA
e-mail: drzimbardo@gmail.com

J. Vittersø (ed.), *Handbook of Eudaimonic Well-Being*, International Handbooks of Quality-of-Life,
DOI 10.1007/978-3-319-42445-3_22

in praxis – heroic phronesis is informed by lived experience and geared toward right and wise action, as well as independent decision-making centred on self-reflection and mindfulness, congruent with the Ancient Greek understanding of the 'good'. This chapter will reveal the heroic life as confluent with the eudaimonic as "a lifestyle characterised by the pursuit of virtue/excellence, meaning/purpose, doing good/making a difference, and the resulting sense of fulfillment or flourishing" (Wong, 2011, p. 70). But perhaps most importantly it offers an interpretation of the eudaimonic, alongside the heroic, as *paradox* – it is process and outcome, suffering and joy, downfall and transcendence, weakness and strength, simultaneously. The pursuit of eudaimonia involves the acknowledgement of the mutual value of these contradictory forces, resulting in a negative rationality approach to well-being that transcends the "tyranny of positivity" (Wong, 2011, p. 69); it sees crisis as a fundamental opportunity for growth, revealing the redemptive quality of phronetic action, and heroic action. This is exemplified in a set of attitudes held by those who hold a stance of heroic readiness or potentiality as part of a journey toward a complex understanding of their own optimal state as humans. This state may be deeply uncomfortable as part of day-to-day lived experience, but also profoundly gratifying and actualizing when observed through the lens of a lifetime's efforts or works (Kohen, 2013).

In this chapter, we explore three major areas where the ideas of heroism and eudaimonia enhance each other and deepen our understanding of the good life, personal well-being, and group flourishing. First, we advance a framework for heroic eudaimonic living and autonomy; we present mounting empirical evidence of the universal potency of heroism and hero stories for personal and community well-being and flourishing. This includes a brief discussion on the relationship between heroic action and phronesis as part of the process of flourishing. Second, we propose that the achievement of heroic eudaimonia and the Good Life is historically and empirically bound to the tragic and the mastery of suffering – the thesis of the tragedy of unrequited heroism, or the costs of not pursuing a heroic path for eudaimonia is presented. Third, we examine the relationship between heroism and an encounter with primordial truth, situations that allow the actor to encounter the sublime. We argue that for some, this encounter is the only moment when fullest self-actualization is possible. In these moments of crisis, heroes must drawn on deep intellectual, emotional, and physical reserves and act in ways that are designed to create optimal outcomes in the midst of crisis. Despite the risks encountered in the heroic moment, this transcendent activity also has a hedonistic element, as the hero enters a state of sublime self-actualization. In this sense, the acceptance even of death can be seen as a hedonistic act, if one views the satisfaction of desire as the highest good and if one, in fact, desires to die well (i.e. to experience *beautiful death*). Finally, this prospect for unification of the competing notions of hedonism and eudaimonia is extended to a discussion on developing a theory of heroic eudaimonia, centred on a summary of the set of hero/eudaimon virtues that we have arrived at through considering this space. The discussion concludes with some final thoughts on heroic eudaimonia as the *summum bonum* of the human pursuit of the path to wholeness and virtue.

22.2 Section 1: The Skill Set of Heroic Eudaimonia

Eudaimonic well-being is understood as the definition of "the good life, to comprise pleasure, a sense of meaningfulness, and a rich psychosocial integration in a person's understanding of himself or herself" (Deci & Ryan, 2008, p. 6). Heroism or a heroic stance is not necessarily a way of being, but a set of skills that can be called on in certain situations to ensure the actor does not violate core principles that express their personal narrative through actions. This is more of a latent than active manifestation. In this sense, what heroism does is *preserve* one's self-respect during and after challenging situations – heroism does not so much push us toward eudaimonia as it ensures that we do *not move away from it* (Kohen, 2013).

Below we offer an outline of some of the core properties of the skill set of heroic eudaimonia:

1. *Instrinsic goal-setting and lived experience.*

   Heroic actions and hero stories carry intrinsic value and inherent self-affirming functions; Allison and Goethals (2015, p. 2) support that "heroes and hero narratives fulfill important cognitive and emotional needs, including the need for wisdom, meaning, hope, inspiration, and growth". This core "epistemic" function of hero stories (Allison & Goethals, 2014, p. 170, 2015) is a central component of eudaimonic well-being; Bauer, McAdams, and Pals (2008) join a string of contemporary authors in supporting the importance of the development of a coherent 'life story' as vital to eudaimonia in the development of intrinsic goals, personal growth, autonomy and community well-being.

   One of the core drivers of heroic well-being is its "energizing" property (Allison & Goethals, 2014, p. 170). The centrality of dynamic personal transformation in well-being is discussed by Ryan and Deci (2000, pp. 68, 74) in their analysis of self-determination as a precursor to "intrinsic motivation, social development and well-being": "By our definition, a basic need, whether it be a physiological need... or a psychological need, is an energizing state that, if satisfied, conduces toward health and well-being but, if not satisfied, contributes to pathology and ill-being". Diener (2000, p. 34) indicates the importance of the self as interpreter and evaluator of personal life narrative in his investigation of "subjective well-being": "This subjective definition of quality of life is democratic in that it grants to each individual the right to decide whether his or her life is worthwhile".

2. *Independent and self-directed behaviour.*

   Autonomy, dynamism and volition are imperative to heroic action. A growing body of work is illustrating the power of the hero's journey model in its use as a counselling and pedagogical tool for self-transformation and heroic leadership as vital to well-being (for examples see: Brown & Moffett, 1999 Busick, 1989; Goldstein, 2005; Halstead, 2000; Robbins, 2005). The autonomous nature of heroism is freedom of choice and a sense of control over one's actions: "Subjectively, the hero is fully invested in the realization of freedom, understood in universal terms" (Merleau-Ponty, 1948; as cited in Smyth, 2010, p. 178). This universality and investment of the hero in freedom is a core propellant of heroic action, and the eudaimonics of heroism. Volition is key – the fundamental stance of heroism is toward action, rather than toward shutting down through psychological defences (e.g. fantasy defense) (Freud, 1959). Where non-heroic actors accept 'fate', heroes literally choose life through their actions; they elect to take life sustaining risks that create possibility, rather than to accept and succumb to situational constraints, even if it signifies their individual death (literally or metaphorically). This is exemplified in the men and women who jumped out of the World Trade Centre complex in New York during the September 11 disaster when the buildings were on fire. Those were arguably heroic acts, because of the exerted volitional control over a situation that was no longer controllable – those individuals fought back against the void, by choosing how they enter it. Presenting this in a way that broadly makes sense and is acceptable however is, admittedly, problematic.

3. *Mindfulness and self-awareness.*

   Mindfulness and the awareness of "an extended time-horizon, not just the present moment" is a crucial aspect of everyday heroism (Franco & Zimbardo, 2006, p. 34). Situational awareness is a vital skill that is astutely trained in individuals in professions that are likely to call for heroic action and immediate responsiveness (such as firefighters and soldiers). A hero *in that moment* is in essence a prior "hero-in-waiting" and "hero-in-training" (Zimbardo, 2015) who has recognised and seized the heroic moment; in the event of an emergency their mindful awareness and training allows them to move, react, perceive, think and feel in a way that is fully situated and immersed in the lived moment.

This heightened mindfulness is not only invaluable in emergency situations, but broader longer-term personal and community efforts to holistic improvement. Much of the efforts of contemporary heroism promotion and education initiatives are focussed on combating the culture of violence and bullying in schools. The Hero Construction Company's[1] story-based material, for example, is strategically developed with the specific aim to change automatic reactive behaviours of students and the broader school community, and to develop more effective, mindful responses to confronting issues such as bullying. This is wise and virtuous heroic well-being based on mindful practices and lived experience; it is "learning how to wisely and effectively stand up, speak out, and take heroic action against injustice of all kinds – bullying, prejudice, unjust authority, and apathy of passive bystanders in emergencies" (Franco & Zimbardo, 2016, p. 516).

4. *Self-efficacy and pro-sociality.*

Allison and Goethals (2015, p. 2) note, "Hero stories provide epistemic benefits by providing scripts for prosocial action, by revealing fundamental truths about human existence, by unpacking life paradoxes, and by cultivating emotional intelligence". The advanced competencies fostered by heroic action and characteristic of heroes – including "moral elevation", healing "psychic wounds" and inspiring "psychological growth" (Allison & Goethals, 2015, p. 2) – lend heroism, at least in part, readily as a superior form of prosocial action. Pallone and Hennessy (1998, p. 208) propose that "heroism emerges from a mix that includes neurogenic impulsivity (but not self-aggrandizement), sensitization to prosocial interpersonal environments, and a (more or less chance) encounter with an opportunity to behave impulsively in prosocial ways". Ryan, Huta, and Deci (2008, p. 139) note that "Studies indicate that people high in eudaimonic living tend to behave in more prosocial ways, thus benefiting the collective as well as themselves"; the demonstrable critical link between prosocial behaviour and heroism suggests a crucial relationship between heroic living and eudaimonic living. The combination of embodied competencies, social relatedness and capacity for both snap and laborious independent thinking, is the a recipe that can result in improved well-being at the personal and collective level.

Eudaimonia also implies that the individual is tied to the polis – this results in a clear interrelationship between individual eudaimonic activity and community well-being. As a deeply timeless social and cultural activity (Allison & Goethals, 2014; Campbell, 1949; Kinsella, 2013; Price, 1978) heroism serves as one of the highest forms of civic virtue. The 'gift' of heroism as the ultimate end result means that the personal benefits are shared with the community and enjoyed in unison; heroic eudaimonia prepares us for the capacity for communication and connectedness at all levels of well-being and interaction.

5. *Prudential wisdom and phronetic action.*

Phronesis or prudence and eudaimonia are the backbone of "virtue ethics" (Tan Bhala, 2009); in "Aristotelian science … the distinctive role of practical wisdom (phronesis) is to use the knowledge of universals provided by science, dialectic, and understanding so as to best promote happiness (eudaimonia)" (Reeve, 1992). But the essence of phronesis can be found in a very simple concept; "Phronetic action and thinking come close to the normal idea of *wisdom* [emphasis added] … phronesis is applied or practical philosophy" (Brier, 2000, p. 448). Allison and Goethals (2015, p. 28) argue that "stories about the rise of heroes, and even the fall of heroes, fulfill an important epistemic function by showing us paths to success as well as paths to ruin". This distinct function of heroism is a guide map on the road to eudaimonia, phronetic action and virtue, and "making the right choices" (Deci & Ryan, 2008, p. 7) that lead to situational or socially optimal, or even *beautiful* outcomes (Sandy, 2011).

[1] See: http://www.heroconstruction.org/

The increasing flurry of research on heroism and heroic action has "brought with it the deepening recognition that heroic action is much more commonplace than one would at first suspect ... This work has brought us closer to an understanding that heroic activity is actually within the grasp of everyone." (Franco & Zimbardo, 2016, pp. 496-497) The ideas of the virtuous mean and phronesis resonate well with the notion of everyday or banal heroism – at a deep level, heroism is highly situated activity that is a response to a set of constraints and possibilities, and cannot occur through the actions of someone from the 'outside'. The everyday is where individuals choose to act heroically, or also recognize that the problem is too complex and elect not to act. Heroic phronesis is "practical wisdom" in every sense; it is bound to our lived experience, our self-determination and autonomy as human-hero actors, and driven by "the acquisition of the highest principles for action in society" (Brier, 2000, p. 451). Heroic action with its inherent epistemic and energizing properties is thus one expression of phronesis – applied or practical philosophy and wisdom – in action.

22.3 Section 2: The Heroic, the Good Life, and the Tragic: Suffering as Pathway to Eudaimonia and the Impacts of Unrequited Heroism

Heroism and heroic acts have been celebrated in all cultures throughout history; the heroic state is undoubtedly an exemplary state of human experience. But what of the costs of pursuing, and perhaps most importantly, *not* pursuing a heroic life, or the 'road less travelled'? Little or no research addresses this important question. Emerging literature is revealing the downsides of heroism, its transience, and the significant risks associated with its enactment (Franco et al., 2011; Goethals & Allison, 2012; Parks, 2016), contributing to more in-depth understandings of the complexity of the phenomenon. This does not, however, illuminate the consequences of unrealised heroism. The adage 'it is the things that we do not do in life that we end up regretting the most' is likely to apply here – this could result in a renewed view of the hero as someone who lives in a way that *defends as best as one can against regret*, opening the door to a deeply fascinating set of questions. If "we are all developmentally equipped to pursue a lifelong hero-like journey" (Allison & Goethals, 2014, p. 175), then denying our very nature stands to have far-reaching consequences; it is possible that we will never be completely fulfilled unless we realise our innate capacity for a heroic life.

Historically the tragic has been bound to the heroic. Tarnas (1996, p. 396) asserts that major philosophical movements in the West are directly associated with the "archetypal sacrifice" of seminal prophetic and heroic figures – in particular, that Christ's sacrifice gave rise to Christianity, Galileo's to modern scientific thought, and Nietzsche's philosophy of nihilism to the postmodern mind. Allison and Setterberg (2015) cite "pain", "suffering" and "sacrifice" as the "Necessary ingredients of heroism" and "opportunities for people to develop an extraordinary life". Findings from a study conducted in 2013 by Zimbardo, Breckenridge and Moghaddam "suggest that the idea of 'altruism born of suffering' (Vollhardt, 2009), may extend to the realm of heroic acts as well" (Franco & Zimbardo, 2016, p. 496). Allison and Goethals (2015, p. 13) note:

> For the hero, according to Rohr (2011), "the way down is the way up" (p. 18). This paradoxical journey is not just reserved for mythic heroes; all human beings face painful challenges that are a necessary path toward personal growth. "Where you stumble," wrote Campbell, "there lies your treasure." (p. 75)

The inextricable link between the tragic and the heroic denotes that living a good life is, in a eudaimonic sense, likely to involve enduring deeply painful experiences. Thus the ability to *endure* is a virtue in the thought-set of eudaimonia. This is "passive heroism" – endurance, fortitude, and so forth – or the ability to bear up under extreme pressure, to *not* act in some situations as a heroic outcome (Zimbardo, 2007; Franco et al. 2011). Denying this process, however, might cause a different and more profound pain for many heroic individuals; that is, they would have felt deeply held principles were abdicated in exchange for the hedonic (in its popular sense). Campbell (1988, p. 113) asserted that the hero's journey involves following our "bliss". This is a statement often misinterpreted as meaning that the heroic life is synonymous with a hedonic life – to achieve heroic well-being we must confront the crisis at its heart, and be deeply cognizant of both the costs of pursuing a heroic life, and especially not pursuing it, firmly embedding the heroic state with the eudaimonic at an even deeper level.

For many, the notion of pursuing a heroic life would not pose a consideration in the slightest from the outset. The grandiose pre-conceptions associated with the word 'hero' are undoubtedly perpetuated by enduring cultural tropes from both historical accounts and contemporary popular culture of victorious heroes and underdogs. A large part of heroism promotion, education and research is consequently justifiably placed in developing the idea of 'everyday heroism', in contrast to these broader historical notions of heroism. Upon closer inspection, the notion of heroism is far more immediate and relevant to our daily lives – put simply, it is a surrender to a higher calling and what we know is right for our immediate circumstances. This 'calling' is very personal and differs for everyone. In a deceptively simple, but deeply profound statement, Campbell (1988) described a hero as someone who gives themselves to something bigger than themselves. Contemporary researchers such as Dik, Shimizu, and O'Connor (2016) are indeed framing heroism as a calling. But like anyone who hears the door knock and does not answer it, we will never know who came calling – and it is not knowing that causes the greatest amount of uncertainty, disempowerment and suffering in many cases. By implication, if a heroic life stands to offer its actors a range of benefits, its opposite state of refusing its call denotes that the individual must suffer the psychological, spiritual and biological costs of this refusal. If the positive state of following a heroic path is heroic well-being, then its opposite is a pathological state of malaise and *dis*-ease (with the emphasis placed on the "natural state of 'ease' being imbalanced or disrupted" by holistic wellness practitioners (Desy, 2015)).

If we think about heroism as fundamentally transformative, maybe one of the 'powers' that heroes gain is the ability to metamorphosize things or to act on the world (even their personal psychological world) in a transformative, creative way. If the hero is the "master of two worlds" (Campbell, 1949), the heroic actor is able to act with a new set of skills borrowed from this dual experience. The effective mastery of pain in all its forms and the achievement of self-transcendence through this uncomfortable process and passage through the 'unknown' world, is thus the pathway to heroic virtue, and heroic eudaimonia.

An important part of this idea is the notion that accepting and confronting our mortality is integral to heroism. Fostering the notion of the banality or everyday heroism in contemporary society denotes that we need to move away from the 'ideal' notion of heroism, and reconceptualise it as something grounded in human weaknesses and flaws, as the road to achieving virtue and excellence. Satisfaction and pleasure are therefore not the only source of the Good Life; paradoxically in this reading, discomfort, pain and dis-ease are. This extends to our ability to face death – both terror management and purpose are as central for eudaimonic well-being (Bowie, 2011; Keyes & Simoes, 2012; Robinson, 1990; Routledge et al., 2010, 2011) as they are to the heroic (Allison, 2014; McCabe, Carpenter, & Arndt, 2015). In their investigation of the "role of mortality awareness in heroic enactment" McCabe et al. (2015, p. 104) have found that:

> after reminders of death and linking pain tolerance to heroism, participants reported less pain on a cold pressor task (CPT). Further, those reminded of death and given false-feedback indicating heroic performance on the CPT, i.e., significant levels of pain tolerance, had lower death thought accessibility.

This emerging empirical research evidences the integral link between facing one's mortality and heroic eudaimonia. As Robinson (1990, p. 18) notes, "The wise man comes to grips with his mortality and recognizes that the prudent life is one that will spare him such pain as might reasonably be avoided"; prudence is a virtue of the heroic that is often overlooked. This heightens our sense of purpose, self-determination and the awareness of the transience of our existence, resulting in a Heideggerian *heroic-being-toward-death*. Herein lies the paradoxical virtue of hero/eudaimon – that in moving to accept death, we affirm life, risking only what we must.

This is a type of "negative rationality" approach to heroic eudaimonia expounded by thinkers such as Popper and Hegel (Agassi, 2014; Agger, 1976). But this negative heroic rationality is not to be confused with martyrdom. 'Sacrifice' has been commonly associated with heroism since the Christian era, a notion which has endured in contemporary observations (Franco et al., 2011; Glazer & Glazer, 1989; Blau, 2013). Nonetheless, the passage through the pain and tragedy, however essential, is necessary in order to achieve deep personal and collective transformation. At its heart, heroism is a core transformative process (Allison & Goethals, 2014, 2015). It therefore requires the acknowledgement of the *outcome* as much as the process, as well as some degree of hedonic experience albeit advanced, in the achievement of that transformation; this is what we have termed *transcendent hedonism*, defined as 'wise pleasure' and satisfaction in a life or set of actions well executed, even if there are steep costs.

22.4 Section 3: Heroism as the Embodiment of the Sublime

Traditionally, "From Aristotle to contemporary positive psychology, well-being or happiness has been usefully proposed to consist of at least two ingredients: hedonia and eudaimonia" (Berridge & Kringelbach, 2011, p. 2). But the two have been conceptually at odds with each other in the Western philosophical tradition, with the hedonic state being synonymous with "a high rate of positive affect and low rate of negative affect" (Wong, 2011, p. 70) and "*outcome*" focused, versus "*content*" and "*processes*" driven eudaimonia (Ryan et al., 2008, p. 140). As we have seen, eudaimonia with its meaningful, purposeful and process-driven orientation fits well with emerging readings of the heroic process.

But hedonism is not completely irrelevant to an analysis of heroic well-being. In many instances of heroism, the appropriation of heroic status is still largely dependent on the outcome. Further, the 'feel-good' sensory pleasures associated with the execution of heroic tasks, and if one is lucky, victory of the heroic outcome and its associated altruistic properties. For example in saving someone's life or shielding someone from a profound injustice are deeply meaningful acts that, even if not taken in the moment for pleasure, ultimately can be reflected on as providing meaning and create powerful forms of epicurean satisfaction. Indeed, heroism is still largely associated with the victor rather than failure, and altruism, though not the same as heroism (Franco et al., 2011), carries a distinct pleasure property. Berridge and Kringelbach (2011, p. 2) argue that "Conceptually, hedonic processing and eudaimonic meaningfulness are very different from each other. Yet, empirically, in real people well-being has been found to involve both together". Deci and Ryan (2008, p. 3) also concur that "the two are highly correlated, and most researchers agree that there will be considerable overlap". If we read heroism as an acquired skill, this is an instinct that is cultivated over time. Situated and embodied heroism aligns with the hedonic in its emphasis of sense experience grounded in our immediate environment and situatedness in the everyday.

Heroic action calls for a heightened awareness, mind-body connection and sense perception of our immediate surroundings and experiences, and an interest in the generation of optimal (perhaps even beautiful), and thus satisfying, outcomes. At times this even means a willingness to engage with things that are "terribly beautiful", i.e. the sublime (Burke, 1998; Kearney, 2003), which carry deep risks for the actor and others in the situation. Encountering these sublime moments of beauty/terror may be pleasurable in and of themselves, as these moments bring one closer to the primordial, unvarnished state of existence, thus offering a transcendental moment of escape from the mundane (Schneeberger, 2011), even though these situations are necessarily bounded in the everyday. Paradoxically, while the hero may be acutely aware that the situation calling for heroic action may push them over the edge, into the void (death, destruction, loss, etc.), for heroes, achieving one's highest state may only be possible when the stakes are so high, thus in part explaining the appetitive desire to enter into the heart of crisis situations.

Thus, for heroic actors, fighting against the void and a complementary knowing, appreciation of, and even communion with the void are necessary antecedents for *entelechy* to be achieved. In this sense, heroes are deeply aware of, and find pleasure in negotiating the edge of the event horizon between entropy and order, between the powers of primordial vastness and the desire to survive in the present finite moment. Where others run away, cower, or pretend nothing is wrong because the crisis is so frightful, for heroes these situations are the conditions under which they feel most alive. Heroes attempt to martial all of their intellectual understanding, physical knowing (Efthimiou, 2016), and emotional insight (Allison & Goethals, 2014, p. 171) to express dominion on the indomitable.

This fullest expression of embodied knowing and action is the achievement of greatness, of one's highest state within the contexts and constraints of daily life; a practical perfection. And thus, the very action of heroic intervention, even if it ultimately fails, can imbue its own form of pleasure. Even in the face of defeat, the hero can be satisfied that all avenues of action were exhausted and that her duty was full discharged. This is ultimately a form of hedonic pleasure in the personal embodiment of ethics, allowing one's mind and body to not just know what the virtue ethics are, but to literally become them. In so doing, one's acts become instantiated in a way that defies the erasure of time and become a guide post to others.

A breadth of research is evidencing the value of embodied practices to well-being in everyday contexts (for examples see: Bunne, 2013; Humberstone, 2015; Impett, Daubenmier, & Hirschman, 2006; Payne, 2014; Sointu, 2006; Van Der Riet, 1999). The sensory basis of heroism is only just beginning to be investigated by researchers. Parks (2016) outlines some of the preliminary findings for the hormonal bases of heroic action; Kafashan, Sparks, Rotella and Barclay (2016) and Preston (in press) are investigating the neurobiological drivers of heroism. Ryan et al. (2008, pp. 140–141) argue for the importance of pleasure to well-being:

> the focus of hedonic research is on a valued but delimited state, namely pleasure. Although pleasure is often demeaned as an important human outcome, it is in our view a very significant one. Pleasure and positive affect are important human experiences not only because they represent intrinsically preferred states, but also because they can facilitate and support other human functions... Moreover, it is clear that pleasure, psychological health, and optimal functioning are inter-correlated.

A heroic act may carry the properties of hedonism. Heroic acts do often involve an apparent element of "impulsivity" (Pallone & Hennessy, 1998, p. 139) (as is characteristic of hedonistic acts), such as throwing oneself in harm's way to save a person from danger. Heroic pleasure is not a self-centred pleasure. It is centred around the 'other', being "in service to others in need" (Franco et al., 2011, p. 101), and surrender of the self to the 'other' – whether it be a person, an ideal, a group or a cause. Campbell (1988) defined a hero as "someone who has given his or her life to something bigger than oneself". There is a satisfaction and an evolved sense of pleasure that comes from heroic nobility, virtue and self-sacrifice, following one's bliss in the Campbellian sense and surrendering to something greater than oneself.

22.5 Discussion: Developing a Framework to Explore Heroic Eudaimonia

A number of researchers are now embarking on the ambitious enterprise of mapping a science of happiness and eudaimonia (Berridge & Kringelbach, 2011; Keyes & Annas, 2009; Layard & Layard, 2011; Deci & Ryan, 2008; Ryff, 2014, Chap. 6, this volume). The epistemic function of heroism opens the door to a phenomenologically informed science of heroic well-being that recognises science, in its mechanistic and Newtonian traditional sense, as but one form of valid empirical knowledge and means of observing our Heidegerrian 'being-in-the-world'.

We propose that an exploration of heroic eudaimonia be based on the conceptual and empirical observation and testing of the central virtues associated with the processes and outcomes of heroism, which we have preliminarily identified in this chapter. In summary, these are: *purposeful sacrifice; embodied mindfulness; mortality awareness; self-leadership; self-efficacy* (e.g. emotional, physical and other intelligence); *social relatedness (or collective consciousness?); prudential wisdom and action; transformative action; redemptive action; resilience* (moral, physical, mental, spiritual etc.); *transcendent hedonism* (or wise pleasure and delayed gratification); and, *paradox regulation.*

The stabilizing view of heroic well-being reveals the hedonic and the eudaimonic as co-requirements for happiness – one defines the other and reflects the human experience in its entirety. As hero-human actors we need to experience true subjective well-being, and both inner and collective balance. In their efforts to develop "a neuroscience of pleasure and well-being" Berridge and Kringelbach (2011, p. 1) "discuss how brains might *connect* hedonia states of pleasure to eudaimonia assessments of meaningfulness, and so *create balanced states of positive well-being* [emphasis added]". Kashdan, Biswas-Dienerb, and King (2008, p. 219) argue for the problematic nature of continuing to make this distinction between hedonic and eudaimonic states of well-being which "does not necessarily translate well to science. Among the problems of drawing too sharp a line between 'types of happiness' is the fact that eudaimonia is not well-defined and lacks consistent measurement"–hence a science of heroic eudaimonia must address this enduring and limiting epistemological divide, and aim to not only reconcile the two perceived competing states, but travel beyond that to consider the relevance of heroism to other forms of happiness, such as "prudential" and "chaironic" (Wong, 2011).

Achieving heroic well-being, and a science of heroic eudaimonia, should thus involve not only reconciling hedonism and eudaimonia, but recognising the presence of different epistemologies of happiness that all lend well to heroism, and the need for their integration, rigorous observation and accumulation of data. The synergy of heroism and heroic well-being with different types of happiness demonstrates the need for a more inclusive balanced approach based on empirical observation and lived experience, and an integrative open and embodied science that critically assesses ancient philosophical traditions and divided epistemologies. The notion of everyday heroism, heroic eudaimonia and heroism science are the balusters on which this union may rest. Heroism offers an avenue not only for the bridging of the hedonic and the eudaimonic notions of well-being, but the basis for the development of a "balanced interactive model of the Good Life" as a carrier of "the four pillars of the good life as meaning, virtue, resilience, and well-being" (Wong, 2011, p. 69).

The mindful and situated approach to everyday heroic eudaimonia arguably offers the welcome "pause" for well-being thinkers called on by Nussbaum (2008, p. S108). Everyday heroism situated in lived experience offers a prime example of this intermission in the field of eudaimonic well-being, and meaningfully reconceptualises it. The heroic life is thus a virtuous life, and by implication, an exemplar of the eudaimonic life. "Happy warriors" (Nussbaum, 2008) can be reframed as 'hero warriors' grounded in heroic resilience through suffering. But "While advocating for more everyday heroism is an easy, positive, and potentially impactful message to send out to citizens and especially our youth, a number of important empirical, philosophical and ethical questions remain" (Franco & Zimbardo, 2016, p. 497). The risk and suffering inextricably bound to the heroic process, stands to be a critical consideration in the eudaimonics of heroism and their impact on heroic self-determination and autonomy, from both a philosophical and empirical standpoint.

It could boldly be said that heroic eudaimonia is the *summum bonum* of the human pursuit. Perhaps its most ambitious offering is the potential for a science of happiness that transcends the knowledge cultures and their traditional boundaries, producing a balanced path to well-being. The hero's journey is an evolutionary process of growth, personal and social evolution, and phronetic wisdom and praxis, ultimately leading to expression of personal perfection in moments of complexity and crisis. We have a duty to ourselves to perceive and live our heroic calling, and be mindful of the consequences of our inaction. As the height of autonomous and civic virtue, heroic phronesis reveals eudaimonia as "life for the hero" (Levit, 2013).

References

Agassi, J. (2014). Karl Raimund Popper (1902–1994). In *Popper and his popular critics* (pp. 37–52). Springer International Publishing.

Agger, B. (1976). Marcuse and Habermas on new science. *Polity, 9*, 158–181.

Allison, S. T. (2014). What is your purpose in life? In *The selected works of Scott T. Allison*. Retrieved from: http://works.bepress.com/scott_allison/9.

Allison, S. T., & Goethals, G. R. (2014). "Now he belongs to the ages": The heroic leadership dynamic and deep narratives of greatness. In G. R. Goethals, S. T. Allison, R. M. Kramer, & D. M. Messick (Eds.), *Conceptions of leadership: Enduring ideas and emerging insights* (pp. 167–183). New York: Palgrave Macmillan.

Allison, S. T., & Goethals, G. R. (2015). Hero worship: The elevation of the human spirit. *Journal for the Theory of Social Behaviour. 46*(2), 187–210. Accepted manuscript.

Allison, S. T., & Setterberg, G. C. (2015). Suffering and sacrifice: The necessary ingredients of heroism. In *Heroes: What they do and why we need them*. Retrieved from: http://blog.richmond.edu/heroes/2015/04/05/suffering-and-sacrifice-the-necessary-ingredients-of-heroism/.

Anderson, J. W. (1986). Military heroism: An occupational definition. *Armed Forces and Society, 12*(4), 591–606.

Bauer, J. J., McAdams, D. P., & Pals, J. L. (2008). Narrative identity and eudaimonic well-being. *Journal of Happiness Studies, 9*(1), 81–104.

Berridge, K. C., & Kringelbach, M. L. (2011). Building a neuroscience of pleasure and well-being. *Psychology of Well-Being, 1*(1), 1–26.

Blau, K. (2013). *Correlates of heroic behavior* (Doctoral dissertation, Palo Alto University).

Bowie, T. (2011). *Mortality, immortality, and meaningfulness in life*. Unpublished PhD thesis, Carleton University, Ottawa.

Brier, S. (2000). Trans-scientific frameworks of knowing: Complementarity views of the different types of human knowledge*. *Systems Research and Behavioral Science, 17*(5), 433–458.

Brown, J. L., & Moffett, C. A. (1999). *The hero's journey: How educators can transform schools and improve learning*. Washington, DC: ASCD.

Bunne, A. (2013). *Exploring embodied well-being*. Unpublished masters thesis, The University of Edinburgh.

Burke, E. (1998). *A philosophical enquiry into the sublime and beautiful*. London: Penguin.

Busick, B. S. (1989). Grieving as a hero's journey. In M. E. Lattanzi-Licht, M. E. Kirschling, & S. J. Fleming (Eds.), *Bereavement care: A new look at hospice and community based services* (pp. 89–126). New York: Haworth Press, Inc.

Campbell, J. (1949). *The hero with a thousand faces*. Princeton, NJ: Princeton University Press.

Campbell, J. (1988). *The power of myth: Joseph Campbell with Bill Moyers*. Apostrophe S Productions, Incorporated and Public Affairs Television Incorporated.

Deci, E. L., & Ryan, R. M. (2008). Hedonia, eudaimonia, and well-being: An introduction. *Journal of Happiness Studies, 9*(1), 1–11.

Desy, P. L. (2015). Dis-ease. *About religion*. Retrieved from: http://healing.about.com/od/energyhealing/g/dis-ease.htm.

Diener, E. (2000). Subjective well-being: The science of happiness and a proposal for a national index. *American Psychological Association, 55*(1), 34.

Dik, B. J., Shimizu, A. B., & O'Connor, W. (2016). Career development and a sense of calling: Contexts for heroism. In S. T. Allison, G. R. Goethals, & R. M. Kramer (Eds.), *Handbook of heroism and heroic leadership* (pp. 316–338). New York: Routledge.

Efthimiou, O. (2016). The hero organism: Advancing the embodiment of heroism thesis in the 21st century. In S. T. Allison, G. R. Goethals, & R. M. Kramer (Eds.), *Handbook of heroism and heroic leadership* (pp. 139–162). New York: Routledge.

Franco, Z., Blau, K., & Zimbardo, P. G. (2011). Heroism: A conceptual analysis and differentiation between

heroic action and altruism. *Review of General Psychology, 15*(2), 99–113.
Franco, Z., & Zimbardo, P. (2006). The banality of heroism. *Greater Good, 3*(2), 30–35.
Franco, Z., & Zimbardo, P. (2016). The psychology of heroism: Extraordinary champions of humanity in an unforgiving world. In A. G. Miller (Ed.), *The social psychology of good and evil* (2nd ed.) (pp. 494–523). New York: The Guilford Press.
Freud, S. (1959). The relation of [he poet to daydreaming. In Collected papers. New York: Basic Books. Vol. IV.
Glazer, M., & Glazer, P. M. (1989). *The whistleblowers: Exposing corruption in government and industry*. New York: Basic Books.
Goethals, G. R., & Allison, S. T. (2012). Making heroes: The construction of courage, competence, and virtue. *Advances in Experimental Social Psychology, 46,* 183.
Goldstein, L. S. (2005). Becoming a teacher as a hero's journey: Using metaphor in preservice teacher education. *Teacher Education Quarterly, 32*(1), 7–24.
Halstead, R. W. (2000). From tragedy to triumph: Counselor as companion on the hero's journey. *Counseling and Values, 44*(2), 100–106.
Hull, C. L. (1943). *Principles of behavior: An introduction to behavior theory*. Appleton-Century: Oxford, England.
Humberstone, B. (2015). Embodiment, nature and well-being. In *Experiencing the outdoors* (pp. 61–72). Rotterdam: SensePublishers.
Igou, E., Ritchie, T., & Kinsella, E. L. (2012). *UL research highlights the importance of heroism in everyday life*. University of Limerick. Retrieved from: http://www.ul.ie/news-centre/news/ul-research-highlights-the-importance-of-heroism-in-everyday-life.
Impett, E. A., Daubenmier, J. J., & Hirschman, A. L. (2006). Minding the body: Yoga, embodiment, and well-being. *Sexuality Research & Social Policy, 3*(4), 39–48.
Kafashan, S., Sparks, A., Rotella, A., & Barclay, P. (2016). Why heroism exists: Evolutionary perspectives on extreme helping. In S. T. Allison, G. R. Goethals, & R. M. Kramer (Eds.), *Handbook of heroism and heroic leadership* (pp. 36–57). New York: Routledge.
Kashdan, T. B., Biswas-Diener, R., & King, L. A. (2008). Reconsidering happiness: The costs of distinguishing between hedonics and eudaimonia. *The Journal of Positive Psychology, 3*(4), 219–233.
Kearney, R. (2003). Terror, philosophy and the sublime. Some philosophical reflections on 11 September. *Philosophy and Social Criticism, 29*(1), 23–51.
Kearney, E. (2014). Canadian gothic: Literature, history and the spectre of self-invention. *The Irish Journal of Gothic and Horror Studies, 13,* 99.
Keyes, C. L., & Annas, J. (2009). Feeling good and functioning well: Distinctive concepts in ancient philosophy and contemporary science. *The Journal of Positive Psychology, 4*(3), 197–201.
Keyes, C. L., & Simoes, E. J. (2012). To flourish or not: Positive mental health and all-cause mortality. *American Journal of Public Health, 102*(11), 2164–2172.
Kinsella, E. L. (2013). *A psychological perspective on the features and functions of heroes*. Unpublished PhD thesis, University of Limerick, Ann Arbor.
Kohen, A. (2013). *Untangling heroism: Classical philosophy and the concept of the hero*. New York: Routledge.
Layard, P. R., & Layard, R. (2011). *Happiness: Lessons from a new science*. London: Penguin.
Levit, L. Z. (2013). Eudaimonia: Life for the hero. *Journal of Modern Foreign Psychology, 2*(1), 69–77.
McCabe, S., Carpenter, R. W., & Arndt, J. (2015). The role of mortality awareness in heroic enactment. *Journal of Experimental Social Psychology*. 61, pp. 104-109. Accepted manuscript.
Merleau-Ponty, M. (1948). *Sens et non-sens [Sense and non-sense]*. Paris: Nagel.
Nussbaum, M. C. (2008). Who is the happy warrior? Philosophy poses questions to psychology. *The Journal of Legal Studies, 37*(S2), S81–S113.
Pallone, N. J., & Hennessy, J. J. (1998). Counterfeit courage: Toward a process psychology paradigm for the "Heroic rescue fantasy". *Current Psychology, 17*(2–3), 197–209.
Parks, C. D. (2016). Accidental and purposeful impediments to heroism. In S. T. Allison, G. R. Goethals, & R. M. Kramer (Eds.), *Handbook of heroism and heroic leadership*. New York: Routledge.
Payne, H. (2014). Authentic movement groups in the development of well-being in our bodymindspirit. In J. Corrigall, H. Payne, & H. Wilkinson (Eds.), *About a body: Working with the embodied mind in psychotherapy* (pp. 162–180). New York: Routledge.
Peterson, C., & Seligman, M. E. (2004). *Character strengths and virtues: A handbook and classification*. New York: Oxford University Press.
Preston, S. (2016). The evolution and neurobiology of heroism. In S. T. Allison, G. R. Goethals, & R. M. Kramer (Eds.), *Handbook of heroism and heroic leadership* (pp. 74-87). New York: Routledge.
Price, R. (1978). *A palpable god*. New York: Atheneum.
Reeve, C. D. C. (1992). *Practices of reason: Aristotle's Nicomachean ethics*. Oxford: Clarendon Paperbacks.
Robbins, R. A. (2005). Harry Potter, ruby slippers and Merlin: Telling the client's story using the characters and paradigm of the archetypal hero's journey. *Seattle University Law Review, 29*(4), 767.
Robinson, D. N. (1990). Wisdom through the ages. *Wisdom: Its Nature, Origins, and Development, 1,* 13–24.
Rohr, R. (2011). *Falling upward*. New York: Jossey-Bass.
Routledge, C., Arndt, J., Wildschut, T., Sedikides, C., Hart, C. M., Juhl, J., et al. (2011). The past makes the present meaningful: Nostalgia as an existential resource. *Journal of Personality and Social Psychology, 101*(3), 638–652.

Routledge, C., Ostafin, B., Juhl, J., Sedikides, C., Cathey, C., & Liao, J. (2010). Adjusting to death: The effects of mortality salience and self-esteem on psychological well-being, growth motivation, and maladaptive behavior. *Journal of Personality and Social Psychology, 99*(6), 897–916.

Ryan, R. M., & Deci, E. L. (2000). Self-determination theory and the facilitation of intrinsic motivation, social development, and well-being. *American Psychologist, 55*(1), 68.

Ryan, R. M., Huta, V., & Deci, E. L. (2008). Living well: A self-determination theory perspective on eudaimonia. *Journal of Happiness Studies, 9*(1), 139–170.

Ryff, C. D. (2014). Psychological well-being revisited: Advances in the science and practice of eudaimonia. *Psychotherapy and Psychosomatics, 83*(1), 10–28.

Sandy, M. (2011). Practical beauty and the legacy of pragmatism: Generating theory for community-engaged scholarship. *Interchange, 42*(3), 261–285.

Schneeberger, A. (2011). Aesthetics of the brink: Environmental crisis and the sublime in Mary Shelley s Frankenstein and Philip K. Dick's do androids dream of electric sheep?

Smyth, B. (2010). Heroism and history in Merleau-Ponty's existential phenomenology. *Continental Philosophy Review, 43*(2), 167–191. doi:10.1007/s11007-010-9138-5.

Sointu, E. (2006). Healing bodies, feeling bodies: Embodiment and alternative and complementary health practices. *Social Theory and Health, 4*(3), 203–220.

Staats, S., Hupp, J. M., & Hagley, A. M. (2008). Honesty and heroes: A positive psychology view of heroism and academic honesty. *The Journal of Psychology, 142*(4), 357–372.

Tan Bhala, K. W. Y. (2009). *Fortifying virtue ethics: Recognizing the essential roles of eudaimonia and phronesis*. Dissertation Available from: University of Kansas.Retrieved from KUSCHOLARWORKS database: https://kuscholarworks.ku.edu/handle/1808/5440

Tarnas, R. (1996). *The passion of the western mind: Understanding the ideas that have shaped our world view* (Vol. 218). New York: Random House.

Van Der Riet, P. (1999). Ethereal embodiment of cancer patients. *The Australian Journal of Holistic Nursing, 6*(2), 20–27.

Vollhardt, J. R. (2009). Altruism born of suffering and prosocial behavior following adverse life events: A review and conceptualization. *Social Justice Research, 22*(1), 53–97.

Walker, L. J., & Frimer, J. A. (2008). Being good for goodness' sake transcendence in the lives of moral heroes. In F. Oser & W. Veugelers (Eds.), *Getting involved: Global citizenship development and sources of moral values* (pp. 309–326). Rotterdam: Sense Publishers.

Wong, P. T. (2011). Positive psychology 2.0: Towards a balanced interactive model of the good life. *Canadian Psychology/Psychologie Canadienne, 52*(2), 69.

Zimbardo, P. (2007). *The lucifer effect: Understanding how good people turn evil*. New York: Random House LLC.

Zimbardo, P. G., Breckenridge, J. N., & Moghaddam, F. M. (2013). "Exclusive" and "Inclusive" visions of heroism and democracy. *Current Psychology, 32*(3), 221–233.

Zimbardo, P. (2015, January 21). *Philip zimbardo and matt langdon at the hero round table 2014: What makes a hero?* [Video file]. Retrieved from https://www.youtube.com/watch?v=ujtkIaAfiSM.

23 The Eudaimonics of Health: Exploring the Promise of Positive Well-Being and Healthier Living

Jay Kimiecik

Does eudaimonia impact one's health? If so, how? Until recently these questions were rarely asked. Despite the World Health Organization's (1948, 1986) definitional attempts to conceptualize health within a holistic, well-being framework, the subjective experience of the individual had been considered irrelevant to one's health (Kimiecik, 2011). The formalization of the positive psychology movement (Seligman & Csikszentmihalyi, 2000), coinciding with other societal and healthcare trends (e.g., wellness), has sparked a new era, one that Breslow (2004) called the "third revolution," which reconceptualizes health as a resource for everyday living fueled by optimal well-being. We are in the very beginnings of this movement and there is much we don't know about the complex connection between positive subjective experience and health. Hence, the general purpose of this chapter is to delve into the dynamics of the relationship between eudaimonia and health. Specifically, to set the groundwork for exploring the relationship between eudaimonia and health, an overview of some of the conceptual/definitional challenges involving these two concepts will be presented. Next, key findings and highlights of selective research that has examined the eudaimonia-health connection across the lifespan will be discussed. Lastly, key issues and future directions for interventions within a eudaimonia-health framework will be presented.

J. Kimiecik (✉)
Department of Kinesiology and Health,
Miami University, Oxford, OH 45056, USA
e-mail: kimiecjc@miamioh.edu

23.1 Conceptual/Definitional Challenges

Because space is limited, the conceptual/definitional examination of both eudaimonia and health will be all to brief. But as Nussbaum (2008, p. S108) points out, it is useful to examine these kinds of concepts at times from a historical, conceptual, or philosophical perspective: "…we had better pause and sort things out before going any further."

23.1.1 Health

Historically, human health in the Western mainstream was, and still is, driven by a biomedical model grounded in physical and pathogenic terms (Antonovsky, 1996; Buchanan, 2000). Out of this model concepts such as disease, illness, prevention, treatment, and compliance emerged (Keyes, 2007; Kimiecik & Lawson, 1996). At its essence, a biomedical perspective views the body as a machine (see Longino, 1997). Disease, which is defined as a disruption in the body's biological processes, is divorced from emotions and spirit (Capra, 1982).

J. Vittersø (ed.), *Handbook of Eudaimonic Well-Being*, International Handbooks of Quality-of-Life,
DOI 10.1007/978-3-319-42445-3_23

Thus, the focus of the biomedical model is on fixing what goes wrong with the body (treatment) and attempting to prevent diseases from manifesting themselves. The biomedical orientation evolved out of Cartesion dualism where, "there is nothing included in the concept of body that belongs to the mind; and nothing in that of mind that belongs to the body" (quoted in Capra, 1982, p. 59). The development of modern medicine was then guided by reductionism and concentrated on smaller and smaller fragments of the body, losing the patient as a human being (Ghane & Sweeny, 2013). In the late 1800s/early 1900s, biomedical science developed vaccines and other treatments for the leading diseases of the times, which were primarily infectious ones. Once these diseases were controlled or eliminated, people started living longer and began to experience chronic degenerative conditions, such as cancer, stroke, and cardiovascular disease. Epidemiologists and other biomedicalists studying the causes or risk factors associated with these leading chronic degenerative diseases found, in general, that lifestyle factors (e.g., behaviors) were major causes of these diseases. More specifically, these studies reported that anywhere from 50 to 70% of contemporary diseases and medical problems were associated with or caused by "modifiable" lifestyle-related factors (Danaei et al., 2009; McGinnis & Foege, 1993).

The epidemiological science that identified this lifestyle-disease relationship spawned a focus on prevention of disease via both secondary and primary prevention (Kaplan, 2000). Secondary prevention is typically based on diagnosis and treatment of an existing condition and treated via surgery or medication, whereas primary prevention emphasizes health behavior change as a means of avoiding or delaying the onset of disease. Kaplan argues that primary prevention should have a bigger long-term public health payoff than secondary prevention. Within this primary prevention approach, health behaviors are defined as any actions (e.g., physical activity) that help individuals minimize the development of risk factors (e.g., high blood pressure) connected to chronic-degenerative disease (e.g., cardiovascular disease). Health promotion emerged out of this pathogenic, prevention model (Antonovsky, 1996) but has attempted to move towards a more holistic, wellness-oriented paradigm as indicated by the editor of the *American Journal of Health Promotion:*

> Health Promotion is the art and science of helping people discover the synergies between their core passions and optimal health, enhancing their motivation to strive for optimal health, and supporting them in changing their lifestyle to move toward a state of optimal health. Optimal health is a dynamic balance of physical, emotional, social, spiritual, and intellectual health. (O'Donnell, 2009, p. iv)

Despite the attempts to shift the focus into the realms of positive health, it has been suggested that the emphasis on risk reduction and disease prevention continues to dominate health promotion and remains even more powerful than 50 years ago (Nettelton, 2006; von Heimburg, 2010). Health promotion, which continues to emphasize biometrics, education, and the prevention of disease, has resulted in a modest impact on long-term health behavior change and health outcomes, and is still quite controversial (Lewis, 2012; Mattke et al., 2013; O'Donnell, 2013). Thus, the biomedical model has fallen short of making significant inroads into helping people live healthier lives. Multiple studies and reviews have highlighted this lack of success for positively influencing behaviors identified as risk factors (e.g., physical inactivity) for chronic degenerative disease (Blanck et al., 2007; Ezzati, Martin, Skjold, Vander Hoorn, & Murray, 2006; Institute of Medicine, 2006; Sapkota, Bowles, Ham, & Kohl, 2005).

A possible reason for this ineffectiveness is that a pathogenic orientation of health disregards essential human dimensions (e.g., mind) and it certainly ignores the positive aspects of health (Antonovsky, 1996; Kimiecik, 2011; von Heimburg, 2010). If the human being is missing from health then by definition so is meaning and purpose (Segar & Richardson, 2014). This point cannot be overstated. Without considering meaning or the lived experiences of individuals and the communities in which they live, the effects of most change attempts will be short-lived because the starting point is focused on disease reduction outcomes rather than the whole person. As Seligman and Csikszentmihalyi (2000) pointed out, a change model grounded in the psychological science of disease and illness cannot move us any closer to preventing these serious problems. Ryff and Singer (1998, p. 3) observed that the central objective of the biomedical model is "returning the body from states of negative functioning back to neutral. *Positive health* has minimal presence in this realm...Unfortunately, the medical profession and culture has equated the task of treating human infirmity with the goal of fostering health."

Certainly there have been attempts within a variety of disciplines inside and outside of medicine to remove health from the biomedical, pathogenic stranglehold and make it more human, holistic, and positive (e.g., Antonovsky, 1996; Mitman, 2005; Seligman, 2008). Wellness surfaced in the late 1950s long before positive psychology formally emerged at the beginning of the new millennium. These newer models were more practitioner-driven with the intent of helping individuals go beyond neutral with respect to their health and explore optimal well-being. In essence, wellness theories or philosophies are holistic and integrative attempting to add *meaning* into health promotion (Arloski, 2007). Over the years, the accepted definition of wellness evolved into the idea that people are holistic beings with physical, mental, spiritual, and social dimensions, and that personal development is based on a potpourri of balance, interdependence, and integration of these dimensions for each individual (see National Wellness, 2009). Baer, Hays, McClendon, McGoldrick, and Vespucci (1998) point out that although the holistic health movement began as a response to the perceived inadequacy of biomedicine, it has been co-opted by biomedicine and may actually be contributing to further medicalization, something that it was trying to change or at least avoid. Similarly, some scholars have commented on the co-option of wellness and its assimilation into the biomedical paradigm, limiting its potential to optimize the quality of people's lives and health behavior change. Fahlberg and Fahlberg (1997) suggest that this co-option of wellness has led to no more than the relief of symptoms with the end goal of health neutral—similar to the biomedical approach. Focusing on health issues without addressing deeper human experience, such as life meaning and purpose, will achieve limited long-term success (Robison, 2004).

Other attempts have called for expanding or reconceptualizing the definition of health to move closer to a well-being ideal. Capra (1982, p. 323) redefined health as "an experience of well-being, resulting from a dynamic balance that involves the physical and psychological aspects of the organism, as well as interactions with its natural and social environments." Pelletier (1994, pp. 15–16) suggested that health is "an inner quality that gives rise to particular health practices but cannot in itself be reduced to those practices...an ongoing process of self-discovery, manifesting a positive influence on the world around us." Buchanan (2000, p. 103) proposes that health be redefined as well-being, which is "living one's life in accordance with values that matter. It is a life of becoming not a discrete fixed outcome." Edington (2009, p. 22) wrote that "health is having the energy, mobility, and independence we need to live the lives we want to lead, fully, and for as long as possible." And more recently, Langeland and Vinje (2013, p. 305), following Antonovsky's (1996) salutogenic model, suggest that health is a "person's subjective experience of being in a state of positive well-being."

In sum, human health traditionally has focused on disease and the physical dimension due to Cartesian dualism (i.e., mind-body split), which led to the emergence and dominance of a biomedical model. Prevention and treatment of disease have focused on risk factors, many of which are lifestyle related. Within this narrow, reductionistic model, there has been very little room for holistic, positive conceptions of health. More recently, holistic health and wellness movements have opened up the possibilities for positive psychology and well-being science to be integrated into health.

23.1.2 Eudaimonia

Much of the holistic health and wellness movement laid the groundwork for integrating well-being into various aspects of health and health promotion (Allen, Carlson, & Ham, 2007). But as Nussbaum (2008) points out, similar to health, well-being and happiness have their own conceptual confusion. As such, well-being may be the new health. Sumner (2002, p. 37) suggests that "Well-being concerns the prudential value of a life" and considers "eudaimonia as more or less equivalent to well-being." This is but one of many views of well-being and epitomizes the definitional/conceptual challenges involving eudaimonia and well-being. Is eudaimonia well-being? Or does eudaimonia lead to enhanced well-being? Is eudaimonia an activity, a state, or an outcome of one's experience? Different conceptualizations and definitions of well-being have been proposed and even within eudaimonistic circles there are differing perspectives. For example, Lambert, Passmore, and Holder (2015) categorize eudaimonic psychological theories of well-being into four major categories: humanistic theories, psychological well-being, self-determination theory, and social well-being. And Huta and Waterman (2014) propose a classification system for different definitions of hedonia and eudaimonia based on degree of centrality of core variables falling into four main categories: (a) orientations, (b) behaviors, (c) experiences, and (d) functioning.

As the reader may surmise, well-being is complex and it is not the purpose of this chapter to wade through the morass of its conceptual, definitional, and operational conundrums. However, the main themes of eudaimonia appear to revolve around the ideas of pursuing excellence or the best within us, true self, actualizing potential, self-realization, and feelings of personal expressiveness (Huta, 2013, Chap. 15, this volume; Huta & Ryan, 2010; Ryan, Huta, & Deci, 2008; Ryff & Singer, 2008; Ryff, Chap. 6, this volume; Vittersø, 2013, Chap. 17, this volume; Waterman, 2013). Henderson and Knight (2012) observe that other constructs have been linked to eudaimonia as well, such as meaning and purpose. Sugarman (2007, p. 179) interprets Aristotle's eudaimonia as a "flourishing state of the soul" and Aristotle considered eudaimonia to be the highest virtue: "and this will be that of the best thing in us." Kimiecik (2010, 2011) suggests that eudaimonia is a subjective experience that is lived and felt, and is very much framed within existential phenomenology (Fahlberg, Fahlberg, & Gates, 1992; Valle, King, & Halling, 1989). As we experience things, we feel them. When individuals in action feel how they want to feel, they experience resonance (Newburg, Kimiecik, Durand-Bush, & Doell, 2002).

In contrast to eudaimonia, hedonia typically refers to happiness, positive emotions, or pleasure. As Nettle (2006, p. 29) suggests, "When people talk of happiness, they generally mean a state involving positive feelings or positive judgments about feelings." Hedonia has also been separated out from subjective well-being, suggesting that positive emotional states or pleasure (hedonia) are linked to the maximization of the good in or satisfaction with one's life (Henderson & Knight, 2012; Vittersø & Søholt, 2011). Not everyone agrees that eudaimonia and hedonia are separate experiences (Kahneman, Diener, & Schwarz, 1999; Kashdan, Biswas-Diener, & King, 2008). However, many scholars do cite Aristotle as coining *eudaimonia* (Deci & Ryan, 2008; Ryan & Martela, Chap. 7, this volume; Norton, 1976; Ryan et al., 2008; Ryff & Singer, 2008; Sugarman, 2007), even though the term had been part of Greek culture several hundred years before his writings (McMahon, 2006). In sum, similar to health, the essence of positive well-being differs depending on who you ask. Typically, however, hedonia and eudaimonia are differentiated and that is the assumption on which this chapter proceeds.

23.2 The Eudaimonia and Health Relationship

This section will take a broad brush to examining the link between eudaimonia and health. As the previous sections indicate, both health and eudaimonia are concepts that have been investigated from many perspectives and the remainder of this chapter will also take that approach by being holistic, multidimensional, and inclusive. Also, due to the potential interaction of eudaimonic and hedonic experience, the role of hedonia in one's health will also be examined to address the triadic relationship among eudaimonia, hedonia, and health.

As indicated in the prior Health section, health has been traditionally defined within a disease model. Hence, in the sections that follow, health is considered a multi-dimensional, biomedical construct (see Howell, Kern, & Lyubormisky, 2007), including physical health or health status (e.g., heart disease), biological and immunological markers (e.g., cortisol levels), risk factors, and health-promoting (e.g., physical activity) and health-risk behaviors (e.g., smoking). Also, as indicated in the previous Eudaimonia section, eudaimonia will be broadly defined and an inclusive approach will be utilized to explore how concepts closely aligned with eudaimonia, such as meaning, purpose, and vitality, may be involved in the well-being-health relationship.

This is a selective review of positive well-being and health as a number of systematic reviews have been done quite well by others (see Chida & Steptoe, 2008; Howell et al., 2007; Ng et al., 2012; Roepke, Jayawickreme, & Riffle, 2014; Jayawickreme & Dahill-Brown, Chap. 31, this volume). Specifically, the link between *eudaimonia and health outcomes and behaviors across the lifespan* will be the primary focus, and will be examined assuming a dynamic, reciprocal relationship. That is, eudaimonia may impact health behavior and health behavior could influence eudaimonia. This is an area that well-being theorists and health professionals have long suggested is ripe for enhanced understanding and intervention (Ryff & Singer, 1998; Kimiecik, 2011; Steger, Fitch-Martin, Donnelly, & Rickard, 2015; Steger, Chap. 11, this volume). All designs of studies will be included as well: correlational, cross-sectional, and prospective, as each may provide an enhanced understanding of this complex relationship.

The next section focuses on studies that utilize definitions of well-being (e.g., happiness, subjective well-being, meaning) that are closely aligned with eudaimonic and hedonic concepts, followed by two sections focused specifically on eudaimonic- and hedonic-based studies examining the link between positive well-being and health outcomes and health behaviors, respectively. The final section discusses issues and interventions.

23.2.1 Well-Being and Health Outcomes/Behaviors

Systematic reviews and meta-analyses conclude that well-being does impact human health (e.g., Howell et al., 2007; Ng et al., 2012; Roepke et al., 2014; Vazquez, Hervas, Rahona, & Gomez, 2009; Veenhoven, 2008). But what kinds of well-being? In Howell and colleagues' review of studies including college students and adults, well-being was defined as subjective well-being (i.e., happiness, life-satisfaction, and positive affect). The primary findings suggest that subjective well-being enhances both short-term and long-term health by strengthening immune functioning and/or buffering the stress response. Happiness as positive affect or positive emotions played a significant role in impacting a variety of health-related variables. Veenhoven's review examined the relationship between happiness and physical health (i.e., absence of illness or defect), defining happiness as overall appreciation of one's life-as-a-whole or how much one likes the life one lives, which parallels the subjective well-being approach adopted by Howell and colleagues. Veenhoven (p. 449) was primarily interested in the happiness-longevity connection and found that happiness strongly predicts longevity in healthy populations, but not in sick populations and advocated for more public health initiatives focused on a "greater happiness of a greater number."

A group of studies has also shown that positive emotions can be enhanced via loving kindness meditation and that these resultant emotions are associated with fewer headaches, less chest pain, congestion, weakness, and enhanced vagal tone, which may be a key factor in regulating physical health (Fredrickson, Cohn, Coffey, Pek, & Finkel, 2008; Fredrickson, Chap. 12, this volume; Kok et al., 2013). Although most studies have found positive emotions to be related to or influencing health, one meta-analysis found little evidence of positive emotions impacting health-related cognitions or actions (Cameron, Bertenshaw, & Sheeran, 2014). These authors suggest that when it comes to people's health, positive affect without meaning or purpose may not be enough for them to activate health goals.

The influence of meaning on health has also been examined (Roepke et al., 2014; Steger et al., 2015). Roepke and colleagues included a variety of definitions of meaning in conducting their systematic review (e.g., a sense of coherence, feelings of purpose and direction). Meaning and purpose were clearly associated with better physical health, especially for those who found and experienced meaning rather than those who were searching for meaning. In addition, individuals with more meaning and purpose were more likely to participate in health-promoting behaviors, such as exercise, and avoid risk-behaviors such as smoking. Steger and colleagues utilized a Meaning in Life model based on Antonovsky's (1987) Sense of Coherence model to examine the meaning-health connection in college students. Their findings suggest that meaning in life significantly influences health by facilitating a more positive orientation towards health, which motivates individuals to avoid risk-taking behavior and increase health-promoting behaviors.

Relatedly, Henderson and colleagues (2013) found that meaning in life was more strongly associated with eudaimonic activity than hedonic activity in adults and proposed a reciprocal relationship that leads to elevating experience. That is, enhanced meaning in one's life may lead to experiencing activities in a more eudaimonic fashion and eudaimonic activity can also enhance meaning. Although not directly connected to health or health behaviors, this dynamic relationship would potentially make the health behavior experience more positive and sustainable. As Steger and associates (2015, p. 594) write, "It seems unrealistic to expect people to labor to adopt healthy lifestyles if they cannot link such efforts to what matters to them."

A review of Self-Determination Theory applied to health contexts found that autonomy, a concept connected to eudaimonia, and autonomy-supportive environments were essential predictors of healthy behaviors (Ng et al., 2012). These authors suggest that autonomy and other intrinsic aspirations may be crucial for long-term maintenance of health behaviors. Autonomy is part of Ryff's (2013) Psychological Well-Being (PWB) model and one of three intrinsic, psychological needs in SDT. Ryan and colleagues (2008, p. 158) claim that "eudaimonia is necessarily rooted in human autonomy." A eudaimonic way of living would more likely encourage autonomy, leading to the internalization of a healthy lifestyle, which Williams and Niemiec (2012) suggest is crucial for the maintenance of behavior change.

In shifting the focus to young people, other aspects of well-being have also been linked to various health behaviors. Carvajal (2012) examined the predictive utility of adolescents' global positive expectancies (GPE), operationalized as dispositional optimism and hope, relating to their health-risk and health-enhancing behaviors. Higher initial levels of GPE predicted healthier food choices and greater physical activity over time. Importantly, GPE did decrease over time suggesting the plasticity and changeability of these global expectancies in young people. Similarly, Hoyt, Chase-Lansdale, McDade, and Adam (2012) found that adolescents who perceived positive well-being (happiness, enjoyment of life, and hopefulness about the future) had a more positive health behavior profile over time. And results from McDade et al. (2011) demonstrate that adolescents who rated their chances to attend college more highly exercised more in early adulthood. These findings suggest that perceived life choices, as reflected in positive expectancies for the future, are motivational and can influence health behavior as one gets older.

In sum, various constructs of well-being—positive emotions, meaning and purpose, autonomy, positive expectancies and hopefulness—conceptually aligned with eudaimonia and hedonia are associated with or influence health outcomes and behaviors for both youth and adults. The next section examines more specifically the eudaimonia/hedonia-health connection.

23.2.2 Eudaimonia/Hedonia and Health Outcomes

Ryff and Singer (1998) were one of the first to write about the possible connection between eudaimonia and healthy living. They suggested that health-promoting behaviors may be more likely to be adopted and maintained by those who demonstrate high levels of life meaning and purpose:

> Taking good care of yourself presupposes that your life is worth taking care of… It is thus attention to the broader context of people's lives and their encounters with core life goods that may illuminate underlying reasons for practicing, or failing to practice, positive health behaviors. (p. 22)

Ryff's studies and others have demonstrated a strong connection between eudaimonia and health (see Ryff, 2013). For example, in a study of older women Ryff, Singer, and Love (2004) found that those with higher levels of eudaimonic well-being—measured with the six dimensions of well-being—had lower levels of daily salivary cortisol, pro-inflammatory cytokines, cardiovascular risk, and longer duration REM sleep. All of these factors are positively linked to long-term physical health. Purpose in life and personal growth were the two major eudaimonic factors involved with this connection, whereas hedonic well-being—measured as positive affect—was minimally related to health markers. Relatedly, in a series of longitudinal studies over several years (Boyle, Barnes, Buchman, & Bennett, 2009; Boyle, Buchman, & Bennett, 2010; Boyle, Buchman, Barnes, & Bennett, 2010), those adults with high purpose in life were less likely to develop disabilities and Alzheimer's disease and lived longer than those with lower levels of life purpose.

Another study with older women participating in the long-term Women's Health Initiative found an association between eudaimonic well-being and healthy survival (Zaslavsky et al., 2014). Those women who scored low on personal growth and purpose in life were more likely to have prevalent mobility disability and disease or incident of death before the age of 85 years. Hence, experiencing meaning, purpose, and direction in life along with putting into action one's personal talents have significant health consequences. Zaslavsky and colleagues suggest that the mechanisms mediating this relationship could be physiological, immunological, and behavioral. Interestingly, a qualitative study examining the role of eudaimonia in older adults' community arts participation (e.g, painting, creative writing, dance/movement) found through interviews that the participants were eager to engage in activities that would provide a sense of life purpose (Swindells et al., 2013). Many of the older adults described a process of losing their life purpose and needing activities to take their minds off of physical and mental pain.

Complementing the eudaimonia-longevity link, a number of studies and reviews support a hedonia-longevity relationship. In an extensive meta-analytic review of longitudinal studies, Lyubormisky, King, & Diener (2005) conclude that people who experience ample positive emotions are less likely to die of certain causes. In a review of prospective studies, Cohen and Pressman (2005) also found an association between trait positive affect and lower morbidity. Results from Steptoe and Wardle (2011) demonstrated that enjoyment of life predicted survival over a 7-year period and more recent work (Steptoe, Oliveira, Kemakakos, & Zaninotto, 2014) found that less positive affective well-being predicted declining physical function, which predicts mortality (Studenski et al., 2011). Lastly, compelling data from a co-twin control study revealed that greater positive affect and life satisfaction predicted increased longevity independent of shared genes and common environment (Sadler, Miller, Christensen, & McGue, 2011).

Taking a deeper look into the biological implications of eudaimonia and hedonia, Fredrickson and colleagues (2013) explored a possible connection with functional genomics. These authors examined whether eudaimonia or hedonia is related to gene expression involved in the body's inflammatory response, which could have implications for long-term health. Measuring both hedonia (e.g., "how often did you feel happy?") and eudaimonia (e.g., "your life has a sense of meaning or direction"), the findings were interpreted to suggest that those adults who were high in eudaimonia had decreased expression of pro-inflammatory genes and reduced expression of genes involved in antibody synthesis, both indicators of positive, molecular health. This finding was picked up by various media sources (e.g., Smith, 2013) as break-through research connecting mind-body mechanisms for long-term health. However, caution is warranted as Coyne (2013) and Brown, MacDonald, Samanta, Friedman, and Coyne (2014) have been critical of both the study's theoretical and methodological approaches, which they feel undermine the study's findings. One of the issues relates to a recurring theme of this chapter: the difficulty of differentiating eudaimonia from hedonia, both conceptually and via self-report measures. Their criticism cuts to the heart of the matter: what is eudaimonia and, subsequently, how should it be measured? Brown and colleagues (2014, p. 12706) state, "This conceptual limitation leads us to question whether there is a scientifically adequate definition and taxonomy of well-being on which to do research in the first place." This is an overly harsh statement on the state of positive well-being research, but as Nussbaum advocated, should definitely give one pause. This academic tit for tat certainly shouldn't stop the burgeoning research on eudaimonic/hedonic well-being but perhaps it will encourage a philosophical sorting things out as to who and what is the Happy Warrior (Nussbauam, 2008). Of course, Nussbaum (2011) herself has added to the conceptual chaos of well-being with her ten central capabilities, under which are subsumed such things as human emotions, affiliation, and physical health. Does such a broad framework add clarification, or create more confusion, to the research and practice focused on the well-being-health relationship?

Boehm and Kubzansky (2012) reviewed studies that examined positive psychological well-being (PPWB) and cardiovascular health (CVD). These authors utilized a eudaimonic/hedonic framework, but similar to the approach of this section, included these two primary PPWB variables within a broad category, which included constructs such as optimism and vitality that may "contain elements of both eudaimonic and hedonic well-being, but are not pure measures of either" (p. 656). Their model capturing this relationship focuses on the restorative processes of PPWB experiences as they relate to health behaviors, biological function, and disease outcomes. Relating to disease outcomes, their review reports that PPWB reduces risk of CVD in healthy populations and slows progression in patient populations, with optimism and vitality providing the strongest protection. Related to biological functioning, findings are less clear with eudaimonia, hedonia, and optimism related to inflammatory markers, autonomic nervous system regulation, and cardiovascular function. Boehm and Kubzansky (2012, p. 680) also suggest that such work has been limited and that "clearly distinguishing between PPWB constructs may provide greater understanding of what aspects are particularly relevant for cardiovascular health," which has been a major theme of this section.

23.2.3 Eudaimonia/Hedonia and Health Behaviors

Another aspect of the well-being-health connection is the potential relationship between positive psychological states and health-promoting behaviors, such as sleep, eating, and physical activity, and risk-behaviors, such as excessive alcohol consumption and smoking. Health behaviors play a crucial role in both short- and long-term physical health (Brady et al., 2013), but many behaviors have been relatively impervious to change for the vast majority of the population (e.g., Reeves & Rafftery, 2005). As suggested earlier, it is highly likely that the relationship between well-being and health behaviors is dynamic and reciprocal. In their thorough review, Boehm and Kubzansky (2012) found eudaimonia (e.g., optimism) and hedonia associated with healthier behaviors. However, they do point out that (1) few studies have examined this relationship as per CVD, and (2) the well-being-health behavior relationship is far less clear than when examining health status and disease outcome variables.

Sleep and well-being is one example of the likelihood of a reciprocal relationship. The results of a longitudinal study (Karlson, Gallagher, Olson, & Hamilton, 2013) showed that insomnia symptoms, even 10 years apart, negatively impacted both subjective well-being (i.e., affect) and eudaimonic well-being (i.e., mastery, self-acceptance). Disturbed sleep results in a lower quality of life experience. But do positive psychological states enhance sleep quality? Results from one longitudinal study (Phelan, Love, Ryff, Brown, & Heidrich, 2010) and two cross-sectional studies (Ryff, Singer, & Love, 2004; Steptoe, O'Donnell, Marmot, & Wardle, 2008) suggest a positive relationship. Using Ryff's 6-dimensional PWB model, these studies found higher eudaimonic well-being associated with enhanced sleep quality. Positive affect was also a well-being factor associated with sleep quality in the Steptoe and colleagues' investigation. These kinds of findings call for more dynamic, complex investigations that include multiple data points so that temporal links between eudaimonia/hedonia and health behaviors can be more clearly delineated (Steptoe et al., 2008).

A dynamic, reciprocal relationship likely exists for most health-promoting or health-risk behaviors in relation to eudaimonia/hedonia (Boehm, Vie, & Kubzansky, 2012). However, the relationship has predominantly been studied with health behavior as the starting point. This is not surprising considering the dominance of the biomedical model of health, where meaning and purpose of the experience are irrelevant. Within a prevention model, health behaviors have been considered lifestyle-related risk factors for chronic degenerative disease and, thus, the primary research orientation has been to study the physical health outcomes of these behaviors. It's only recently, with the influx of positive psychology and positive youth development (PYD) models, that mental health or psychological well-being has been considered important as both an antecedent and consequence of health behaviors (see Boehm & Kubzansky, 2012; Ng et al., 2012; Schwartz, Pantin, Coatsworth, & Szapocznik, 2007). In short, the primary emphasis has been to examine well-being as an outcome or dependent variable. This is particularly true with studies that have examined the relationship between exercise or physical activity and positive well-being.

For years, the primary call from health professionals and kinesiology researchers has been for people to exercise and much time and effort has been spent on creating a prescriptive approach to physical activity based on guidelines continually revised and updated by expert-based organizations, such as the Centers for Disease Control and American College of Sports Medicine (e.g., Pate et al., 1995). Although these guidelines for physical activity have changed over the years (see Pate, 2012), the primary focus is on how much is enough (i.e., frequency, intensity, duration) for reducing risk of chronic degenerative disease. And the assumption is—no matter the recommendation—that people need to be pushed to adhere to an exercise regimen so they reach target thresholds of intensity (Ekkekakis, 2009). This mindset of experts in charge and that experts know what is best for people is firmly entrenched within the health and fitness professions (Kimiecik & Lawson, 1996), and trickles down to children and adolescents with similar guidelines for physical activity for these age groups as well (Sallis & Patrick, 1994; U.S. Department of Health and Human Services, 2008). But according to research on adults reviewed by Ekkekakis (p. 882) the prescription-based approach is unnecessary:

> It appears that, when most adults are allowed to self-select their exercise intensity (assuming the activity is framed as 'exercise'), they choose a level within the range considered safe and effective for the development and maintenance of cardiorespiratory fitness.

Even when positive well-being has been considered relevant, it's been as a potential benefit of physical activity participation, asking the question, "If you regularly move your body, does that experience positively impact your mental health?" Reviews show generally that it does (e.g., Biddle & Asare, 2011). Much of the research has focused on physical activity's impact on hedonic or subjective well-being (e.g., life satisfaction, positive affect). The assumption is that participation in regular physical activity will enhance mood or decrease stress and anxiety, and, typically, the literature supports these assumptions across the lifespan (Ekkekakis & Backhouse, 2009). It has also been shown that acute physical activity has the most significant effect on mood for adult women with the lowest levels of positive affect before exercising (Gauvin, Rejeski, & Norris, 1996). The worse you feel before exercise the better you feel afterwards. And some studies have found that even short, brisk walks of 10–15 min can elevate one's affective state (Ekkekakis, Hall, Van Landuyt, & Petruzzello, 2000). These findings support the general consensus in the well-being literature that enhanced hedonic well-being is an immediate, short-term outcome of physical activity participation (Huta & Ryan, 2010; Lyubomirsky, Sheldon, & Schkade, 2005).

Some recent work has begun to examine the role of eudaimonia within physical activity contexts. In general, results of these studies indicate that the *quality* of the physical activity experience is related to well-being outcomes. This is significant because generally in health and fitness the physical activity experience has been overshadowed by the admonition of *just do it*. Results of a study by Ferguson, Kowalski, Mack, Wilson, & Crockers (2012) indicate that participation in health-enhancing physical activity (HEPA) in and of itself was unrelated to eudaimonic well-being in young women. However, when participants experienced HEPA in both eudaimonic and hedonic ways (via motives) resultant eudaimonic well-being was enhanced, suggesting that the quality of the HEPA experience is more relevant to eudaimonic well-being than is the quantity (frequency/duration). When it comes to eudaimonic well-being it may not be how much physical activity you do but how you do it and experience it that are the critical factors. In a related study with young adults, Sylvester, Mack, Busseri, Wilson, and Beauchamp (2012) found that perceived HEPA effort was a consistent predictor of positive affect, satisfaction, and personal expressiveness, whereas frequency and duration were unrelated to either hedonic or eudaimonic well-being. Thus, the quality, not the quantity, of HEPA is significantly related to positive well-being. Extending this work to multiple health behaviors, Pressman and colleagues (2009) found that individuals who had high quality (i.e., enjoyable) of experience across myriad leisure activities had better psychological and physical functioning.

Studies are also beginning to examine the psychological mechanisms involved in the HEPA-eudaimonic/hedonic well-being relationship. Sylvester and colleagues (2012) found that perceptions of autonomy mediated the impact of HEPA on hedonic well-being, whereas an experience of relatedness mediated the link with personal expressiveness. Mack et al. (2011) examined similar possibilities in individuals living with osteopenia. Results suggest that perceptions of competence and autonomy linked engagement in leisure-time physical activity with both hedonic and eudaimonic motives for well-being. These findings support Ryan and colleagues' (2008) contention that self-determination, exemplified by the fulfillment of the three universal psychological needs, plays a significant role in how and if physical activity participation relates to positive well-being. When physical activity is experienced as intrinsic (high quality), well-being outcomes, such as positive affect, feelings of personal growth, and personal expressiveness, will result. It is difficult to tease out the roles of and relationship between hedonic well-being and eudaimonic well-being in physical activity contexts, but both seem relevant to this health behavior. However, results of a study by Lee, Sirgy, Yu, and Chalamon (2015) found that personal expressiveness associated with college students' physical activity had a direct and positive effect on hedonic well-being. This finding supports the conclusions of Henderson and colleagues (2013, p. 334): "…eudaimonic activities are more likely to be simultaneously experienced as hedonic. Therefore, if aiming to increase both hedonia and eudaimonia in life, targeting eudaimonic activity may be more effective in this regard." Future work within health behavior change should investigate this possibility.

When it comes to health-promoting behavior, such as exercise, it seems likely that both pleasure and meaning are necessary for adopting and maintaining (Segar & Richardson, 2014). Very little work has examined the role of positive well-being in this process and is probably the next exciting research venue to explore (Boehm & Kubzansky, 2012). From a hedonic perspective, exercise needs to be experienced as pleasant or most people will not continue, making all the wonderful physiological and psychological benefits moot (Ekkekakis, 2013). When the exercise experience is hedonic, positive affect will result. Fredrickson (2003) has demonstrated the value of positive emotions for many life endeavors as they can help individuals build personal resources, such as creative thinking, and make them more resilient and optimistic. Thus, perhaps an hedonic exercise experience can enhance motivation and the person's ability to continue to participate. This becomes a crucial point. Is positive affect alone enough for individuals to continue to be attracted to and participate in physical activity? Fredrickson (2001) also suggested that positive meaning in one's experiences can enhance positive emotions. This may be the role that eudaimonia plays in sustaining health behaviors. Huta and Ryan (2010) propose that eudaimonia is more connected to engagement in longer term actions and experiences. And Steger, Kashdan, and Oishi (2008) found that today's eudaimonic activities have a sustained positive association with the next day's well-being. They suggest that eudaimonic activities have deeper and more meaningful effects than hedonic behaviors and that pleasure-seeking may be a poor long-term strategy for experiencing enduring well-being.

Thus, when an individual approaches a health behavior, such as exercise, in a way that connects to a deeper personal meaning (eudaimonia) he/she is likely to experience it as a eudaimonic activity. As results from studies reviewed here show, along with the fulfillment of intrinsic needs, this internal process enhances positive well-being. As Henderson and colleagues (2013, p. 333) state, "Having a sense of meaning may therefore be a necessary prerequisite for eudaimonic activity to ensue." This eudaimonic approach to and experience with a behavior would also likely lead to a more enjoyable, pleasurable physical activity experience as reflected in positive affect. This makes sense because if people are always guided by their feelings, they are at the mercy of whether they are feeling good or bad at any one moment. For example, when people are experiencing negative affect they may be attracted to health-risk behaviors, such as consuming high-fat foods (Salovey, Rothman, Detweiler, & Steward, 2000) as a temporary escape or to "feel" better (Baumeister, 1991). These are very challenging health moments (e.g., "should I exercise right now?") as recent research suggests that the affective system drives decisions whose outcomes and targets are closer to the present (Chang & Pham, 2013). However, a strong eudaimonic identity (Waterman & Schwartz, 2013) may help individuals avoid these emotional landmines by swaying the decision making to a process of ideas, thoughts, and feelings about the movement experience connected to eudaimonic self-expression, competence, or achieving self-concordant goals (Sheldon & Elliot, 1999; Sheldon, Chap. 36, this volume). Of course, future research will need to sort out the roles of both eudaimonia and hedonia pertaining to health-promoting behavior such as physical activity. Because there is conceptual and empirical overlap between these two aspects of experience (Huta, 2013; Waterman, 1993), it is likely that a synergistic relationship exists. Henderson and Knight (2012, p. 216) write: "it is likely that too much hedonia or eudaimonia will be detrimental to well-being, and that optimal experiences of well-being will be associated with striking a balance between the two." Similarly, Henderson and colleagues (p. 334) state: "behaving hedonically and eudaimonically is associated with various well-being benefits." Only future research can help decipher the balance and synergy between hedonia and eudaimonia and their influence on health behaviors.

The final point of discussion relates to the typical research approach undertaken when studying the adoption and maintenance of health behaviors. The vast majority of this work has focused on the social cognitive determinants specifically connected to the health behavior of interest. For example, researchers study people's attitudes toward physical activity or food consumption. They might also assess individuals' self-efficacy for exercising or whether they are intrinsically or extrinsically motivated to eat healthy foods (Dishman, Heath, & Lee, 2013). These approaches would be labeled contextual or situational whereby the independent variables are tied directly to the behavior of interest. Even research that has adopted a positive well-being approach is primarily contextual/situational. For example, the Lee, Sirgy, Yu, and Chalamon (2015) study assessed self-expressiveness and hedonic enjoyment associated with the exercise experience itself. A primary assumption guiding this work is that motivation or well-being assessed at the contextual or situational level will better predict functioning or behavior in a specific context (Vallerand & Lalande, 2011; Vallerand, Chap. 13, this volume). To understand healthy eating, for example, one must assess motivation or well-being relating to that behavior. This approach certainly has merit. The challenge, however, is that contextual/situational measures of intrapersonal processes must be developed for every behavior, which seems inefficient and unwieldy. Within research studying adolescent health behavior, this approach has been criticized. Flay (2002) has suggested that health-risk behavior change approaches for adolescents based on this proximal model of targeting each specific behavior have been less effective than broad, comprehensive PYD-based programs. Hence, research or practice that begins to include global, positive intrapersonal processes, such as eudaimonic well-being, and their relation to adolescent health-promoting behavior could contribute to the development of more sustainable, comprehensive, multimodal PYD experiences for adolescents and their communities.

Examining the impact of eudaimonic well-being assessed at the global or higher-order level and its impact on varying health behaviors could be a fruitful research endeavor. Ryan and colleagues (2008) and Huta (2013) suggest that eudaimonic living—seeking to find and use the best in oneself—focuses individuals on what is intrinsically worthwhile to human beings, which would lead to enhanced vitality and self-determination, reflected through intrinsic motivation. These broad, internal characteristics—eudaimonic well-being, subjective vitality, and intrinsic motivation—may also be involved in the process of directing people into adopting and sustaining health-promoting behavioral routines (Kimiecik, 2011). Some of this kind of research has been conducted within the framework of PYD and health behaviors of adolescents. An example of a top-down approach is the study by Hoyt and colleagues (2012) mentioned earlier. In this study, positive well-being was prospectively measured by asking adolescents a number of questions about whether they have good qualities; have a lot to be proud of; happiness; hopefulness about the future, and so forth. The researchers then examined the effects of this positive well-being composite over time on specific health-risk and health-promoting behavior. Another study found that both adolescent boys and girls with a profile high in generalized autonomy, competence, and relatedness were more physically active and consumed healthier foods than boys and girls who scored low on these global, intrapersonal processes (Kimiecik & Horn, 2016). And results from Schwartz and colleagues (2011) indicate that emerging adults who were high in eudaimonic well-being—those who perceived themselves as doing well in life with a clear sense of meaning and purpose—were least likely to engage in health-risk behaviors, such as drug use.

In sum, the results of studies examining the link between positive well-being and health/risk behaviors suggest a promising path. However, the dynamic, reciprocal nature of the relationship makes studying these processes very complex. Much of the research has focused on how health behaviors may impact eudaimonic or hedonic well-being, but studies are also beginning to examine the front-end influence of positive well-being on healthy living. Teasing out the nature of the interactive relationship among eudaimonia, hedonia, and health behavior would make a significant contribution to this literature. Lastly, examining positive well-being's role in health behavior change from various levels of analysis—situational, contextual, and global—would also be a useful undertaking.

23.3 Issues and Interventions

This selective review suggests that positive well-being is associated with myriad aspects of health. This section first highlights the key issues and then discusses some future directions relating to interventions targeting the eudaimonia-health relationship.

23.3.1 Issues

The first issue pertains to the conceptual/definitional confusion surrounding both health and eudaimonia. These are complex constructs and multiple definitions and conceptualizations are to be expected. But when researchers are attempting to tease out the roles of and relationships among eudaimonia, hedonia, and human health, different studies using different conceptualizations and measurements make it very challenging to compare and decipher the results across studies. Perhaps as this area of research matures this issue will sort itself out.

Second, however positive well-being and health are defined and measured, there seems to be a moderate relationship, although many of the studies are cross-sectional limiting strong conclusions. Despite this design limitation, subjective and hedonic well-being (e.g., happiness, positive affect) are either associated with, or influence, the disease and illness aspects of health. Similarly, eudaimonic-related constructs, such as meaning and optimism, have been found to be associated with or influence health status. In some studies, measures of eudaimonia, such as personal growth and purpose in life, have been significantly linked to biological and immunological health-protective processes, whereas hedonia has not. The dynamic, reciprocal interactions between eudaimonia and hedonia are clearly evident when examining positive well-being and health behaviors, such as sleep, physical activity, and food consumption.

Third, just what is the role of eudaimonia and hedonia in the health process, especially relating to the motivation for and participation in varying health behaviors? My own biases and experiences (as well as the literature) have led me to view eudaimonia as the cornerstone of a healthy living process. A higher-order, global sense or feel of interest, engagement, and personal expressiveness (a eudaimonic way of being) may be at the core for both initiating and maintaining healthy living. When one has this spark, daimon, central inner force, or self-identified core passion (Coatsworth & Sharp, 2013; Norton, 1976; Waterman, 2013), health behaviors are likely to become more naturally connected to the eudaimonic self. And when eudaimonic individuals begin to move their bodies or start eating a healthier diet, these behaviors will be experienced as eudaimonic activities, making them easier to maintain over time—the health behavior experience will be more connected to the self. Literature (some reviewed earlier) supports this possibility as intrinsic motivation and flow have been found to be subjective experience mediators of health behaviors and well-being outcomes. For instance, a study found that flow states in teenagers were associated with higher satisfaction with life, hedonic balance, and psychological well-being (Bassi, Steca, Monzani, Greco, & Delle Fave, 2014). In addition, when health behaviors, such as physical activity or food consumption, are perceived to satisfy intrinsic needs (i.e., autonomy, competence, and relatedness), the quality of the experience is heightened. This internalization process results in greater hedonic and edudaimonic well-being, and likely enhances motivation to maintain these health behaviors—the positive cycle of healthy living continues via a very positive feedback loop. Thus, this eudaimonic way of being, which may also include aspects of what Csikszentmihalyi (1990) has labeled an autotelic personality or meta flow skills (Csikszentmihalyi & Nakamura, 1989) may predispose individuals to healthier living.

Fourth, a focus on eudaimonia as the spark for healthy living does not discount the relevance of hedonia. As reviewed here and elsewhere (e.g., Boehm & Kubzansky, 2012; Vazquez et al., 2009), positive affective states have a moderate association with healthy living as they can influence motivation to partake in varying health behaviors (front end) as well as be positively impacted by health behavior participation (back end). If hedonic well-being is related to more immediate circumstances as some well-being theorists suggest, then we need to pay closer attention to its role in the health behavior experience. If a health behavior experience produces negative feelings or is neutral with respect to emotions, these experiences could override the eudaimonic influence. For example, if an individual starts to eat more fruits and vegetables as a means to gain energy to perform better at work (eudaimonia) and the feelings are negative, the behavior may be discontinued as the behavioral decision may be influenced by the immediate, affective experience (Chang & Pham, 2013). On the positive side, simple positive affective messages can motivate participation in health behaviors, such as physical activity (Conner, Rhodes, Morris, McEachan, & Lawton, 2011; Gellert, Ziegelmann, & Schwarzer, 2012).

To optimize the health behavior-well-being connection, it is likely that both eudaimonia *and* hedonia need to be involved in the behavior change process, and future research should begin to more closely examine the interactional possibilities. Overemphasis on hedonic experiences may not motivate sustainable change without any connection to deeper meaning (Steger et al., 2015), and an unbalanced emphasis on eudaimonia may discount the pleasurable/enjoyable aspects of the experience itself (e.g., purpose without pleasure). This calls for the balanced approach where both eudaimonia and hedonia are actively integrated into a health behavior change process, leading to sustainable change and optimal well-being. In fact, Henderson and Knight (2012) have suggested that flourishing may be the dynamic balance between and interaction of purpose and pleasure. And Seligman's (2011) PERMA model suggests that flourishing includes both positive emotions and eudaimonic-like concepts, such as engagement and meaning. Related to flourishing, Su, Tay, and Diener (2014, p. 256) have developed a dispositional measure of what they call thriving that "denotes the state of positive functioning at its fullest range," and incorporates both eudaimonic ("my life has a clear sense of purpose") and hedonic ("I feel happy most of the time") measures. Studies indicate that both flourishing and thriving are connected to health outcomes. For example, Keyes (2007) found that people who flourish (a combination of eudaimonic and hedonic well-being) had the least incidence of chronic physical conditions, such as high blood pressure, arthritis, and back problems. Results from Su and colleagues indicated that thriving predicted physical health, health behaviors, and health-related quality of life. Future research will need to conceptually consider the similarities and differences among eudaimonia, flourishing, and thriving, and further explore the influence of a eudaimonic-hedonic balance on health behavior change.

23.3.2 Eudaimonic Interventions and Health Behavior Change

Evidence indicates that despite all of the positive research linking positive well-being to health, few people are flourishing. Data from Keyes (2007) shows that only 17% of the U.S. adult population is categorized as flourishing, which is why it is not too surprising that so many people struggle with sustaining health behavior change. If a relatively strong well-being-health behavior-well-being connection exists and people aren't flourishing, the chances of long-term success are minimal. This leads to a discussion of interventions.

Space does not allow for an in-depth philosophical discussion of well-being intervention (see Kimiecik, 2011), but two aspects will be addressed here: (1) positive well-being interventions, and (2) positive well-being interventions connected to health behavior change. Much of the recent work on positive well-being has focused on utilizing positive activity intervention

(PAI) to enhance positive emotions, thoughts, and behaviors (see Layous & Lyubomirsky, 2014). These activities range from performing random acts of kindness to counting your blessings to positive reflection. In general, results suggest that PAIs—if practiced regularly—may trigger upward spirals of positive emotions, thoughts, and behaviors, perhaps via the satisfaction of the three basic psychological needs of autonomy, competence, and relatedness. Much of the focus of this PAI work has been on enhancing subjective or hedonic well-being, which seems to be moderately effective, although the key words are *if practiced regularly*. Intentionality and effort are required for maintenance of these happiness-enhancing techniques (Layous & Lyubomirsky, 2014).

The danger, of course, is that in the context of attempting to enhance people's happiness and/or hedonic experiences, the agentic feel of one's eudaimonia may be relegated to the back seat as it has been within the biomedical approach to health enhancement. Short-term hedonic enhancement at the expense of long-term eudaimonia may not lead to sustainable flourishing. It is possible that if people give themselves up to the techniques and the know how of hedonia that they will surrender much of their agentic freedom and choice to the experts offering the PAI (Sugarman, 2007), moving them further away from creating and internalizing a eudaimonic way of being—their true nature. The PAI-hedonic-enhancement approach is eerily similar to health behavior change approaches immersed in the biomedical/prevention paradigm—in both cases, experts are prescribing what should be done with the expectation that the prescribee need only adhere to the regimen offered to reap the benefits. The result could be the same—people knowing what they should do but little long-term action taking place, resulting in feelings of inadequacy, guilt, and shame.

A eudaimonic way of living is not about technique, know how, or strategy. To discover core passions or a central inner force or to feel personally expressive and vital requires some freedom, autonomy, and choice (Williams & Niemiec, 2012). It seems unlikely that PAIs will lead to this transformative, eudaimonic self. Nettle (2006, p. 20) points out that eudaimonia is a "different entity or experience from typical perspectives of happiness…everyone's potential is different." Prescribing hedonia could squelch or cloak eudaimonic experiences, which some have suggested is the driving force to optimal well-being (Coatsworth & Sharp, 2013; Deci & Ryan, 2008; Steger et al., 2015; Vittersø & Søholt, 2011; Waterman & Schwartz, 2013). To help people experience their own, unique eudaimonia, we need to take to heart what Norton (1976, p. 222) writes: "If we are to recognize eudaimonia in others, we must avoid substituting our own feelings with respect to where they are and what they are doing."

This potential conflict between hedonic-enhancing activities and a eudaimonic way of being could have implications for positive well-being enhancement as a mechanism for health behavior change. For example, many of the positive psychological well-being enhancement strategies (e.g., letters of gratitude, kindness) to catalyze health behavior change advocated by Boehm and colleagues (2012) are similar to the aforementioned PAIs. Caution is warranted with mindfulness as well, as results from several studies indicate an increase in primarily positive emotions (hedonia) (Boehm & Kubzansky, 2012). Also, a systematic review and meta-analysis of meditation programs found no effect or insufficient evidence for changing positive mood (Goyal et al., 2014). In general, a mindfulness-based approach to health behavior change targets a heightened awareness between thought and emotion. Will this process impact or elevate eudaimonia? Are targeting thoughts and feelings the path to enlightenment and change? Coates (2012) points out that the idea of changing behavior by changing our thinking and emotions is grounded in a rational model of Cartesian philosophy and not at all how people behave or change. When it comes to health behavior change, Oz (2011 p. 432) states "people do not change their minds based on what they know, they change based on what they feel."

There has been a spattering of eudaimonic-based interventions designed to enhance positive well-being. In clinical environments, well-being therapy, framed within Ryff's multidimensional model of psychological well-being, has been used effectively as a form of treatment with patients with affective disorders or depression (Fava & Ruini, 2003). For example, Moeenizadeh and Salagame (2010) found well-being therapy more effective than cognitive behavioral therapy in improving psychological well-being in patients with symptoms of depression. The well-being therapy intervention process is based on the six dimensions of Ryff's positive well-being model with 8–12 sessions and includes self-observation, structured diaries, and interaction between patients and therapists.

Ruini and colleagues (2009) adapted the well-being therapy implemented in clinical settings to a non-clinical, school environment focusing on adolescents. Results from this brief intervention of six weekly sessions indicated that personal growth and autonomy were positively impacted for the youth in the well-being group when compared to a placebo-control group. In addition, the well-being group also experienced greater decreased distress, and these changes persisted at a 6-month followup. In another study, a self-discovery process grounded in flow, personal expressiveness, and self-actualization was utilized with emerging adults over an 8-week period (Schwartz, Kurtines, & Montgomery, 2005). Grounded in Friere's (1973) transformative pedagogy where facilitator and participant learn together, individuals were encouraged to identify their unique potentials and to formulate goals and ideals corresponding to those potentials. Results, although modest, showed an increase in personal expressiveness via the self-discovery process.

These eudaiomic-based interventions show promise for enhancing positive well-being. More research needs to compare and contrast the long-term positive well-being effects of interventions grounded in both the simple PAI approach (Lyubomirsky & Layous, 2013) and the eudaimonic-enhancement models (e.g., well-being therapy). Few of the interventions reviewed here examined how and if enhancing eudaimonia may increase the likelihood that individuals engage in healthy behaviors (as proposed by Boehm et al., 2012; Kimiecik, 2011). However, an interesting intervention study by Falk and colleagues (2015) found that individuals who practiced a self-affirmation process connecting to and expressing personal values and life purpose were more open to health-related physical activity messages and increased physical activity 1 month following the intervention.

Also, Lewis, Kimiecik, Horn, Zullig, and Ward (2014) implemented an intervention where university employees participated in the Well-Being Way (WBW), an 8-week eudaimonic-enhancement experience specifically designed to help participants explore and experience how they want to feel and make more natural connections to high quality living. The WBW attempts to emphasize each individual's unique gifts (eudaimonia) with ample opportunities for sharing, interactive activities, dialogue, discussion, and reflection. The results indicate that participation in the WBW experience, as compared to a control group, was strongly linked to increased subjective vitality. In addition, before the WBW experience participants averaged 6200 steps "typical of daily activity excluding volitional sports/exercise and might be considered 'low active'" (see Tudor-Locke & Bassett, 2004, p. 6). Following immersion in the WBW process, participants significantly increased their steps to an average of nearly 7800, which placed them in a new average daily step category that is indicative of, "some volitional activities and might be considered 'somewhat active'" (Tudor-Locke & Bassett, 2004, p. 6).

Lastly, Kimiecik (2010) describes an intervention attempt with high school freshman over a 2-year period emphasizing the global, intrapersonal processes of eudaimonic well-being and self-determination as the conceptual underpinnings of the program experience. Trained college mentors partnered with teachers and worked within freshman classrooms once a week for 12 weeks to deliver a well-being curriculum comprised of playful activities designed to foster personal expressiveness, relatedness, autonomy, competence, and subjective vitality. Students completed self-reported pre and post measures of eating behavior and physical activity. The only focus on these health behaviors was if they were discussed during the group activities or debriefing following each experience. Data analyses will determine if this eudaimonic-enhancement process impacted positive well-being and if it played a role in changing students' health-promoting behaviors.

23.4 Conclusion

To conclude, we are in the very beginning stages of an exciting time whereby the theory and practice of positive well-being is being studied in many different, creative ways. Although this research is infused with some conceptual and definitional confusion, the "third revolution" advocated by Breslow (2004) is well on its way. There is no doubt that both future eudaimonic- and hedonic-oriented research will begin to illuminate the nature of the connection between one's subjective experience and health, ultimately helping people transcend disease and move toward an *experience* of optimal health as a resource for everyday living.

References

Allen, D., Carlson, D., & Ham, C. (2007). Well-being: New paradigms of wellness—Inspiring positive health outcomes and renewing hope. *The Art of Health Promotion, 21*, 1–9.

Antonovsky, A. (1987). *Unraveling the mystery of health*. San Francisco: Jossey-Bass.

Antonovsky, A. (1996). The salutogenic model as a theory to guide health promotion. *Health Promotion International, 11*(1), 725–733.

Arloski, M. (2007). *Wellness coaching for lasting lifestyle change*. Duluth, MN: Whole Person Associates.

Baer, H., Hays, J., McClendon, N., McGoldrick, N., & Vespucci, R. (1998). The holistic health movement in the San Francisco bay area: Some preliminary observations. *Social Science in Medicine, 47*, 1495–1501.

Bassi, M., Steca, P., Monzani, D., Greco, A., & Delle Fave, A. (2014). Personality and optimal experience in adolescence: Implications for well-being and development. *Journal of Happiness Studies, 15*, 829–843.

Baumeister, R. F. (1991). *Escaping the self: Alcoholism, spirituality, masochism, and other flights from the burden of selfhood*. New York: Basic Books.

Biddle, S., & Asare, M. (2011). Physical activity and mental health in children and adolescents: A review of reviews. *British Journal of Sports Medicine, 45*, 886–895.

Blanck, H., Gillespie, C., Khan, L., Serdula, M., Solera, M., Mokdad, A., et al. (2007). Fruit and vegetable consumption among adults: United States, 2005. *Morbidity and Mortality Weekly Reports, 56*, 213–217.

Boehm, J., & Kubzansky, L. (2012). The heart's content: The association between positive psychological well-being and cardiovascular health. *Psychological Bulletin, 138*, 655–691.

Boehm, J., Vie, L., & Kubzansky, L. (2012). The promise of well-being interventions for improving health risk behaviors. *Current Cardiovascular Risk Reports, 6*, 511–519.

Boyle, P., Barnes, L., Buchman, A., & Bennett, D. (2009). Purpose in life is associated with mortality among community-dwelling older persons. *Psychosomatic Medicine, 71*(5), 574–579.

Boyle, P., Buchman, A., Barnes, L., & Bennett, D. (2010). Effect of a purpose in life on risk of incident Alzheimer disease and mild cognitive impairment in community-dwelling older persons. *Archives of General Psychiatry, 67*(3), 304–310.

Boyle, P., Buchman, A., & Bennett, D. (2010). Purpose in life is associated with a reduced risk of incident disability among community-dwelling older persons. *American Journal of Geriatric Psychiatry, 18*(12), 1093–1102.

Brady, T. J., Murphy, L., O'Colmain, B. J., Beauchesne, D., Daniels, B., Greenberg, M., … Chervin, D. (2013). A meta-analysis of health status, health behaviors, and health care utilization outcomes of the chronic disease self-management program. *Preventing Chronic Disease, 10*, doi: http://dx.doi.org/10.5888/pcd10.120112.

Breslow, L. (2004). Perspectives: The third revolution in health. *Annual Review of Public Health, 25*, xiii–xviii.

Brown, N., MacDonald, D., Samanta, M., Friedman, H., & Coyne, J. (2014). A critical reanalysis of the relationship between genomics and well-being. *Proceedings of the National Academy of Sciences, 111*, 12705–12709.

Buchanan, D. (2000). *An ethic for health promotion: Rethinking the sources of human well-being*. New York: Oxford University Press.

Cameron, D., Bertenshaw, E., & Sheeran, P. (2014). The impact of positive affect on health cognitions and behaviours: A meta-analysis of the experimental evidence. *Health Psychology Review*. http://dx.doi.org/10.1080/17437199.2014.923164.

Capra, F. (1982). *The turning point: Science, society, and the rising culture*. New York: Simon and Schuster.

Carvajal, S. (2012). Global positive expectancies in adolescence and health-related behaviours: Longitudinal

models and latent growth and cross-lagged effects. *Psychology and Health, 27*, 916–937.
Chang, H., & Pham, M. (2013). Affect as a decision-making system of the present. *Journal of Consumer Research, 40*(1), 42–63.
Chida, Y., & Steptoe, A. (2008). Positive psychological well-being and mortality: A quantitative review of prospective observational studies. *Psychosomatic Medicine, 70*, 741–756. doi:10.1097/PSY.0b013e31818105ba.
Coates, J. (2012). *The hour between dog and wolf: Risk taking, gut feelings and the biology of boom and bust*. New York: The Penguin Press.
Coatsworth, J., & Sharp, E. (2013). Discovering positive lives and futures: Adolescent eudaimonic expression through activity involvement. In A. Waterman (Ed.), *The best within us: Positive psychology perspectives on eudaimonia* (pp. 249–268). Washington, DC: The American Psychological Association.
Cohen, S., & Pressman, D. (2005). Positive affect and mental health. *Current Directions in Psychological Science, 15*, 122–125.
Conner, M., Rhodes, R. E., Morris, B., McEachan, R., & Lawton, R. (2011). Changing exercise through targeting affective or cognitive attitudes. *Psychology & Health, 26*(2), 133–149.
Coyne, J. (2013). Letter to editor: Highly correlated hedonic and eudaimonic wellbeing thwart genomic analysis. *Proceedings of the National Academies of Sciences, 110*(45), E4183.
Csikszentmihalyi, M. (1990). *Flow: The psychology of optimal experience*. New York: Harper Row.
Csikszentmihalyi, M., & Nakamura, J. (1989). The dynamics of intrinsic motivation: A study of adolescents. *Research on Motivation in Education, 3*, 45–71.
Danaei, G., Ding, E. L., Mozaffarian, D., Taylor, B., Rehm, J., Murray, C. J., et al. (2009). The preventable causes of death in the United States: Comparative risk assessment of dietary, lifestyle, and metabolic risk factors. *PLoS Medicine, 6*(4), e1000058.
Deci, E., & Ryan, R. (2008). Hedonia, eudaimonia, and well-being: An introduction. *Journal of Happiness Studies, 9*, 1–11.
Dishman, R., Heath, G., & Lee, I. (2013). Adopting and maintaining a physically active lifestyle. In R. Dishman, G. Heath, & I. Lee (Eds.), *Physical activity epidemiology* (pp. 503–553). Champaign, IL: Human Kinetics.
Edington, D. (2009). *Zero trends: Health as a serious economic strategy*. Ann Arbor, MI: Health Management Research Center.
Ekkekakis, P. (2009). Let them roam free? Physiological and psychological evidence for the potential of self-selected exercise intensity in public health. *Sports Medicine, 39*(10), 857–888.
Ekkekakis, P. (2013). Redrawing the model of the exercising human in exercise prescriptions: From headless manikin to a creature with feelings! In J. M. Rippe (Ed.), *Lifestyle medicine* (2nd ed., pp. 1421–1433). Boca Raton, FL: CRC Press.
Ekkekakis, P., & Backhouse, S. H. (2009). Exercise and psychological well-being. In R. Maughan (Ed.), *Olympic textbook of science in sport* (pp. 251–271). Hoboken, NJ: Wiley-Blackwell.
Ekkekakis, P., Hall, E. E., Van Landuyt, L. M., & Petruzzello, S. J. (2000). Walking in (affective) circles: Can short walks enhance affect? *Journal of Behavioral Medicine, 23*(3), 245–275.
Ezzati, M., Martin, H., Skjold, S., Vander Hoorn, S., & Murray, C. (2006). Trends in national and state-level obesity in the USA after correction for self-report bias: Analysis of health surveys. *Journal of the Royal Society of Medicine, 99*, 250–257.
Fahlberg, L. L., & Fahlberg, L. A. (1997). Wellness re-examined: A cross-cultural perspective. *American Journal of Health Studies, 13*, 8–17.
Fahlberg, L. L., Fahlberg, L. A., & Gates, W. (1992). Exercise and existence: Exercise behavior from an existential-phenomenological perspective. *The Sport Psychologist, 6*, 172–191.
Falk, E. B., O'Donnell, M. B., Cascio, C. N., Tinney, F., Kang, Y., Lieberman, M., … Strecher, V. (2015). Self-affirmation alters the brain's response to health messages and subsequent behavior change. *Proceedings of the National Academies of Sciences, 112*(7), 1977–1982.
Fava, G., & Ruini, C. (2003). Devleopment and characteristics of a well-being enhancing psychotherapeutic strategy: Well-being therapy. *Journal of Behavior Therapy and Experimental Psychiatry, 34*, 45–63.
Ferguson, L., Kowalski, K., Mack, D., Wilson, P., & Crocker, P. (2012). Women's health-enhancing physical activity and eudaimonic well-being. *Research Quarterly for Exercise and Sport, 83*, 451–463.
Flay, B. R. (2002). Positive youth development requires comprehensive health promotion programs. *American Journal of Health Behavior, 26*(6), 407–424.
Fredrickson, B. (2001). The role of positive emotions in positive psychology: The broaden-and-build theory of positive emotions. *American Psychologist, 56*, 218–226.
Fredrickson, B. L. (2003). The value of positive emotions. *American Scientist, 91*, 330–335.
Fredrickson, B. L., Cohn, M. A., Coffey, K. A., Pek, J., & Finkel, S. M. (2008). Open hearts build lives: Positive emotions, induced through loving-kindness meditation, build consequential personal resources. *Journal of Personality and Social Psychology, 95*, 1045–1062.
Fredrickson, B. L., Grewen, K. M., Coffey, K. A., Algoe, S. B., Firestine, A. M., Arevalo, J. M. G., et al. (2013). A functional genomic perspective on human well-being. *Proceedings of the National Academy of Sciences, 110*, 13684–13689.
Friere, P. (1973). *Education for critical consciousness*. New York: Seabury Press.
Gauvin, L., Rejeski, W. J., & Norris, J. L. (1996). A naturalistic study of the impact of acute physical activity

on feeling states and affect in women. *Health Psychology, 15*(5), 391–397.

Gellert, P., Ziegelmann, J. P., & Schwarzer, R. (2012). Affective and health-related outcome expectancies for physical activity in older adults. *Psychology & Health, 27*(7), 816–828.

Ghane, A., & Sweeny, K. (2013). Embodied health: A guiding perspective for research in health psychology. *Health Psychology Review, 7*, S159–S184.

Goyal, M., Singh, S., Sibinga, E., Gould, N., Rowland-Seymour, A., Sharma, R., … Haythornthwaite, J. (2014). Meditation programs for psychological stress and well-being: A systematic review and meta-analysis. Kah *JAMA Internal Medicine, 174*, 357–368.

Henderson, L. W., & Knight, T. (2012). Integrating the hedonic and eudaimonic perspectives to more comprehensively understand wellbeing and pathways to well-being. *International Journal of Wellbeing, 2*, 196–221.

Henderson, L. W., Knight, T., & Richardson, B. (2013). An exploration of the well-being benefits of hedonic and eudaimonic behavior. *The Journal of Positive Psychology, 8*, 322–336.

Howell, R., Kern, M., & Lyubormisky, S. (2007). Health benefits: Meta-analytically determining impact of well-being on objective health outcomes. *Health Psychology Review, 1*, 1–54.

Hoyt, L. T., Chase-Lansdale, P. L., McDade, T. W., & Adam, E. K. (2012). Positive youth, healthy adults: Does positive well-being in adolescence predict better perceived health and fewer risky health behaviors in young adulthood? *Journal of Adolescent Health, 50*(1), 66–73.

Huta, V. (2013). Pursuing eudaimonia versus hedonia: Distinctions, similarities, and relationships. In A. S. Waterman (Ed.), *The best within us: Positive psychology perspectives on eudaimonia* (pp. 139–158). Washington, DC: APA Books.

Huta, V., & Ryan, R. (2010). Pursuing pleasure or virtue: The differential and overlapping well-being benefits of hedonic and eudaimonic motives. *Journal of Happiness Studies, 11*, 735–762.

Huta, V., & Waterman, A. (2014). Eduaimonia and its distinction from hedonia: Developing a classification and terminology for understanding conceptual and operational definitions. *Journal of Happiness Studies, 15*, 1425–1456.

Institute of Medicine. (2006). *Sleep disorders and sleep deprivation: An unmet public health problem.* Washington, DC: National Academies Press.

Kahneman, D., Diener, E., & Schwarz, N. (1999). *Well-being: The foundations of hedonic psychology.* New York: Russell Sage.

Kaplan, R. (2000). Two pathways to prevention. *American Psychologist, 55*, 382–396.

Karlson, C., Gallagher, M., Olson, C., & Hamilton, N. (2013). Insomnia symptoms and well-being: Longitudinal follow-up. *Health Psychology, 32*, 311–319.

Kashdan, T., Biswas-Diener, R., & King, L. (2008). Reconsidering happiness: The cost of distinguishing between hedonics and eudaimonia. *The Journal of Positive Psychology, 3*, 219–233.

Keyes, C. (2007). Promoting and protecting mental health as flourishing: A complementary strategy for improving national mental health. *American Psychologist, 62*, 95–108.

Kimiecik, J. (2010). Reflecting on a well-being enhancement experience with ninth graders in a public school: The why, what, and how of a screaming heart. *Education in a Democracy: A Journal of the NNER, 2*, 95–124.

Kimiecik, J. (2011). Exploring the promise of eudaimonic well-being within the practice of health promotion: The "how" is as important as the "what". *Journal of Happiness Studies, 12*, 769–792.

Kimiecik, J., & Horn, T. (2016). The big motivational picture: Examining the relationship between positive intrapersonal processes and adolescent health-promoting behaviors. *Applied Developmental Science*, doi:10.1080/10888691.2016.1158651.

Kimiecik, J., & Lawson, H. (1996). Toward new approaches for exercise behavior change and health promotion. *Quest, 48*, 102–125.

Kok, B. E., Coffey, K. A., Cohn, M. A., Catalino, L. I., Vacharkulksemsuk, T., Algoe, S. B., et al. (2013). How positive emotions build physical health: Perceived positive social connections account for the upward spiral between positive emotions and vagal tone. *Psychological Science, 24*, 1123–1132.

Lambert, L., Passmore, H., & Holder, M. (2015). Foundational frameworks of positive psychology: Mapping well-being orientations. *Canadian Psychology, 56*, 311–321.

Langeland, E., & Vinje, H. (2013). The significance of salutogenesis and well-being in mental health promotion: From theory to practice. In C. Keyes (Ed.), *Mental well-being: International contributions to the study of positive mental health* (pp. 299–330). New York: Springer.

Layous, K., & Lyubomirsky, S. (2014). The how, why, what, when, and who of happiness: Mechanisms underlying the success of positive interventions. In J. Gruber & J. Moscowitz (Eds.), *Positive emotion: Integrating the light sides and dark sides* (pp. 473–495). New York: Oxford University Press.

Lee, D., Sirgy, M., Yu, G., & Chalamon, I. (2015). The well-being effects of self-expressiveness and hedonic enjoyment associated with physical exercise. *Applied Research in Quality of Life, 10*, 141–159.

Lewis, A. (2012). *Why nobody believes the numbers: Distinguishing fact from fiction in population health management.* New York: Wiley.

Lewis, P., Kimiecik, J., Horn, T., Zullig, K., & Ward, R. (2014). Can becoming my self influence my health?: Exploring the effects of a eudaimonic well-being enhancement process on psychological indicators of

well-being and physical activity. *Applied Research in Quality of Life, 9*, 643–665.
Longino, C. (1997, December). Beyond the body: An emerging medical paradigm, *American Demographics*, pp. 1–3. Retrieved June 10, 1999, from http://www.deomographics.com.
Lyubomirsky, S., & Layous, K. (2013). How do simple positive activities increase well-being? *Current Directions in Psychological Science, 22*, 57–62.
Lyubomirsky, S., Sheldon, K. M., & Schkade, D. (2005). Pursuing happiness: The architecture of sustainable change. *Review of General Psychology, 9*, 111–131.
Lyubormisky, S., King, L., & Diener, E. (2005). The benefits of frequent positive affect: Does happiness lead to success? *Psychological Bulletin, 131*, 8-3-855.
Mack, D., Gunnell, K., Wilson, P., Gilchrist, J., Kowalski, K., Crocker, P., … & Adachi, J. (2011). Physical activity in individuals living with osteopenia: Associations with psychological need satisfaction and motives for well-being. *The Shield, 6*, 26–41.
Mattke, S., Hangsheng, L., Caloyeras, J., Huang, C., Van Busum, K., Khodyakov, D., et al. (2013). *Workplace wellness programs study*. Santa Monica, CA: Rand Corporation.
McDade, T., Chyu, L., Duncan, G., Hoyt, L., Doane, L., & Adam, E. (2011). Adolescents expectations for the future predict health behaviors in early adulthood. *Social Science & Medicine, 73*, 391–398.
McGinnis, J., & Foege, W. (1993). Actual causes of death in the United States. *JAMA, 270*, 2207–2212.
McMahon, D. (2006). *The pursuit of happiness. A history from the Greeks to the present*. London: Allen Lane.
Mitman, G. (2005). In search of health: Landscape and disease. *Environmental History, 10*, 184–210.
Moeenizadeh, M., & Salagame, K. (2010). The impact of well-being therapy on symptoms of depression. *International Journal of Psychological Studies, 2*, 223–230.
National Wellness Institute. (2009). *Defining wellness*. Retrieved November 24, 2009, from http://www.nationalwellness.org/index.php?id_tier=2&id_c=26.
Nettelton, S. (2006). *The sociology of health and illness* (2nd ed.). Cambridge, MA: Polity Press.
Nettle, D. (2006). *Happiness: The science behind your smile*. New York: Oxford University Press.
Newburg, D., Kimiecik, J., Durand-Bush, N., & Doell, K. (2002). The role of resonance in performance excellence and life engagement. *Journal of Applied Sport Psychology, 14*, 249–267.
Ng, J., Ntoumanis, N., Thogersen-Ntoumani, C., Deci, E., Ryan, R., Duda, J., et al. (2012). Self-determination theory applied to health contexts: A meta-analysis. *Perspectives on Psychological Science, 7*, 325–340.
Norton, D. (1976). *Personal destinies*. Princeton, NJ: Princeton University Press.
Nussbauam, M. (2008). Who is the happy warrior? Philosophy poses questions to psychology. *Journal of Legal Studies, 37*, S81–S113.
Nussbaum, M. (2011). *Creating capabilities: The human development approach*. Cambridge, MA: Belknap.
O'Donnell, M. (2009). Definition of health promotion. *American Journal of Health Promotion, 24*, iv.
O'Donnell, M. (2013). Editor's notes. *American Journal of Health Promotion, 28*, iv–vi.
Oz, M. (2011). Healthcare peer-to-peer: Boots on the ground in the battle for a healthier nation. *Childhood Obesity, 7*, 431–433.
Pate, R. (2012). Historical perspectives on physical activity, fitness, and health. In C. Bouchard, S. Blair, & W. Haskell (Eds.), *Physical activity and health* (pp. 21–37). Champaign, IL: Human Kinetics.
Pate, R. R., Pratt, M., Blair, S. N., Haskell, W. L., Macera, C. A., Bouchard, C., … Wilmore, J. H. (1995). Physical activity and public health. *JAMA, 273*(5), 402–407.
Pelletier, K. (1994). *Sound mind, sound body*. New York: Simon & Schuster.
Phelan, C., Love, G., Ryff, C., Brown, R., & Heidrich, S. (2010). Psychosocial predictors of changing sleep patterns in aging women: A multiple pathway approach. *Psychology and Aging, 25*, 858–866.
Pressman, S., Matthews, K., Cohen, S., Martire, L., Scheier, M., Baum, A., et al. (2009). Association of enjoyable leisure activities with psychological and physical well-being. *Psychosomatic Medicine, 71*, 725–732.
Reeves, M., & Rafftery, A. (2005). Healthy lifestyle characteristics among adults in the United States, 2000. *Archives of Internal Medicine, 165*, 854–857.
Robison, J. (2004). Reinventing the profession. *Absolute Advantage, 6*, 7–11.
Roepke, A., Jayawickreme, E., & Riffle, O. (2014). Meaning and health: A systematic review. *Applied Research in Quality of Life, 9*, 1055–1079.
Ruini, C., Ottolini, F., Tomba, E., Belaise, C., Albieri, E., Visani, D., … Fava, G. (2009). School intervention for promoting psychological well-being in adolescence. *Journal of Behavioral Therapy and Experimental Psychiatry, 40*, 522–532.
Ryan, R., Huta, V., & Deci, E. (2008). Living well: A self-determination theory perspective on eudaimonia. *Journal of Happiness Studies, 9*, 139–170.
Ryff, C. D. (2013). Eudaimonic well-being and health: Mapping consequences of self-realization. In A. S. Waterman (Ed.), *The best within us: Positive psychology perspectives on eudaimonia* (pp. 77–98). Washington, DC: American Psychological Association.
Ryff, C. D., & Singer, B. (1998). The contours of positive human health. *Psychological Inquiry, 9*, 1–28.
Ryff, C., & Singer, B. (2008). Know thyself and become what you are: A eudaimonic approach to psychological well-being. *Journal of Happiness Studies, 9*, 13–39.
Ryff, C. D., Singer, B. H., & Love, G. D. (2004). Positive health: Connecting well-being with biology.

Philosophical Transactions of the Royal Society of London B, 359, 1383–1394.

Sadler, M., Miller, C., Christensen, K., & McGue, M. (2011). Subjective well-being and longevity: A co-twin study. *Twin Research and Human Genetics, 14*, 249–256.

Sallis, J. F., & Patrick, K. (1994). Physical activity guidelines for adolescents: consensus statement. *Pediatric Exercise Science, 6*, 302–314.

Salovey, P., Rothman, A. J., Detweiler, J. B., & Steward, W. T. (2000). Emotional states and physical health. *American Psychologist, 55*(1), 110–121.

Sapkota, S., Bowles, H., Ham, S., & Kohl, H. (2005). Adult participation in recommended levels of physical activity: United States 2001 and 2003. *Morbidity and Mortality Weekly Reports, 54*, 1208–1212.

Schwartz, S., Kurtines, W., & Montgomery, M. (2005). A comparison of two approaches for facilitating identity exploration processes in emerging adults: An exploratory study. *Journal of Adolescent Research, 20*, 309–345.

Schwartz, S. J., Pantin, H., Coatsworth, J. D., & Szapocznik, J. (2007). Addressing the challenges and opportunities for today's youth: Toward an integrative model and its implications for research and intervention. *The Journal of Primary Prevention, 28*(2), 117–144.

Schwartz, S., Waterman, A., Vazsonyi, A., Zamboanga, B., Whitbourne, S., Weisskirch, R., … Ham, L. (2011). The association of well-being with health risk behaviors in college-attending young adults. *Applied Developmental Science, 15*, 20–36.

Segar, M., & Richardson, C. (2014). Prescribing pleasure and meaning: Cultivating walking motivation and maintenance. *American Journal of Preventive Medicine online*, http://ds.doi.org/10.1016/j.amepre.2014.07.001.

Seligman, M. E. P. (2008). Positive health. *Applied Psychology: An International Review, 57*, 3–18. doi:10.1111/j.1464-0597.2008.00351.x.

Seligman, M. (2011). *Flourish: A visionary new understanding of happiness and well-being*. New York: Free Press.

Seligman, M., & Csikszentmihalyi, M. (2000). Positive psychology: An introduction. *American Psychologist, 55*, 5–14.

Sheldon, K., & Elliot, A. (1999). Goal striving, need satisfaction, and longitudinal well-being: The self-concordant model. *Journal of Personality and Social Psychology, 76*, 482–497.

Smith, E. (2013, August). Meaning is healthier than happiness. *Atlantic*. Retrieved from http://www.theatlantic.com/health/archive/2013/08/meaning-is-healthier-than-happiness/278250/. Accessed 15 Jul 2016.

Steger, M., Fitch-Martin, A., Donnelly, J., & Rickard, K. (2015). Meaning in life and health: Proactive health orientation links meaning in life to health variables among American undergraduates. *Journal of Happiness Studies, 16*, 583–597.

Steger, M., Kashdan, T., & Oishi, S. (2008). Being good by doing good: Daily eudaimonic activity and well-being. *Journal of Research in Personality, 42*, 22–42.

Steptoe, A., O'Donnell, K., Marmot, M., & Wardle, J. (2008). Positive affect, psychological well-being, and good sleep. *Journal of Psychosomatic Research, 64*, 409–415.

Steptoe, A., Oliveira, C., Kemakakos, P., & Zaninotto, P. (2014). Enjoyment of life and declining physical function at older ages: A longitudinal study. *Canadian Medical Association Journal, 186*, E150–E156.

Steptoe, A., & Wardle, J. (2011). Positive affect measured using ecological momentary assessment and survival in older men and women. *Proceedings of the National Academy of Sciences USA, 108*, 18244–18248.

Studenski, S., Perera, S., Patel, K., Rosano, C., Faulkner, K., Inzitari, M., … Guralnik, J. (2011). *JAMA, 305*, 50–58.

Su, R., Tay, L., & Diener, E. (2014). The development and validation of the Comprehensive Inventory of Thriving (CIT) and the Brief Inventory of Thriving (BIT). *Applied Psychology: Health and Well-Being, 6*, 251–279.

Sugarman, J. (2007). Practical rationality and the questionable promise of positive psychology. *Journal of Humanistic Psychology, 47*, 175–197.

Sumner, L. (2002). Happiness now and then. In L. Jost & R. Shiner (Eds.), *Eudaimonia and well-being: Ancient and modern conceptions*. Kelowna: Academic Printing & Publishing.

Swindells, R., Lawthom, R., Rowley, K., Siddiquee, A., Kilroy, A., & Kagan, C. 2013. Eudaimonic well-being and community arts participation. *Perspectives in Public Health, 133*, 60–65.

Sylvester, B., Mack, D., Busseri, M., Wilson, P., & Beauchamp, M. (2012). Health-enhancing physical activity, psychological needs satisfaction, and well-being: Is it how often, how long, or much effort that matters? *Mental Health and Physical Activity, 5*, 141–147.

Tudor-Locke, C., & Bassett, D., Jr. (2004). How many steps/day are enough? Preliminary pedometer indices for public health. *Sports Medicine, 34*, 1–8.

U.S. Department of Health and Human Services. (2008). *2008 Physical activity guidelines for Americans*. Washington, DC: US Department of Health and Human Services.

Valle, R. S., King, M., & Halling, S. (1989). An introduction to existential-phenomenological thought in psychology. In R. Valle & S. Halling (Eds.), *Existential-phenomenological perspectives in psychology* (pp. 3–16). New York: Plenum Press.

Vallerand, R., & Lalande, D. (2011). The MPIC model: The perspective of the hierarchical model of intrinsic and extrinsic motivation. *Psychological Inquiry, 22*, 45–51.

Vazquez, C., Hervas, G., Rahona, J., & Gomez, D. (2009). Psychological well-being and health. Contributions of

positive psychology. *Annuary of Clinical and Health Psychology, 5*, 15–27.
Veenhoven, R. (2008). Healthy happiness: Effects of happiness on physical health and the consequences of preventive health care. *Journal of Happiness Studies, 9*, 449–469.
Vittersø, J. (2013). Feelings, meanings, and optimal functioning: Some distinctions between hedonic and eudaimonic well-being. In A. S. Waterman (Ed.), *The best within us: Positive psychology perspectives on eudaimonia* (pp. 39–55). Washington, DC: APA Books.
Vittersø, J., & Søholt, Y. (2011). Life satisfaction goes with pleasure and personal growth goes with interest: Further arguments for separating hedonic and eudaimonic well-being. *Journal of Positive Psychology, 6*, 326–335.
von Heimburg, D. (2010). *Public health and health promotion: A salutogenic approach*. Unpublished masters thesis, Norwegian University of Science and Technology.
Waterman, A. (1993). Two conceptions of happiness: Contrasts of personal expressiveness (eudaimonia) and hedonic enjoyment. *Journal of Personality and Social Psychology, 64*, 678–691.
Waterman, A. (2013). Introduction: Considering the nature of a life well lived—Intersections of positive psychology and eudaemonist philosophy. In A. Waterman (Ed.), *The best within us: Positive psychology perspectives on eudaimonia* (pp. 3–17). Washington, DC: The American Psychological Association.
Waterman, A., & Schwartz, S. (2013). Eudaimonic identity theory. In A. Waterman (Ed.), *The best within us: Positive psychology perspectives on eudaimonia* (pp. 99–118). Washington, DC: The American Psychological Association.
Williams, G., & Niemiec, C. (2012). Positive affect and self-affirmation are beneficial, but do they facilitate maintenance of health behavior change? *Archives of Internal Medicine, 172*, 327–328.
World Health Organization (WHO). (1948). *Constitution of the World Health Organization*. Geneva: WHO Basic Documents.
World Health Organization (WHO). (1986). *The Ottawa charter*. Geneva: WHO.
Zaslavsky, O., Rillamas-Sun, E., Fugate Woods, N., Cochrane, B., Stefanick, M., Tindle, H., … LaCroix, A. (2014). Association of the selected dimensions of eudaimonic well-being with healthy survival to 85 years of age in older women. *International Psychogeriatrics, 26*, 2081–2091.

Eudaimonia, Aging, and Health: A Review of Underlying Mechanisms

24

Anthony D. Ong and Alicia Patterson

> If happiness is activity in accordance with virtue, it is reasonable that it should be in accordance with the highest virtue; and this will be that of the best thing in us. – Aristotle (*Nicomachean Ethics*)

24.1 Eudaimonic Approach to Well-Being

More than two millennia after Aristotle wrote *Nicomachean Ethics*, scientific research on well-being has proliferated. Over the past four decades interest in well-being has been driven by two major philosophical perspectives, one emphasizing *hedonia* or happiness and the other emphasizing *eudaimonia* or self-actualization (Ryan & Deci, 2001; Waterman, 1993). These perspectives have shaped varying accounts of what constitutes quality living, flourishing, and the good life. Whereas hedonic well-being (sometimes called experienced happiness) emphasizes the affective quality of an individual's everyday experience, eudaimonic well-being (sometimes called evaluative well-being) emphasizes an individual's global judgments about life as a whole (Kahneman & Riis, 2005). Ryff and colleagues (Keyes, Shmotkin, & Ryff, 2002; Ryff, 1995; Ryff & Singer, 1998) operationalize eudaimonia as a multidimensional construct consisting of six distinct psychological well-being (PWB) components: a positive attitude toward oneself and one's past life (self-acceptance), high quality, satisfying relationships with others (positive relations with others), a sense of self-determination and freedom from norms (autonomy), having life goals and a belief that one's life is meaningful (purpose in life), the ability to manage life and one's surroundings (environmental mastery), and being open to new experiences and making use of one's personal talents and potential (personal growth).

Psychological studies of adult development and aging suggest that the arc of eudaimonic well-being (as indexed by Ryff's PWB measures) in adulthood and later life is marked by divergent trajectories. While personal growth and purpose in life decline with advancing age, self-acceptance, environmental mastery, and positive relationships appear to increase or at least remain fair stable by later adulthood (Ryff & Singer, 1998, 2008). Much of the existing literature has focused on identifying the health correlates of eudaimonia (Boehm & Kubzansky, 2012; Ryff, 2014; Ryff, Friedman, Fuller - Rowell et al., 2012;

A.D. Ong (✉)
Department of Human Development, Cornell University, Ithaca, NY, USA
e-mail: ado4@cornell.edu

A. Patterson
Department of Philosophy, Cornell University, Ithaca, NY, USA
e-mail: aep95@cornell.edu

J. Vittersø (ed.), *Handbook of Eudaimonic Well-Being*, International Handbooks of Quality-of-Life,
DOI 10.1007/978-3-319-42445-3_24

Ryff, Friedman, Morozink, & Tsenkova, 2012). In this chapter, we review the biobehavioral and psychosocial mechanisms that may account for the relationship between eudaimonia and health in later adulthood. Although the literature is not without theoretical gaps and methodological inconsistencies, overall, the data suggests that evaluative or eudaimonic well-being is associated with favorable health outcomes in later life, the net effect of which may be to slow or delay the rate of functional decline in physiological resilience.

24.1.1 Underlying Mechanisms

Increasing evidence suggests that independent of hedonic well-being, measures of eudaimonic well-being are associated with better health outcomes in later adulthood. A recent integrative review (Boehm & Kubzansky, 2012) documented robust associations between measures of eudaimonia and improved health. Across cross-sectional and large scale prospective epidemiological studies, significant aspects of adult health predicted by eudaimonic well-being include self-reported health, physiological responses, physical functioning, disease severity, and mortality (see also Steptoe, Deaton, & Stone, 2015).

Associations between the broad category of eudaimonic well-being and adult health outcomes raise the question of mechanisms underlying these effects. A number of candidate pathways linking eudaimonia to adult health have been identified (Ryff, Singer, & Love, 2004; Ryff et al., 2006), but with few exceptions, the evidence base to date includes few formal tests of mechanistic hypotheses. In what follows, we review evidence for three intermediate pathways linking eudaimonic well-being to morbidity and mortality: health behaviors, biological function, and stress-buffering effects.

Restorative and Deteriorative Health Behaviors

Health habits are heavily implicated in the development of acute and chronic health conditions. Moreover, because the effects of negative health behaviors, such as poor nutrition, a sedentary lifestyle, and reduced sleep accumulate with age, older adults are at greater risk for chronic and acute health disorders (Adler & Matthews, 1994). Importantly, individual differences in eudaimonic well-being may directly impact health by affecting the initiation and maintenance of restorative health practices over time. Summative reviews (e.g., Boehm & Kubzansky, 2012; Ryff, 2014) indicate that eudaimonic well-being is associated with greater health-enhancing behaviors, such as better diet, regular exercise, and improved sleep. In an illustrative study, Steptoe and associates (2008) used data from a cross-sectional study of 736 adults (58–72 years) and reported an association between eudaimonic well-being (measured by environmental mastery, autonomy, self-acceptance, and purpose in life) and good or restorative sleep that was independent of age, sex, employment status, and psychological distress. Longitudinal studies corroborate the correlational link between eudaimonia and sleep. For example, in a prospective study of 115 adult women (55–84 years), Phelan, Love, Ryff, Brown, and Heidrich (2010) found that higher levels of environmental mastery, personal growth, purpose in life, and self-acceptance at baseline were associated with improved sleep patterns at follow-up (8 and 10 years later), controlling for initial sleep quality.

In addition to being associated with restorative health behaviors, findings suggest that eudaimonic well-being is inversely associated with deteriorative health practices (e.g., cigarette smoking, alcohol consumption, inactive or sedentary life style). Again, the strongest evidence comes from prospective investigations that examine how initial eudaimonic well-being is subsequently related to deteriorative health processes over time. For instance, in a longitudinal study spanning 20 years, Gale, Batty, and Deary (2008) reported that greater locus of control (mastery) in childhood was associated with a reduced risk of smoking during adulthood. In contrast, evidence from longitudinal studies of alcohol consumption and physical activity is mixed. For example, in longitudinal analyses, eudaimonic well-being (e.g., control/mastery) is inversely associated with alcohol dependence (Twisk, Snel, Kemper, & van Mechelen, 1998) and positively related with subsequent physical activity (Gale et al., 2008), although null associations have also been reported (Adalbjarnardottir & Rafnsson, 2001; Williams, Gagne, Mushlin, & Deci, 2005).

In sum, although longitudinal evidence suggests that higher levels of eudaimonic well-being is associated with health-enhancing behaviors, recent systematic and narrative reviews (Boehm & Kubzansky, 2012; Steptoe et al., 2015) report that the effects of positive mental health or eudaimonic well-being on morbidity and mortality persist even after controlling for health behaviors, such as smoking and exercise, suggesting that there may be more than one explanatory pathway through which eudaimonia may exert influence on adult health outcomes.

Biological Functioning

Progress has also been made at understanding the correlates of eudaimonic well-being at the biological level. Findings regarding biological function, however, vary across studies, reflecting the different study designs (longitudinal vs. cross-sectional), populations sampled (healthy vs. patient), and specific biological system under consideration. The limited number of longitudinal studies have reported inverse associations between evaluative well-being and coronary calcification, lipids, body mass index (BMI), and allostatic load (Gale et al., 2008; Matthews, Owens, Edmundowicz, Lee, & Kuller, 2006; Twisk et al., 1998; Zilioli, Slatcher, Ong, & Gruenewald, 2015), with other studies reporting null associations between eudaimonic well-being and cardiovascular and metabolic functioning (Gale et al., 2008; Tsenkova, Love, Singer, & Ryff, 2007). In contrast, cross-sectional evidence generally suggests an association between eudaimonic well-being and smaller waist circumference, lower levels of plasma triglycerides, interleukin-6, and lower daily cortisol; greater levels of dehydroepiandosterone sulfate and high-density lipoprotein cholesterol; lower concentrations of inflammatory markers C-reactive protein and fibrinogen); and higher body mass index and resting blood pressure (Friedman, Hayney, Love, Singer, & Ryff, 2007; Ryff et al., 2004; Steptoe, Demakakos, de Oliveira, & Wardle, 2012), although mixed findings have also been reported (Boehm & Kubzansky, 2012; Ryff, 2014; Ryff et al., 2006).

Increasing attention has also focused on the neural correlates of eudaimonic well-being, with initial evidence showing that those with higher profiles of eudaimonia (e.g., personal growth, positive relations and purpose in life) have differential brain responses to negative (less amygdala activation and increased ventral anterior cingulated cortex activation) and positive stimuli (sustained activation of the ventral striatum and dorsolateral prefrontal cortex) and show greater insular cortex volume, a region of the brain associated with higher-order functions (Heller et al., 2013; Lewis, Kanai, Rees, & Bates, 2014; Urry et al., 2004; van Reekum et al., 2007). Finally, measures of eudaimonic (but not hedonic) well-being have been recently linked with down regulation of proinflammatory genes and increased expression of antibody synthesis genes (Fredrickson et al., 2013), although the hedonic and eudaimonic well-being measures showed high positive correlations as in previous studies (Kashdan, Biswas-Diener, & King, 2008; Steptoe et al., 2012).

While the adult literature is limited and includes relatively few prospective longitudinal studies, the available data provide promising evidence that eudaimonic well-being may alter disease vulnerability by modulating the prolonged activation of biological systems. Overall, findings suggest that the link between eudaimonia and health may be particularly important at older ages when the accrual of physiological deficits increases vulnerability to disease, although more research on age differences in the association between eudaimonia and biological processes is clearly needed.

Stress-Buffering Effects

Individual differences in stressor exposure have long been suspected as contributing to age-related differences in vulnerability to illness and premature mortality. In an influential review, Cohen and Williamson (1991) proposed that stress may interact with age to precipitate dysregulation in immune functioning. Subsequent reviews (e.g., Kiecolt-Glaser & Glaser, 2001) have supported the hypothesis that differential exposure to stressors contributes to, and hastens, age-related declines in physical health. However, not all aging individuals evidence maladaptive functioning in the face of hardship and adversity. Empirical evidence from studies of community-dwelling older adults indicates eudaimonia may play an important role in facilitating resilient adaptation to various targeted life challenges, including socioeconomic adversity (Chen, Miller, Lachman, Gruenewald, & Seeman, 2012; Lachman, Agrigoroaei, Murphy, & Tun, 2010), the experience of abuse in childhood (Greenfield & Marks, 2010; Pitzer & Fingerman, 2010), the death of a loved one (Ong, Fuller-Rowell, & Bonanno, 2010; Ong, Fuller-Rowell, Bonanno, & Almeida, 2011) the onset of a major illness (Costanzo, Ryff, & Singer, 2009; Pudrovska, 2010), as well as the normative challenges of aging, including overall declines in physical health (Cotter & Lachman, 2010; Friedman & Ryff, 2012), mental health (Choi & Kim, 2011; Greenfield & Marks, 2004), and cognitive functioning (Boyle, Barnes, Buchman, & Bennett, 2009; Seeman et al., 2011).

Overall, the vast majority of studies documenting stress-buffering effects of eudaimonic well-being are cross-sectional, making it difficult to assess the causal direction. Thus, although the available evidence suggests that eudaimonia may be a protective resource in old age, more research investigating the prospective, longitudinal links between eudaimonia, stress, and health among vulnerable older people is urgently needed.

24.2 Intervention Studies

Turning to intervention studies, a key question is whether eudaimonia (i.e., flourishing) can be promoted among older persons. To date, a range of psychosocial interventions have been developed to promote eudaimonic well-being in adult populations. Ryff (2014) reviewed relevant clinical interventions to enhance well-being of those suffering from diverse psychiatric and chronic conditions such as major depression (Fava et al., 2004), anxiety disorder (Ruini & Fava, 2009), cyclothymic disorder (Fava, Rafanelli, Tomba, Guidi, & Grandi, 2011), rheumatoid arthritis (Pradhan et al., 2007), schizophrenia (Johnson et al., 2011), and posttraumatic stress (Feder et al., 2013). Among the important methodological issues identified in previous intervention studies include differences in the duration of interventions and frequency of the interventions sessions, potential for regression toward the mean and selection bias in nonrandomized controlled trials, the need to match interventions to specific therapies and population characteristics, and the relative paucity of well-controlled randomized control trials.

In general, intervention studies suggest that eudaimonic well-being may have lasting implications for physical health, but additional long-term studies are needed to determine whether well-being interventions that foster eudaimonia afford protection against the health challenges of aging. Likewise, there is a need for better-designed well-being interventions (e.g., cognitive behavioral therapy, loving-kindness meditation) that target vulnerable older people. Specific groups of older adults who might benefit from targeted well-being interventions might include the functionally disabled, the hearing and cognitive impaired, as well as the "oldest-old" (cf. Cohen-Mansfield & Perach, 2015; Ong, Uchino, & Wethington, 2016), who are at heightened risk for loneliness and social isolation due to decreasing opportunities for social connection.

24.3 Future Directions

Data reviewed above demonstrate that core dimensions of eudaimonic well-being (positive relations with others, personal growth, purpose in life, environmental mastery, self-acceptance, and autonomy) have benefits on downstream behavioral, psychosocial, and biological processes, as well as on meaningful disease endpoints in later life such as morbidity and mortality. Research on eudaimonia and aging is still in its early phases, however, and several important questions remain. Below we highlight several critical but, as yet, unresolved issues for future research.

A key question for future research is the extent to which measures of eudaimonic and hedonic well-being (e.g., life satisfaction, positive affect) influence different behavioral and biological pathways or exert different effects on the same pathways. This is made challenging by the ongoing discussion about the extent to which these measures can be meaningfully distinguished (Kashdan et al., 2008; Springer & Hauser, 2006).

Second, the limited longitudinal work suggests that there may be bidirectional relationships between eudaimonic well-being and various risk factors (e.g., initial health status, health behaviors, depression). However, with few exceptions, long-term investigations of eudaimonia and mental and physical health have rarely been examined. In addition to providing a more rigorous assessment of mechanistic pathways, prospective, multi-wave, longitudinal studies are critically important in advancing the science of eudaimonia and health because they (a) allow for tests of theoretical models that assume stability of relations over time, (b) help address questions regarding duration of eudaimonia and whether sustained eudaimonia over time is associated with health outcomes above and beyond a single report, and (c) provide evidence against reverse-causality arguments, which posit that individuals who are ill may also report less eudaimonic well-being.

Finally, it is possible that various dimensions of positive mental health or flourishing are confounded with unmeasured variables Recent reviews (e.g., Boehm & Kubzansky, 2012) have advocated testing the association between positive psychological well-being and health through careful statistical control of potential confounds (e.g., physical symptoms and health), as well as closely related psychological constructs (e.g., optimism, vitality, and other measures of positive psychological well-being). Although statistical controls are invaluable in nonexperimental research, such adjustments may obscure the identification of potential mechanisms of change. Thus, observational studies that attempt to substantiate a causal link between eudaimonia and health should apply statistical controls in a theory-driven manner. Other methodological challenges concern the measurement of eudaimonic well-being. The vast majority of included studies relied on self-report measures, with few studies examining the effects of manipulated eudaimonic well-being (e.g., purpose in life, autonomy) on physical health outcomes. Furthermore, considering the significant heterogeneity across studies in measures of positive psychological well-being (Boehm & Kubzansky, 2012; Hutcheon, Chiolero, & Hanley, 2010), measurement error remains an issue that may contribute to biases associated with effect estimation.

24.4 Concluding Remarks

Twenty-three centuries have passed since Aristotle's formulation of the good life. In his *Nicomachean Ethics*, Aristotle stated that the highest of all goods achievable by human action was "eudaimonia," a property of evaluative well-being arrived at through virtuous living in accordance with reason and rationality. Although the eudaimonic perspective on well-being has had a significant impact on humanistic and existential psychology (Allport, 1961; Frankl & Lasch, 1959; Maslow, 1968; Rogers, 1962), until recently, there has been little empirical support for these ideas. Foundational evidence for the adaptive function of eudaimonia is now beginning to accrue, however. Taken together, the available data indicate that there is no single answer to the question of how eudaimonia influences health outcomes in later adulthood. Instead, findings suggest that health behaviors, physiological systems, and stress-buffering may be among the key pathways underlying disparities in physical health, psychological well-being, and even longevity in later life. Future work building on these findings will require greater attention to the interaction between eudaimonic well-being and the presence of decreasing physiological resilience with aging. Targeted prevention and intervention strategies that enhance eudaimonia, particularly among the most vulnerable, are likely to play an important role in preventing serious physical illness, minimizing the burden of stress, and improving overall functioning in older adults.

References

Adalbjarnardottir, S., & Rafnsson, F. D. (2001). Perceived control in adolescent substance use: Concurrent and longitudinal analyses. *Psychology of Addictive Behaviors, 15*, 25–32.

Adler, N., & Matthews, N. (1994). Health psychology: Why do some people get sick and some stay well? *Annual Review of Psychology, 45*, 229–259.

Allport, G. W. (1961). *Pattern and growth in personality*. Oxford, UK: Holt, Reinhart and Winston.

Boehm, J. K., & Kubzansky, L. D. (2012). The heart's content: The association between positive psychological well-being and cardiovascular health. *Psychological Bulletin, 138*, 655–691.

Boyle, P. A., Barnes, L. L., Buchman, A. S., & Bennett, D. (2009). Purpose in life is associated with mortality among community–dwelling older persons. *Psychosomatic Medicine, 71*, 574–579.

Chen, E., Miller, G. E., Lachman, M. E., Gruenewald, T. L., & Seeman, T. E. (2012). Protective factors for adults from low-childhood socioeconomic circumstances: The benefits of shift-and-persist for allostatic load. *Psychosomatic Medicine, 74*, 178–186.

Choi, N., & Kim, J. M. (2011). The effect of time volunteering and charitable donations in later life on psychological wellbeing. *Ageing and Society, 31*, 590–611.

Cohen, S., & Williamson, G. M. (1991). Stress and infectious disease in humans. *Psychological Bulletin, 109*, 5–24.

Cohen-Mansfield, J., & Perach, R. (2015). Interventions for alleviating loneliness among older persons: A critical review. *American Journal of Health Promotion, 29*, 109–125.

Costanzo, E. S., Ryff, C. D., & Singer, B. H. (2009). Psychosocial adjustment among cancer survivors: Findings from a national survey of health and well-being. *Health Psychology, 28*, 147–156.

Cotter, K. A., & Lachman, M. E. (2010). Psychosocial and behavioural contributors to health: Age-related increases in physical disability are reduced by physical fitness. *Psychology & Health, 25*, 805–820.

Fava, G. A., Rafanelli, C., Tomba, E., Guidi, J., & Grandi, S. (2011). The sequential combination of cognitive behavioral treatment and well-being therapy in cyclothymic disorder. *Psychotheray and Psychosomatics, 80*, 136–143.

Fava, G. A., Ruini, C., Rafanelli, C., Finos, L., Conti, S., & Grandi, S. (2004). Six-year outcome of cognitive behavior therapy for prevention of recurrent depression. *American Journal of Psychiatry, 161*, 1872–1876.

Feder, A., Ahmad, S., Lee, E. J., Morgan, J., Singh, R., Smith, B. W., et al. (2013). Coping and PTSD symptoms in Pakistani earthquake survivors: Purpose in life, religious coping and social support. *Journal of Affective Disorder, 147*, 156–163.

Frankl, V. E., & Lasch, I. (1959). *Man's search for meaning: An introduction to logotherapy*. Boston: Beacon Press.

Fredrickson, B. L., Grewen, K. M., Coffey, K. A., Algoe, S. B., Firestine, A. M., Arevalo, J. M. G., et al. (2013). A functional genomic perspective on human well-being. *PNAS Proceedings of the National Academy of Sciences of the United States of America, 110*, 13684–13689.

Friedman, E. M., Hayney, M., Love, G. D., Singer, B. H., & Ryff, C. D. (2007). Plasma interleukin-6 and soluble IL-6 receptors are associated with psychological well-being in aging women. *Health Psychology, 26*, 305–313.

Friedman, E. M., & Ryff, C. D. (2012). Living well with medical comorbidities: A biopsychosocial perspective. *The Journals of Gerontology: Series B: Psychological Sciences and Social Sciences, 67B*, 535–544.

Gale, C. R., Batty, G. D., & Deary, I. J. (2008). Locus of control at age 10 years and health outcomes and behaviors at age 30 years: The 1970 British Cohort Study. *Psychosomatic Medicine, 70*, 397–403.

Greenfield, E. A., & Marks, N. F. (2004). Formal volunteering as a protective factor for older adults' psychological well-being. *Journals of Gerontology. Series B Psychological Sciences and Social Sciences, 59B*, S258–S264.

Greenfield, E. A., & Marks, N. F. (2010). Identifying experiences of physical and psychological violence in childhood that jeopardize mental health in adulthood. *Child Abuse & Neglect, 34*, 161–171.

Heller, A. S., van Reekum, C. M., Schaefer, S. M., Lapate, R. C., Radler, B. T., Ryff, C. D., et al. (2013). Sustained striatal activity predicts eudaimonic well-being and cortisol output. *Psychological Science, 24*, 2191–2200.

Hutcheon, J. A., Chiolero, A., & Hanley, J. A. (2010). Random measurement error and regression dilution bias. *BMJ, 340*, c2289.

Johnson, D. P., Penn, D. L., Fredrickson, B. L., Kring, A. M., Meyer, P. S., Catalino, L. I., et al. (2011). A pilot study of loving-kindness meditation for the negative symptoms of schizophrenia. *Schizophrenia Research, 129*, 137–140.

Kahneman, D., & Riis, J. (2005). Living, and thinking about it: Two perspectives on life. In F. A. Huppert,

N. Baylis, & B. Keverne (Eds.), *The science of well-being* (pp. 285–304). Oxford, UK: Oxford University Press.

Kashdan, T. B., Biswas-Diener, R., & King, L. A. (2008). Reconsidering happiness: The costs of distinguishing between hedonics and eudaimonia. *Journal of Positive Psychology, 3*, 219–233.

Keyes, C. L., Shmotkin, D., & Ryff, C. D. (2002). Optimizing well-being: The empirical encounter of two traditions. *Journal of Personality and Social Psychology, 82*, 1007–1022.

Kiecolt-Glaser, J. K., & Glaser, R. (2001). Stress and immunity: Age enhances the risks. *Current Directions in Psychological Science, 10*, 18–21.

Lachman, M. E., Agrigoroaei, S., Murphy, C., & Tun, P. A. (2010). Frequent cognitive activity compensates for education differences in episodic memory. *American Journal of Geriatric Psychiatry, 18*, 4–10.

Lewis, G. J., Kanai, R., Rees, G., & Bates, T. C. (2014). Neural correlates of the 'good life': Eudaimonic well-being is associated with insular cortex volume. *Social Cognitive and Affective Neuroscience, 9*, 615–618.

Maslow, A. H. (1968). *Toward a psychology of being* (2nd ed.). New York: Van Nostrand.

Matthews, K. A., Owens, J. F., Edmundowicz, D., Lee, L., & Kuller, L. H. (2006). Positive and negative attributes and risk for coronary and aortic calcification in healthy women. *Psychosomatic Medicine, 68*, 355–361.

Ong, A. D., Fuller-Rowell, T. E., Bonanno, G. A., & Almeida, D. M. (2011). Spousal loss predicts alterations in diurnal cortisol activity through prospective changes in positive emotion. *Health Psychology, 30*, 220–227.

Ong, A. D., Fuller-Rowell, T. E., & Bonanno, G. A. (2010). Prospective predictors of positive emotions following spousal loss. *Psychology and Aging, 25*, 653–660.

Ong, A. D., Uchino, B., & Wethington, E. (2016). Loneliness and health in older adults: A review and synthesis. *Gerontology, 62*, 443–449.

Phelan, C. H., Love, G. D., Ryff, C. D., Brown, R. L., & Heidrich, S. M. (2010). Psychosocial predictors of changing sleep patterns in aging women: A multiple pathway approach. *Psychology and Aging, 25*, 858–866.

Pitzer, L. M., & Fingerman, K. L. (2010). Psychosocial resources and associations between childhood physical abuse and adult well-being. *Journals of Gerontology. Series B, Psychological Sciences and Social Sciences, 65B*, 425–433.

Pradhan, E. K., Baumgarten, M., Langenberg, P., Handwerger, B., Gilpin, A. K., Magyari, T., et al. (2007). Effect of mindfulness-based stress reduction in rheumatoid arthritis patients. *Arthritis & Rheumatism-Arthritis Care & Research, 57*, 1134–1142.

Pudrovska, T. (2010). What makes you stronger: Age and cohort differences in personal growth after cancer. *Journal of Health and Social Behavior, 51*, 260–273.

Rogers, C. R. (1962). The interpersonal relationship: The core of guidance. *Harvard Educational Review, 32*, 416–429.

Ruini, C., & Fava, G. A. (2009). Well-being therapy for generalized anxiety disorder. *Journal of Clinical Psychology, 65*, 510–519.

Ryan, R. M., & Deci, E. L. (2001). On happiness and human potentials: A review of research on hedonic and eudaimonic well-being. *Annual Review of Psychology, 52*, 141–166.

Ryff, C. D. (1995). Psychological well-being in adult life. *Current Directions in Psychological Science, 4*, 99–104.

Ryff, C. D. (2014). Psychological well-being revisited: Advances in the science and practice of eudaimonia. *Psychotherapy and Psychosomatics, 83*, 10–28.

Ryff, C., Friedman, E., Fuller - Rowell, T., Love, G., Miyamoto, Y., Morozink, J., et al. (2012). Varieties of resilience in midus. *Social and Personality Psychology Compass, 6*, 792–806.

Ryff, C. D., Friedman, E. M., Morozink, J. A., & Tsenkova, V. (2012). Psychological resilience in adulthood and later life: Implications for health. In B. Hayslip Jr. & G. C. Smith (Eds.), *Annual review of gerontology and geriatrics, Vol 32: Emerging perspectives on resilience in adulthood and later life* (Vol. 32, pp. 73–92). New York: Springer Publishing Co.

Ryff, C. D., Love, G. D., Urry, H. L., Muller, D., Rosenkranz, M. A., Friedman, E. M., et al. (2006). Psychological well-being and ill-being: Do they have distinct or mirrored biological correlates? *Psychotherapy and Psychosomatics, 75*, 85–95.

Ryff, C. D., & Singer, B. (1998). The contours of positive human health. *Psychological Inquiry, 9*, 1–28.

Ryff, C. D., & Singer, B. (2008). Know thyself and become what you are: A eudaimonic approach to psychological well-being. *Journal of Happiness Studies, 9*, 13–39.

Ryff, C. D., Singer, B. H., & Love, G. D. (2004). Positive health: Connecting well-being with biology. *Philosophical Transactions of the Royal Society of London, 359*, 1383–1394.

Seeman, T. E., Miller-Martinez, D. M., Merkin, S. S., Lachman, M. E., Tun, P. A., & Karlamangla, A. S. (2011). Histories of social engagement and adult cognition: Midlife in the U.S. study. *The Journals of Gerontology: Series B: Psychological Sciences and Social Sciences, 66B*, 141–152.

Springer, K. W., & Hauser, R. M. (2006). An assessment of the construct validity of Ryff's scales of psychological well-being: Method, mode, and measurement effects. *Social Science Research, 35*, 1080–1102.

Steptoe, A., Deaton, A., & Stone, A. A. (2015). Psychological well-being, health and ageing. *Lancet, 385*, 640–648.

Steptoe, A., Demakakos, P., de Oliveira, C., & Wardle, J. (2012). Distinctive biological correlates of positive psychological well-being in older men and women. *Psychosomatic Medicine, 74*, 501–508.

Steptoe, A., O'Donnell, K., Marmot, M., & Wardle, J. (2008). Positive affect, psychological well-being, and good sleep. *Journal of Psychosomatic Research, 64*, 409–415.

Tsenkova, V. K., Love, G. D., Singer, B. H., & Ryff, C. D. (2007). Socioeconomic status and psychological well-being predict cross-time change in glycosylated hemoglobin in older women without diabetes. *Psychosomatic Medicine, 69*, 777–784.

Twisk, J. W., Snel, J., Kemper, H., & van Mechelen, W. (1998). Relation between the longitudinal development of personality characteristics and biological and lifestyle risk factors for coronary heart disease. *Psychosomatic Medicine, 60*, 372–377.

Urry, H. L., Nitschke, J. B., Dolski, I., Jackson, D. C., Dalton, K. M., Mueller, C. J., et al. (2004). Making a life worth living: Neural correlates of well-being. *Psychological Science, 15*, 367–372.

van Reekum, C. M., Urry, H. L., Johnstone, T., Thurow, M. E., Frye, C., Jackson, C. A., et al. (2007). Individual differences in amygdala and ventromedial prefrontal cortex activity are associated with evaluation speed and psychological well-being. *Journal of Cognitive Neuroscience, 19*, 237–248.

Waterman, A. S. (1993). Two conceptions of happiness: Contrasts of personal expressiveness (eudaimonic) and hedonic enjoyment. *Journal of Personality and Social Psychology, 62*, 678–691.

Williams, G. C., Gagne, M., Mushlin, A., & Deci, E. L. (2005). Motivation for behavior change in patients with chest pain. *Health Education, 105*, 304–321.

Zilioli, S., Slatcher, R. B., Ong, A. D., & Gruenewald, T. (2015). Purpose in life predicts health locus of control and allostatic load ten years later. *Journal of Psychosomatic Research, 79*, 451–457.

Wholeness and Holiness: The Spiritual Dimension of Eudaimonics

25

Kenneth I. Pargament, Serena Wong, and Julie J. Exline

Robert Oxnam was a broken man. He stumbled through life disoriented, spinning from role to role while in the grips of alcoholism, bulimia, and depression. In coping with childhood trauma, his personality split into separate identities. He describes these fragmented experiences living with multiple personality disorder, now known as dissociative identity disorder, in his memoir, *A Fractured Mind* (2005). During the course of his therapy, Oxnam delved inward and united parts of himself that were previously divided. The process of integration was only partially successful by the end of his narrative; yet Oxnam's three remaining personalities agreed to live alongside each other, re-oriented to a shared search for significance within one body. Today he is President Emeritus of the Asia Society, an accomplished scholar on China, and an artist.

Although most people's experiences of brokenness are less dramatic, there are numerous examples of individuals who turn their lives around and experience growth. Some commit themselves to a healthier lifestyle. Others shift careers in pursuit of something more meaningful. Still others embrace a worldview that transforms their lives. How do we understand this type of profound change for the better? Over the past 50 years, theorists have offered a number of valuable frameworks for understanding growth and well-being (e.g., Tedeschi & Calhoun, 2004, on post-traumatic growth; Ryff, 1989, Chap. 6, this volume, on well-being; Peterson & Seligman, 2004, on character strengths and virtues; Vittersø, 2013, on functional well-being). In this chapter, we suggest another potentially valuable construct for understanding eudaimonics, one with deep ties to the concept of spirituality and one which holds important theoretical, empirical, and practical implications for the ways we consider people at their best. Our focus here is on the concept of wholeness, its relationship to eudaimonic well-being, and its particular links to spirituality (i.e., holiness).

Central to various conceptualizations of eudaimonia is the notion of the well-functioning person (e.g., Vittersø, 2013, Chap. 17, this volume). In these conceptualizations of well-functioning, we can identify streams of thought that are highly resonant with the notion of wholeness. For instance, in his classical work, *The Varieties of Religious Experience*, William James (1902) identified the unification of the divided self as the critical task in the achievement of optimal functioning. However, in many writings about well-being, concepts of wholeness and brokenness have not been fully articulated. In this chapter,

K.I. Pargament (✉) • S. Wong
Bowling Green State University,
Bowling Green, OH, USA
e-mail: kpargam@bgsu.edu; swong@bgsu.edu

J.J. Exline
Case Western Reserve University,
Cleveland, OH, USA
e-mail: julie.exline@case.edu

J. Vittersø (ed.), *Handbook of Eudaimonic Well-Being*, International Handbooks of Quality-of-Life,
DOI 10.1007/978-3-319-42445-3_25

we suggest the value of moving wholeness from the background to the foreground of attempts to understand eudaimonic well-being. Doing so, we will note, has some important advantages. For instance, whereas eudaimonic well-being tends to be conceptualized and evaluated largely in subjective terms (Besser-Jones, this volume), the concept of wholeness calls for a multi-level systems understanding and assessment, one which taps into the interplay among cognitive, behavioral, relational, affective, and motivational dimensions of human functioning.

Concepts of wholeness as key to "the good life" are perhaps most fundamentally rooted in the religions of the world. That people are in some ways broken is a precept fundamental to the great religious traditions. And each tradition offers an antidote to our brokenness that involves a movement toward greater wholeness. In this vein, it is interesting to note that the term "holy" is an etymological descendant of the Old English word *hālig*, which translates into wholeness, health, and happiness (New World Encyclopedia, 2008). For example, according to Jewish mystical tradition, in the creative process, God withdrew to form a finite space or vessel within the infinite realm and then injected a ray of divine light into this vessel (Frankel, 2005). However, the vessel was unable to fully contain this light and shattered. In this sense, the universe was broken from its inception. It is up to humankind to repair the damage by acts of caring, compassion, and justice that bring wholeness and healing back to a fragmented world. According to classical Christian thought, sin and death were brought into the world when Adam and Eve ate from the fruit of the tree that had been forbidden to them by God. In doing so, they lost their free and unrestricted access to God (Smith, 1958). This breach was ultimately repaired through the sacrifice of Jesus Christ on the cross, who is said to offer a connection to God to all those who accept him as savior. Nontheistic religions also provide guidelines for approaching greater wholeness. According to Buddhist philosophy, suffering is a natural state of imperfection, or brokenness, th at is fundamental to human existence. The Mahayana tradition tells how Buddha provided a solution to suffering for the Dragon King through wholesome ways of action, which serve as ethical practices that move individuals toward enlightenment, an ideal state of completeness (Bhikkhu, 1985). As illustrated above, the search for wholeness is an essential motive underlying religion. Johnson (1955, p. 49), wrote, "The finite person is ever fragmentary and incomplete. But in knowing this he transcends the fleeting moment, looks before and after, and longs for Someone greater and more complete to answer his loneliness."

More recently, some psychologists have also stressed the movement from brokenness to wholeness as an essential developmental task. For instance, Palmer (2004) maintains that each of us contains an inner wholeness. Yet internal and external constraints prevent us from realizing this wholeness and, as a result, we experience the pain of disconnectedness from our authentic selves and disconnection from others. People face the developmental challenge of overcoming this division by rediscovering and cultivating their true spirit. Fowler (1981) also proposes a shift in development, and faith development in particular, over the lifespan from less to greater wholeness. He describes the movement from undifferentiated, literal, and socially conventional stages of faith to more individually reflective and ultimately universalizing stages which place the emphasis on inclusive visions of humanity. Such broad perspectives, as we will explain further, are signals of wholeness. Building on this tradition of work, this chapter will consider some of the more recent contributions of theory, research, and practice to our understanding of wholeness, holiness, and eudaimonic well-being.

As a prelude to this discussion, it is important to note that our exploration of wholeness and holiness rests on some assumptions, previously articulated by Pargament in 1997, 2011, and 2013: Humans are proactive beings, motivated to seek out and foster a relationship with whatever they may hold to be of value or significance in life. People do not approach this search for significance empty-handed; they are guided by an orienting system. The orienting system refers to an individual's general framework of values, beliefs, practices, emotions, and relationships that offer direction and stability in the search for significance. Think of the orienting system as a "general way of viewing and dealing with the world," a blueprint that provides a design for living and aids in helping the individual come to terms with life's transitions and traumas (Pargament, 1997, p. 99). This orienting system is also embedded in and shaped by a larger sociocultural context. But not all orienting systems are equivalent. They can vary in their strength, their capacity to help people negotiate life's demands and realize their goals. Individuals with stronger orienting systems are better equipped to face life's challenges, while those with more limited orienting systems are more vulnerable in the face of transitions and trauma. Pargament has stressed that the key to a stronger orienting system lies not in one particular value, belief, or practice; rather it involves the degree to which the individual's life framework is well-integrated, whole, and cohesive.

Pargament and Mahoney (2005) also make the assumption that people are spiritual beings, fundamentally concerned about aspects of life they hold sacred. By sacred, they are referring not only to concepts of divinity, God, and higher powers, but also to other life domains that have been imbued with divine-like qualities, such as transcendence, ultimacy, and boundlessness. Once sanctified, a practice can become a ritual, a thought can become a religious belief, a dramatic event can become a miracle, relationships can become a religious congregation, a goal can become a life vocation. And these expressions of spirituality can be fully interwoven into the individual's orientation to life. In fact, as we will see, spirituality often serves as an integrative dimension in the orienting system, a force for wholeness that provides the individual with higher-order overarching values and an ultimate source of meaning that organizes lower-order goals and gives life a consistent unifying direction. Thus, the pursuit of wholeness and holiness can go hand-in-hand for some individuals. At the same time, we will acknowledge the darker side to spirituality; spirituality can be a force for disharmony, disintegration, and brokenness. And that darker potential must also enter into any discussion of wholeness and holiness.

With these assumptions in mind, we now turn our attention to what it means to be whole in terms of one's orienting system, drawing on both psychological and spiritual contributions. Because wholeness, like spirituality, is a multifaced numinous construct, our analysis will be illustrative rather than comprehensive. We will consider the meaning of wholeness and zero in on five sets of elements that distinguish greater wholeness vs. greater brokenness in the orienting system (see Pargament, 1997, for further discussion): (a) deeply purposive vs. aimless; (b) broad and deep vs. narrow and shallow; (c) flexible and enduring vs. rigid and unstable; (d) balanced, cohesive, and discerning vs. imbalanced, incohesive, and non-reflective; (e) benevolent and life-affirming vs. non-benevolent and life-limiting. Our discussion of these five sets of elements will place particular emphasis on spiritual contributions to wholeness and brokenness. We will then discuss how people may grow to achieve greater wholeness in their lives, emphasizing the vital role that spiritual struggles can play in this process. We will conclude by summarizing points of convergence and divergence between wholeness and varying conceptualizations of eudaimonia, along with reflections on the utility of wholeness in distinguishing between eudaimonic and hedonic approaches to well-being.

25.1 Elements of Wholeness and Brokenness

How do we best describe wholeness? The term "whole" may seem overwhelming, encompassing virtually anything and everything. In speaking about wholeness, we turn away from the simplicity of a single key or set of keys that may unlock the mystery of well-being. Instead, we have to grapple with life in its greater complexity, the fact that we are biological, psychological, social, and spiritual beings. The language of wholeness speaks to the quality of the interplay between all of the bits and pieces that make up a life. It calls for a different language. In this discussion of wholeness we will use terms such as breadth, depth, connectedness, cohesiveness, balance, and harmony. The converse of wholeness, brokenness, calls for its own language as well, including terms such as shallowness, narrowness, disconnection, fragmentation, imbalance, and discord. Perhaps, in its most basic form, wholeness has to do with how well we put our lives together. Of course, we can put our lives together in many ways; there are, in short, many ways to be whole. We are left then with the challenging question of how to evaluate the degree to which a life is well put together.

In this chapter we consider five sets of elements that distinguish greater wholeness from greater brokenness. These elements are different yet interconnected. You might think of them as indicators of the degree to which orienting systems are more or less whole or broken. Like eudaimonic well-being, we will see that signals of wholeness are often related to other signs of health and well-being, whereas aspects of brokenness are associated with signs of poorer health and deep despair. However, wholeness and brokenness cannot be equated with life satisfaction and dissatisfaction respectively. Although optimal functioning tends to facilitate pleasurable experiences and feelings, the modest correlations reported in empirical studies suggest that neither wholeness nor eudaimonia are fully captured by measures of life satisfaction or positive emotions. Rather, wholeness and eudaimonia involve the processes of balancing joy and pain, growth and struggle, throughout one's life (Pargament, 1997; Vittersø, 2013).

As a prelude to this discussion, it is important to emphasize that, although it is useful to contrast the elements of wholeness and brokenness, the reality is that each of us is in part whole and in part broken. Wholeness is always a work in progress; no one can achieve full wholeness because we remain human, finite, and flawed. The challenge in the search for significance is to become as whole as possible in the context of our human woundedness, limitations, frailties, and struggles. Wholeness and brokenness then are not two black-and-white options for living. They are interrelated. In fact, as we will see later in the chapter, human weakness, vulnerability, and brokenness can become a spur to greater wholeness.

25.1.1 Purposive vs. Aimless

Wholeness is marked by a deep sense of purpose and direction in life. Vittersø (2013) similarly regards meaning as an element of optimal functioning, adding that a meaningful life is not necessarily a happy one. The quality of purposiveness within an orienting system is encapsulated by 13-year-old Anne Frank's (2010, p. 214) declaration: "I know what I want, I have a goal, an opinion, I have a religion and love. Let me be myself and then I am satisfied." Her diary reveals a clear, guiding vision of herself and her life within the chaotic context of the Nazi regime bent on its destructive agenda beyond her hiding space. When the orienting system is purposive, the search for significance becomes itself significant. Life is made meaningful. This element is also found in eudaimonic identity theory (Waterman, 1993), where purposiveness gives way to feelings of personal expressiveness.

Spirituality is often intimately involved in the articulation of human purpose (Pargament, 1997). Theologian Paul Tillich (1957) defined faith as "the state of being ultimately concerned" and "the centered movement of the whole personality toward something of ultimate meaning and significance" (p. 123). Building on this perspective, Emmons (1999, 2005) conducted research in which he asked people to define their key goals or strivings in life. Individuals who reported a higher proportion of spiritual strivings in their list of goals manifested less conflict among their goals as a whole and a greater purpose in life. Thus, spirituality appeared to serve as a higher-order framework of meaning providing people with an overarching organization to lower-level goals and values by bringing them into the realm of the sacred. Other studies have also shown that having an ultimate concern has important implications for well-being (Ryff, 1989; Zika & Chamberlain, 1992). In a national U. S. survey of older adults, Krause (2003) found that those who experienced greater meaning in life derived from religion reported greater life satisfaction, self-esteem, and optimism. Generally, people who infuse their goals with sacred purpose also endorse greater levels of investment and commitment to those strivings, and benefit from increased meaning in life and positive emotions (Mahoney et al., 2005; Martos, Kézdy, & Horváth- Szabó, 2011; Todd, Houston, & Odahl-Ruan, 2014; Todd, McConnell, & Suffrin, 2014).

On the dark side, however, people who struggle to find an ultimate meaning experience lower levels of life satisfaction and poorer mental health, including more depressive symptoms, generalized anxiety, anger, and loneliness (Exline, Pargament, Grubbs, & Yali, 2014). Like those drifting on a boat rudderless at sea, people who are unable to discover or construct a greater meaning to their lives find themselves totally at the mercy of the larger forces that surround them. Aimless and facing an existential void, individuals become more likely to fill that void with unsatisfactory substitutes, such as devotion to destructive leaders or addictions to drugs, alcohol, sex, gambling, and materialism (Faigin, Pargament, & Abu-Raiya, 2014).

25.1.2 Broad and Deep vs. Narrow and Shallow

An orienting system that is whole is broad and deep. Breadth is the orienting capacity to encompass the full range of challenges and transitions that life brings. Depth refers to the ability to see more deeply into life, and to be able to grapple with complex, intense, and paradoxical experiences. Spiritual and political leader Mahatma Gandhi exhibited both of these qualities in his personal vision for religious pluralism in India, proclaiming, "I want the cultures of all the lands to be blown about my house as freely as possible. But I refuse to be blown off my feet by any." As this quote highlights, Gandhi was able to perceive other people, including those from faiths outside of his own, as spiritual beings. His capacity to see the sacred in the stranger was, in turn, linked with a spirituality marked by tremendous breath and openness to engaging others. Indeed, interfaith engagement represents one pathway to a broader and deeper orienting system (Patel, 2012). In this vein, Mayhew (2014) conducted a longitudinal national survey in which he linked college students' interfaith activities with more appreciative attitudes towards other beliefs, a more pluralistic orientation toward other religions, and greater time spent reflecting upon their religious perspective in relation to those of others. This suggests that when individuals adopt a mindset of religious pluralism, faith deepens and perspective expands.

In contrast, a less whole or well-integrated orienting system is narrow and shallow. This lack of range and depth tends to cause problems for individuals and those around them. For instance, Phillips (1997) introduced the problem of "small gods" – one-dimensional, underdeveloped representations of the sacred. Gods can become too small in many possible ways: when they are perceived as purely punitive beings lacking mercy or compassion, when they are viewed as indulgent deities that fail to challenge individuals to live better lives, when they are seen as passively removed from the affairs of this world, or when they offer love and protection only to those who affirm a particular religious identification. These limited representations of the sacred fail to equip people with the full range of resources needed to handle life's complex problems (Pargament, 2011). Moreover, small gods can cause problems for others. Unfortunately, in the world today, there is no shortage of religious groups that define those who fall outside the protective shield of their own religious umbrella and exclusivist gods, as transgressors, ungodly, and even evil (Doehring, 2013).

Rather than being limited to any one religious group, religious exclusivism can be found among most major religious traditions, including Christians, Jews, Muslims, Hindus, and Buddhists. Followers of Nichiren Buddhism, for instance, believed solely in the teachings of the Lotus scripture and forcefully proselytized these beliefs in Japan during the Kamakura period (Anesaki, 1916). Another example that is salient today would be the Islamic State's efforts to force its radical version of Islam on other people. Using meta-analysis, Hall, Matz, and Wood (2010) have shown that measures of religious exclusivism predict greater right-wing authoritarianism, which is in turn linked to greater prejudice toward out-group members such as sexual minorities (Laythe, Finkel, Bringle, & Kirkpatrick, 2002), African Americans (Brandt & Reyna, 2014) Jews (Pargament, Trevino, Mahoney, & Silberman, 2007), and Muslims (Abu-Raiya, Pargament, Mahoney, & Trevino, 2008). According to Abu-Raiya, Pargament, Mahoney, and Trevino (2011), prejudice comes from the perception of having one's sacred values threatened by the out-group. And once others are defined as dangerous outsiders rather than fellow children of God, the stage is set for acts of violence justified in the name of the most sacred ideals. Based on content analyses of interviews with college students, Hunsberger and Jackson (2005) have also posited that people with highly exclusivist orientations tend to think less complexly about existential or religious topics, which impedes their capacity to integrate challenging experiences into their religious schemas. In this way, the prejudice and bigotry generated by exclusivist orienting systems could be explained, in part, by a narrow perspective of the sacred which can lead in turn to the inhumane treatment of those who do not believe in that same God.

25.1.3 Flexible and Enduring vs. Rigid and Unstable

Whole orienting systems are also flexible and enduring. They are able to adapt to changing environments, while maintaining a level of continuity and lasting commitment to the pursuit of significant ends (Pargament, Desai, & McConnell, 2006). Without flexibility and openness to change, the individual would be fixed and frozen, unable to learn from experience, grow, and mature. Without continuity, the individual would be subject to the whims of changing times, moods, and circumstances, disconnected from any guiding commitment that might sustain an enduring sense of identity. A study by McIntosh, Inglehart, and Pacini (1990) provides a case in point. They identified college students who scored highly on both a measure of religious flexibility and a measure of religious commitment. Compared to other religious orientations, these highly religiously flexible and committed students manifested greater well-being, better adjustment to life events, and fewer physical health symptoms. Flexible and enduring orienting systems also help generate new solutions to problems while sustaining the individual's underlying approach to life. Religious purification, a form of religious coping, involves this type of change; the individual experiences the profound benefit of spiritual cleansing while maintaining a commitment to a religious worldview (Pargament, 1997). Consider this example from a Christian woman who spoke about her changes in faith after she was raped:

> [God had] given me a chance to cleanse myself and to renew myself. ...Now, after the incident I have a much, much deeper understanding of why I go to church to practice my religion. ... I'm able to live my life daily in a new way, a new purpose and with so much more meaning. (de Castella & Simmonds, 2013, p. 544–547)

When stressors threaten the stability of the orienting system, flexibility and continuity help people find new ways to preserve their relationship with the sacred rather than losing faith and significance in their journey. Similarly, Waterman (1993) discusses the practical difficulties associated with self-realization and how individuals approach eudaimonia by navigating alternative pathways and demonstrating persistence in the pursuit of their goals. As outlined in Vittersø's (2013) functional well-being approach, personal growth requires effort and endurance, often in the absence of pleasure.

Orienting systems that are less whole are marked by rigidity and/or instability in the pursuit of significant goals. Religious scrupulosity provides a case in point. The problem here is a rigid spiritual system characterized by religious obsessions and compulsions. In fact, this problem has been labeled a sub-type of obsessive-compulsive disorder, characterized by excessive concern with adherence to religious rules (Greenberg & Huppert, 2010). Sadly, the adherence to these rigid rules, though founded on deep commitment, is ultimately unstable for it interferes with the ability to pursue and reach the more elevated goals of spiritual life. Thus, a religious individual so concerned with the laws of religious purity (e.g., washing hands) may miss attending religious services in which he/she feels a deep connection to God. Scrupulosity has been associated with lower levels of spiritual well-being, life satisfaction, and self-esteem and higher levels of anxiety and depression (Allen & Wang, 2014; Greenberg & Huppert, 2010).

25.1.4 Balanced, Cohesive, and Discerning vs Unbalanced, Incohesive, and Non-reflective

A great piece of music is more than a random set of notes, tempos, and volumes. A composer puts these and other elements of music together to create a work that has its own distinctive integrity and wholeness. Consider how a celebrated composer's repertoire also fits together authentically and cohesively; a piece by Bach sounds different from a piece by Stravinsky. Composing calls for discernment on the part of the musical creator – the ability to find the right response to the right challenge in the right context at the right time. These same abilities are essential elements of a whole orienting system and wisdom (Kitchener & Brenner, 1990; Sternberg, 2004) more generally. In an orienting system of greater wholeness, the individual is able to use his/her discernment to put the diverse pieces of life together into a cohesive pattern. This can be a challenging process, given life's competing demands: how to balance role commitments to work and family, how to integrate desires for personal autonomy and social intimacy, how to make a mark on the world while coming to terms with human limitations and finitude. Some empirical research suggests that people who are able to integrate these competing desires and demands have higher levels of well-being and less stress and depression (Ménard & Brunet, 2011; Ryan, LaGuardia, & Rawsthorne, 2005; Ryan & Martela, Chap. 7, this volume).

Balance, cohesion, and discernment are also emphasized in diverse religious traditions. In the *Serenity Prayer*, the final line ("God grant me the serenity to accept things I cannot change, Courage to change things I can, and wisdom to know the difference") is an appeal to God for the wisdom to discern between the changeable and unchangeable aspects of one's life. Moreover, Taoist teachings are primarily concerned with harmony and balance, symbolized by the opposing *yin and yang* energies (Tzu, 2012). In fact, the Taoist practice of *tai chi*, a martial art known for its calm, meditative movements, is empirically linked with various health benefits, including psychological well-being (Wang et al., 2010), improved cognitive functioning (Wayne et al., 2014), and better sleep-quality in older adults (Du et al., 2015). Wallace and Shapiro (2006) also provide an excellent conceptualization of well-being, informed by Buddhist principles, as four types of mental balance: Conative balance is maintained through wholesome intentions that contribute to the long-term welfare of oneself and others; attentional balance is the capacity for sustained focus and awareness; cognitive balance comes from an undistorted view of the world; and affective balance is rooted in stable and appropriate emotional reactions. In addition to balance within each area, we suggest that balance among all life domains, including the spiritual, is essential to a whole orienting system. For instance, work-life balance is associated with better physical and mental health, higher levels of life and job satisfaction, and lower levels of anxiety and depression (Haar, Russo, Suñe, & Ollier-Malaterre, 2014; Lunau, Bambra, Eikemo, van der Wel, & Dragano, 2014).

In contrast, individuals with more broken orienting systems have difficulty negotiating competing demands, roles, needs, and challenges. They may lack a capacity to reflect on themselves and their lives, and as a result, are unable to succeed in pulling the disparate pieces together into a cohesive pattern. Recall the dramatic case of Robert Oxnam who, prior to treatment, was unable to integrate his different personalities into a unifying, overarching identity. Palmer (2004) described his own battle negotiating his desires for success as an academic psychologist with his more deeply felt desire to explore spirituality and well-being. For many years, he hid his "true self." Waterman (1993) might conceptualize the way in which Palmer had been living as lacking in authenticity and failing to reflect his *daimon*, or his guiding spirit. But confronted with periods of depression, Palmer engaged in reflective soul-searching and transformed his life to one more consistent with his sacred aspirations. Or consider how people can lose their balance in the religious realm, by conflating religious teachings with self-serving beliefs. One active street criminal justified his violent behavior on religious grounds, saying he's "giving punishment to them for Jesus" (Topalli, Brezina, & Bernhardt, 2012, p. 12). Indeed, research has shown that people who are low in mindfulness tend to exhibit poorer coping mechanisms (Pepping, O'Donovan, Zimmer-Gembeck, & Hanisch, 2014) and act less ethically (Ruedy & Schweitzer, 2010). Conversely, mindfulness interventions have led to improved well-being and decreased stress in both clinical and non-clinical samples (Gu, Strauss, Bond, & Cavanagh, 2015). Through the practice of nonjudgmental focus on one's present thoughts and emotions, individuals seem better equipped to find their inner balance.

25.1.5 Benevolent and Life-Affirming vs. Non-benevolent and Life-Limiting

Orienting systems that are more whole are also benevolent and life-affirming. Many religious traditions describe a loving, caring God or benevolent force at play in the universe. A number of empirical studies have found clear connections between these divine beliefs and feelings, greater well-being, and lower distress (Hall & Fujikawa, 2013; Krause, Emmons, & Ironson, 2015). Conversely, negative beliefs and emotions related to God have been consistently linked with anxiety, depression, and poorer health. For instance, belief in a cruel God is predictive of greater anger at God (Exline, Grubbs, & Homolka, 2015), and people who experience more anger at God tend to be more prone to physical symptomatology and emotional distress (Exline, Park, Smyth, & Carey, 2011).

Another outgrowth of the benevolent worldviews of major religious traditions is the virtue of having compassion for oneself and others. The world's religions directly promote the virtue of benevolence in their teachings. The word *mudita*, from Buddhist philosophy, refers to the unselfish joy that arises from others' happiness. Similarly, the *Rig Veda*, an ancient Hindu text, says "The person who is always involved in good deeds experiences incessant divine happiness." Benevolence thrives within the large and growing number of faith-based charities around the world. Spirituality may also indirectly encourage goodwill. In an experiment that involved anonymously leaving money for a stranger, theists acted less selfishly when primed with spiritual words, such as "divine," "sacred," or "God" (Shariff & Norenzayan, 2007). In other words, theists who are exposed to religious content tend to act in ways that benefit others rather than themselves (Shariff, Willard, Andersen, & Norenzayan, 2015).

Individuals are rewarded for the good behavior that may have been prompted in part by their spirituality. This affirmation is often experienced as "warm fuzzies," or feelings of positivity and warmth from helping others. For example, spending money on others rather than oneself tends to make the spender happier (Dunn, Gilbert, & Wilson, 2011). Volunteer work is also associated with health and well-being, particularly among older adults (Jenkinson et al., 2013; Kumar, Calvo, Avendano, Sivaramakrishnan, & Berkman, 2012). In addition, compassion for oneself is associated with well-being and better interpersonal relationships (Neff, 2009). The spirit of benevolence is captured by the 14th Dalai Lama (1998): "If you want others to be happy, practice compassion. If you want to be happy, practice compassion." As such, the element of benevolence fits with Vittersø's (2013; Chap. 17, this volume) notions that people who are living the good life are more motivated to help others and promote happiness as a result of their optimal functioning.

On the other hand, non-benevolent and life-limiting systems seem to cripple the spirit, particularly when intense feelings of guilt and shame are directed inward. Marya Hornbacher (1999) writes poignantly about how these moral emotions fueled her eating disorders:

> I wanted to kill the me underneath. That fact haunted my days and nights. When you realize you hate yourself so much, when you realize that you cannot stand who you are, and this deep spite has been the motivation behind your behavior for many years, your brain can't quite deal with it.

Such feelings, left unresolved, have strong linkages with depression (Kim, Sangmoon, Thibodeau, & Jorgensen, 2011; Zahn et al., 2015) and spiritual struggles of a moral nature (Exline et al., 2014; Murray & Ciarrocchi, 2007). More specifically, religious guilt and shame due to perceived wrongdoing are tied to suicidality (Exline, Yali, & Sanderson, 2000). Similarly, Worthington and Langberg (2012) have proposed that guilt, shame, and perceived moral failure give rise to self-condemnation. They highlight self-forgiveness as a pathway to greater wholeness, a process that involves an appeal to God, grounded in the Christian notions of boundless mercy and the inevitability of human failings. In this sense, spirituality can act as a benevolent and life-affirming force in the lives of those who bear the weight of traumatic experiences.

25.2 Re-orientation and the Cultivation of Wholeness Through Struggles

Our description of the elements that distinguish greater wholeness from greater brokenness may leave the impression that wholeness and the orienting system are static and unchanging. That is not the case. The movement toward wholeness is an ongoing process. And this process of change is not necessarily pain or stress-free. Stimulated in part by internal developmental transitions and by external events, major and minor, people experience times of tension, conflict, and struggle which may serve as precursors to changes in the orienting system and wholeness. Of particular importance here are spiritual struggles, defined as tensions and conflicts around sacred matters with respect to the supernatural, other people and institutions, and within oneself (Exline, 2013; Pargament, Murray-Swank, Magyar, & Ano, 2005). Spiritual struggles have to do with the most fundamental issues of life – questions of ultimate meaning, good and evil, religious doubts, intimacy, the divine and one's relationship with a higher power (Exline et al., 2014). These struggles are fundamentally dis-orienting; they shake people to their very core. A number of studies have linked struggles in the spiritual domain to psychological, social and physical signs of distress (Exline, 2013). But distress and dis-orientation are not the end of the story.

As people struggle, they try to re-orient themselves to the challenges posed by internal transitions and external events. Although popular culture has sentimentalized the value of difficult life experiences, as we hear in statements such as "no pain, no gain" and "suffering builds character," it must be stressed that efforts to re-orient following difficult life experiences are not necessarily successful. Some people experience only pain, suffering, and brokenness through their struggles. In this regard, higher levels of spiritual struggles have been associated with decline in immune functioning (Trevino et al., 2010), increases in depression (e.g., Pirutinsky, Rosmarin, Pargament, & Midlarsky, 2011), and even greater risk of dying (Pargament, Koenig, Tarakeshwar, & Hahn, 2001).

It is true, however, that spiritual struggles can be a source of growth and greater wholeness. Fowler (1981) speaks to this point in his theory of faith development, "Growth and development in faith also result from life crises, challenges, and the kinds of disruptions theologians call revelation. Each of these brings disequilibrium and requires changes in our ways of seeing and being in faith" (pp. 100–101). Empirical studies have shown some ties between spiritual struggles and reports of growth following trauma and major life events (e.g., Gall, Charbonneau, & Florack, 2011; Magyar-Russell, Pargament, Trevino, & Sherman, 2013; Trevino, Archambault, Schuster, Richardson,

& Moye, 2012). This aligns with Vittersø's (2013) functional well-being perspective, wherein personal growth results from successful adaptation to the unknown, and is an essential element for optimal functioning. We suspect this growth is manifested by shifts in orienting systems that become more whole; that is, more deeply purposive, broader and deeper, more flexible, more coherent and discerning, and more benevolent and life-affirming. In support of this notion, Desai and Pargament (2015) compared college students following a period of spiritual struggle who experienced growth or decline. Those who reported greater growth were able to find greater meaning from their struggle, were able to draw on more positive religious coping resources, had a more secure relationship with God, and had integrated religion more fully into their lives.

It is important to add that the relationship between brokenness and wholeness is neither simple nor straightforward. As we noted earlier, according to most religious traditions, brokenness is part of the human condition. And there is a fluid relationship between wholeness and brokenness, as Frankel (2005) described: "Just when things seem to be falling apart or ending, new life is often generated, and just when we think we have it all together, things often fall apart" (p. 16). Brokenness, in particular, creates opportunities for greater wholeness. Writing to this point from a spiritual perspective, Harvey (1991) said: "The heart must break to become large... when the heart is broken, then God can put the whole universe in it" (p. 54). The condition of brokenness then offers the potential for re-orientation, fundamental shifts in one's approach to life that can lead even the most shattered individual toward greater wholeness.

25.3 Wholeness, Optimal Functioning, and Eudaimonic Well-Being

There are several areas where wholeness and eudaimonia intersect. Wholeness as optimal functioning can produce eudaimonic well-being. As Johnson (1955, p. 98) has stated, "Integration of the personality means the effective coordination of interest, emotions, and intentions. The unified harmonious functioning of all one's powers brings a sense of well-being." We have further illustrated how several elements of a whole orienting system overlap with Vittersø's (2013) principles underlying the functional well-being approach to eudaimonia and the components of optimal functioning: (a) autonomy, (b) social relations, (c) meaning, and (d) personal growth. In particular, both wholeness and functional well-being are concerned with the breadth of experiences and balance of emotions. William James (1902, p. 333) has similarly noted the important role of these elements:

> Excess, in human faculties, means usually one-sidedness or want of balance; for it is hard to imagine an essential faculty too strong, of other faculties equally strong be there to cooperate with it in action. Strong affections need a strong will; strong active powers need a strong intellect; strong intellect needs strong sympathies to keep life stead. If the balance exist, no one faculty can possibly be too strong – we only get the strong all-around character… spiritual excitement takes pathological forms whenever other interests are too few and the intellect too narrow.

Additionally, both wholeness and eudaimonia are value-laden in their conceptualizations and largely process-focused, whereas hedonic well-being is outcome-focused (Besser-Jones, 2016). Another point of convergence in our conceptualizations of wholeness and eudaimonia can be found in Besser-Jones' (2014) organismic integration theory, which underscores people's innate drive to organize and integrate experiences, resulting in better functioning.

However, a major point of divergence between wholeness as optimal functioning and eudaimonic well-being is that the former encompasses both objective and subjective elements while the latter emphasizes the subjective, "feeling" component. Wholeness is not limited to feelings and emotions. The orienting system includes cognitive, behavioral, relational, motivational as well as affective aspects of life, and negative feelings do not necessarily signal a lack of wholeness. For instance, a whole person living through a broken time may display an abundance of sorrow. In fact, the inability to experience sorrow in times of tragedy may be a sign of brokenness. Wholeness as optimal functioning also differs from Waterman's (1993) conceptualization of eudaimonia in that wholeness considers the degree of integration among domains rather than separately assessing functioning within each domain. In other words, the wholeness framework is holistic rather than domain-specific.

Because the wholeness framework encompasses both objective and subjective assessment of functioning, it is useful in distinguishing between eudaimonic and hedonic approaches to well-being. The hedonic lifestyle is reflected in elements of a broken orienting system. Non-benevolence, imbalance, and shallowness, for instance, are manifest in narcissistic or extremely self-centered behaviors. Although narcissism is associated with higher scores on measures of life satisfaction, life expectancy, psychological well-being, and social skills (Aghababaei & Blachnio, 2015; Jonason, Baughman, Carter, & Parker, 2015), it damages interpersonal relationships in the long run. Lyons and Hughes (2015) observed that narcissistic persons engage in more malicious forms of gossip intended to negatively influence others. People who feel more narcissistically entitled also tend to be more easily offended and unforgiving (Exline, Baumeister, Bushman, Campbell, & Finkel, 2004). A disproportionate focus on hedonic pursuits corrupts the spirit and one's personal identity, leading to greater fragmentation. Indicators of a broken orienting system function as signals of this disintegration. Perhaps unsurprisingly, narcissism is inversely related to religiosity (Watson, Hood, Morris, & Hall, 1986). The disfigured portrait of Dorian Gray, from Oscar Wilde's literary classic, captures the spiritual damage that results from a lifetime of hedonic pursuits (Jonason et al., 2015). As illustrated, whole and broken elements of an orienting system are linked to eudaimonic and hedonic lifestyles, respectively, and the latter may not function optimally.

Moreover, the traditional view of optimal functioning focuses on the development and pursuit of goals that are meaningful to the individual (Vittersø, 2013). From the wholeness perspective, however, certain pathways and destinations are neither healthy nor eudaimonic. Consider the goals of materialism or instant gratification, which may be perceived as meaningful, and the pathways of self-deception or "winning at all costs." From a wholeness perspective, these would be viewed as signs of dis-integration in the orienting system. As such, wholeness departs from other definitions of optimal functioning in that it evaluates both the pathways and destinations set by individuals in terms of multiple criteria (e.g., life-affirming vs. life-limiting; broad and deep vs. narrow and shallow).

25.4 Conclusion

In this chapter, we focused on one critical aspect of optimal functioning, wholeness, and its relationships to eudaimonia and holiness. As seen in the lives of Robert Oxnam, Anne Frank, Gandhi, and the Dalai Lama, there are many pathways towards wholeness, and each person's journey is different. Wholeness does not translate into blandness or uniformity across personalities. Rather, people move toward wholeness in ways which incorporate their particular quirks, idiosyncrasies, and frailties into their orienting systems. Orienting systems of greater wholeness are deeply purposive, broad and deep, flexible and enduring, balanced, cohesive, and discerning, and benevolent and life-affirming. More broken systems, in contrast, are aimless, narrow and shallow, rigid and unstable, imbalanced, incohesive, and non-reflective, and non-benevolent and life-limiting. We also focused on the points of convergence and divergence between wholeness and eudaimonic well-being. Wholeness facilitates both the subjective feelings of eudaimonic well-being and the objective assessment of functioning. As the wholeness framework rests on a systems-based conceptualization of optimal functioning, it calls for holistic rather than domain-specific assessment. Elements of wholeness versus brokenness can also signal eudaimonic and hedonic approaches to well-being, respectively. Furthermore, wholeness expands upon optimal functioning in its evaluation of both pathways and destinations set by the individual by criteria that go beyond the subjective sense of meaningfulness. Finally, we considered ways that spirituality can facilitate both wholeness and brokenness. When the power of spirituality is harnessed for good, it promotes the ingredients of wholeness and well-being. Yet spirituality can also be expressed in ways that lead to greater brokenness. Even so, brokenness is not necessarily the last chapter of the story. Spiritual struggles and the problems that ensue can lead to fundamental re-orientation and subsequent transformation and growth toward greater wholeness over time.

Moreover, our conceptualization of wholeness as optimal functioning has practical relevance. As described here, wholeness involves the interplay among cognitive, affective, behavioral, relational, and motivational dimensions of life. It follows that efforts to facilitate optimal functioning must go beyond an exclusive focus on subjective appraisals to encompass the complex interplay among the various ingredients that make up a whole life. Furthermore, by attending to sacred aspects of the personal search for significance, we may enhance the impact of our efforts to help people "live the good life," and promote the well-being of society as a whole. Promising steps have already been taken to facilitate greater wholeness through psychospiritual interventions (Pargament, 2011), interfaith initiatives in higher education (Patel & Meyer, 2011), and holistic healthcare (Balboni et al., 2007, 2011).

Thinking of wholeness as a key dimension of well-being does add some complexity to our jobs as researchers and practitioners. As we have described it here, wholeness is a dynamic, multi-dimensional, and multi-layered construct. But the concept of wholeness is also one that resonates with efforts to understand and improve people's lives in all of their richness and fullness. We believe a focus on wholeness adds an important dimension to current approaches to understanding optimal functioning and eudaimonic well-being. Our understanding of wholeness, in turn, can be enriched by attending to spirituality; wholeness and holiness are intimately related and any attempt to cultivate wholeness that overlooks the spiritual dimension, we believe, is likely to be incomplete. Our take-home point is this: wholeness and holiness are important elements of eudaimonia and deserve further attention from researchers and practitioners.

References

Abu-Raiya, H., Pargament, K. I., Mahoney, A., & Trevino, K. (2011). On the links between perceptions of desecration and prejudice toward religious and social groups: A review of an emerging line of inquiry. *Implicit Religion, 14*(4), 455–482. doi:10.1558/imre.v14i4.455.

Abu-Raiya, H., Pargament, K. I., Mahoney, A., & Trevino, K. (2008). When Muslims are perceived as a religious threat: Examining the connection between desecration, religious coping, and anti-Muslim attitudes. *Basic and Applied Social Psychology, 30*(4), 311–325. doi:10.1080/01973530802502234.

Aghababaei, N., & Błachnio, A. (2015). Well-being and the Dark Triad. *Personality and Individual Differences, 86*, 365–368. doi:10.1016/j.paid.2015.06.043.

Allen, G. E., & Wang, K. T. (2014). Examining religious commitment, perfectionism, scrupulosity, and well-being among LDS individuals. *Psychology of Religion and Spirituality, 6*(3), 257. doi:10.1037/a0035197.

Anesaki, M. (1916). *Nichiren: The Buddhist prophet*. Cambridge, MA: Harvard University Press.

Balboni, T. A., Balboni, M., Paulk, M. E., Phelps, A., Wright, A., Peteet, J., et al. (2011). Support of cancer patients' spiritual needs and associations with medical care costs at the end of life. *Cancer, 117*(23), 5383–5391. doi:10.1002/cncr.26221.

Balboni, T. A., Vanderwerker, L. C., Block, S. D., Paulk, M. E., Lathan, C. S., Peteet, J. R., et al. (2007). Religiousness and spiritual support among advanced cancer patients and associations with end-of-life treatment preferences and quality of life. *Journal of Clinical Oncology, 25*(5), 555–560. doi:10.1200/JCO.2006.07.9046.

Besser-Jones, L. (2014). *Eudaimonic ethics: The philosophy and psychology of living well* (Vol. 27). New York: Routledge.

Bhikkhu, S. (1985). *The giving rise of the ten kinds of mind of the Bodhisattva/the discourse on the ten wholesome ways of action*. Kuala Lumpur, Malaysia: Syarikat Dharma.

Brandt, M. J., & Reyna, C. (2014). To love or hate thy neighbor: The role of authoritarianism and traditionalism in explaining the link between fundamentalism and racial prejudice. *Political Psychology, 35*(2), 207–223. doi:10.1111/pops.12077.

Dalai, L., & Cutler, H. C. (1998). *The art of happiness: A handbook for living*. New York: Riverhead Books.

de Castella, R., & Simmonds, J. G. (2013). "There's a deeper level of meaning as to what suffering's all about": Experiences of religious and spiritual growth following trauma. *Mental Health, Religion & Culture, 16*(5), 536–556. doi:10.1080/13674676.2012.702738.

Desai, K. M., & Pargament, K. I. (2015). Predictors of growth and decline following spiritual struggle. *The International Journal for the Psychology of Religion, 25*, 42–56. doi:10.1080/10508619.2013.847697.

Doehring, C. (2013). An applied integrative approach to exploring how religion and spirituality contribute to or counteract prejudice and discrimination. In K. I. Pargament, A. Mahoney, & E. P. Shafranske (Eds.), *APA handbook of psychology, religion, and spirituality (Vol 2): An applied psychology of religion and spirituality* (pp. 389–403). Washington, DC: APA Press.

Du, S., Dong, J., Zhang, H., Jin, S., Xu, G., Liu, Z., et al. (2015). Taichi exercise for self-rated sleep quality in older people: A systematic review and meta-analysis. *International Journal of Nursing Studies, 52*(1), 368–379. doi:10.1016/j.ijnurstu.2014.05.009.

Dunn, E. W., Gilbert, D. T., & Wilson, T. D. (2011). If money doesn't make you happy, then you probably aren't spending it right. *Journal of Consumer Psychology, 21*(2), 115–125. doi:10.1016/j.jcps.2011.02.002.

Emmons, R. A. (1999). *The psychology of ultimate concerns: Motivation and spirituality in personality*. New York: Guilford.

Emmons, R. A. (2005). Striving for the sacred: Personal goals, life meaning, and religion. *Journal of Social Issues, 61*(4), 731–745. doi:10.1111/j.1540-4560.2005.00429.x.

Exline, J. J. (2013). Religious and spiritual struggles. In K. I. Pargament, A. Mahoney, & E. P. Shafranske (Eds.), *APA handbook of psychology, religion, and spirituality (Vol 1): Context, theory, and research* (pp. 459–475). Washington, DC: APA Press.

Exline, J. J., Baumeister, R. F., Bushman, B. J., Campbell, W. K., & Finkel, E. J. (2004). Too proud to let go: Narcissistic entitlement as a barrier to forgiveness. *Journal of Personality and Social Psychology, 87*(6), 894. doi:10.1037/0022-3514.87.6.894.

Exline, J. J., Grubbs, J. B., & Homolka, S. J. (2015). Seeing God as cruel or distant: Links with divine struggles involving anger, doubt, and fear of God's disapproval. *The International Journal for the Psychology of Religion, 25*(1), 29–41. doi:10.1080/10508619.2013.857255.

Exline, J. J., Pargament, K. I., Grubbs, J. B., & Yali, A. M. (2014). The religious and spiritual struggles scale: Development and initial validation. *Psychology of Religion and Spirituality, 6*(3), 208. doi:10.1037/a0036465.

Exline, J. J., Park, C. L., Smyth, J. M., & Carey, M. P. (2011). Anger toward God: Social-cognitive predictors, prevalence, and links with adjustment to bereavement and cancer. *Journal of Personality and Social Psychology, 100*, 129–148. doi:10.1037/a0021716.

Exline, J. J., Yali, A. M., & Sanderson, W. C. (2000). Guilt, discord, and alienation: The role of religious strain in depression and suicidality. *Journal of Clinical Psychology, 56*(12), 1481–1496. doi:10.1002/1097-4679.

Faigin, C. A., Pargament, K. I., & Abu-Raiya, H. (2014). Spiritual struggles as a possible risk factor for addictive behaviors: An initial empirical investigation. *The International Journal for the Psychology of Religion, 24*, 201–214. doi:10.1080/10508619.2013.837661.

Fowler, J. W. (1981). *Stages of faith: The psychology of human development and the quest for meaning*. San Francisco: Harper Collins.

Frank, A. (2010). *The diary of a young girl*. New York: Alfred A. Knopf.

Frankel, E. (2005). *Sacred therapy: Jewish spiritual teachings on emotional healing and inner wholensss*. Boston: Shambhala.

Gall, T. L., Charbonneau, C., & Florack, P. (2011). The relationship between religious/spiritual factors and perceived growth following a diagnosis of breast cancer. *Psychology and Health, 26*, 287–305.

Greenberg, D., & Huppert, J. D. (2010). Scrupulosity: A unique subtype of obsessive-compulsive disorder. *Current Psychiatry Reports, 12*, 282–289.

Gu, J., Strauss, C., Bond, R., & Cavanagh, K. (2015). How do mindfulness-based cognitive Therapy and mindfulness-based stress reduction improve mental health and wellbeing? A systematic review and meta-analysis of mediation studies. *Clinical Psychology Review, 37*, 1–12. doi:10.1016/j.cpr.2015.01.006.

Haar, J. M., Russo, M., Suñe, A., & Ollier-Malaterre, A. (2014). Outcomes of work–life balance on job satisfaction, life satisfaction and mental health: A study across seven cultures. *Journal of Vocational Behavior, 85*(3), 361–373. doi:10.1016/j.jvb.2014.08.010.

Hall, T. W., & Fujikawa, A. M. (2013). God image and the sacred. In K. I. Pargament, A. Mahoney, & E. P. Shafranske (Eds.), *APA handbook of psychology, religion, and spirituality (Vol 1): Context, theory, and research* (pp. 277–292). Washington, DC: APA Press.

Hall, D. L., Matz, D. C., & Wood, W. (2010). Why don't we practice what we preach? A meta-analytic review of religious racism. *Personality and Social Psychology Review, 14*(1), 126–139. doi:10.1177/1088868309352179.

Harvey, A. (1991). *Hidden journey: A spiritual awakening*. New York: Penguin Books.

Hornbacher, M. (1999). *Wasted: A memoir of anorexia and bulimia*. New York: Harper Collins.

Hunsberger, B., & Jackson, L. M. (2005). Religion, meaning, and prejudice. *Journal of Social Issues, 61*(4), 807–826. doi:10.1111/j.1540-4560.2005.00433.x.

James, W. (1902). *The varieties of religious experience*. Cambridge, MA: Harvard University Press.

Jenkinson, C. E., Dickens, A. P., Jones, K., Thompson-Coon, J., Taylor, R. S., Rogers, M., … & Richards, S. H. (2013). Is volunteering a public health intervention? A systematic review and meta-analysis of the health and survival of volunteers. *BMC Public Health, 13*(1), 773. doi:10.1186/1471-2458-13-773.

Johnson, P. (1955). *The psychology of religion*. Nashville, TN: Abingdon Press.

Jonason, P. K., Baughman, H. M., Carter, G. L., & Parker, P. (2015). Dorian Gray without his portrait: Psychological, social, and physical health costs associated with the Dark Triad. *Personality and Individual Differences, 78*, 5–13. doi:10.1016/j.paid.2015.01.008.

Kim, S., Thibodeau, R., & Jorgensen, R. S. (2011). Shame, guilt, and depressive symptoms: a meta-analytic review. *Psychological Bulletin, 137*(1), 68. doi:10.1037/a0021466.

Kitchener, K. S., & Brenner, H. G. (1990). Wisdom and reflective judgment: Knowing in the face of uncertainty. In R. J. Sternberg (Ed.), *Wisdom: Its nature, origins, and development* (pp. 212–229). New York: Cambridge University Press.

Krause, N. (2003). Religious meaning and subjective well-being in late life. *The Journals of Gerontology Series B: Psychological Sciences and Social Sciences, 58*(3), S160–S170. doi:10.1093/geronb/58.3.S160.

Krause, N., Emmons, R. A., & Ironson, G. (2015). Benevolent images of God, gratitude, and physical health status. *Journal of Religion and Health*, 1–17. doi:10.1007/s10943-015-0063-0

Kumar, S., Calvo, R., Avendano, M., Sivaramakrishnan, K., & Berkman, L. F. (2012). Social support, volunteering and health around the world: Cross-national evidence from 139 countries. *Social Science & Medicine, 74*(5), 696–706. doi:10.1016/j.socscimed.2011.11.017.

Laythe, B., Finkel, D. G., Bringle, R. G., & Kirkpatrick, L. A. (2002). Religious fundamentalism as a predictor of prejudice: A two-component model. *Journal for the Scientific Study of Religion, 41*(4), 623–635. doi:10.1111/1468-5906.00142.

Lunau, T., Bambra, C., Eikemo, T. A., van der Wel, K. A., & Dragano, N. (2014). A balancing act? Work–life balance, health and well-being in European welfare states. *The European Journal of Public Health, 24*(3), 422–427. doi:10.1093/eurpub/cku010.

Lyons, M. T., & Hughes, S. (2015). Malicious mouths? The Dark Triad and motivations for gossip. *Personality and Individual Differences, 78*, 1–4. doi:10.1016/j.paid.2015.01.009.

Magyar-Russell, G., Pargament, K. I., Trevino, K. M., & Sherman, J. E. (2013). Religious and spiritual appraisals and coping strategies among patients in medical rehabilitation. *Research in the Social Scientific Study of Religion, 24*, 92–135.

Mahoney, A., Pargament, K. I., Cole, B., Jewell, T., Magyar, G. M., Tarakeshwar, N., et al. (2005). A higher purpose: The sanctification of strivings in a community sample. *The International Journal for the Psychology of Religion, 15*(3), 239–262. doi:10.1207/s15327582ijpr1503_4.

Martos, T., Kézdy, A., & Horváth-Szabó, K. (2011). Religious motivations for everyday goals: Their religious context and potential consequences. *Motivation and Emotion, 35*(1), 75–88. doi:10.1007/s11031-010-9198-1.

Mayhew, M. J. (2014). *Interfaith effectiveness* [PowerPoint slides]. Retrieved from the U.S. Department of Education Center for Faith-based and Neighborhood Partnerships site: http://www.ed.gov/edblogs/fbnp/files/2013/07/Mayhew-Presentation.pdf

McIntosh, D. N., Inglehart, M. R., & Pacini, R. (1990). *Flexible and central religious belief systems and adjustment to college.* Paper presented at the meeting of the Midwestern Psychological Association, Chicago, IL.

Ménard, J., & Brunet, L. (2011). Authenticity and well-being in the workplace: A mediation model. *Journal of Managerial Psychology, 26*(4), 331–346. doi:10.1108/02683941111124854.

Murray, K., & Ciarrocchi, J. W. (2007). The dark side of religion, spirituality, and the moral emotions: Shame, guilt, and negative religiosity as markers for life dissatisfaction. *Journal of Pastoral Counseling, 42*, 22–41. doi:33363020.

Neff, K. D. (2009). Self-compassion. In M. R. Leary & R. H. Hoyle (Eds.), *Handbook of individual differences in social behavior* (pp. 561–573). New York: Guilford Press.

New World Encyclopedia. (2008). Holy. In *New World Encyclopedia.* Retrieved from http://www.newworldencyclopedia.org/entry/Holy

Oxnam, R. (2005). *A fractured mind: My life with multiple personality disorder*. New York: Hyperion.

Palmer, P. J. (2004). *A hidden wholeness: The journey toward an undivided life*. San Francisco: Jossey-Bass.

Pargament, K. I. (1997). *The psychology of religion and coping: Theory, research, practice*. New York: Guilford Press.

Pargament, K. I. (2011). *Spiritually integrated psychotherapy: Understanding and addressing the sacred.* New York: Guilford Press.

Pargament, K. I. (2013). Searching for the sacred: Toward a nonreductionistic theory of spirituality. In K. I. Pargament, J. J. Exline, & J. W. Jones (Eds.), *APA handbook of psychology, religion, and spirituality* (pp. 257–273). Washington, DC: APA Press.

Pargament, K. I., Desai, K. M., & McConnell, K. M. (2006). Spirituality: A pathway to posttraumatic growth or decline? In L. G. Calhoun & R. G. Tedeschi (Eds.), *Handbook of posttraumatic growth: Research and practice* (pp. 121–137). New York: Lawrence Erlbaum Associates.

Pargament, K. I., Koenig, H. G., Tarakeshwar, N., & Hahn, J. (2001). Religious struggle as a predictor of mortality among medically ill elderly patients: A 2-year longitudinal study. *Archives of Internal Medicine, 161*, 1881–1885. doi:10.1001/archinte.161.15.1881.

Pargament, K. I., & Mahoney, A. (2005). Sacred matters: Sanctification as a vital topic for the psychology of religion. *The International Journal for the Psychology of Religion, 15*(3), 179–198. doi:10.1207/s15327582ijpr1503_1.

Pargament, K. I., Murray-Swank, N., Magyar, G., & Ano, G. (2005). Spiritual struggle: A phenomenon of interest to psychology and religion. In W. R. Miller & H. Delaney (Eds.), *Judeo-Christian perspectives on psychology: Human nature, motivation, and change* (pp. 245–268). Washington, DC: APA Press.

Pargament, K. I., Trevino, K., Mahoney, A., & Silberman, I. (2007). They killed our Lord: The perception of Jews as desecrators of Christianity as a predictor of anti-Semitism. *Journal for the Scientific Study of Religion, 46*(2), 143–158. doi:10.1111/j.1468-5906.2007.00347.x.

Patel, E. (2012). *Sacred ground: Pluralism, prejudice, and the promise of America*. Boston: Beacon.

Patel, E., & Meyer, C. (2011). The civic relevance for interfaith cooperation for colleges and universities. *Journal of College and Character, 12*(1), 1764. doi:10.2202/1940-1639.

Pepping, C. A., O'Donovan, A., Zimmer-Gembeck, M. J., & Hanisch, M. (2014). Is emotion regulation the process underlying the relationship between low mindfulness and psychosocial distress? *Australian Journal of Psychology, 66*(2), 130–138. doi:10.1111/ajpy.12050.

Peterson, C., & Seligman, M. E. (2004). *Character strengths and virtues: A handbook and classification*. New York: Oxford University Press.

Phillips, J. B. (1997). *Your God is too small*. New York: Touchstone Books.

Pirutinsky, S., Rosmarin, D. H., Pargament, K. I., & Midlarsky, E. (2011). Does negative religious coping accompany, precede, or follow depression among Orthodox Jews? *Journal of Affective Disorders, 132*, 401–405. doi:10.1016/j.jad.2011.03.015.

Ruedy, N. E., & Schweitzer, M. E. (2010). In the moment: The effect of mindfulness on ethical decision making. *Journal of Business Ethics, 95*(1), 73–87. doi:10.1007/s10551-011-0796-y.

Ryan, R. M., LaGuardia, J. G., & Rawsthorne, L. J. (2005). Self-complexity and the authenticity of self-aspects: Effects on well being and resilience to stressful events. *North American Journal of Psychology, 7*(3), 431–448. Retrieved from http://www.selfdeterminationtheory.org/SDT/documents/2005_RyanLaGuardiaRawsthorne_NAJP.pdf

Ryff, C. D. (1989). Happiness is everything, or is it? Explorations on the meaning of psychological well-being. *Journal of Personality and Social Psychology, 57*(6), 1069. doi:10.1037/0022-3514.57.6.1069.

Shariff, A. F., & Norenzayan, A. (2007). God is watching you priming God concepts increases prosocial behavior in an anonymous economic game. *Psychological Science, 18*(9), 803–809. doi:10.1111/j.1467-9280.2007.01983.x.

Shariff, A. F., Willard, A. K., Andersen, T., & Norenzayan, A. (2015). Religious priming: A meta-analysis with a focus on prosociality. *Personality and Social Psychology Review*. doi:10.1166/1088868314568811.

Smith, H. (1958). *The world's religions*. New York: Harper Collins.

Sternberg, R. J. (2004). What is wisdom and how can we develop it? *The Annals of the American Academy of Political and Social Science, 591*(1), 164–174. doi:10.1177/0002716203260097.

Tedeschi, R. G., & Calhoun, L. G. (2004). Posttraumatic growth: Conceptual foundations and empirical evidence. *Psychological Inquiry, 15*(1), 1–18. Retrieved from http://www.jstor.org/stable/20447194

Tillich, P. (1957). *Dynamics of faith*. New York: HarperCollins.

Todd, N. R., Houston, J. D., & Odahl-Ruan, C. A. (2014). Preliminary validation of the Sanctification of Social Justice Scale. *Psychology of Religion and Spirituality, 6*(3), 245. doi:10.1037/a0036348.

Todd, N. R., McConnell, E. A., & Suffrin, R. L. (2014). The role of attitudes toward white privilege and religious beliefs in predicting social justice interest and commitment. *American Journal of Community Psychology, 53*(1–2), 109–121. doi:10.1007/s10464-014-9630-x.

Topalli, V., Brezina, T., & Bernhardt, M. (2012). With God on my side: The paradoxical relationship between religious belief and criminality among hardcore street offenders. *Theoretical Criminology, 17*(1), 49–69. doi:10.1177/1362480612463114.

Trevino, K. M., Archambault, E., Schuster, J., Richardson, P., & Moye, J. (2012). Religious coping and psychological distress in military veteran cancer survivors. *Journal of Religion and Health, 51*, 87–98.

Trevino, K., Pargament, K. I., Cotton, S., Leonard, A. C., Hahn, J., Caprini-Faigin, C. A., et al. (2010). Religious coping and physiological, psychological, social and spiritual outcomes in patients with HIV/AIDS: Cross-sectional and longitudinal findings. *AIDS and Behavior, 14*, 379–389. doi:10.1007/s10461-007-9332-6.

Tzu, L. (2012). *Lao-tzu's Taoteching: With selected commentaries from the past 2,000 years*. Port Townsend, WA: Copper Canyon Press.

Vittersø, J. (2013). Functional well-being: Happiness as feelings, evaluations and functioning. In S. A. David, I. Boniwell, & A. Conley Ayers (Eds.), *The Oxford handbook of happiness* (pp. 227–244). Oxford, UK: Oxford University Press.

Wallace, B. A., & Shapiro, S. L. (2006). Mental balance and well-being: Building bridges between Buddhism and Western psychology. *American Psychologist, 61*(7), 690. doi:10.1037/0003-066X.61.7.690.

Wang, C., Bannuru, R., Ramel, J., Kupelnick, B., Scott, T., & Schmid, C. H. (2010). Tai Chi on psychological well-being: Systematic review and meta-analysis. *BMC Complementary and Alternative Medicine, 10*(1), 23. doi:10.1186/1472-6882-10-23.

Waterman, A. S. (1993). Two conceptions of happiness: Contrasts of personal expressiveness (Eudaimonia) and hedonic enjoyment. *Journal of Personality and Social Psychology, 64*, 678–691.

Watson, P. J., Hood, R. W., Morris, R. J., & Hall, J. R. (1986). The relationship between religiosity and narcissism. *Counseling and Values, 31*(2), 179–184. doi:10.1002/j.2161-007X.1986.tb00490.x.

Wayne, P. M., Walsh, J. N., Taylor-Piliae, R. E., Wells, R. E., Papp, K. V., Donovan, N. J., et al. (2014). Effect of Tai Chi on cognitive performance in older adults: Systematic review and meta-Analysis. *Journal of the American Geriatrics Society, 62*(1), 25–39. doi:10.1111/jgs.12611.

Worthington, E. L., Jr., & Langberg, D. (2012). Religious considerations and self-forgiveness in treating complex trauma and moral injury in present and former soldiers. *Journal of Psychology and Theology, 40*(4), 274. doi: 84442312.

Zahn, R., Lythe, K. E., Gethin, J. A., Green, S., Deakin, J. F. W., Young, A. H., et al. (2015). The role of self-blame and worthlessness in the psychopathology of major depressive disorder. *Journal of Affective Disorders, 186*, 337–341. doi:10.1037/a0021466.

Zika, S., & Chamberlain, K. (1992). On the relation between meaning in life and psychological well-being. *British Journal of Psychology, 83*(1), 133–145. doi:10.1111/j.2044-8295.1992.tb02429.x.

Positive Interventions That Erode the Hedonic and Eudaimonic Divide to Promote Lasting Happiness

26

Dianne A. Vella-Brodrick

26.1 Introduction

The desire to live the 'good life' of health and happiness is strong for countless individuals. However, happiness can be an elusive and unsustainable goal. It is for this reason that interest in the field of positive psychology – which focuses on promoting optimal states of functioning and flourishing – continues to burgeon across the globe. There is considerable hope that this scientific discipline will provide direction to the average and not so average person on how to attain the good life. In fact, such is the anticipation and enthusiasm, that the application of positive psychology can at times precede the scientific verification. While there is some merit to proactively pursuing well-being, adopting an ad hoc and intuitive approach can hamper progress and undermine the scientific basis underpinning positive psychology. This is especially true in light of findings indicating that subjective accounts do not always align with scientific findings and can be laden with biases (Wilson & Gilbert, 2003, 2005). For example, it has been found that individuals are generally unreliable forecasters of what will make them happy, particularly in relation to long term happiness. This occurs because there are biases associated with recall, salience and current mood that influence decision-making (Wilson & Gilbert, 2003, 2005). Hence, there is a pronounced level of responsibility felt by those working in the area of positive psychology to contribute scientific knowledge on factors for promoting the 'good' life, and to translate these findings into reliable and practical well-being interventions.

The aim in this chapter is to briefly discuss the broad characteristics of a good life, and to underscore the importance of a multi-faceted well-being framework that accurately represents the good life as it plays out in the real world, in its many and varied forms. I will then provide an overview of some core interventions designed to achieve these positive qualities and in so doing, I will critique what I see as the often arbitrary and simplified divisions between eudaimonia and hedonia. The focus will then shift to a discussion about the relevance of intervention content, delivery processes and individual and environmental factors for intervention success. Here I will refer to some of the research I have conducted with colleagues and students and the insights gained along the way. It will be argued that the characteristics of the intervention alone, are not sufficient to predict whether or not it will be effective – the system within which the positive intervention is embedded is equally as important.

D.A. Vella-Brodrick (✉)
Melbourne Graduate School of Education, Centre for Positive Psychology, University of Melbourne, Melbourne, Victoria, Australia
e-mail: dianne.Vella-Brodrick@unimelb.edu.au

J. Vittersø (ed.), *Handbook of Eudaimonic Well-Being*, International Handbooks of Quality-of-Life,
DOI 10.1007/978-3-319-42445-3_26

26.2 Characteristics That Contribute to Lasting Happiness

I will start by asking: what exactly do we mean by the 'good' life? Frequently reported answers are *happiness* and *health*. This sounds simple enough, but on closer inspection, the terms health and happiness are also unclear. These desirable states and outcomes need to be clearly operationalised and accurately measured so that any changes that occur in well-being can be tracked in response to interventions. At face value happiness is often linked with having heightened positive emotions such as joy and excitement. Along these lines, the scientific field of inquiry known as 'subjective well-being' has focused largely on measuring life satisfaction and affect (high positive and low negative affect) using standardised self-report scales (Diener, 1994; Diener, Emmons, Larsen, & Griffin, 1985; Diener, Suh, Lucas, & Smith, 1999). To date, those working in positive psychology have focused predominantly on studying *subjective well-being*, with many adopting positive affect and life satisfaction as the main well-being variables of interest. Although this narrow focus on hedonic aspects of well-being has enabled a deep understanding to be gained about factors contributing to a satisfying and emotionally gratifying life, the full breadth of the well-being experience has not been covered, raising concerns that targeting hedonic aspects of happiness alone could result in adversities rather than benefits. Although experiencing sensory and hedonistic pleasures such as eating a delicious meal, receiving a massage and going shopping can be highly enjoyable, once the stimulus is removed there can be feelings of regret or a desire for more. Ultimately this can lead to a desire for constantly increasing amounts of the stimulus to achieve the same level of satisfaction; a phenomenon referred to as the 'hedonic treadmill' (Diener, Lucas, & Scollon, 2006). For some individuals, this relentless desire for sensory gratification can ultimately lead to addiction and ill health. At an optimal level, however, positive emotions, mood and affect can produce desirable outcomes. For example, Fredrickson (2001) has found that positive emotions can be highly beneficial in helping to broaden and build experiences and resources such as social networks and intellectual capital, and can create increased perceptions of oneness across different cultures (Fredrickson, 2004; Waugh & Fredrickson, 2006; Fredrickson, Chap. 12, this volume). The issue is not so much that positive emotions are not useful and important, but rather that they are not the full complement of ingredients necessary for well-being, particularly if the aim is to achieve *lasting* happiness. To get a more complete understanding of happiness many scholars have adopted a dual category approach to happiness (Kashdan, Biswas-Diener, & King, 2008) which distinguishes between hedonic and eudaimonic characteristics. The former aligns with sensory gratification, positive emotions and life satisfaction, while the latter aligns with allegedly higher level qualities such as growth, life meaning and transcendence.

Although there has been a longstanding fascination, largely by philosophers, with trying to find the optimal formula for happiness including the role of both hedonic and eudaimonic qualities, a rigorous scientific process of investigation was not evident in those early years of investigation. It was not until the late 1950s that psychology scholars began formally studying the constituents of *positive* mental health. One of the forerunners, Jahoda (1958), identified the importance of positive attitudes towards self, mastery, independent thinking, authentic functioning and the realisation of potentials for good mental health. Her work was later refined by Ryff (1989) who found empirically that eudaimonic aspects of well-being, such as self-acceptance, positive relations with others, autonomy, environmental mastery, purpose in life and personal growth, were fundamental to *psychological well-being*. Ryff also developed a corresponding measure, the Ryff Scales of Psychological Well-Being, which provided an alternative measure of happiness to that offered in the field of subjective well-being (see also Ryff, Chap. 6, this volume).

These empirical developments have led to a number of well-being frameworks comprising both hedonic and eudaimonic factors such as positive emotions, quality relationships, fostering hope and meaning through the aspiration and attainment of goals, being authentic and living life to the fullest. Examples include Orientations to Happiness (Peterson, Park, & Seligman, 2005), PERMA (Seligman, 2011) and Complete Mental Health (Keyes, 2002). These contemporary frameworks better represent the complex and multi-faceted nature of well-being and have incited the development of corresponding measures such as the PERMA Profiler (Kern, Waters, Adler, & White, 2015), the Mental Health Continuum (Keyes, 2002) and the Eudaimonic and Hedonic Happiness Inventory (Delle Fave, Brdar, Freire, Vella-Brodrick, & Wissing, 2011). Diener et al. (2010) have also recently developed the Flourishing Scale which assesses social-psychological prosperity and is intended to complement subjective well-being questionnaires. There are now also scales which are specifically designed to measure eudaimonia or central components thereof. For example the Questionnaire for Eudaimonic Well-Being developed by Waterman et al. (2010) has a clear focus on eudaimonia and Steger, Frazier, Oishi, and Kaler's (2006) Meaning in Life Questionnaire specifically assesses a pivotal component of eudaimonia; meaning. Therefore, contemporary understandings of well-being and the 'good' life, include a synthesis of many hedonic and eudaimonic components which can now be measured with scales that are suitably aligned (see also Steger, Chap. 11, this volume).

26.3 Eroding the Hedonic and Eudaimonic Divide

The parallel streams of measuring well-being – subjective and psychological well-being, also referred to as hedonic and eudaimonic approaches respectively– prompted scholars such as Waterman (1993), Huta and Ryan (2010), Huta, Chap. 15, (this volume), and Keyes, Shmotkin and Ryff (2002) to explore the extent to which eudaimonia and hedonia differed. Collectively these findings led to the understanding that eudaimonia provides unique value beyond hedonia in fostering well-being and therefore should not be neglected. A recent study by Baumeister, Vohs, Aaker, and Garbinsky (2013) also supported this position. These authors compared the predictors of (a) being happy (hedonia) and (b) finding life meaningful (eudaimonia), and found that while there were some overlapping aspects, there were also some important differences. The primary differences related to time perspective with happiness being linked with a 'right now' orientation and meaningfulness being associated with a more integrated account of the past, present and future. Happiness was associated with taking rather than giving, while the reverse was found for meaning. Meaningfulness was associated with higher levels of personal identity and self-expression, as well as with higher levels of worry, stress and anxiety compared with happiness. What is evident is that higher levels of both eudaimonia and hedonia correlate differentially with aspects of well-being and mental health and that both elements have important roles to play in relation to heightened levels of well-being.

Preliminary empirical studies examining the relative contributions of hedonic and eudaimonic qualities have confirmed that a full and satisfying life requires both elements. For example, Peterson et al. (2005) have identified in their Orientations to Happiness framework, three distinct pathways to happiness; pleasure, engagement and meaning. To live the 'full life', it is believed that one needs to have elements of all three orientations; with engagement and meaning being especially critical for life satisfaction (Peterson et al., 2005; Vella-Brodrick, Park, & Peterson, 2009). There does however, appear to be a hierarchy of importance with eudaimonic aspects such as engagement and meaning, taking centre stage for optimal well-being. This is consistent with one perspective that the ultimate life goal is to live a virtuous life; one which is synonymous with eudaimonic qualities, and then sensory and emotional happiness will follow (e.g., hedonia is experienced as a byproduct) (Ryff, 1989; Ryan & Deci, 2001; Ryan & Martela, Chap. 7, this volume).

This perspective assumes however, that the divide between hedonia and eudaimonia is clear, real and possibly even sequential. This may not be the case. For example, through a series of six studies with sufficiently large samples, there is evidence to suggest that positive moods may be conducive to reports of higher life meaning and may incite awareness of meaning-relevance for specific situations (King, Hicks, Krull, & Del Gaiso, 2006). Mood has also been found to play an important role in assessing perceived level of authenticity (a eudaimonic quality), with participants feeling more authentic when in a positive mood compared with being in a negative mood (Lenton, Slabu, Sedikides, & Power, 2013). Therefore, the sequence of achieving well-being in terms of which comes first and whether or not one is a byproduct of the other, is not clear. One reason for this is that the boundaries for these two 'categories' of happiness are not always clear. For example, Kashdan et al. (2008) have claimed that there is no single framework that adequately incapsulates the fundamentals of eudaimonia, other than the common element of *excluding* an explicit affective component (see also Ward & King, Chap. 35, this volume). Similarly, Huta and Waterman (2014) have asserted that the eudaimonic category is not sufficiently contained and includes virtually anything that is not classified as hedonic such as self-acceptance, flow, autonomy, relatedness, environmental mastery, personal growth and meaning. It would seem then that for eudaimonia, there is greater inclusion and heterogeneity of characteristics by default rather than by a clear set of criteria. Hedonia on the other hand is a slightly more well considered and contained factor. A further point to note is that in the real world eudaimonia and hedonia can be experienced as an eclectic mix and are at times inseparable. Individuals are unlikely to use a dual category approach for understanding and describing their well-being and happiness experiences. For example an individual might describe at one time point feeling both joy and contentment or sadness and personal growth. This organic and dynamic account deserves to be captured and reported without being reduced to one of two broad categories which have been created largely by scholars.

Collectively these findings suggest that labelling happiness experiences as either eudaimonic or hedonic may be superficial and unrealistic. As per Kashdan et al.'s (2008) recommendation perhaps we should forego using these broad labels in favour of clear facet descriptors. Happiness includes many diverse characteristics that can each provide incremental value. To achieve long lasting happiness the focus may need to be on nurturing the full range of characteristics through well planned positive interventions.

26.4 What Do We Know About the Characteristics of Effective Positive Interventions?

26.4.1 Aligning Inputs and Outputs

There are two important interdependent components of a positive intervention; the content (inputs) and the anticipated and actual outcomes (outputs). Much of the emphasis tends to be placed on the nature and content of the positive intervention and less on clarifying the end goal beyond broad terms such as happiness and well-being. Both components are important as will be outlined in the following section.

In the 1970s Fordyce was among the first to conduct work on positive interventions. He was heavily invested in the development and evaluation of programs to increase happiness (Fordyce, 1977, 1983). The 14 Fundamentals for Happiness program included ideologies and practices such as; keep busy and active, interact with others, stop worrying, stay in the moment and prioritize the attainment of happiness. Finding meaning in your work and being yourself were also important elements of the program that went beyond subjective well-being and into the realm of eudaimonia. These studies found that compared with a placebo control group, those who completed the 14 Fundamentals for Happiness program reported significant boosts to their happiness, some showing effects up to 28 month later. This provided initial evidence that happiness could be improved through intentional strategies and more specifically through an extensive program that involved a combination of hedonic and eudaimonic activities. Considerable thought was placed on inputs by way of developing a thorough program that strategically sought to attain happiness. The Architecture of Sustainable Change model explicates the important role of volition and strategy (Lyubomirsky, Sheldon, & Schkade, 2005). While this model acknowledges the contribution of genetics and situational variables in determining happiness levels, it also recognises that there is scope to enhance happiness levels through volitional activities. This perspective was instrumental in paving the way for the development of positive psychology interventions – deliberate strategies which target feelings, cognitions and behaviours, for improving well-being (Sin & Lyubomirsky, 2009).

Leading scholars within positive psychology have embraced this opportunity to develop and empirically investigate the efficacy of a number of positive interventions designed to enhance well-being. A seminal study by Seligman, Steen, Park and Peterson (2005) examined the effects of five positive psychology interventions (the gratitude visit, three good things in life, you at your best, using signature strengths in a new way, and identifying signature strengths) on well-being and depression in comparison to a placebo control condition. The findings indicated that three of these interventions not only enhanced well-being post intervention but also decreased symptoms of depression. The authors concluded that "Positive interventions can supplement traditional interventions that relieve suffering and may someday be the practical legacy of positive psychology." (p. 410). The outputs focused on the dual model of mental health espoused by Keyes (2007) in that the interventions were assessed in terms of reducing ill-health as well as fostering happiness (subjective well-being). From this point forward the development and dissemination of well-being programs incorporating positive interventions proliferated. There was however, a preoccupation with assessing intervention outcomes in terms of subjective well-being and depression with less attention on eudaimonic characteristics.

Giannopoulos and Vella-Brodrick (2011) recognised the scarcity of research exploring a combination of hedonic and eudaimonic activities and subsequently modified the three good things intervention originally developed by Seligman et al. (2005) into four separate interventions; (a) three pleasurable things (b) three engaging things (c) three meaningful things and (d) one pleasurable, one engaging and one meaningful thing. The results indicated that individuals who were assigned to an activity that differed from their preferred orientation to happiness, reported the greatest improvements in well-being. This was especially pronounced for those with a dominant pleasure orientation. Well-being was assessed using the composite score of the MHC-SF (Keyes, 2009). This 14-item scale measures (a) emotional well-being (positive affect and satisfaction with life); (b) social well-being (one item on each of the facets of social acceptance, social actualisation, social contribution, social coherence and social integration); and (c) psychological well-being as described in Ryff's (1989) model (one item for each of autonomy, environmental mastery, personal growth, positive relations with others, purpose in life and self-acceptance). What can be drawn from this study is that if the aim is to achieve more complete well-being which incorporates emotional, social and psychological components, then the prescribed activities for improving well-being need to correspond with the end goal and should be equally comprehensive. While individuals may have a natural tendency towards a specific pathway to happiness, such as pleasure, there are certain happiness pathways, such as engagement and meaning that are thought to be essential for genuine and enduring happiness. The aim therefore, is to develop a variety of activities that nurture the full range of happiness and to use measures which assess the same constructs. This will help to determine if the outcomes have aligned with the program goals. For example a 5-week program might include: savouring, active constructive responding, best possible self, strengths spotting in others and loving kindness meditation. Such a program is likely to heighten positive feelings and cognitions but also social connection and meaning. Using a single measure of well-being which assesses for example, life satisfaction will not assess the full anticipated effects of the program.

It is acknowledged, however, that attempting to decipher between hedonic and eudaimonic activities and their likely outcomes can be difficult. A single activity may produce emotions and thoughts that characterise numerous aspects of well-being that span across both categories. For instance having a delicious meal with friends may satisfy the tastebuds (hedonia), result in lots of stimulating conversation (hedonia and eudaimonia) and incite feelings of connection and gratitude (eudaimonia); all of which contribute to a heightened sense of well-being. However, what is especially important is the interpretation of that event by the individual involved in terms of the ratio of hedonia and eudaimonia ascribed. More work is needed to avoid making these assumptions and to instead understand the individual experience resulting from the positive interventions.

26.4.2 Importance of the Individual Experience

In future work the individual experience of the intervention needs to be examined more fully and incorporated in interpretations of evaluations. To illustrate, Owens and Patterson (2013) adapted a gratitude and 'best possible self' (BPS) intervention for children aged 5–11 years. They were instructed to draw what they are grateful for (gratitude) or a time in the future when they are at their best (BPS). The children were also asked to complete measures of positive and negative affect, satisfaction with life and self-esteem pre and post intervention. The BPS condition resulted in increased levels of self-esteem in comparison to the control group who were simply asked to "draw a picture of something you did today". It is noteworthy though, that gratitude and BPS interventions are generally designed to promote personal growth and quality relationships and hence have eudaimonic characteristics. However, when the gratitude drawings were analysed into themes, there was a wide range of responses, with the most common ones being sport, friends and family, and pets. Some focused on material hedonistic aspects such as "a new shirt" or having a "ton of money", while others focused on eudaimonic characteristics of being happy such as because "I am helping people" or planting seeds to "help the earth".

The importance of understanding the individual experience of an intervention is also evident in a study by Steger et al. (2013) whereby 86 participants were asked to depict via 9–12 photographs, what makes their life feel meaningful. After a week, participants were asked to rank each photo they had taken in terms of greatest importance to their meaning in life and to write a description of what each photo represented and why this holds meaning for them. Improvements in meaning in life, life satisfaction, and positive affect were reported post intervention – factors associated with both hedonia and eudaimonia. The researchers described auto-photography as a sophisticated way of understanding the various sources of meaning in life for individuals. For some people meaning can be ascribed to materialistic and sensory factors and for others it is represented in relationships with others, nature and a higher entity. This method while quite time intensive can capture more subtle and complex facets underlying meaning and also illustrates the cross-permeation of hedonic and eudaimonic aspects in the way humans experience the world. Adopting a bottom-up rather than top-down perspective can offer less restricted insights garnered by standardised measures which have a tendency to focus on dichotomised conceptualisations of fundamental and complex constructs. The work by Delle Fave, Brdar, Freire, Vella-Brodrick and Wissing (2011) also demonstrates this point. In their study asking 666 participants from 7 countries about their experiences of happiness using open ended questions, it was found that the most common definitions of happiness offered by participants were associated with psychological balance and harmony. This was confirmed with a further study including 2799 adults from 12 countries (Delle

Fave et al., 2016). According to study participants, harmony which entailed emotional stability, being in tune with the universe and balancing desires and achievements, was identified as central to happiness. Not only is it necessary to develop interventions that might impact the full well-being spectrum but it is also necessary to develop assessment tools that will capture subtle changes and underlying processes across the full well-being spectrum and to incorporate qualitative methods into study designs, even if it means studying a smaller group in more detail.

26.5 Assessing Intervention Processes

A study by Monshat et al. (2013) has focused on delivering a quality intervention and detailed assessment of the participant experience. A small group of participants completed six weekly 90 min group mindfulness sessions delivered by an academic who is also a primary care physician with over 20 years' experience in teaching mindfulness. In addition to the face to face mindfulness sessions, audio-recorded instructions and handouts with information about how to apply mindfulness skills to everyday life were provided to participants to supplement the meditation practice. Through the use of focus group, interview, and written and online feedback, an iterative approach to data collection and analysis was attained along with a richness of data that included considerable depth and breadth of the program experience. This level of detail provided insights into not just the outcome but the underlying mechanisms of the program that can influence the outcome. Through this study it was identified that participants typically progress through three core phases as they undergo the mindfulness program; first they experience emotional distress in response to examining their life circumstances, then they use mindfulness as a stress management and relaxation technique which helps them to feel more control over their emotional responses, and finally they come to realise the utility of mindfulness in clearing the mind, self-reflection and better understanding the self. This leads to heightened feelings of confidence and competence. It is plausible that during phase 1 when distress is experienced that individuals may discontinue the activity. It is responsible practice to understand the types of experiences that seemingly 'positive' interventions can harness and to avoid making assumptions that everyone will have positive experiences along the entire journey. These real insights enable researchers and practitioners to be better prepared for any adverse reactions and to develop strategies to minimise harm and maximise benefits for program participants. However, not all interventions will be received in the same way or will be suited to everyone. While it is helpful to detect general patterns of experiences and strategies for responding to these, understanding individual responses is also important particularly if the interventions are intended to be applied with individual clients. Hence an exploration of 'fit' factors is necessary.

26.5.1 Level of Fit

Although there is meta-analytical evidence (Bolier et al., 2013; Sin & Lyubomirsky, 2009) and general consensus that positive psychology interventions are generally beneficial, there are circumstances which heighten the likelihood of a positive outcome. As stated previously, it is therefore necessary to understand the underlying mechanisms that contribute to the intervention effects. Ironically these factors are rarely measured and considered, or at least they are not reported, in many evaluation studies. One set of factors refers to person-activity fit (Sheldon & Lyubomirsky, 2007). This can include a range of individual factors relating to individual readiness and openness such as level of motivation, efficacy beliefs and skill, interest and effort. Demographic factors such as age, gender, education level and culture, as well as activity characteristics such as type of activity (e.g., writing, self-reflection, time required, type of well-being targeted) can also contribute to the activity experience and success. One example relates to a study comparing the effects of two strengths interventions; one focused on using five lesser strengths in a new way and the other focused on using five signature strengths in a new way (Proyer, Wellenzohn, Gander, & Ruch, 2015). It was found that baseline levels of strengths was a pivotal factor. If both the signature and lesser strengths were relatively high then the benefits to happiness and depression were similar for the two interventions, however those with comparatively lower levels of strengths were found to benefit more from working on signature strengths. They also found that high levels of certain strengths, such as persistence, moderated the effects of the intervention.

Proyer et al. (2015) also examined four fit-factors; *preference* (how much they liked and felt they benefitted from the intervention), *continued practice* (level of voluntary practice), *effort* (measured in terms of following instructions and making time for the activity) and *early reactivity* (how quickly they perceived positive effects from the intervention). They found with their sample of 165 women, that all factors differentially influenced happiness and depressive symptom ratings. What these researchers concluded was that "the way people *think* about positive psychology interventions, the way they *work* with them, and the way they *react* to them play a role in predicting well-being at a later point in time", (p. 121) even after 3.5 years. Therefore the human element associated with a positive psychology intervention cannot be ignored. What individuals bring to the table and what they experience and interpret from participating in an intervention will contribute to the success of the intervention.

26.5.2 Enhancing Well-Being at the Group Level

Fit factors can be applied not just to individuals but also to systems. Heightened attention on eudaimonic facets of well-being has fostered an increased interest in promoting health in more diverse ways than for individual benefit alone. There is a shift from focusing predominantly on what will make an individual happy, to the exploration of how individuals can contribute to the well-being of others and on group well-being. For example the work of Quinlan, Swain, Cameron & Vella-Brodrick (2014) examined the effects of a classroom-based strengths intervention on outcome variables such as class cohesion, relatedness and engagement. This *Awesome Us* program was developed for students aged between 9 and 12 years and comprised six 90 min sessions and one follow up session 1 month later. The session content was developed around strengths recognition and goal setting. A battery of standardised scales was used to assess class cohesion and engagement, need satisfaction, strengths use and subjective well-being. Participants who completed the strengths program reported significantly higher class cohesion and relatedness need satisfaction and lower levels of class friction compared with the control group participants. Program participants also reported higher levels of strengths use, positive affect, classroom engagement and autonomy need satisfaction. Importantly, this study is among the first to examine classroom outcomes in response to a strengths program and provides initial support for the use of strengths interventions to improve class climate. This is an example of working towards developing a suite of interventions that can target different outcomes across various systems such as classrooms. Another approach is to develop interventions that focus on different but interdependent dimensions within the individual (e.g., physical health, social, psychological).

26.5.3 Whole Person Interventions in Supportive Contexts

My own research examining the effects of positive education on multidimensional well-being has uncovered the importance of a comprehensive, multipronged approach to promoting and evaluating school-based well-being programs (see Vella-Brodrick, Rickard, & Chin, 2013). For example, the Year 9 Geelong Grammar School (GGS) Timbertop program which includes 60 min of positive education per week over the school year has produced some highly favourable well-being results as determined by both quantitative and qualitative data. More specifically, compared with best-matched control participants from other schools, GGS students completing the Year 9 Timbertop program significantly increased their well-being, post intervention. Examples of areas where they improved include; satisfaction with life, meaning, strengths knowledge and use, optimism, autonomy, gratitude, school enjoyment, physical health and relatedness. It is not surprising that such beneficial outcomes resulting from the Timbertop program were reported given the environmental context in which the program was delivered and the commitment of GGS to delivering the best quality program. First GGS invested in whole school positive psychology training. This enabled the delivery of positive education via a well-trained and dedicated team of staff who form part of a supportive infrastructure. Moreover the positive education program was embedded within a larger outdoor health education program which included hiking, solo camps, cross country running and time in nature. It fostered camaraderie and team cohesion whilst encouraging students to pursue and meet challenges they never thought were possible. This example highlights the need for intervention readiness and preparation, whether on an individual level or on a large organisation or community level. Furthermore, this example demonstrates that positive interventions can have greater impact if embedded within a comprehensive health and well-being program that includes physical activity, psychosocial growth potential and relating to fundamental aspects such as nature. It is critical to develop programs that include multidisciplinary perspectives and take into account nutrition, physical activity, sleep, leisure activities and psychological well-being. For example, the biopsychosocial model developed by Engel (1977) asserts that biological, psychological (e.g., thoughts, emotions, behaviors) and social (socio-economic, socio-environment, culture) elements all contribute to healthy human functioning. Despite recognition of the importance of multiple factors for good health and well-being, seldom are these integrated into a coherent program. So while I argue in this chapter for the erosion of boundaries around hedonia and eudaimonia, I also advocate a similar position for physical and psychological health. Developing interventions or programs that work on both of these interdependent dimensions and add incremental effects may boost levels of well-being.

As with all subjective states, well-being rests on biological foundations. Any attempts to modify well-being must therefore consider the underlying mechanisms supporting this subjective state. The success or otherwise of well-being interventions will ultimately depend on the plasticity of these systems. Interventions that permeate deeply to the biological foundations of well-being are likely to have more sustained effects (see Rickard & Vella-Brodrick, 2014). By including biomarkers of well-being such as cortisol and heart rate variability, interventions which have an impact on these substrates, and subsequently the interventions which may have greater longevity can be identified. Some leading examples of multi-level assessments of well-being involving psychophysiological/biological indices include work by Ryff and Singer (1998), Davidson et al. (2003) and Kok et al. (2013). Interventions with particular characteristics associated with hedonia or eudaimonia may produce deeper changes at the biological level.

26.6 Summary and Recommendations

Positive interventions have the scope to improve the full spectrum of well-being if some careful thought is placed into the intervention design, support infrastructure and end user experiences and requirements. A goal of positive interventions is to enable individuals and groups to experience multiple pathways for well-being which include a combination of eudaimonic and hedonic facets. To thrive, individuals need to be malleable to their circumstances by having a comprehensive response repertoire. Providing a diverse set of interventions that can satisfy sensory needs, trigger joy and laughter and foster personal insight and growth as well as pro-social behaviours suggests that the likelihood of achieving deep and authentic happiness is vastly improved.

The development of a wide number and range of strategies means that there is more variety to maintain interest and to align with person-environment characteristics.

It is also important to align inputs, outputs and processes such that more will be known about not only the effectiveness of an intervention but also the underlying mechanisms for their success or otherwise. Another key point is that the divide between hedonic and eudaimonic interventions is meaningless without the subjective experiences of the user. The aim is to encourage the user of an intervention to optimise each activity by deriving all they can from the experience in terms of basic happiness, personal meaning and service to others. It is this combination of outcomes that makes for the 'good life'.

Acknowledgement I would like to thank Jessie Sun and Hayley Jach for their assistance with editing this chapter.

References

Baumeister, R. F., Vohs, K. D., Aaker, J. L., & Garbinsky, E. N. (2013). Some key differences between a happy life and a meaningful life. *The Journal of Positive Psychology*, *8*(6), 505–516. http://dx.doi.org/10.1080/17439760.2013.830764

Bolier, L., Haverman, M., Westerhof, G. J., Riper, H., Smit, F., & Bohlmeijer, E. (2013). Positive psychology interventions: A meta-analysis of randomized controlled studies. *BMC Public Health*, *13*(1), 119. http://dx.doi.org/10.1186/1471-2458-13-119

Davidson, R. J., Kabat-Zinn, J., Schumacher, J., Rosenkranz, M., Muller, D., Santorelli, S. F., …& Sheridan, J. F. (2003). Alterations in brain and immune function produced by mindfulness meditation. *Psychosomatic Medicine*, *65*(4), 564–570. http://dx.doi.org/10.1097/01.psy.0000077505.67574.e3.

Delle Fave, A., Brdar, I., Freire, T., Vella-Brodrick, D., & Wissing, M. P. (2011). The eudaimonic and hedonic components of happiness: Qualitative and quantitative findings. *Social Indicators Research*, *100*(2), 185–207. http://dx.doi.org/10.1007/s11205-010-9632-5

Delle Fave, A., Brdar, I., Wissing, M. P., Araujo, U., Castro Solano, A., Freire, T., … & Soosai-Nathan, L. (2016). Lay definitions of happiness across nations: The primacy of inner harmony and relational connectedness. *Frontiers in Psychology*, *7*, 30. http://dx.doi.org/10.3389/fpsyg.2016.00030.

Diener, E. (1994). Assessing subjective well-being: Progress and opportunities. *Social Indicators Research*, *31*(2), 103–157. http://dx.doi.org/10.1007/BF01207052

Diener, E., Emmons, R., Larsen, J., & Griffin, S. (1985). The satisfaction with life scale. *Journal of Personality Assessment*, *49*(1), 71–75. http://dx.doi.org/10.1207/s15327752jpa4901_13

Diener, E., Lucas, R. E., & Scollon, C. N. (2006). Beyond the hedonic treadmill: Revising the adaptation theory of well-being. *The American Psychologist*, *61*(4), 305–314. http://dx.doi.org/10.1037/0003-066X.61.4.305

Diener, E., Suh, E. M., Lucas, R. E., & Smith, H. L. (1999). Subjective well-being: Three decades of progress. *Psychological Bulletin*, *125*(2), 276–302. http://dx.doi.org/10.1037/0033-2909.125.2.276

Diener, E., Wirtz, D., Tov, W., Kim-Prieto, C., Choi, D., Oishi, S., & Biswas-Diener, R. (2010). New well-being measures: Short scales to assess flourishing and positive and negative feelings. *Social Indicators Research*, *97*(2), 143–156. http://dx.doi.org/10.1007/s11205-009-9493-y

Engel, G. L. (1977). The need for a new medical model: A challenge for biomedicine. *Science*, *196*(4286), 129–136. http://dx.doi.org/10.1126/science.847460

Fordyce, M. W. (1977). Development of a program to increase personal happiness. *Journal of Counseling Psychology*, *24*(6), 511–521. http://dx.doi.org/10.1037/0022-0167.24.6.511

Fordyce, M. W. (1983). A program to increase happiness: Further studies. *Journal of Counseling Psychology*, *30*(4), 483–498. http://dx.doi.org/10.1037/0022-0167.30.4.483

Fredrickson, B. L. (2001). The role of positive emotions in positive psychology. The broaden-and-build theory of positive emotions. *The American Psychologist*, *56*(3), 218–226. http://dx.doi.org/10.1037/0003-066X.56.3.218

Fredrickson, B. L. (2004). The broaden-and-build theory of positive emotions. *Philosophical Transactions of the Royal Society of London. Series B, Biological Sciences*, *359*(1449), 1367–1378. http://dx.doi.org/10.1098/rstb.2004.1512

Giannopoulos, V. L., & Vella-Brodrick, D. A. (2011). Effects of positive interventions and orientations to happiness on subjective well-being. *The Journal of Positive Psychology*, *6*(2), 95–105. http://dx.doi.org/10.1080/17439760.2010.545428

Huta, V., & Ryan, R. M. (2010). Pursuing pleasure or virtue: The differential and overlapping well-being benefits of hedonic and eudaimonic motives. *Journal of Happiness Studies*, *11*(6), 735–762. http://dx.doi.org/10.1007/s10902-009-9171-4

Huta, V., & Waterman, A. S. (2014). Eudaimonia and its distinction from hedonia: Developing a classification and terminology for understanding conceptual and operational definitions. *Journal of Happiness Studies*, *15*(6), 1425–1456. http://dx.doi.org/10.1007/s10902-013-9485-0

Jahoda, M. (1958). Current concepts of positive mental health. *American Anthropologist, 61.* http://dx.doi.org/10.1037/11258-000

Kashdan, T. B., Biswas-Diener, R., & King, L. A. (2008). Reconsidering happiness: The costs of distinguishing between hedonics and eudaimonia. *The Journal of Positive Psychology*, *3*(4), 219–233. http://dx.doi.org/10.1080/17439760802303044

Kern, M. L., Waters, L. E., Adler, A., & White, M. A. (2015). A multidimensional approach to measuring well-being in students: Application of the PERMA framework. *The Journal of Positive Psychology*, *10*(3), 262–271. http://dx.doi.org/10.1080/17439760.2014.936962

Keyes, C. L. M. (2002). The mental health continuum: From languishing to flourishing in life. *Journal of Health and Social Behavior*, *43*(2), 207–222. http://dx.doi.org/10.2307/3090197

Keyes, C. L. M. (2007). Promoting and protecting mental health as flourishing: A complementary strategy for improving national mental health. *American Psychologist*, *62*(2), 95–108. http://dx.doi.org/10.1037/0003-066X.62.2.95

Keyes, C. (2009). Brief description of the mental health continuum short form (MHC-SF). *American Journal of Public Health*, *100*(12), 2366–2371. http://dx.doi.org/10.2105/AJPH.2010.192245

Keyes, C. L. M., Shmotkin, D., & Ryff, C. D. (2002). Optimizing well-being: The empirical encounter of two traditions. *Journal of Personality and Social Psychology*, *82*(6), 1007–1022. http://dx.doi.org/10.1037/0022-3514.82.6.1007

King, L. A., Hicks, J. A., Krull, J. L., & Del Gaiso, A. K. (2006). Positive affect and the experience of meaning in life. *Journal of Personality and Social Psychology*, *90*(1), 179–196. http://dx.doi.org/10.1037/0022-3514.90.1.179

Kok, B. E., Coffey, K. A, Cohn, M. A, Catalino, L. I., Vacharkulksemsuk, T., Algoe, S. B., … & Fredrickson, B. L. (2013). How positive emotions build physical health: Perceived positive social connections account for the upward spiral between positive emotions and vagal tone. *Psychological Science*, *24*(7), 1123–1132. http://dx.doi.org/10.1177/0956797612470827.

Lenton, A. P., Slabu, L., Sedikides, C., & Power, K. (2013). I feel good, therefore I am real: Testing the causal influence of mood on state authenticity. *Cognition & Emotion*, *27*(7), 1202–1224. http://dx.doi.org/10.1080/02699931.2013.778818

Lyubomirsky, S., Sheldon, K. M., & Schkade, D. (2005). Pursuing happiness: The architecture of sustainable change. *Review of General Psychology*, *9*(2), 111–131. http://dx.doi.org/10.1037/1089-2680.9.2.111

Monshat, K., Khong, B., Hassed, C., Vella-Brodrick, D., Norrish, J., Burns, J., & Herrman, H. (2013). "A conscious control over life and my emotions:" Mindfulness practice and healthy young people. A qualitative study. *Journal of Adolescent Health*, *52*(5), 572–577. http://dx.doi.org/10.1016/j.jadohealth.2012.09.008

Owens, R. L., & Patterson, M. M. (2013). Positive psychological interventions for children: A comparison of gratitude and best possible selves approaches. *The Journal of Genetic Psychology*, *174*(4), 403–428. http://dx.doi.org/10.1080/00221325.2012.697496

Peterson, C., Park, N., & Seligman, M. E. P. (2005). Orientations to happiness and life satisfaction: The full life versus the empty life. *Journal of Happiness Studies*, *6*(1), 25–41. http://dx.doi.org/10.1007/s10902-004-1278-z

Proyer, R. T., Wellenzohn, S., Gander, F., & Ruch, W. (2015). Toward a better understanding of what makes positive psychology interventions work: Predicting happiness and depression from the person × Intervention fit in a follow-up after 3.5 years. *Applied Psychology: Health and Well-Being*, *7*(1), 108–128. http://dx.doi.org/10.1111/aphw.12039

Quinlan, D. M., Swain, N., Cameron, C., & Vella-Brodrick, D. A. (2014, October). How "other people matter" in a classroom-based strengths intervention: Exploring interpersonal strategies and classroom outcomes. *The Journal of Positive Psychology*, *10*(1), 1–13. http://dx.doi.org/10.1080/17439760.2014.920407.

Rickard, N. S., & Vella-Brodrick, D. A. (2014). Changes in well-being: Complementing a psychosocial approach with neurobiological insights. *Social Indicators Research*, *117*(2), 437–457. http://dx.doi.org/10.1007/s11205-013-0353-4

Ryan, R., & Deci, E. (2001). On happiness and human potentials: A review of research on hedonic and eudaimonic well-being. *Annual Review of Psychology*, *52*, 141–166. http://dx.doi.org/10.1146/annurev.psych.52.1.141

Ryff, C. D. (1989). Happiness is everything, or is it? Explorations on the meaning of psychological well-being. *Journal of Personality and Social Psychology, 57*, 1069–1081.

Ryff, C. D., & Singer, B. (1998). The contours of positive human health. *Psychological Inquiry*, *9*(1), 1–28. http://dx.doi.org/10.1207/s15327965pli0901_6

Seligman, M. E. P. (2011). *Flourish: A visionary new understanding of happiness and well-being*. New York: Free Press.

Seligman, M. E. P., Steen, T. a, Park, N., & Peterson, C. (2005). Positive psychology progress: Empirical validation of interventions. *The American Psychologist*, *60*(5), 410–421. http://dx.doi.org/10.1037/0003-066X.60.5.410

Sheldon, K. M., & Lyubomirsky, S. (2007). Is it possible to become happier? (And if so, how?). *Social and Personality Psychology Compass*, *1*(1), 129–145. http://dx.doi.org/10.1111/j.1751-9004.2007.00002.x

Sin, N. L., & Lyubomirsky, S. (2009). Enhancing well-being and alleviating depressive symptoms with positive psychology interventions: A practice-friendly meta-analysis. *Journal of Clinical Psychology*, *65*(5), 467–487. http://dx.doi.org/10.1002/jclp.20593

Steger, M. F., Frazier, P., Oishi, S., & Kaler, M. (2006). The meaning in life questionnaire: Assessing the presence of and search for meaning in life. *Journal of Counseling Psychology*, *53*(1), 80–93. http://dx.doi.org/10.1037/0022-0167.53.1.80

Steger, M. F., Shim, Y., Rush, B. R., Brueske, L. A., Shin, J. Y., & Merriman, L. A. (2013). The mind's eye: A photographic method for understanding meaning in people's lives. *The Journal of Positive Psychology*, *8*(6), 530–542. http://dx.doi.org/10.1080/17439760.2013.830760

Vella-Brodrick, D. A., Park, N., & Peterson, C. (2009). Three ways to be happy: Pleasure, engagement, and meaning – Findings from Australian and US samples. *Social Indicators Research*, *90*(2), 165–179. http://dx.doi.org/10.1007/s11205-008-9251-6

Vella-Brodrick, D. A., Rickard, N. S., & Chin, T.-C. (2013). *Evaluation of youth-led programs run by The Reach Foundation*. Melbourne, Australia: Monash University.

, A. S. (1993). Two conceptions of happiness: Contrasts of personal expressiveness (eudaimonia) and hedonic enjoyment. *Journal of Personality and Social Psychology*, *64*(4), 678–691. http://dx.doi.org/10.1037/0022-3514.64.4.678

Waterman, A. S., Schwartz, S. J., Zamboanga, B. L., Ravert, R. D., Williams, M. K., Bede Agocha, V., … & Brent Donnellan, M. (2010). The questionnaire for eudaimonic well-being: Psychometric properties, demographic comparisons, and evidence of validity. *The Journal of Positive Psychology*, *5*(1), 41–61. http://dx.doi.org/10.1080/17439760903435208.

Waugh, C. E., & Fredrickson, B. L. (2006). Nice to know you: Positive emotions, self-other overlap, and complex understanding in the formation of a new relationship. *The Journal of Positive Psychology*, *1*(2), 93–106. http://dx.doi.org/10.1080/17439760500510569

Wilson, T. D., & Gilbert, D. T. (2003). Affective forecasting. *Advances in Experimental Social Psychology*, *35*, 345–411. http://dx.doi.org/10.1016/S0065-2601(03)01006-2

Wilson, T. D., & Gilbert, D. T. (2005). Affective forcasting: Knowing what to want. *Current Directions in Psychological Science*, *14*(3), 131–134. http://dx.doi.org/10.1111/j.0963-7214.2005.00355.x

Part IV

Eudaimonia and the Society

Eudaimonia and Culture: The Anthropology of Virtue

27

Francis Mckay

27.1 Introduction

> Culture... is the quintessence of all the natural goods of the world and of those gifts and qualities which, while belonging to man, lie beyond the immediate sphere of his needs and wants. All that is good in this sense, all man's gifts and faculties are not necessarily useful in a practical way; though there is no denying that they belong to a truly human life, not strictly speaking necessary, even though he could not do without them. (Pieper, 2009, p. 16)

There have been roughly two general stages in the theorization of eudaimonia. The first is found in the long history of virtue ethics in Western philosophy, a history which had an extended influence in Ancient, Medieval and Renaissance ethical thinking, witnessed a decline during the enlightenment, and reemerged during the mid to late twentieth century in Anglo-American philosophy.[1] What is common to this first stage is a general definition of eudaimonia as composed of three related terms: "virtue," "wisdom," and "flourishing well-being" (Annas, 2011, p. 1; Hursthouse, 1999, pp. 9–13). The second stage, by contrast, is found in the burgeoning empirical studies on what is now called "subjective well-being" (SWB), particularly those works dealing with the concepts of flourishing, fulfilling, or satisfying lives. Such studies appeared mostly at the end of the twentieth century, and they were largely under the purview of the quantitative social sciences, most notably, economics, psychology, neuroscience, and social survey research.[2] What is common to this second stage is a greater reliance on empirical research methods as a way of understanding the elements of eudaimonia (especially as it is considered at the level of the population), and thus a greater engagement with public policy, insofar as the knowledge produced about eudaimonia is hoped to steer political decision making in a direction more conducive to

[1]There are many reasons cited for the apparent decline in virtue ethics in the modern period (see Frede, 2013; MacIntyre, 2007; Schneewind, 1990; Slote, 2015 for important contributions). Regardless of the causes, however, it is generally recognized that Aristotelian ethics played a less obvious role in the modern period until its reemergence in the twentieth century. This resurgence of virtue was largely credited to Anscombe's classic paper "Modern Moral Philosophy" (1958), but her views were developed, challenged, and extended by a range of philosophers from the 1970s onwards, for instance, Geach (1977), Foot (1978), Williams (1981, 1985), Nussbaum (1986, 1994), Taylor (1989), Slote (1992), Annas (1993), McDowell (1998), and Hursthouse (1999).

[2]For an early summary of works in this area see, for instance, Ryan and Deci (2001). For more recent examples, see Huppert and So (2013), Lewis, Kanai, Rees, and Bates (2014), and Vittersø and Søholt (2011).

F. Mckay, PhD (✉)
University of Chicago, Chicago, IL, USA
e-mail: francismckay@uchicago.edu

J. Vittersø (ed.), *Handbook of Eudaimonic Well-Being*, International Handbooks of Quality-of-Life,
DOI 10.1007/978-3-319-42445-3_27

the flourishing of the population at the local, national, and international level.

Both phases are welcome for a number reasons. Not only do they provide a set of conceptual tools for understanding and refining the notion of eudaimonia, they also open it up to rigorous empirical methods, interdisciplinary dialogue, and political interventions. In the transition from philosophical virtue ethics to the quantitative study of subjective well-being, however, an important element of the first stage has been overlooked, namely, the role of culture as an essential foundation for the realization of eudaimonia. Though not always recognized as an essential component of eudaimonia, at the latter end of the twentieth century, virtue ethicists increasingly came to see culture as a necessary condition for acquiring virtue and wisdom and, thus, for achieving a flourishing life. As Mattingly puts it, "Philosophy's virtue ethics provides conceptual support for a historically and culturally shaped understanding of ethics grounded in social practice" (2014, p. 39). By contrast, one can find few discussions in the quantitative investigations of subjective well-being on the necessary historical situatedness of eudaimonia.

The reason for this overlooking of culture no doubt stems from the knowledge-production practices contained within the social sciences themselves. The specific epistemic art of the quantitative social sciences is largely to abstract and reduce the complexity of historical specificities, and to bracket cultural situatedness, in order to provide an account composed of basic key values that can be found across all cultures.[3] This is not a problem per se. One could argue, in fact, that it is precisely the job of those sciences to bracket as many particularities as possible in order to obtain a framework for thinking about eudaimonia (or any other phenomenon) that applies cross-culturally. I suspect, however, the time has come for integration, and that integration, I argue, can come from the qualitative social sciences such as history and anthropology.

In this paper, I therefore argue for the need of a third phase in research on eudaimonia, what I call a "critical eudaimonics."[4] Such a project reintroduces culturally situated understandings of eudaimonia through thick historical and ethnographic descriptions of virtue, wisdom and flourishing well-being to highlight the conditions in which people actually cultivate eudaimonia in everyday life. Moreover, the reason such a stage is needed is because, as I will argue, the elements of eudaimonia (virtue, wisdom, flourishing happiness) do indeed have a cultural history, and that cultural history provides the material, conceptual, and practical resources people draw on in navigating and evaluating "the good life." To put it simply, the relationship between culture and eudaimonia is one which is necessary: culture provides resources for eudaimonia, and without the "gifts" of culture (as Pieper puts it in the lead quote), there would be nothing for human beings to draw upon in order to start the process of cultivating eudaimonia in their everyday lives.

To make the case for eudaimonia and culture, the paper proceeds in three parts. Parts one and two offer an account of eudaimonia, comparing Aristotle's understanding of it with Alasdair MacIntyre's theory of virtue to provide a brief intellectual history for how modern moral philosophers came to see eudaimonia as necessarily possessing a cultural history. Part three then turns to recent understandings of virtue in anthropology, and my own ethnographic research on compassion, to offer a definition of eudaimonia fit for the qualitative social sciences.

27.2 Aristotle

In the *Nicomachean Ethics* (hereafter referred to as NE), Aristotle followed the Greek tradition in conceiving of virtue as an excellence. As he says, "every virtue causes that of which it is a virtue to

[3] A good example here is Peterson and Seligman's *Character Strengths and Virtues: A Handbook and Classification* (2004). This alternative DSM offers a taxonomy of virtues, which although developed initially from historical accounts of the virtues, abstracts from that to provide a universal framework that applies cross-culturally.

[4] I owe my thanks to John Tresch for suggesting this term to me.

be in a good state, and to perform its characteristic activity well" (NE ii.6 1106a15; trans. Crisp). But what exactly does it mean to do an activity well (postponing, for later, the question of what is specifically meant by characteristic activity)? To do something well, according to Aristotle, is to do it "at the right time, about the right things, towards the right people, for the right end, and in the right way" (NE ii.6 1106b20). It is, thus, about rightness of action. And so, the question becomes, what is rightness of action in that case? As he clarifies, it is about achieving the mean between two extremes. Any action, Aristotle notes, can be done in extremes: "fear, confidence, appetite, anger, pity, and in general pleasure and pain can be experienced too much or too little, and in both ways not well" (NE ii.6 1106b17). A virtuous action, however, avoids these extremes and, instead, hits the mean between them.

Exercising virtue in this way is, as Aristotle points out, hard to achieve, and there are two things that make it so. First, as he says, the mean "is not one single thing, nor is it the same for all" (NE ii.6 1106a32). What counts as too much of an action in one context, might be just the right amount in another, or even for another person in the same situation (MacIntyre, 2007, p. 154). Second, following from this, there are no rules one can rely on to ascertain what the mean is and so engage in right action. Rather, figuring out the mean—that is, figuring out what a particular situation requires in terms of right action—requires one to think about *that* situation and to make a judgment about it. So how does one judge? As Aristotle says, "one should rationally choose the mean" (NE vi.1 1138b18). It is, then, the virtuous exercise of this capacity for rational thinking, what he calls practical reason (or practical wisdom, *phronesis*), that allows one to judge well.

There are three key elements to Aristotelian practical reason: desire, deliberation, and a rational choice based upon that deliberation. First, let us take desire: for Aristotle, all desires aim at what is seemingly good for a person. But desires might also be mistaken about the good. People desire all kinds of things and not always what is best for them. Hence, Aristotle distinguishes between what one thinks (pre-reflexively) is good for oneself, and what actually is (and one knows is) good for oneself (MacIntyre, 2007, p. 150). Given this discrepancy, however, one needs a way of distinguishing which desires are the "correct" ones, i.e., which desires genuinely aim at the agent's good, and which do not. For that one needs deliberation.

In deliberation, one rationally judges whether something is good for oneself or not. Such deliberation is holistic and teleological. It is not, in other words, concerned merely with individual decisions, such as what I should have for lunch today, or how I should complete a particular task, but with what I should aim for in life in general, "what conduces to living well as a whole," as he says (NE vi.5, 1140a25). Since, however, what is good for a whole life determines the particular decisions one needs to make in that life, deliberation also entails rationally appraising the means for achieving that end (NE vi.9, 1142b30). Once the agent has deliberated about the ends and means of his or her life, a "rational choice" is then made based upon that practically wise understanding, leading to action (NE vi.10 11439).

Significantly, this rational choice has all the force of logical necessity. As MacIntyre points out, practical wisdom is a kind of "teleo-logic," which takes the form of a practical syllogism, in which the action (the conclusion) is entailed by the premises and the reasoning about those premises (which was provided by the deliberation on desires) (2007, pp. 161–162). Thus, practical wisdom, one might say, is the intellectual virtue of correctly appraising and enacting the good life, insofar as it provides true premises, valid reasoning, and, therefore, sound conclusions about what is in one's best interests. But to be clear, as Aristotle points out, practical reason is not "scientific knowledge" (NE vi.5 1140b). What prevents it from being so is the fact that judgment concerning "the good" is irreducible. Just because one might know what the good is through deliberation, does not mean one can deduce from that what one should do on any particular occasion. There are no formalized rules for how to live the good life. Rather, knowledge of how to proceed toward the good relies on judgment, and good judgment comes from virtue, specifically the intellectual virtue of practical reason, something which itself comes only from experience or from the teachings of other experienced and practically wise persons (NE vi.8 1142a).

If practical reason involves an understanding of the good, what is that conception of the good which is revealed through it? Aristotle is not interested in just any kind of good, but what is *ultimately* good for a person. And what is ultimately good for a person is a person's telos (his final end). Evidence that human beings have an end is revealed through their behavior, which exhibits a series of nested goals: one does *a* to get *b*, and one gets *b* to achieve *c*, and so on. There must be, then, some point at which those nested goals reach terminus in an end point that provides the ultimate context for all the other actions. Such is the final cause of one's actions for Aristotle.

This raises a problem, however: if ends are nested, how can one discern what the end in question is? That is, how does one know a specific value under interrogation is actually the final end and not simply another means masquerading as an end? There needs to be, it seems, criteria for distinguishing sub-goals from final ends. These criteria Aristotle finds in what he calls completeness and self-sufficiency, the former referring to the fact that the good needs to be pursued for its own sake and the latter to the fact that the good should be "unimprovable," as Crisp puts it, by the addition of any other good (2000, p. xii; NE x.2 1172b30).[5]

As it turns out, however, most goods are not like this according to Aristotle. For instance, all extrinsic goods (such as wealth and material objects generally) are never valued for their own sake, but because they enable the acquisition of other goods. They are incomplete and cannot be the ultimate good. By contrast, what Aristotle calls intrinsic goods, though they are valued for their own sake (for that is the definition of an intrinsic good), tend only to be complete in a qualified sense. Although they are pursued for their own sake (and in that sense complete), they are also sometimes valued because they enable the acquisition of other intrinsic goods (and are therefore qualifiedly complete). In this category Aristotle puts virtue in general, because it is valued in itself, but also allows the agent to acquire other intrinsic goods.

There is, however, a category of good which is "always worth choosing in itself and never for the sake of something else" (NE i.7 1097b). This latter good he calls "complete without qualification" (NE i.7 1097b35) or happiness (eudaimonia) for short:

> Happiness in particular is believed to be complete without qualification, since we always choose it for itself and never for the sake of anything else. Honour, pleasure, intellect, and every virtue we do indeed choose for themselves (since we would choose each of them even if they had no good effects), but we choose them also for the sake of happiness, on the assumption that through them we shall live a life of happiness; whereas happiness no one chooses for the sake of any of these nor indeed for the sake of anything else. (NE i.7 1097b)

In addition to being complete without qualification, happiness is also self-sufficient, for when one is happy, one tends not to ask for anything else to improve the situation.

There are two things to note about Aristotle's conception of eudaimonia at this point. The first point concerns the relation between virtues and the ultimate good. As mentioned, virtues are intrinsic goods, but they also have instrumental value, for they allow one to reach the ultimate good of happiness. Indeed, that is the primary function of the virtues. They are, as MacIntyre puts it, "precisely those qualities the possession of which will enable an individual to achieve *eudaimonia* and the lack of which will frustrate his movement toward that *telos*" (MacIntyre, 2007, p. 148). The second point follows from this and concerns the distinction between happiness and teleology. Human beings are by nature teleological for Aristotle. Often, however, humans are unclear about what their final goal is and so one needs criteria by which to recognize what genuinely counts as a final end—found in

[5]In regards to self-sufficiency, if one thinks a life of pleasure is the ultimate good, but one also thinks such a life would be better if one was also wise, then pleasure cannot have been that good, since it would not be self-sufficient, i.e., it would be improved by the other good of wisdom.

the conditions of completeness without qualification and self-sufficiency.

In this view, happiness is, for Aristotle, a kind of folk psychological category for a universal aspiration for teleology. This subtle distinction between happiness and teleology matters because happiness, as a general psychological term, is polyvalent. Sometimes it is used to refer to what provides completeness and self-sufficiency to life, but other times it can be used to describe ways of life possessing intrinsic goods that are only qualifiedly complete or sometimes ways of life obsessed with achieving merely extrinsic goods, as when one confuses happiness with honor, pleasure, or wealth. In such instances, one does not have teleological happiness but, rather, social norms masquerading as ends.

That the ultimate good is eudaimonia, however, does not tell us what it is exactly. To understand that, one needs to return to the notion introduced at the beginning of this section, namely, that of a "characteristic activity." For Aristotle, the characteristic activity of human beings is the capacity for reason, since it is what separates humans from animals and plants (NE i.7 1098a). He also acknowledges, however, that there are two ways in which reason may be exercised. It may be practical, that is, applied to particulars, or it may be theoretical, that is, applied to universals. As such, each application of reason has its own corresponding virtue. In the former case, there is, as has been said already, practical reason (*phronesis*). In the latter case, there is what Aristotle calls intellectual wisdom (*sophia*)—the ability to reason well about non-practical matters. As noted, practical reason cannot be the ultimate good, because it is only qualifiedly complete. It is not just for its own sake, but also for the sake of something else. Hence, one's telos must be found in intellectual wisdom. And since the exercise of that virtue comes through contemplation, it is contemplation that Aristotle says represents the most complete and self-sufficient life. As he puts it, "contemplation alone seems to be liked for its own sake, since nothing results from it apart from the fact that one has contemplated, whereas from the practical virtues, to a greater or lesser extent, we gain something beyond the action" (NE x.7 1177b).

27.3 MacIntyre

Aristotle's conception of eudaimonia is grounded in what MacIntyre calls a "metaphysical biology" (2007, p. 148). It is biological insofar as human beings, by virtue of their nature as a species, do have a final cause, and it is metaphysical insofar as that final cause is found in an activity that is seemingly disengaged from the practical affairs of life. This last point comes from the fact that Aristotle sees in intellectual activity a kind of activity that is most godlike. As he says,

> Such a life is superior to one that is simply human, because someone lives thus, not in so far as he is a human being, but in so far as there is some divine element within him. (NE x.7 1177b26-31)

The contemplative life is thus the most divine life; through it, humans share in the divine. Contemplation, however, is also remarkably impractical and apolitical. As MacIntyre says, "the metaphysical contemplation… which furnishes man with his specific and ultimate telos… is nothing other than thought timelessly thinking itself and conscious of nothing but itself" (2007, p. 158). Such a conception of teleology runs counter to modern thought in a variety of ways. For instance, grounding teleology in biology goes against the presuppositions of modern biology and evolutionary theory, as well as post-modern rejections of grand narratives, while the specific image of metaphysical contemplation is ill-fitted to "secular" Western thought, which is largely skeptical about notions of the divine. The question, then, is whether Aristotle's account still has any use. That is, if Aristotle offers the first systematic account of eudaimonia, but his conception relies on premises fundamentally at odds with contemporary thought, how can one think about eudaimonia without that framework? In short, how does one think about virtue, practical wisdom, and flourishing in the absence of his metaphysical biology? This is the challenge that MacIntyre takes up, offering a conception of teleology, and thus eudaimonia, that is grounded in history and culture.[6] Essential to his argument is a definition of virtue in terms of practice, narrative, and tradition.

Practice-based virtues are what allow the practitioner to acquire "the goods" belonging to a practice (MacIntyre, 2007, p. 191). Practice-based virtues are similar to what one might call a skill, and indeed, recent authors have argued similarly (Annas, 2011; Widlok, 2004). Such a definition of virtue is multi-faceted. What constitutes a virtue depends on the practice, and since practices are multiple, so too are the virtues needed to acquire the goods associated with those practices. In being multiple, however, they are also disunited. That is, there are many different kinds of practices (playing football or the piano, engaging in politics or science, etc.) and the virtues required by each of these practices may often be very different in kind or even incompatible with one another—for instance, as "justice and compassion" might be incompatible with each other in legal practice (Lambek, 2008, p. 145). That said, there is, MacIntyre notes, another level of virtue development, which although related to these practical virtues, also goes beyond them. These are the virtues relative to the whole of life and which MacIntyre finds grounded in narrative and tradition.

In order to have virtues relative to the whole of life, there needs to be some conception of the "whole of life" in the first place, to which the virtues can apply. In the absence of a metaphysical biology, MacIntyre thus turns to what he sees as the universal capacity for narrative to highlight how such a unified notion of the self is possible. By narrative, MacIntyre is referring to the fact that human beings conceive of themselves and their agency in terms of narrative, that is, as having a beginning, middle, and end. All intelligible human actions are thus what he calls "enacted narratives" (2007, p. 211), and these enacted narratives are "teleological" in nature:

> We live out our lives, both individually and in our relationships with each other, in the light of certain conceptions of a possible shared future, a future in which certain possibilities beckon us forward and others repel us, some seem already foreclosed and others perhaps inevitable. There is no present which is not informed by some image of some future and an image of the future which always presents itself in the form of a *telos*—or of a variety of ends or goals—towards which we are either moving or failing to move in the present. (2007, pp. 215–216)

As he also notes, however, narratives involve unpredictability: "it is crucial that at any given point in an enacted dramatic narrative we do not know what will happen next" (2007, p. 215). Hence life involves both a move toward a telos, and the inevitable disclosure that the path there is uncertain, filled with mystery and sometimes even great pain through the various obstacles that prevent one from reaching the good. This is where the virtues acquire their significance. The virtues that are relative to life as opposed to practice are those dispositions that provide the agent with a knowledge of what the good life is as well as the means for achieving it. In his words, the virtues

> sustain us in the relevant kind of quest for the good, by enabling us to overcome the harms, dangers, temptations and distractions which we encounter, and which will furnish us with increasing self-knowledge and increasing knowledge of the good. (MacIntyre, 2007, p. 219)

Though the virtues facilitate the development of an understanding of the means and ends of life, it does not occur blindly. The virtues relative to the whole of life thus require a conception, however preliminary, of the ends of life. This is because without an early conception of the good to begin with, the agent would not be able to take the first step towards it and engage in the deliberation over the viability of that good or how to achieve it. As he says, "Without those moral particularities to begin from there would never be anywhere to begin; but it is in moving forward from such particularity that the search for the good, for the universal, consists" (2007, p. 221). The important point to note is that one acquires that conception not by inventing it oneself. Moral

[6] In his later writings, MacIntyre defends a biological and metaphysical conception of teleology. I will not address those arguments here, but for those interested see *Dependent Rational Animals* (1999).

particularities are socially and historically grounded. Consequently, one acquires it from what MacIntyre calls a "tradition," which provides the moral agent with the conceptual and practical resources for imagining possible means and ends of life.

What is a tradition exactly? MacIntyre describes it as a "historically extended, socially embodied argument, and an argument precisely in part about the goods which constitute that tradition" (2007, p. 222).[7] By the term "argument," however, MacIntyre is not referring to the vexed attempt to prove others wrong, but to an ongoing dialogue about what the proper goods are for life. This argument may occur over long stretches of time. As he says, "Within a tradition the pursuit of goods extends through generations, sometimes through many generations" (2007, p. 222). It is, then, a living discussion, and one not fixed but mutable. Accordingly, the conception of the good life will likely shift over time, especially as it responds to changing historical circumstance. Part of this change comes from the fact that all traditions have room for critique within them, and thus the extension or challenge of whatever conceptions of the good they articulate. In his words, "all reasoning takes place within the context of some traditional mode of thought, transcending through criticism and invention the limitations of what had hitherto been reasoned in that tradition" (2007, p. 222).

Examples of traditions are wide ranging. It may apply to the world's religious traditions (Christianity, Islam, Hinduism, Buddhism, Judaism, and so on). Equally, it may include the tradition of western politics as a shared discourse about what the democratic good is. Similarly both philosophy and science represent traditions (and their sub-divisions, traditions also), while education, healthcare, and agriculture may also represent traditions of thinking about the good life. As he says, "when an institution—a university, say, or a farm, or a hospital—is the bearer of a tradition of practice or practices, its common life will be partly, but in a centrally important way, constituted by a continuous argument as to what a university is and ought to be or what good farming is or what good medicine is" (2007, p. 222). So it seems that many things constitute a tradition for MacIntyre. But the important point is that virtue ethics always takes place within some tradition, which provides the conceptual and practical resources practitioners draw upon in their pursuits of the good life.

27.4 The Anthropology of Virtue

This idea of MacIntyre's, that virtue, practical reason, and the good life acquire meaning only through a "tradition" in which they are embedded, has led to a more general claim in philosophy and anthropology about the need to contextualize virtue in its historical and ethnographic context. This foregrounding of culture and history as a necessary component of the good life has, in fact, been for many a defining feature of modern virtue ethics, the element that distinguishes it from other moral theories such as utilitarianism and deontology, both of which are said to reject historically situated ethics in favor of a universal moral system of rational principles.[8] Consequently, the emphasis given to culture and history has also inspired a view that moral philosophy needs the tools of the qualitative social sciences, in order to carry out the project of a "situated virtue ethics." As Laidlaw says, "it has been natural for virtue ethicists to express the view that philosophy requires 'a dimension of social explanation' (Williams, 1985, p. 131) or 'an ethnographic stance' (Williams, 1986, pp. 203–204), or presupposes 'interpretive ethnography' (Moody-Adams, 1997, p. 169), or should be 'descriptive anthropology' (Baier, 1985, p. 232)" (2014, pp. 47–48).

Over the past 10 years, the call for a culturally situated virtue ethics has been explored through

[7] It is hard to say what a moral tradition is beyond this. As Porter acknowledges, "even though MacIntyre discusses tradition extensively, he never defines the term… nor does he situate his account of tradition in the context of other recent discussions" (2003, p. 36).

[8] See Martha Nussbaum (1999) for an exception to this view.

an emerging anthropology of virtue (see, for instance, Asad, 1993; Hirschkind, 2006; Laidlaw, 2014; Lambek, 2000, 2008, 2010; Mahmood, 2005; Mattingly, 2010, 2014; Pandian, 2009; Robbins, 2004, 2013; Widlok, 2004, 2012). The field owes much to Aristotle, though it is an Aristotle that has been filtered through the works of MacIntyre and Foucault.[9] Thus, from Aristotle, it acquires the concepts of "virtue," "practical reason," and "flourishing" well-being as key components of the good life; from MacIntyre it takes the notions of "narrative" and "tradition" in order to place those concepts found in Aristotle into their historical and cultural context; while from Foucault it borrows from the language of discourse, techniques of power, and techniques of the self to situate virtue ethics not just in relation to history and culture, but to power too (Laidlaw, 2014, p. 48; Mattingly, 2014, p. 35).

In so doing, however, a debate has also opened up in the anthropology of virtue around two different ways of thinking about practical reason. The first is what one might call the "discursive tradition" approach. This approach sees practical reason primarily in terms of habits, which are themselves replications of structures found in a tradition. The second is the "ordinary ethics" approach. Although not blind to the importance of habit and tradition, this approach gives greater weight to the faculty of deliberative judgment in practical reason, arguing for a constantly vigilant subject who draws upon a fragmented set of cultural resources in figuring out the path to the good life. Let me take each in turn.

The first stems from the writings of Talal Asad, who coined the term "discursive tradition" and those followers of his who have extended his insights. For Asad, a discursive tradition is an authoritative epistemic and moral framework, one that provides the context in which practices of virtue acquire their meaning and standards of performance. As he says, "A tradition consists essentially of discourses that seek to instruct practitioners regarding the correct form and purpose of a given practice" (Asad, 2009, p. 14). There are two important points about discursive traditions. First, they are situated in a time and place. As he says, they "relate conceptually to a *past* (when the practice was instituted, and from which the knowledge of its point and proper performance has been transmitted) and a *future* (how the point of that practice can best be secured in the short or the long term, or why it should be modified or abandoned), through a *present* (how it is linked to other practices, institutions, and social conditions)" (Asad, 2009, p. 14). Second, they are "authoritative." They instruct practitioners on the "correct forms" of the good life, and they possess a variety of resources for that end: institutions; moral exemplars, teachers and general authority figures; texts (canonical writings plus commentaries on those writings); actual techniques of the self intended to embody the virtues (for instance, prayers, imitations of moral exemplars, study of texts); conceptual frameworks for understanding the relative value of competing virtues (tables and hierarchies of virtue), and so on. All of these, moreover, are oriented in terms of a specific conception of the good-life, which the tradition holds as the telos of self-disciplinary practices and which practitioners reflect upon and adopt as the ends of their practical reason.[10]

All this is not a problem in itself. A tradition's collective practical reason, as the historical sedimentation of thinking about a way of life, does indeed provide important resources that practitioners draw upon in developing practical reason. In the hands of some of Asad's followers, however, this idea of a discursive tradition shapes a unique interpretation of practical reason itself. For instance, here is what Mahmood has to say on the subject, using the practices of virtue cultivation

[9] I have not discussed Foucault in this essay as his role has been discussed extensively elsewhere (cf. Laidlaw, 2014; Mattingly, 2014).

[10] Thus, as Asad points out, in the tradition of Christianity, there is the institution of the medieval monastery or the Church itself (as well as the ritual practices that occur within those institutions: sermons, liturgies, etc.); the moral exemplar of Jesus Christ and the authority figures of the Church Fathers; the canonical texts (the Bible or the Rule of St. Benedict); commentaries written about these foundational texts; and the practices of faith, hope, charity, humility, prudence, obedience, and so on, that allow one to embody the virtues of that tradition.

amongst the members of the women's mosque movement in Egypt as illustration:

> Even though I focus on the practices of the mosque participants, this does not mean that their activities and the operations they perform on themselves are products of their independent wills; rather, my argument is that these activities are the products of authoritative discursive traditions whose logic and power far exceeds the consciousness of the subjects they enable... The women are summoned to recognize themselves in terms of the virtues and codes of these traditions, and they come to measure themselves against the ideals furbished by these traditions; in this important sense, the individual is contingently made possible by the discursive logic of the ethical traditions she enacts. (2005, p. 32)

On first glance, it may seem that Mahmood here is simply arguing for the important role traditions have in cultivating virtue. She goes beyond that, however, to argue that discursive traditions are authoritative to the point that practical reason becomes synonymous with habit. She draws upon Aristotle's notion of habitus to explain:

> Habitus... is concerned with ethical formation and presupposes a specific pedagogical process by which a moral character is acquired. In this understanding, both vices and virtues—insofar as they are considered to be products of human endeavor, rather than revelatory experience or natural temperament—are acquired through the repeated performance of actions that entail a particular virtue or vice, until all behavior comes to be regulated by the habitus. Thus habitus in this tradition of moral cultivation implies a quality that is acquired through human industry, assiduous practice, and discipline such that it becomes a permanent feature of a person's character. Premeditated learning is a teleological process aimed at making moral behavior a *nondeliberative* aspect of one's disposition. (2001, p. 838; my italics)

Thus, in Mahmood's view, the subject's practical reason finds its fulfilment, if performed diligently, in a nondeliberative habit.

Contrast this, however, with what Laidlaw says on the matter: "for Aristotle the cultivation of virtuous dispositions is not the same as the inculcation of bodily reflexes, and so despite Mahmood's own protestations to the contrary... what she describes is closer to Bourdieu's habitus than it is to Aristotle's hexis... The habit of thinking of habit as un-thinking is not an Aristotelian one" (2014, p. 75). Laidlaw's point is that Mahmood has misinterpreted Aristotle here. Practical reason is not mere habit, he says. Rather, it involves deliberation and judgment. This, then, is where the problem emerges according to the ordinary ethics approach. In the sophistication by which discursive traditions apparently map out paths to the good life, and through the authority they are said to possess on the matter, they take the burden of practical reason off the subject (at least to some degree), and place it in the hands of the tradition itself, which comes to represent a kind of collective practical reason concerning the means and ends of life and which the subject then internalizes by participating in the way of life it advocates. Thus, the capacity of practical reason (as the art of appraising and enacting the good life) becomes de-psychologized, relocated, and reified in the tradition itself, the structures of which the practitioner embodies by habitually following its teachings.

In contrast to this view, however, there is the "ordinary ethics" approach to practical reason. It argues two things. First, it distances itself from the role of habit to foreground the irreducibility of deliberation in navigations of the good life. As Mattingly states:

> people do not deliberate about everything all of the time. Any adequate virtue ethics that takes moral experience seriously must recognize the importance of its habitual and nondeliberative aspects... However, if moral life concerns ongoing attempts to realize ground projects, if we take the *temporality* of morality seriously, in other words, then we can see that small moments and routine activities that, at first glance, appear repetitious, prereflective, or inconsequential come to take on depth as episodes in unfolding narratives of moral striving and as part of conscious commitments to realize particular versions of the good life. (2014, p. 205)[11]

Second, the ordinary ethics approach also departs from the discursive tradition view by situating virtue ethics not in a "tradition" as such, but in

[11]A similar point is made by Lambek when he says: "Practice theory needs to attend to more than power, habit, or competitions of honor and taste and should attend to reasoned judgment as developed in recent accounts of Aristotle's *Ethics*" (2000, p. 310).

the broader domain of culture instead. The concept of tradition, it is said, implies a degree of coherence that may be lacking in everyday commitments to virtue. As Pandian puts it, "certain postulates in MacIntyre's work concerning the necessary coherence of a vital moral tradition—the unity of its canonical foundations, of its narratives of selfhood, and of its collective practices—ought to be loosened for a fuller realization of this possibility" (2008, p. 466). To focus just on that concept of tradition, then, would be to overlook the variety of everyday cultural resources that people draw upon in their deliberations about the good life.

In the next section, I look further at the role of practical reason in terms of these two ideals. My argument will be that one need not think of virtue practices in such a dualistic manner (tradition encouraging habitus, everyday life providing an arena for deliberation). Rather, in contrast to the discursive tradition approach, I want to argue that practical reason, in the form of deliberative judgment, can be cultivated through tradition. To make this case, I focus exclusively on one person, Jay, who dedicated much of his life to balancing the system of modern Buddhist virtue ethics against his existential and mental health concerns. Jay's example is not a story about the large transformations brought about by the commitment to virtue—that is a subject deserving more extensive treatment elsewhere. Rather, it is about a singular moment of judgment, a brief act of micro-virtue, which I hope acts like a refined lens to magnify the realm of culture in even the simplest or mundane of activities, and thus to show how a habituated affect is transformed into a historically specific form of deliberative practical reason.

27.5 Tradition and Everyday Virtue Ethics

I first met Jay in August 2013. At that time, he had recently become a father, and had gone back to school at the age of 41 in order to train to become a therapist. Jay was not interested in just any kind of therapy, however. Rather, he was exclusively focused on becoming a "contemplative psychotherapist," and had consequently signed up for the only course that offered that opportunity in the US, at Naropa University's department of psychology. His reasons for choosing this path in particular stemmed from his own personal commitment to Buddhism, which had been growing steadily in him since he was an undergraduate student in psychology in his early twenties. From one perspective, his interest was an academic one. As he told me,

> While I was in college, my sister was doing meditation and would talk to me about Buddhist ideas. I didn't know much about Buddhism, but talking to her took it from this place of "I would never do this strange, oriental practice" to "this is pretty cool stuff." As a result, I took a class at the university on Buddhism and started meditating as well. At some point I realized: my god, this is psychology.

From another perspective, his interest was a way of exploring what the good in life might be.

> Buddhism started this process of me thinking about how to see the world and how to be in it. Until that time, I had been Christian. But, for me, what the Buddha had to say in his teachings and the approach of the religion, it just seemed more truthful to me. There wasn't a whole lot of power play or unnecessary psychological garbage, which I felt growing up with Christianity.

How did the tradition support him in this regard? By the time I met Jay, he had been heavily invested in the teachings and practices of modern Buddhism for around 20 years and had acquired an appreciation for a wide variety of its offerings during that time. What seemed to motivate Jay most of all, however, was the primacy given to compassion in that framework. As he put it, "In Buddhism, love and compassion are the central tenets. My brain agrees that that's the way to go." Compassion was not the telos of this framework, however; that was reserved for the third noble truth: the cessation of suffering and thus the realization of long-term well-being. Nevertheless, compassion was the most direct means to that end. "Compassion," he said, was "*the* path to happiness." What he found in the surrounding tradition of American Buddhism, then, was a set of resources that gave him hope for embodying that virtue and achieving that happiness.

It would be useful to pause on this idea of cultivating compassion for a moment to see clearly the challenge confronting Jay (or anyone, for that matter). Early in childhood, most people acquire some capacity for compassion on account of the cultural instruction they receive in moral sentiments while growing up. They thus acquire general expectations for what compassion might be and for when it is needed. In that pre-reflective habitus, compassion is often understood to be a "feeling," one which might also be conflated with a variety of other moral sentiments like sympathy, pity, empathy, and so on (that is, if the person has not taken the time to reflect on the subtle distinctions between those capacities).

Attached to this "feeling" might also be an embodied understanding of the standards for when and how to express that compassion. I do not mean to say that Jay completely lacked this important cultural knowledge, but it was also no doubt true, as I found out, that he saw himself as struggling to exercise those moral sentiments due to his uncertain emotional life. The reason for this struggle came from the fact that, around the same time as he was introduced to Buddhism, Jay was diagnosed with having "manic depression," what is now called "bipolar disorder."

> It started when I was 22. Back then it was everything from beautiful visions, to sheer terror. It was paradoxical. I'd feel good, even though I was messed up inside. What I was getting from the inside was not coherent. And on the outside, people were totally thinking there was something very wrong with me.

Given his new diagnosis, his interest in Buddhism turned out to be fortuitous, for at the time, it seemed to offer him a way to navigate his illness experience. As he summarily put it, "One reason I am able to function is that I've been involved in meditation." That said, it was also true that despite his commitment to meditation, Jay had been in and out of the hospital over the years, and that, in addition to meditating, he had also been taking mood stabilizers and seeing a therapist for nearly two decades in order to get some control over his emotional life.

Given these difficulties balancing his moods, how could Jay transform his everyday understanding of compassion into compassion as a virtue? What exactly would it take not only to feel compassion, but to embody it to the point of excellence, such that it could orient a way of life in which Jay would be flourishing through the moral sentiments? Moreover, even if Jay had not had any of these difficulties, the challenge would be no less significant. There is, after all, a big difference between simply having the capacity for compassion in an everyday sense, and raising the standing of compassion in one's hierarchy of values such that it operates as the direct means to the ends of life. The solution to such a problem is not a simple one. On the contrary, it actually motivates a whole series of difficult questions, such as: what is specifically meant by compassion (how does it differ from seemingly similar moral sentiments such as sympathy, pity, empathy, and so on)? What constitutes an act of compassion (is compassion merely having a feeling of concern or does one need to actually interact with the object of compassion in some way)? If one does interact with the object of compassion, how does one know that the interaction in question is really a compassionate one (that is, how does one discern compassionate actions from actions that could be taken another way—is, for instance, punishing a child when he misbehaves an act of compassion or one of cruelty)? Continuing that line of thought, can there be forms of "compassion" which are not actually virtues, but vices (is indulging a child by giving him whatever he wants whenever he wants it an example of compassion as a vice, being kind "to a fault" so to speak)? Moreover, how wide is the scope of compassion (does it apply only to oneself, to family members, to one's countrymen, to all humans, or to all living beings)? And are there any limits to who can embody that compassion (can anyone adopt it—for instance, including those diagnosed with "affective disorders," as Jay was—or is it reserved for only a select few, a moral elite, who specialize in it and take on the burden of helping others for the sake of everyone else)?

All these questions about the meaning of compassion, which arise as a consequence of taking compassion seriously as a virtue, came up for Jay. Moreover, it was in the tradition of modern

American Buddhism that he explored the answers to those questions, by participating in its way of life and drawing on its numerous resources so as to think through the meaning of compassion and what it takes to enact it. In that regard, there were numerous offerings available to him: the various texts of Buddhist metaphysics, epistemology and ethics—an expansive written and oral tradition that stretched as far back as the canonical writings of Buddhism, to the more recent commentaries by the leading figures of the modern mindfulness movement. In those works, Jay found frameworks for thinking about moral agency and advice on how this framework could be applied to everyday life. In addition to those texts, there were also moral exemplars—persons, real or fictional, who illustrated through their character the possibility that such a framework could be actualized in one's life, and who offered guidance through their example and teachings. For Jay, one important exemplar was the living embodiment of compassion himself, the fourteenth Dalai Lama, whom he greatly admired for being able to embody the moral virtues. But there were numerous other examples too: the Buddha, the founding figures of the different varieties of Buddhism, the authors of canonical texts and their commentaries, numerous longtime practitioners and teachers in positions of authority dotted across the landscape of American Buddhism.

Besides exemplars, there were also the institutions where those figures resided, where their teachings were given, and where communities of practitioners could gather in order to acquire and internalize the Dharma (for instance, monasteries, retreat centers, stress reduction clinics, wellness centers in schools and universities, bookshops, meditation centers, and so on). For Jay, the contemplative life had been found largely at meditation centers and retreats in the past, and they provided him with periodic and fragmentary access to the institutional and communal resources of the contemplative life. Now at Naropa, that way of life was woven into every aspect of the curriculum, providing him with long-term access to his tradition and to a community that seemed to be dedicated to the same path as he was.

The most salient resource, however, besides the texts, exemplars, and institutions, was the practice of mindfulness meditation. It was through mindfulness that one "discovered," he said, the truth of the Dharma, and thus the answers to questions about the meaning of compassion. How did mindfulness do this exactly? In order to answer that question, it is important to say a little on the practice of mindfulness as encountered by Jay at Naropa.

27.5.1 Naropa

The view of mindfulness adopted at Naropa was inspired by its founder, Chögyam Trungpa Rinpoche, a Tibetan monk who came to the US after fleeing Tibet during the Uprising of 1958. During the 1970s, Trungpa Rinpoche founded his own modernized—he called it "secular"—version of Buddhism called Shambhala Buddhism, which he taught to the countercultural communities in and around Boulder, CO. Essential to his teachings was the practice of mindfulness meditation. For Trungpa, mindfulness meant gently watching-without-judging the objects of consciousness, being fully aware of the contents of experience, without rejecting any of it as foreign, inappropriate, or blameworthy. As he put it, "Mindfulness is taking an interest in precision of all kinds, in the simplicity of the breath, of walking, of the sensations of the body, of the experiences of the mind—of the thought process and memories of all kinds" (Trungpa, 2003, p. 20). It is that same view which still inspires the work at Naropa today. As one professor put it,

> The technical meaning of mindfulness is the ability to put your mind on an object and keep it there. In a more general sense, it is paying attention without judging. Or, since you can't stop your mind from judging, at least not showing you're judging. The point is to recognize our judgments as judgments and not to impose them on others. That's mindfulness: being present, simply paying attention to details moment by moment, as they arise and dissolve.

It is not possible to detail everything involved in mindfulness practice, but there is a common feature said to be an essential outcome of the practice, namely, the dissolution of habits. Habits were considered by some, in fact, as the very opposite of mindfulness. As one teacher put it,

> What is mindlessness? It's operating out of habit. That's what it is. Operating out of habitual states of mind, which when unexamined feel perfectly normal and accurate, but which are largely learned and lead to all kinds of suffering through reactivity.

Mindfulness, then, is said to break down those "reactive" habits. By inviting the meditator to "simply observe" those patterns, mindfulness opens up a space between cognitive habits and the tendency to enact whatever behaviors were ordinarily projected by those habits.

> It's a matter of bringing awareness to habits; we keep expanding the arena of our awareness without shutting down into habit. As you observe them, you realize that those habitual states of mind cease to have control over you. And as you experience whatever the states of mind or habits are, you start to see that you're not controlled by them, as there's a spaciousness around them.

The next step was to learn how to read that "space" opened up between thought and action in terms of affect, and of compassion in particular.

> We spend much of our lives saying "this is ok, but that's not ok," or "I'll do that, but not this." That's the kind of reactivity I'm talking about. But when you start to rest and relax in this open way, any state of mind can arise, and there's a sense of growing ok-ness about it all, basic ok-ness. And then it just starts to expand like that; a basic ok-ness that you could also call great compassion and great joy.

At Naropa, mindfulness practices were constantly embedded in a discourse that directed the practitioner to read that space of interiority in terms of compassion. To that end there were explicit meditations on compassion. Here contemplatives turned their attention to the feeling of compassion itself, using imagery of loved ones and memories of compassionate moments, to relive that sentiment in one's body and use it as an object of mindfulness practice. An important practice in this regard was Tonglen meditation, which involved visualizing an image of suffering as one breathed in, and then imagining the release of that pain as one released the breath. One contemplative, Diane, described what she did as follows:

> Tonglen instruction—that's breathing in the pain and breathing out the medicine. I remember during a three week retreat I was given that instruction, and when that happened, it was so easy to breathe in the pain of someone I really cared about, and breathe out the remedy or medicine. It was a powerful experience. I can't remember what I did the first time, because it was such a long time ago, but what I do now is… I do it in different ways… I see that person, I visualize them. For instance, with my father, who had a lot of heart issues, I would breathe in what I thought was his pain based on how he described it, and I would feel it in my heart. Then I would breathe out relaxation for him or kindness. Sometimes I would breathe in physical pain and emotional pain. I would just work on those different levels. And I would actually feel it. It's very much based on feeling for me. And if it isn't, then it's only mental and not much happens for me. So yeah, it's about feeling it. I would then do the same practice for others, imaging strangers in similar pains, or even my enemies. If someone who I didn't get along with set me off, I could breathe in some kind of pain and breathe out the antidote. And this leads to a kind of emotional generosity that allows me to think about other beings who I don't even know who have heart issues.

In Tonglen, then, by progressing through different types of objects of suffering (oneself, family members, enemies, strangers), a practitioner widens the scope of compassion. In so doing, he or she learns about—and comes to embody—the meaning of compassion as an ethical virtue: the wish to limit or end the suffering of all beings, and the commitment to which marks the ideal of the Bodhisattva.

Compassion was not just an ethical virtue, however, but an epistemic one too. That is, it included not merely a desire to end the suffering of all beings, but the knowledge of how to do that.

> Paul: When you have that quality of non-struggle, you know much better what to do in the relative world of appearances because you're not fixed in your views. You're able to respond to the relative world of appearances, not based on your memorization of different categories, but based on what needs to happen. Compassion is the capacity to tend to what needs to happen in the relative world based on the clarity of your mind, or heart, or whatever you want to call it.

In compassion, then, one knows what the goal of life is (to end suffering), but one also knows how to act so as to bring that about. This knowledge is not one based in habit, but in reflection on the nature of suffering and a judgment about how to work with that. This knowledge is described as an effortless knowing of what to do, which led to the required action through that knowledge.

27.5.2 Jay's Hospitalization

When I first met Jay, he was doing well. Granted, he had his ups and downs, but for the most part, things were progressing well for him—not only did he gain great fulfillment from being a father, he was steadily realizing his goal of becoming a therapist and was connecting to a tradition of modern Buddhism through which he was exploring his conceptions of the good life. If to flourish is, as Mattingly says (2014, p. 9), to live a good life, or at least to be in reach of the resources for imagining and actualizing what a good life could be, then Jay seemed to be flourishing.

Several months later, however, Jay was in the hospital, recovering from a "manic episode," as he put it, which had left him "delusional," and "incapacitated." It is unclear, he told me, what the precise cause had been. He admitted that he had stopped taking his medication (against the advice of his doctor) just prior to the event, but he was in general ambivalent about whether this was significant or not. Whatever the reason, the effects were dramatic. "My life was utterly destroyed," he said, "and now I have to start from scratch again. I lost everything: my home, wife, car, possessions."

After he recovered, Jay and I talked about his experiences. He told me about the progression leading up to the event: how he had become increasingly "delusional," convinced that he was a person of great importance—a third party candidate, as he said, for the presidency, and someone who the secret service was protecting. He told me about how, after he recovered, he was embarrassed about these delusions, and at having been so "irrational" for so long: "Delusions are embarrassing. You come back to reality and realize what you did and said, and you're embarrassed that that's what you thought or did. I just lost touch with reality at some point. How the hell was I thinking that way for so long?"

As he was telling me all this, it struck me how disconnected he felt from his tradition. Not only had he needed to drop out of school because of the hospitalization, meaning he had no contact with either the community of Buddhist practitioners at Naropa or the material resources of the university, but he also lost connection to his mindfulness practice. "Mindfulness is largely gone in extreme states," he said. "That's what happened to me, I lost that awareness. I used to meditate an hour a day, I couldn't do that now." In fact, so severe was his situation, all he could do each day was to manage himself little by little: he would merely take his medications, eat, sleep, talk with his doctors, rest and so on.

As he continued his story, however, it also became clear that things were not as bleak as they seemed, for something of his tradition had still remained with him:

> There were times when I was just delusional, and my awareness sensors and stuff were "out there," making me vulnerable to all the stuff going on. But this was combined with a sense of the people, places, and things around me that marked this particular cluster of symptoms as having an awareness. I was delusional at the hospital and had a number of things going through my head, like turning off lights and screwing with the night person's system, but I still remember the cops coming to take me and put me in the ambulance. In the past, that awareness and that maintaining of consciousness would have gone away with these delusional stories I had going on in my head. But I really remember quite well a lot of what actually happened. And that was not common in my earlier experiences.

It was not, however, this continued sense of "awareness" that intrigued me the most, but a more subtle capacity, of which even he had not considered the value. Expanding on the story about the importance of compassion to his recovery, he told me of another occasion when he used that same compassion with a fellow patient.

> I was in a group therapy session at the hospital and the man who sat next to me was telling the group about his life. He started to tear up, so I reached out to him, and held his hand for a while. We're not supposed to do that. We're not supposed to touch each other in the room. That's kinda against the rules. But afterward, the guy told me how much he appreciated it. It's funny though, because at the time I just knew that was what he needed. Even though we're not supposed to do things like that in the group meetings, I just knew I needed to hold his hand to show him someone cared.

This act of reaching out may seem like a relatively trivial detail, a small act of courtesy given to a fellow patient. But given Jay's state during the recovery period, it reveals something much more significant than that. Despite the fact that Jay was still struggling with his own rationality, and was reliant on the care of others, he still possessed some resources, however partial, for virtuous compassion.

Where did this compassion come from? It might seem that this was a case of emulation, Jay exhibiting the same compassion his caregivers had shown him during his illness episode. Yet this could not have been the case—Jay understood that touching broke the rules, and he had not witnessed such behavior in his doctors. The compassion he had admired in them had been their ability to listen and understand where he was coming from without judging him. Neither was this an expression of habit for Jay. On the contrary, this reaching out was out of the ordinary for him. Something he had not done before. It was also apparently not an explicit calculation either. Even disregarding the fact that Jay considered his own abilities to think clearly had been impoverished due to his illness, there was no deduction that could have led him from the premises "I must minimize suffering" to the conclusion, "I must hold this person's hand." Too many other possibilities were available for such a deduction to occur. Jay did not seem to know what lead him to choose holding his fellow patient's hands—Jay would only say that he "just knew." In other words, he made an almost imperceptibly quick judgment about what was needed, and acted upon it. And by his account, it was the right judgment to make, confirmed by the warm thanks his neighbor gave him afterward for showing such kindness and for alleviating his pain.

Jay's moment of compassion, though a brief and arguably insignificant one, highlights something important about the relationship between culture and practical reason. Jay initially found the conditions for virtue, wisdom, and well-being in modern American Buddhism, a tradition that he had been dedicated to for many years and which, when I met him, had led him on a path that seemed to be nourishing him in numerous ways, providing him with resources for navigating his eudaimonic concerns. As a result of his hospitalization, however, both the inner and outer resources of his tradition were largely stripped away from him. Unable to connect with the community of contemplatives, and unable to meditate, he relied largely on the support of the hospital staff in navigating his illness. Stripped of both his inner and outer contemplative resources, and entertaining a series of "delusions," his practical reason had been impoverished to the point that others had to be responsible for his overall well-being and to make judgments on his behalf. He was far from flourishing. At the same time, however, he was not completely without support, for in his embodied memory lingered a kind of affective knowledge about how to act for the sake of the good of others.

What can be seen in his decision to hold his neighbor's hand was a small act of compassion, and a kind of practical reason: a compassion-infused practical reason, which he obtained from his earlier training in mindfulness, and which he continued to have access to despite the loss of a range of other faculties. Through the memory of his tradition, Jay could be seen to artfully appraise the means and ends of life—if only for a moment—not through reason or habit or emulation, but through the virtuous application of an affective practical reason, a culturally specific form of practical reason deeply connected with a cultivated sense of compassion. Practical reason thus became, in his hands, an ethico-affective capacity, and a joint epistemic and moral virtue, grounded in the moral sentiment of compassion, by which he momentarily, yet still artfully, appraised the means and end of life.

27.6 Conclusion

My point in this paper is to highlight the necessity of culture in thinking about the good life. If the path to eudaimonic well-being comes through virtue, particularly through the virtue of practical reason, then it is only within culture that such virtues gain meaningful content. It is not enough to say, for instance, that compassion is important for happiness, for to do so says nothing about the meaning of compassion, nor how it is cultivated and practiced, nor how it is connected to flourishing. Such explanations are instead found in the wider symbolic world in which people live, and in tradition in particular, a sub-domain of culture in which thinking about the good life is refined through extensive and sustained investigations of the good. Indeed, for Jay, it was through the tradition of modern American Buddhism that he discovered practices and insights about compassion that provided him with resources and capacities for cultivating virtue, despite the enormous personal challenges he faced in that regard. Without that, he had few means for virtue development. Though the care of his mental health professionals and his medications were no doubt important for bringing him back to what he saw as a state of health, and though during his hospitalization he was no doubt far from flourishing, it was, nevertheless, only through the lingering memory of his tradition that he had access to any potential virtue. What can one learn from this? If I am correct, then there are methodological consequences for the future investigation of eudaimonic well-being. It is not enough, I would argue, to conduct laboratory experiments, or large-scale social surveys, on what is abstractly called eudaimonic well-being. One likely needs that, but one also needs history and ethnography, to see how particular good lives are built: in short, one needs not a science of eudaimonia, but a "critical eudaimonics," grounded in thick description, in order to locate the conditions in which the good life is meaningfully possible.

References

Annas, J. (1993). *The morality of happiness*. New York: Oxford University Press.

Annas, J. (2011). *Intelligent virtue*. Oxford, UK: Oxford University Press.

Anscombe, G. E. M. (1958). Modern moral philosophy. *Philosophy, 33*, 1–19.

Aristotle. (2000). *Nicomachean ethics*. Cambridge, UK: Cambridge University Press.

Asad, T. (1993). *Genealogies of religion: Discipline and reasons of power in Christianity and Islam*. Baltimore: Johns Hopkins University Press.

Asad, T. (2009). The idea of an anthropology of Islam. *Qui Parle, 17*(2), 1–30.

Foot, P. (1978). *Virtues and vices and other essays in moral philosophy*. Berkeley, CA: University of California Press.

Frede, D. (2013). The historic decline of virtue ethics. In D. C. Russell (Ed.), *The Cambridge companion to virtue ethics* (pp. 124–148). Cambridge, UK: Cambridge University Press.

Geach, P. T. (1977). *The virtues*. Cambridge, UK: Cambridge University Press.

Hirschkind, C. (2006). *The ethical soundscape: Cassette sermons and Islamic counterpublics*. Columbia, NY: Columbia University Press.

Huppert, F. A., & So, T. T. C. (2013). Flourishing across Europe: Application of a new conceptual framework for defining well-being. *Social Indicators Research, 110*(3), 837–861. doi:10.1007/s11205-011-9966-7.

Hursthouse, R. (1999). *On virtue ethics*. Oxford, UK: Oxford University Press.

Laidlaw, J. (2014). *The subject of virtue: An anthropology of ethics and freedom*. Cambridge, UK: Cambridge University Press.

Lambek, M. (2000). The anthropology of religion and the quarrel between poetry and philosophy. *Current Anthropology, 41*(3), 309–320. doi:10.1086/300143.

Lambek, M. (2008). Value and virtue. *Anthropological Theory, 8*(2), 133–157. doi:10.1177/1463499608090788.

Lambek, M. (2010). *Ordinary ethics: Anthropology, language, and action*. New York: Fordham University Press.

Lewis, G. J., Kanai, R., Rees, G., & Bates, T. C. (2014). Neural correlates of the 'Good Life': Eudaimonic well-being is associated with insular cortex volume. *Social Cognitive and Affective Neuroscience, 9*(5), 615–618. doi:10.1093/scan/nst032.

MacIntyre, A. C. (2007). *After virtue: A study in moral theory*. Notre Dame, IN: University of Notre Dame Press.

Mahmood, S. (2001). Rehearsed spontaneity and the conventionality of ritual: Disciplines of ṣalat. *American Ethnologist, 28*(4), 827–853.

Mahmood, S. (2005). *Politics of piety: The Islamic revival and the feminist subject*. Princeton, NJ: Princeton University Press.

Mattingly, C. (2010). *The paradox of hope journeys through a clinical borderland*. Berkeley, CA: University of California Press.

Mattingly, C. (2014). *Moral laboratories: Family peril and the struggle for a good life*. Berkeley, CA: University of California Press.

McDowell, J. (1998). *Mind, value, and reality*. Cambridge, MA: Harvard University Press.

Nussbaum, M. C. (1986). *The fragility of goodness: Luck and ethics in Greek tragedy and philosophy* (Cambridge paperback library). Cambridge, UK: Cambridge University Press.

Nussbaum, M. C. (1994). *The therapy of desire: Theory and practice in Hellenistic ethics*. Princeton, NJ: Princeton University Press.

Nussbaum, M. C. (1999). Virtue ethics: A misleading category? *The Journal of Ethics, 3*(3), 163–201.

Pandian, A. (2008). Tradition in fragments: Inherited forms and fractures in the ethics of South India. *American Ethnologist, 35*(3), 466–480. doi:10.1111/j.1548-1425.2008.00048.x.

Pandian, A. (2009). *Crooked stalks: Cultivating virtue in South India*. Durham, NC: Duke University Press.

Peterson, C., & Seligman, M. E. P. (Eds.). (2004). *Character strengths and virtues a handbook and classification*. Oxford, UK: Oxford University Press.

Pieper, J. (2009). *Leisure: The basis of culture; The philosophical act*. San Francisco: Ignatius Press.

Porter, J. (2003). Tradition in the recent work of Alasdair MacIntyre. In M. C. Murphy (Ed.), *Alasdair MacIntyre* (pp. 38–69). Cambridge, UK: Cambridge University Press.

Robbins, J. (2004). *Becoming sinners Christianity and moral torment in a Papua New Guinea Society*. Berkeley, CA: University of California Press.

Robbins, J. (2013). Beyond the suffering subject: Toward an anthropology of the good. *Journal of the Royal Anthropological Institute, 19*(3), 447–462. doi:10.1111/1467-9655.12044.

Ryan, R. M., & Deci, E. L. (2001). On happiness and human potentials: A review of research on hedonic and eudaimonic well-being. *Annual Review of Psychology, 52*(1), 141–166. doi:10.1146/annurev.psych.52.1.141.

Schneewind, J. B. (1990). The misfortunes of virtue. *Ethics, 101*, 42–63.

Slote, M. A. (1992). *From morality to virtue*. Oxford, UK: Oxford University Press.

Slote, M. A. (2015). Virtue's turn and return. *Dao, 14*(3), 319–324. doi:10.1007/s11712-015-9449-7.

Taylor, C. (1989). *Sources of the self: The making of the modern identity*. Cambridge, MA: Harvard University Press.

Trungpa, C. (2003). In G. Carolyn Rose (Ed.), *The collected works of Chögyam Trungpa* (Vol. 2). Boston: Shambhala.

Vittersø, J., & Søholt, Y. (2011). Life satisfaction goes with pleasure and personal growth goes with interest: Further arguments for separating hedonic and eudaimonic well-being. *The Journal of Positive Psychology, 6*(4), 326–335. doi:10.1080/17439760.2011.584548.

Widlok, T. (2004). Sharing by default?: Outline of an anthropology of virtue. *Anthropological Theory, 4*(1), 53–70. doi:10.1177/1463499604040847.

Widlok, T. (2012). Virtue. In F. Didier (Ed.), *A companion to moral anthropology*. Chichester, UK: Wiley-Blackwell.

Williams, B. (1981). *Moral luck: Philosophical papers, 1973–1980*. Cambridge, UK: Cambridge University Press.

Williams, B. (1985). *Ethics and the limits of philosophy*. Cambridge, MA: Harvard University Press.

28 Eudaimonic Well-being: A Gendered Perspective

Leah J. Ferguson and Katie E. Gunnell

28.1 Eudaimonic Well-being: A Gendered Perspective

> "The part can never be well unless the whole is well." Plato

The World Health Organization (2001) defines health as "a state of complete physical, mental, and social well-being and not merely the absence of disease or infirmity" (p. 1). The quote to start this chapter reminds us how intimately connected the various aspects of our health are; thus, the importance of our psychological health to our overall health is paramount. Psychological health can be partitioned into "well-being" and "illbeing". Focusing on the well-being aspect of our psychological health, in this chapter we address gender differences in psychological well-being.[1] The inherent importance of gender when discussing well-being cannot be ignored, as gender is inextricably connected to our daily life and the core of our being. The woman who works tirelessly to become junior partner at her law firm only to make less money than the men in her office may question the pursuit of her goal, just as the man who takes paternity leave to be a stay-at-home father may experience alienation and guilt because many societies tend to view women as primary child caregivers. Gender has an impact on our well-being. In discussing gender differences in this chapter, we outline two traditions of well-being that will continue to surface in this Handbook: *hedonic well-being* and *eudaimonic well-being*. Consideration for both forms of well-being is crucial for a more comprehensive understanding to overall psychological health in both women and men.

28.2 Two Traditions of Well-being

Prior to the recognition of positive psychological well-being, our understanding of psychological health focused on the negative side of psychological functioning. Central to this focus on

[1] Our presentation of gender differences in well-being stems largely from a perspective of gender categorized as either "woman" or "man". In this chapter we adopt this simplified gender division because many researchers examining eudaimonic well-being have employed this dichotomy. That said, we acknowledge that gender is a fluid construct that goes beyond these categories. In the "moving forward" section of our chapter we offer potential avenues for future research to focus on the conceptualization and operationalization of gender in the well-being literature.

L.J. Ferguson (✉)
College of Kinesiology, University of Saskatchewan, Saskatoon, SK, Canada
e-mail: leah.ferguson@usask.ca

K.E. Gunnell
The Healthy Active Living and Obesity Research Group, The Children's Hospital of Eastern Ontario, Research Institute, Ottawa, ON, Canada
e-mail: KGunnell@cheo.on.ca

J. Vittersø (ed.), *Handbook of Eudaimonic Well-Being*, International Handbooks of Quality-of-Life,
DOI 10.1007/978-3-319-42445-3_28

illbeing was the idea that a person was considered mentally healthy if s/he did not suffer from negative psychological symptoms such as anxiety, depression, disability, loneliness, and mood disorders. Under this historical conceptualization of psychological health, a woman diagnosed with diabetes could be classified as having poor psychological health. Today, we know that people can live with various physical and psychological disorders and still have good overall psychological health. In fact, under our modern conceptualization of psychological health, well-being is not limited to the absence of psychological maladies; rather, it includes the presence of an array of positive aspects of functioning such as positive affect, purpose in life, and social contribution (Cowen, 1991; Keyes, 2007; Ryan, Huta, & Deci, 2008). The shift to consider positive aspects of psychological functioning has had important implications for the advancement of psychology and practice. Under the historical conceptualization of psychological health, people were treated from a disease perspective with the intent to understand a disorder and how to repair or alleviate it (Seligman & Csikszentmihalyi, 2000). With the emergence of positive psychology, researchers began to recognize the importance of understanding why and how people experience *positive* aspects of mental health. Researchers invested in the positive approach to psychological health identified characteristics of positive mental health (Jahoda, 1958), studied the positive potential – or self-actualization – of human beings (Maslow, 1968), conceptualized optimal psychological functioning and development (Ryff, 1989, Chap. 6, this volume), as well as outlined a framework for a science of positive psychology (Seligman & Csikszentmihalyi, 2000).

Initial research couched within the positive psychology movement (Seligman & Csikszentmihalyi, 2000) largely conceptualized well-being as *hedonic well-being*. The hedonic approach to positive psychological well-being reflects the view that well-being consists of maximizing happiness and experiencing pleasure while avoiding displeasure (Ryan & Deci, 2001; Ryan & Martela, Chap. 7, this volume). More specifically, hedonic well-being typically consists of three main components: the presence of positive affect, the absence of negative affect, and satisfaction with one's life (Diener, Suh, Lucas, & Smith, 1999). As such, if a person is attempting to maximize hedonic well-being, that person will typically do things that make her/him happy and feel good. However, it has been argued that some sources that could produce pleasurable feelings characteristic of hedonic well-being may not be beneficial for overall psychological health. For example, a person who has just taken addictive illicit drugs could display high hedonic well-being (i.e., high pleasure), yet that person could be taking drugs to alleviate symptoms of severe depression. Therefore, although the person would score high on a measure of hedonic well-being after taking the drugs, the high hedonic well-being score may not be indicative of good psychological health (Ryan & Huta, 2009). Furthermore, a prominent characteristic of hedonic well-being is that it can be a passive condition that is not necessarily associated with the pursuit and achievement of important goals and purposes in life (Chatzisarantis & Hagger, 2007).

An alternative way to conceptualize positive psychological well-being is through the eudaimonic tradition. *Eudaimonic well-being* is characterized as fulfilling or realizing one's true nature and potential. Heavily influenced by Aristotle, whom wrote about eudaimonic well-being in his *Nicomachean Ethics*, eudaimonic well-being focuses explicitly on individuals' development and self-realization, and is thought to reflect optimal psychological functioning at one's highest potential (Ryan & Deci, 2001; Ryff, 1989, 1995). Although there is no consensus as to exactly what eudaimonic well-being is or how best to measure it (see Kashdan, Biswas-Diener, & King, 2008; Ward & King, Chap. 35, this volume; Kimiecik, 2011, Chap. 23, this volume; Nussbaum, 2008), eudaimonic well-being differs from the happiness, pleasure, or enjoyment that characterize hedonic well-being because the main themes of eudaimonic well-being revolve around ideas of flourishing, human potential, and purpose in life (Kimiecik, 2011). Generally speaking, individuals who have eudaimonic well-being find life not only enjoyable (stemming from the hedonic tradition of well-being), but they also find meaning, value, and worth in life. Unlike hedonic well-being, eudaimonic well-being is associated with active pursuits and achievements of goals (Chatzisarantis & Hagger, 2007), and is reflective of living in accordance with one's excellences towards one's potential. In contrast to the happiness and pleasure that is implicit to hedonic well-being, eudaimonic well-being will most certainly include instances of challenge and difficulty while individuals strive to reach their potential and purpose in life.

Within the eudaimonic tradition of well-being there exists different approaches as to how human potential is conceptualized and operationalized. Although a review of each theory of eudaimonic well-being is beyond the scope of this chapter, we will outline two prominent theories that informed our discussion on gender differences in eudaimonic well-being. We present these differing approaches not to prescribe how best to conceive of eudaimonic well-being, but to further highlight the complexity that exists when considering well-being from a gendered perspective. Readers are encouraged to read Huta (2013) for a more detailed summary of various eudaimonic well-being theories, such as those proposed by Martin Seligman (2002) and Joar Vittersø (2003, Chap. 1, this volume).

One conceptualization of eudaimonic well-being stems from Waterman's (1990, 1993) personal expressiveness research. In Waterman's conceptualization of eudaimonia, individuals' efforts to live in accord with their daimon (or true self) and to realize human potentials should give rise to eudaimonia. These efforts are personally expressive; thus Waterman uses personal expressiveness as an indicator of eudaimonia. Waterman and colleagues (2010) were able to empirically demonstrate that personally expressive feelings emerged during activities that involved pursuits to reach one's best potential and purpose in life. Waterman (1990, 1993) outlined six criteria for personal expressiveness: (1) an unusually intense involvement in an undertaking, (2) a feeling of a special fit or meshing with an activity that is not characteristic of most daily tasks, (3) a feeling of intensely being alive, (4) a feeling of being complete or fulfilled while engaged in an activity, (5) an impression that this is what the person was meant to do, and (6) a feeling that this is who one really is. Since his early research on personal expressiveness, Waterman has recently developed a questionnaire for eudaimonic well-being (i.e., the Questionnaire for Eudaimonic Well-Being; Waterman et al., 2010) as an outcome comprised of six subscales (self-discovery, perceived development of one's best potential, sense of purpose and meaning in life, investment of significant effort in pursuit of excellence, intense involvement in activities, an enjoyment of activities as personally expressive) rooted in eudaimonic philosophy.

Another approach to the eudaimonic tradition of well-being offered by Carol Ryff (1989, 1995) operates from the position that eudaimonic well-being is a multidimensional outcome that an individual arrives at. Ryff contends and has found empirical support to demonstrate that eudaimonic well-being consists of six aspects that define what it means to be fully functioning at one's highest potential. To this end, an individual experiences eudaimonic well-being when s/he (1) is autonomous, (2) has mastery over one's environment, (3) feelings of continued growth and development, (4) positive relationships with others, (5) purpose and meaning in life, and (6) acceptance of oneself. These dimensions of eudaimonic well-being represent points of convergence between various theories on psychological functioning including mental health, clinical psychology, and life span development. For Ryff and her colleagues, the six dimensions constitute eudaimonic well-being; that is, the dimensions define what it means to be eudaimonically-well.

28.3 Gender and Hedonic Well-being

A scan of the hedonic well-being literature presents inconclusive evidence on differences between men and women on indices of hedonic well-being, namely positive affect, negative affect, and satisfaction with life. There is some evidence to suggest that women have lower positive affect and higher negative affect than men (Ahrens & Ryff, 2006; Rhoes & Pivik, 2011); however, there are also instances of women reporting higher positive affect than men (Fujita, Diener, & Sandvik, 1991). Nevertheless, more often than not gender differences do not emerge on positive affect and negative affect (Herzog, Rodgers, & Woodworth, 1982; Perez, 2012; Ryff, 1989). There are also conflicting findings when it comes to satisfaction with life: men have been found to score higher on measures of life satisfaction than women (Ryff, 1989), but there is also evidence to support women reporting higher levels of satisfaction with life (Philippe, Vallerand, & Lavigne, 2009). It has also been found that no gender differences exist on life satisfaction, and has been concluded that the similarities between women and men on this component of hedonic well-being are striking (Diener & Diener, 1995; Herzog et al., 1982). The conflicting findings in the literature make it difficult to arrive at a definitive conclusion regarding differences between women and men on hedonic well-being.

28.4 Gender and Eudaimonic Well-being

Differences between women and men on eudaimonic well-being are equivocal: few differences have been found between women and men, the gender differences have been minimal, or the evidence to support gender differences is conflicting across the literature (Kokko, Korkalainen, Lyyra, & Feldt, 2013; Perez, 2012; Philippe et al., 2009; Robitschek & Keyes, 2009; Roothman, Kirsten, & Wissing, 2003; Ryff & Singer, 1998; Schutte, Wissing, & Khumalo, 2013). Here we highlight some results from the literature that have demonstrated evidence for differences between genders on indicators of eudaimonic well-being. It is worth noting that some of the components contain research findings that conflict with one another; that is, some researchers have found that women score higher on a specific component of eudaimonic well-being, whereas others have found that men score higher on the same component. We return to this issue at the end of the chapter when considering the unclear nature of these research findings overall.

28.5 Waterman's Indicators of Eudaimonic Well-being

Personal Expressiveness In his research on the pursuit or experience of eudaimonic well-being, Waterman and his colleagues have found conflicting results. For example, women have reported significantly higher scores on measures of personal expressiveness than men in some instances (Waterman et al., 2010), whereas no gender differences have emerged on personal expressiveness in other instances (Schwartz, Mullis, Waterman, & Dunham, 2000). Interestingly, when women have reported higher levels of personal expressiveness than men, they do not differ from men on a measure of self-realization (Waterman, 2007), which Waterman (1993) regards as a component of optimal psychological functioning.

Questionnaire for Eudaimonic Well-being Although Waterman and colleagues (2010) explicitly indicated that based on theory they did not expect gender differences on their questionnaire for eudaimonic well-being, results from two studies demonstrated that females reported higher mean levels of eudaimonic well-being compared to males. No gender differences were noted in another study using the same questionnaire (Schutte et al., 2013).

28.6 Ryff's Conceptualization of Eudaimonic Well-being

Autonomy Men tend to report greater levels of autonomy than women (Ahrens & Ryff, 2006; Perez, 2012). Gender differences on autonomy may at least partially be attributed to socialization processes whereby, as Perez contends, men have traditionally been taught or trained to be more independent than women. This socialization process may be influencing men in such a way that they demonstrated greater scores on autonomy compared to women. Conversely, Perez proposed that women rely more on expectations of others and tend to conform to social pressures to act and think in certain ways compared to men. Women have been found to have their autonomy compromised in their daily lives, particularly those who experience some form of discrimination (e.g., being treated with disrespect, insulted, or threatened; Ryff, Keyes, & Hughes, 2003). However, autonomy may be impacted by educational attainment and multiple role occupancy (e.g., spouse, employee, friend, social organization member). Well-educated women with multiple roles report higher levels of autonomy, whereas men with less education and high role occupancy tend to have diminished autonomy (Ahrens & Ryff, 2006).

Environmental Mastery Women report lower environmental mastery compared to men (Ahrens & Ryff, 2006), and their low levels of mastery are magnified for women who experience discrimination (Ryff et al., 2003). Men's ability to maintain a sense of empowerment and competency has been shown to be an important predictor of their resilience to face psychosocial stressors (Boardman, Blalock, & Button, 2008). Perez (2012) contends that men may be more oriented toward mastery and exploration of the world than women, who are more oriented toward interpersonal relationships.

Personal Growth Although the majority of researchers have found that gender is a poor predictor of personal growth, some evidence suggests that women have a trend toward greater personal growth than men (Ryff, 1989, 1995; Vleioras & Bosma, 2005). This finding, however, is dubious when additional factors are taken into consideration, such as discrimination; women with high levels of discrimination in their daily lives, such as being insulted, threatened, or harassed, have their sense of growth compromised (Ryff et al., 2003).

Positive Relations with Others The positive relatedness component of eudaimonic well-being has the most unequivocal research findings, with women consistently reporting more positive relations with others compared to men (Ahrens & Ryff, 2006; Perez, 2012; Ryff, 1989, 1995; Ryff & Keyes, 1995; Ryff & Singer, 2002; Vleioras & Bosma, 2005). This form of interpersonal well-being is the lowest rated dimension for men, although they have qualitatively indicated that relatedness is a critical aspect of optimal psychological functioning (Ryff & Singer, 2002). One way to interpret this gender difference is that women's development may be more focused on interpersonal relations than is men's (Boardman et al., 2008; Ryff, 1989). There may be substantial differences in the way men and women process and understand the social and personal aspects of their relationships with other people (Perez, 2012), causing women to be more inclined towards engaging in relationships than their men counterparts. These findings support evolutionary theory that women are predisposed to engage in caring, nurturing, and intimate relationships (Perez, 2012).

Purpose in Life Women have reported higher purpose in life than men, suggesting that they have clearer goals and sense of direction in life (Perez, 2012; Vleioras & Bosma, 2005). Women may hold beliefs that give them life purpose and provide direction towards goals, aims, and objectives. These gender differences could be attributed to developmental patterns of the brain, as achieving a sense of purpose requires mental maturity and women tend to reach full brain development maturity earlier than men (Lenroot et al., 2007).

Self-acceptance Women have been found to have lower self-acceptance than men (Ahrens & Ryff, 2006; Ryff et al., 2003), and the low levels of self-acceptance are amplified among women who experience perceived discrimination (Ryff et al., 2003). Boardman et al. (2008) found that self-acceptance plays an important role for both women and men in that it operates as a mechanism towards resilience against psychosocial stressors.

28.7 Gender Differences and the Measurement of Well-being

The largely equivocal findings outlined above about the gender differences in well-being[2] could be caused by lack of measurement validity inherent in questionnaires used to assess well-being. Implicit in the testing of gender differences on indicators of well-being is the critical role of measurement validity. Without evidence that the questionnaires used to measure markers of well-being demonstrate score validity (i.e., scores reflect the intended interpretations based on theory; Messick, 1995), it is difficult to know if results are characteristic of an underlying phenomenon or if measurement error is introducing bias into the results. Indeed, unless researchers specifically examine their instruments for *measurement invariance*, it is impossible to know if women and men are responding to questionnaire items in the same way and on the same scale. Measurement invariance helps researchers determine if questionnaire items are operating with the same meaning and on the same metric between two subgroups, such as women and men (Wu, Li, & Zumbo, 2007). It is possible, for instance, that some researchers have demonstrated that men have higher mean levels of certain indicators of well-being because the instruments were biased towards men or women. For example, when a man reads a questionnaire item his response may be scaled differently than the response a woman would provide, making a comparison on their respective mean scores ambiguous. Very few researchers assessing gender differences in well-being have tested measurement invariance, which leads to unclear and weak conclusions (Horn, 1991; Wu et al., 2007). A recent systematic review by Chinni and Hubley (2014) found that only 34.8 % of validation articles on the satisfaction with life questionnaire tested invariance, and only half of those studies investigated gender invariance. Findings from Chinni and Hubley's systematic review highlight the need for a more rigorous investigation to determine if women and men respond to questionnaire items in manners such that scores from these questionnaires can be interpreted with greater confidence.

Researchers could also examine validity evidence based on response processes. For example, a think-a-loud protocol could be used whereby responders are asked to verbalize exactly what they are thinking when they are reading and answering questionnaire items. Examining response processes and potential differences when interpreting and responding to questionnaire items between women and men may shed light on possible gender differences when responding to questions. It is conceivable, for example, that women and men respond to questionnaire items in socially desirable ways. Women may provide a certain response to an item because they believe the item should be true for them because of their gender rather than because they feel the item is true for them personally. Similarly, men may not endorse certain items because they feel that the items contain feminine qualities they do not want to be seen as endorsing. Adopting a think-a-loud protocol to investigate response processes is one way to integrate the element of reflection into our understanding of well-being (Nussbaum, 2008). There is a clear need for future research examining the validity evidence for well-being indicators to determine if researchers can even examine gender differences using the same questionnaires for women and men.

[2]Given the scope of this chapter and our decision to focus on certain conceptualizations of hedonic and eudaimonic well-being, we have not outlined results from literatures that extend beyond these conceptualizations of well-being. Indeed, our intent was not to provide an exhaustive review of the literature on gender differences across a wide range of well-being indicators. Rather, we hoped to provide a "highlight reel" of some general trends in the literature that are specific to hedonic and eudaimonic well-being to generate discourse. Those who are interested in broader contexts of well-being may wish to extend their review of gender differences to other conceptualizations of well-being. For example, gender differences have been noted on social integration and distress in the workplace (Pugliesi, 1995), as well as on self-esteem, happiness, and loneliness among older adults (Pinquart & Sörensen, 2001).

28.8 Moving Forward

In addition to the need for proper examination of the psychometric properties of well-being instruments, including a rigorous investigation of gender invariance and biased responding, much conceptualizing is to be explored regarding eudaimonic well-being for women and men. Though researchers apply theoretical frameworks of eudaimonic well-being to guide their research, it is possible that women and men have varying meanings of eudaimonic well-being and may experience or fulfill their potential differently. This is a particularly relevant possibility when taking into consideration the inconclusive research findings on gender differences in eudaimonic well-being; that is, while some evidence suggests that women score higher on certain components of eudaimonic well-being and men score higher on other components, the majority of findings across the literature tend to conflict with one another. Perhaps our theories of eudaimonic well-being need to be reconsidered and developed with a gender lens, whereby the framework differs for women and men. Just as Aristotle noted the tremendous importance of qualitative distinctions among elements of human life (Nussbaum, 2008), qualitative research that explores meanings and experiences of eudaimonic well-being for women and men may shed light on diverse and multiple understandings of this phenomenon. Bauer, McAdams, and Pals (2008) suggest exploring conceptions and experiences of eudaimonic well-being through life narratives whereby individuals construct and reflect on life stories (see also Bauer, Chap. 10, this volume). Adopting a life narrative approach may capture the complexity and richness in interpreting eudaimonic well-being in women and men's life. Consideration for potential qualitative differences between women and men's eudaimonic well-being will ensure our theoretical frameworks resonate with and are reflective of the intended population.

The literature we presented in this chapter depicts a simplistic view of gender. That is, research on well-being typically includes the classification of study participants as women or men, and statistical analyses are subsequently employed to test for differences between these dichotomous categories on indicators of well-being. Though much information has been generated from this quantitative research approach, it is nevertheless limiting when taking into account the complexity of our psychological constructs of interest. Consideration for our larger social and cultural contexts when investigating gender and well-being is needed. Going beyond the dichotomous approach to gender as woman or man and exploring the fluidity of gender would provide a much more nuanced understanding of eudaimonic well-being. Qualitative research may provide a useful platform to study the complexity of our psychological phenomena and generate knowledge on gender and well-being that is not restricted to simplistic categories. For instance, social norms around femininity and masculinity may shape how women and men define and/or experience gender, and in turn well-being. Using qualitative research methods, investigators can explore the meaning individuals ascribe to gender, their experiences of gender, and how gender shapes their experiences of well-being. In turn, qualitative methods can be used to help alleviate some tensions in the literature that critique hedonic frameworks of well-being as being of limited scope and a fallible indicator of optimal functioning (Ryff & Singer, 1998), and eudaimonic well-being conceptualizations as being overly prescriptive and value-laden in defining well-being (Diener et al., 1999; Kashdan et al., 2008).

28.9 Concluding Remarks

It is imperative to know how we conceptually define well-being in order to understand well-being, and eventually enhance well-being (Ryan & Deci, 2001). This is certainly true when taking a gendered perspective to well-being: attempting to change the lives of women and men for the better through the promotion of well-being necessitates a firm grasp of well-being for each gender (or the varying shades of gender). Expanding on Martha Nussbaum's (2008) sentiment that we are riddled with well-being conception confusion and need to pause to sort things out, we suggest a second pause is warranted to more pointedly consider how gender is connected with well-being. As the literature covered in this chapter suggests, gender differences in well-being are equivocal. The inconsistent research findings can, in our opinion, be attributed to the omission of gender in our theoretical frameworks and conceptual models of well-being. Science and knowledge can be advanced by explicit consideration and integration of gender into the theories and models that drive research on well-being. Including a gendered lens at the fundamental level of our research would most assuredly result in expanding our knowledge of women and men's psychological profiles. From an optimist's perspective, the varied findings on gender differences in well-being imply that there is much to be discovered. We have only begun to uncover a rich area of knowledge on the psychological strengths and vulnerabilities of women and men's well-being.

Acknowledgements We would like to thank Erica V. Bennett for her guidance and insightful comments regarding the fluidity of gender when investigating well-being.

References

Ahrens, C. J. C., & Ryff, C. D. (2006). Multiple roles and well-being: Sociodemographic and psychological moderators. *Sex Roles, 55*, 801–815. doi:10.1007/s11199-006-9134-8.

Bauer, J. J., McAdams, D. P., & Pals, J. L. (2008). Narrative identity and eudaimonic well-being. *Journal of Happiness Studies, 9*, 81–104. doi:10.1007/s10902-006-9021-6.

Boardman, J. D., Blalock, C. L., & Button, T. M. M. (2008). Sex differences in the heritability of resilience. *Twin Research and Human Genetics: The Official Journal of the International Society for Twin Studies, 11*, 12–27. doi:10.1375/twin.11.1.12.

Chatzisarantis, N. L. D., & Hagger, M. S. (2007). The moral worth of sport reconsidered: Contributions of recreational sport and competitive sport to life aspirations and psychological well-being. *Journal of Sports Sciences, 25*, 1047–1056. doi:10.1080/02640410600959954.

Chinni, M. L., & Hubley, A. M. (2014). A research synthesis of validation practices used to evaluate the satisfaction with life scale (SWLS). In B. D. Zumbo & E. K. H. Chan (Eds.), *Validity and validation in social, behavioral, and health sciences* (pp. 35–66). Cham, Switzerland: Springer International Publishing.

Cowen, E. L. (1991). In pursuit of wellness. *American Psychologist, 46*, 404–408.

Diener, E., & Diener, M. (1995). Cross-cultural correlates of life satisfaction and self-esteem. *Journal of Personality and Social Psychology, 68*(4), 653–663. http://doi.org/10.1037/0022-3514.68.4.653.

Diener, E., Suh, E. M., Lucas, R. E., & Smith, H. L. (1999). Subjective well-being: Three decades of progress. *Psychological Bulletin, 125*, 276–302.

Fujita, F., Diener, E., & Sandvik, E. (1991). Gender differences in negative affect and well-being: The case for emotional intensity. *Journal of Personality and Social Psychology, 61*, 427–434. doi:10.1037/0022-3514.61.3.427.

Herzog, A. R., Rodgers, W. L., & Woodworth, J. (1982). *Subjective well-being among different age groups*. Ann Arbor, MI: University of Michigan Institute for Social Research.

Horn, J. L. (1991). Discussion of the issues of factorial invariance. In L. M. Collins & J. L. Horn (Eds.), *Best methods for the analysis of change* (pp. 114–125). Washington, DC: American Psychological Association.

Huta, V. (2013). Eudaimonia. In I. Boniwell, S. A. David, & A. C. Ayers (Eds.), *Oxford handbook of happiness* (pp. 201–213). Oxford, UK: Oxford University Press.

Jahoda, M. (1958). *Current concepts of positive mental health*. New York: Basic Books.

Kashdan, T. B., Biswas-Diener, R., & King, L. A. (2008). Reconsidering happiness: The costs of distinguishing between hedonics and eudaimonia. *The Journal of Positive Psychology, 3*, 219–233. doi:10.1080/17439760802303044.

Keyes, C. L. M. (2007). Promoting and protecting mental health as flourishing: A complementary strategy for improving national mental health. *American Psychologist, 62*, 95–108. doi:10.1037/0003-066X.62.2.95.

Kimiecik, J. (2011). Exploring the promise of eudaimonic well-being within the practice of health promotion: The "how" is as important as the "what". *Journal of Happiness Studies, 12*, 769–792. doi:10.1007/s10902-010-9226-6.

Kokko, K., Korkalainen, A., Lyyra, A. L., & Feldt, T. (2013). Structure and continuity of well-being in mid-adulthood: A longitudinal study. *Journal of Happiness Studies, 14*, 99–114. doi:10.1007/s10902-011-9318-y.

Lenroot, R., Gogtay, N., Greenstein, D., Molloy Wells, E., Wallace, G., Clasen, L., … & Giedd, J. (2007). Sexual dimorphism of brain developmental trajectories during childhood and adolescence. *Neuroimage, 36*, 1065–1073. doi:10.1111/j.1365-2958.2010.07165.x.Characterization.

Maslow, A. H. (1968). *Toward a psychology of being* (2nd ed.). New York: Van Nostrand.

Messick, S. (1995). Validity of psychological assessment: Validation of inferences from persons' responses and performances as scientific inquiry into score meaning. *American Psychologist, 50*, 741–749. doi:10.1037//0003-066X.50.9.741.

Nussbaum, M. C. (2008). Who is the happy warrior? Philosophy poses questions to psychology. *The Journal of Legal Studies, 37*, S81–S113. doi:10.1086/587438.

Perez, J. A. (2012). Gender difference in psychological well-being among Filipino college student samples. *International Journal of Humanities and Social Science, 2*, 84–93.

Philippe, F. L., Vallerand, R. J., & Lavigne, G. L. (2009). Passion does make a difference in people's lives: A look at well-being in passionate and non-passionate individuals. *Applied Psychology: Health and Well-Being, 1*,3–22.doi:10.1111/j.1758-0854.2008.01003.x.

Pinquart, M., & Sörensen, S. (2001). Gender differences in self-concept and psychological well-being in old age: A meta-analysis. *Journal of Gerontology, 56*, 195–213.

Pugliesi, K. (1995). Work and well-being: Gender differences in the psychological consequences of employment. *Journal of Health and Social Behavior, 36*, 57–71.

Rhoes, N., & Pivik, K. (2011). Age and gender differences in risky driving: The roles of positive affect and risk perception. *Accident Analysis & Prevention, 43*, 923–931. doi:10.1016/j.aap.2010.11.015.

Robitschek, C., & Keyes, C. L. M. (2009). Keyes's model of mental health with personal growth initiative as a parsimonious predictor. *Journal of Counseling Psychology, 56*, 321–329. doi:10.1037/a0013954.

Roothman, B., Kirsten, D. K., & Wissing, M. P. (2003). Gender differences in aspects of psychological well-being. *South African Journal of Psychology, 33*, 212–218. doi:10.1177/008124630303300403.

Ryan, R. M., & Deci, E. L. (2001). On happiness and human potentials: A review of research on hedonic and eudaimonic well-being. *Annual Review of Psychology, 52*, 141–166.

Ryan, R. M., & Huta, V. (2009). Wellness as healthy functioning or wellness as happiness: The importance of eudaimonic thinking (response to the Kashdan et al. and Waterman discussion). *The Journal of Positive Psychology, 4*, 202–204. doi:10.1080/17439760902844285.

Ryan, R. M., Huta, V., & Deci, E. L. (2008). Living well: A self-determination theory perspective of eudaimonia. *Journal of Happiness Studies, 9*, 139–170. doi:10.1007/s10902-006-9023-4.

Ryff, C. D. (1989). Happiness is everything, or is it? Explorations on the meaning of psychological well-being. *Journal of Personality and Social Psychology, 57*, 1069–1081. doi:10.1037/034645.

Ryff, C. D. (1995). Psychological well-being in adult life. *Current Directions in Psychological Science, 4*, 99–104.

Ryff, C. D., & Keyes, C. L. (1995). The structure of psychological well-being revisited. *Journal of Personality and Social Psychology, 69*, 719–727. doi:10.1037/0022-3514.69.4.719.

Ryff, C. D., Keyes, C. L. M., & Hughes, D. L. (2003). Status inequalities, perceived discrimination, and eudaimonic well-being: Do the challenges of minority life hone purpose and growth? *Journal of Health and Social Behavior, 44*, 275–291.

Ryff, C. D., & Singer, B. (1998). The contours of positive health. *Psychological Inquiry: An International Journal for Advancement of Psychology Theory, 9*, 1–28. doi:10.1207/s15327965pli0901.

Ryff, C. D., & Singer, B. (2002). From social structure to biology. In C. R. Snyder & S. J. Lopez (Eds.), *Handbook of positive psychology* (pp. 541–555). Oxford, UK: Oxford University Press.

Schutte, L., Wissing, M. P., & Khumalo, I. P. (2013). Further validation of the questionnaire for eudaimonic well-being (QEWB). *Psychology of Well-Being: Theory, Research and Practice, 3*(3), 1–22. http://doi.org/10.1186/2211-1522-3-3.

Schwartz, S. J., Mullis, R. L., Waterman, A. S., & Dunham, R. M. (2000). Ego identity status, identity style, and personal expressiveness: An empirical investigation of three convergent constructs. *Journal of Adolescent Research, 15*, 504–521. doi:10.1177/0743558400154005.

Seligman, M. E. P. (2002). *Authentic happiness: Using the new positive psychology to realize your potential for lasting fulfillment*. New York: Free Press.

Seligman, M. E. P., & Csikszentmihalyi, M. (2000). Positive psychology: An introduction. *American Psychology, 55*, 5–14. doi:10.1037//0003-066X.55.1.5.

Vittersø, J. (2003). Flow versus life satisfaction: A projective use of cartoons to illustrate the difference between the evaluation approach and the intrinsic motivation approach to subjective quality of life. *Journal of Happiness Studies, 4*, 141–167.

Vleioras, G., & Bosma, H. A. (2005). Are identity styles important for psychological well-being? *Journal of Adolescence, 28*, 397–409. doi:10.1016/j.adolescence.2004.09.001.

Waterman, A. S. (1990). The relevance of Aristotle's conception of eudaimonia for the psychological study of happiness. *Theoretical & Philosophical Psychology, 10*, 39–44. doi:10.1037/h0091489.

Waterman, A. S. (1993). Two conceptions of happiness: Contrasts of personal expressiveness (eudaimonia) and hedonic enjoyment. *Journal of Personality and Social Psychology, 64*, 678–691. doi:10.1037/0022-3514.64.4.678.

Waterman, A. S. (2007). Doing well: The relationship of identity status to three conceptions of well-being.

Identity: An International Journal of Theory and Research, 7, 289–307. doi:10.1080/15283480701600769.
Waterman, A. S., Schwartz, S. J., Zamboanga, B. L., Ravert, R. D., Williams, M. K., Bede Agocha, V., … & Brent Donnellan, M. (2010). The questionnaire for eudaimonic well-being: Psychometric properties, demographic comparisons, and evidence of validity. *The Journal of Positive Psychology, 5*, 41–61. doi:10.1080/17439760903435208.
WHO. (2001). *Basic documents* (43rd ed., p. 1). Geneva, Switzerland: World Health Organization.
Wu, A. D., Li, Z., & Zumbo, B. D. (2007). Decoding the meaning of factorial invariance and updating the practice of multi-group confirmatory factor analysis: A demonstration with TIMSS data. *Practical Assessment, Research & Evaluation, 12*, 1–26.

Sentimental Hedonism: Pleasure, Purpose, and Public Policy

29

Paul Dolan and Laura Kudrna

29.1 Introduction

Subjective well-being or 'happiness' is no longer solely the remit of philosophers and psychologists. Government and non-government organisations around the world now utilise, or advocate utilising, happiness measures to inform and appraise public policies, as well as monitor national well-being (Dolan & Metcalfe, 2012; Oishi & Diener, 2014). The UK's HM Treasury uses happiness measures to conduct cost benefit analyses (Fujiwara, 2010). Following from the influential Stigliz Commission (Stiglitz et al. 2009), the US National Academy of Sciences (2014) recommended that statistical agencies collect happiness data alongside traditional economic indicators to more fully understand how well people's lives are going. Internationally, the United Nations defined a new economic paradigm as "one that has as its goal human happiness and the well-being of all life on earth" (United Nations, 2012, p. 10), and the Organisation for Economic Co-operation and Development (2015) includes happiness in its "Better Life Index", which compares well-being across countries.

Research into the causes and consequents of happiness shapes policy discussions. For example, in its annual report to Congress on the Benefits and Costs of Federal Regulations, the US Office of Management and Budget (2013) highlighted the relationship of GDP and income with happiness - an area in which there is a plethora of research (Diener, Ng, Harter, & Arora, 2010). The UK employment minister commented positively on a report from the Department for Business, Innovation and Skills suggesting that employee happiness is conducive to economic growth (Bryson, Forth, & Stokes, 2014; Clarke, 2014). German Chancellor Angela Merkel held a forum on happiness, 'What Matters to People - Well-being and Progress', where she highlighted that economic growth doesn't "prioritize what is really most important to people" (Ellyatt, 2013). There are two main issues in happiness research, however, that remain unclear and/or underdeveloped. These issues are preventing a useful translation of psychological happiness research into other disciplines and domains, including public policy.

The fundamental question is how to measure happiness. As Robinson (2013) notes in her discussion of the use of happiness in cost benefit analysis (see also Adler, 2012), the ambiguity in the literature surrounding the meaning and measurement of happiness is a barrier to the application of happiness research in policy. This concern is not unfounded. Many researchers are unclear about what their various measures of happiness capture and there is no obvious consensus about

P. Dolan (✉) • L. Kudrna
London School of Economics, London, UK
e-mail: L.Kudrna@lse.ac.uk

J. Vittersø (ed.), *Handbook of Eudaimonic Well-Being*, International Handbooks of Quality-of-Life,
DOI 10.1007/978-3-319-42445-3_29

which one(s) should be used (Brown, MacDonald, Samanta, Friedman, & Coyne, 2014). Searching for 'happiness' in an academic database results in articles measuring a range of emotions, 'life satisfaction', 'meaning in life', and many more happiness-related terms using a variety of scales. As a practical matter, it is typically prohibitively expensive to include many measures of happiness in large-scale surveys and so only one or a few may be selected. Even if many were included, it would be challenging to aggregate or weight the results for use in policy appraisal, where single index measures are often required. The different definitions and measures of happiness are not situated within any consistent framework and this is seriously hindering progress in advancing our understanding of happiness and its aetiology.

Moreover, different dimensions of happiness have different determinants (Luhmann, Hofmann, Eid, & Lucas, 2012). As Oishi and Diener (2014) note, "Cognitive evaluation of life (e.g., Cantril's Self-anchoring Scale, General Life Satisfaction) appears to reflect economic conditions fairly well… In contrast, affective aspects of well-being (emotional experiences) appear to capture conditions of life associated with time (e.g., free time)" (p. 200). Similarly, Luhmann et al., (2012) show that life events, such as marriage and unemployment, have dissimilar impacts upon cognitive and affective well-being. After marriage, people have higher cognitive well-being but not higher affective well-being. After becoming unemployed, people's cognitive well-being fully adapts after about 3 years, whereas affective well-being remains low even several years later on. Thus the research on cognitive well-being would suggest that marriage is more important for happiness than unemployment, whereas the research on affective well-being would suggest the opposite. As the authors note, this raises the question: "What is more important, increasing [affective well-being] or increasing [cognitive well-being]? This is a philosophical problem that can turn into a political issue as soon as public policy interventions are affected." (p. 23). We aim to stimulate debate on this question of what kind of happiness should be prioritized in policy.

To address these issues, this article suggests how to classify the many different measures of happiness according to only two dimensions in order to simplify the discussion. These dimensions have been discussed in previous literature (Dolan, 2014), although not coherently classified in this way. The first dimension is the *level* at which happiness is being assessed: either in terms of cognitive "evaluations", which is how people think about their lives, or "experiences", which is how people feel during the experience of their lives (Kahneman & Riis, 2005; Robinson & Clore, 2002). The second dimension is the *type* of happiness being assessed: either "pleasure", and related positive and negative emotions like joy, pain, and worry, or "purpose", and related positive and negative experiences like meaning, pointlessness and futility (Aristotle, 2002; Bentham, 1907). Previously, experiences have been referred to as affective well-being (Luhmann et al., 2012). Following the US National Academy of Sciences (2014), we consider affective well-being to include not only positive and negative emotions, but also positive and negative experiences more generally, including meaningfulness. Even if self-reports of experiences must contain some element of evaluations due to the act of reporting, we are persuaded by arguments made by philosophers of emotions like Dokic and Lemaire (2015) who show that there are experiences that exist independently of evaluations.

Existing efforts to classify happiness measures have contributed greatly to the proposed classification herein. Diener (2000), for example, was a pioneer in distinguishing between affective and cognitive well-being, which Kahneman and Riis (2005) later referred to as evaluations and experiences. Here, we emphasize the evaluation and experience terminology because experiences can encompass more than affect, including experiences of purpose and pointlessness, which may not be affective (Biswas-Diener, Kashdan, & King, 2009). Ryff and Keyes (1995) contributed significantly to our conceptualization of evaluations of purpose with their investigation of the construct "Purpose in Life". Yet a focus on evaluations of purpose neglects whether the activities of our lives feel worthwhile and meaningful.

Our original contribution here is to emphasize that purpose resides in people's experiences; that is, experiences can *feel* purposeful, worthwhile, fulfilling and meaningful. And they can do so independently of the cognitive evaluations of purpose e.g. purpose in life. Academics thus far who have discussed and investigated the experiential component of purpose do not go far enough because they have not analysed measures that truly capture it. For example, Hicks, Cicero, Trent, Burton, & King (2010) measure feelings of meaning with measures that capture understanding and sense-making, e.g. "I struggle to make sense of the events" (p. 972; see also Ward and King, Chap. 35, this volume). We argue that understanding and sense-making are predictors or consequents of experiences of meaning, not experiences of meaning in themselves. Steger, Kashdan, & Oishi's (2008) 'Daily Meaning Scale' has two items: "how meaningful does your life feel" and "how much do you feel your life has purpose?" (p. 27). Such measures combine evaluations and experiences of meaning by asking about both life and feelings, whereas we emphasize solely experiences (see also Nelson, Kushlev, English, Dunn, & Lyubomirsky, 2013). Our view also differs conceptually from academics like Baumeister (1991), who views meaning as a superordinate concept to purpose, values, efficacy and self-worth, because we consider meaning and purpose to be synonyms and values, efficacy and self-worth to be antecedents and/or consequents of experiences of meaning.

We do not presently investigate in detail the separateness or relatedness of the various dimensions of happiness (Busseri & Sadava, 2011). Instead, we emphasize that these distinctions between the dimensions of happiness matter because, as noted earlier, the determinants of happiness differ depending on which level and type of happiness is being measured. For example, as people earn more than $75,000 each year they become increasingly more satisfied with their lives in an evaluative sense, but they do not report feeling any happier in an experiential sense (Kahneman & Deaton, 2010). So our conclusions about how circumstances of life affect happiness depend critically on the level at which happiness are measured. And whilst working is experienced as one of the least pleasurable activities, it is also experienced as one of the most purposeful (White & Dolan, 2009). So our conclusions about how the activities we engage in affect happiness depend critically on the type of happiness being measured.

In what follows, we will set out more clearly the conceptual and empirical differences between the two main dimensions of happiness. Experiences of purpose have been most overlooked in the literature to date and so we additionally present a brief summary of some fresh evidence from data on time use.

Following from the discussion of the dimensions of happiness and their differing determinants, we then address the second issue and consider which level of happiness is more important for determining the degree to which someone is happy (Dolan & Metcalfe, 2012). The aim is not to reinvigorate well-rehearsed debates about hedonism (Crisp, 2006; Nozick, 1977; Smart, Quinton, & Williams, 1974); rather, it is to consider whether evaluations or experiences are a better indicator of how well our lives are going. This then informs the practical task of selecting happiness indicators in research and policy. We define the rich array of feelings we experience as 'sentiments' and put forward 'sentimental hedonism': an account of happiness that emphasizes experiences of happiness containing assessments of both pleasure and purpose.

It is worth emphasizing that this article is not intended to be a descriptive account of what people do or how they think and feel. Rather, it is an attempt to clarify ambiguities in the academic literature on happiness for policy purposes, as well as an invitation to reflect on how we can better understand what we measure when we research 'happiness', and what we should be paying more attention to when we do so. Our main conclusions are that it is incumbent on those who use happiness measures to be clear about how they define happiness, that we should work towards improving our understanding of experiences of purpose in particular, and that the debate about what sort of happiness should be our primary aim should continue.

29.2 Two Dimensions to Happiness

As alluded to above, we suggest that measures of happiness can be categorised according to two dimensions. The first is the level at which happiness is being tapped into. On the one hand, we can elicit relatively high level evaluations that capture cognitive judgments about life overall or certain aspects of life such as work or relationships (Kahneman & Krueger, 2006). A typical question would ask something along the lines of "Overall, how happy are you these days?", which clearly requires an evaluation of overall happiness. Alternatively, we can tap into relatively low level experiences that capture people's assessments of how they feel on a moment-to-moment basis (Kahneman, Krueger, Schkade, & Schwartz, 2004; Scollon, Kim-Prieto, & Diener, 2003). A typical question would ask something along the lines of "How happy do you feel right now"? It has long been recognized that evaluations and experiences are separate constructs even though they are not always treated as such (Campbell, Converse, & Rodgers, 1976; Kahneman & Riis, 2005; Pavot & Diener, 1993; Weiss, 2002).

We reach different conclusions about who is happiest and what makes people happy if we use evaluative measures as compared to experiential ones. We would conclude that retirement makes people unhappy from evaluative but not experiential questions, and that marriage doesn't affect happiness at all if we looked only to experiential questions rather than evaluative ones (Luhmann et al., 2012). Middle age is usually the most miserable time of life according to evaluative measures of life satisfaction, but studies of experiences of happiness have shown that younger people are actually less happy than middle aged people (Blanchflower & Oswald, 2008; Carstensen et al., 2011). So, young people can seemingly look forward to better experiences of happiness with age but not better evaluations of their lives. Unemployed people are much less satisfied with their lives than the employed but their day-to-day experiences of pleasure are similar to the employed because they have more free time (Knabe, Rätzel, Schöb, & Weimann, 2010). Our conclusions about the impact of unemployment beyond its economic consequences will therefore depend greatly on the level at which happiness is conceptualised and measured.

The second dimension that happiness measures can be categorized according to is the type of happiness being assessed. On the one hand, there are assessments of what we shall call pleasure. We use this term as shorthand for a range of adjectives associated with positive and negative hedonic feelings, such as joy, contentment, anger, worry, stress and sadness (Watson & Tellegen, 1985). The idea of hedonic happiness is most closely associated with the famous utilitarian philosopher Jeremy Bentham (1907). Assessments of pleasure can also be at the evaluative level, such as when people are asked how happy they feel overall. On the other hand, we can tap into a different type that we shall refer to as purpose. Under this heading sits adjectives associated with positive and negative feelings that are non-hedonic, such as purpose, fulfillment, meaning, pointlessness and futility. The idea of non-hedonic happiness, which can be called eudemonic happiness, is associated with the ancient Greek philosopher Aristotle who postulated that the ultimate good is a virtuous life that contains worthwhile activities (Aristotle, 2002). As with pleasure, assessment of purpose can be at the evaluative level, such as when people are asked how much purpose they have in their lives.

The determinants of happiness again differ depending on whether happiness is measured with a hedonic or non-hedonic type of question. For example, studies investigating the effect of having children on evaluations and experiences of pleasure show that their effect is, at best, neutral (Dolan, Peasgood, & White, 2008; Hansen, 2012). Yet children are associated with more purpose, both in people's evaluations and in their experiences (Burton, 1998; White & Dolan, 2009). In addition, watching TV would appear better for happiness than working from the data on experiences of pleasure, whereas the opposite would be concluded from the data on experiences of purpose (White & Dolan, 2009). And people who volunteer do not necessarily report experiencing more pleasure than those who don't, but they do report higher evaluations of purpose (Son & Wilson, 2012). Just as if we looked only to evaluations or only to experiences of happiness, if we looked only at pleasure or purpose, we would reach different conclusions about who is happiest and what makes them so.

Combining the evaluative and experiential levels of happiness with the pleasure and purpose types of happiness, leads to a 2×2 typology of measures of happiness, as shown in Table 29.1. Later we will describe data that have been used previously to show the distinct factor structures of pleasure and purpose (White & Dolan, 2009), which complement extensive previous work distinguishing evaluations from experiences (Kahneman & Riis, 2005; Robinson & Clore, 2002). There are certainly further typologies within some of these categories, such as positive and negative affect within experiences of pleasure (Watson & Tellegen, 1985), and judgments about the pleasure or purpose associated with various domains of life, such as work or relationships, within the evaluation categories. Here we focus on the higher level differences between overall categories. Note also that we have excluded all behavioral conceptualization of happiness from these dimensions, taking the view that activities and behaviors – or perceptions of them – like goal-setting and socializing are determinants of happiness, rather than happiness itself (Ryff & Keyes, 1995; Ryff, Chap. 6, this volume).

Table 29.1 also shows that some measures are 'other' or combinations of the level of happiness. For example, the question, "How happy did you feel yesterday?" is evaluative in the sense that it asks for a cognitive judgment about the whole of yesterday, but is also experiential because it asks about feelings. Students who were asked the 'happy yesterday' question, and who also filled out a diary of yesterday's activities and reported how happy they felt during them, recollected feeling happier yesterday than shown in the aggregated average daily happiness scores from their diaries (Tadić, Braam, Van Vliet, & Veenhoven, 2013). Other studies have shown that evaluations of experiences like these tend to be more intense for negative as well as positive emotions, such that people also recall feeling worse than the average of their experiences of negative emotion across a given time period (Christodoulou, Schneider, & Stone, 2012; Miron-Shatz, Stone, & Kahneman, 2009).

The question, "How worthwhile are the things that you do in your life?" is also both evaluative and experiential: it is evaluative in the sense that it requires a judgment about the worthwhileness of things in general, and also experiential because it asks about doing things rather than life overall. In nationally representative data from the Office for National Statistics in the UK, there are no differences in how worthwhile employed and unemployed groups consider the things they do in their life to be, and there are also no differences by education level (Deeming, 2013). Yet other research has found that people who are unemployed report lower evaluations of purpose in life than the employed and also that people with higher education report better evaluations of purpose in life (Ryff, Keyes, & Hughes, 2003). It would seem that people who find their life to be purposeful are not the same people who find the things that they do in their life to be purposeful, although, as with all between-group comparisons discussed, it is also possible that these differ-

Table 29.1 The two dimensions of happiness

Type Level	"Pleasure"	"Purpose"	Combinations and other
Evaluation	"How happy are you with your life overall?"	"How worthwhile is your life overall?"	"How satisfied are you with your life overall?"
Experience	"How much pleasure do you feel right now?"	"How much purpose do you feel right now?"	"How satisfied are you right now?"
Combinations and other	How happy did you feel yesterday?	How worthwhile are the things that you do in your life?	"How satisfied were you yesterday?"

ences can be attributed to differences between the samples rather than differences between the measures.

Further measures reflect combinations of the type of happiness. As noted by several scholars, one of the most widely used happiness questions asks about overall life satisfaction (Aknin, Dunn, Sandstrom, & Norton, 2013; Jivraj, Nazroo, Vanhoutte, & Chandola, 2014). At the time of writing, about 10 % of the publications on Google Scholar containing the word 'happiness' also contain the phrase 'life satisfaction', which is indicative of its prevalence. Life satisfaction is clearly an evaluative question, requiring a cognitive judgment about life overall, but it is unclear whether it is about pleasure or purpose, as the term 'satisfaction' could refer to one or the other, or to both in some combination. That life satisfaction is not clearly about either pleasure or purpose is part of what makes the existing conceptualisations and measures of happiness so confusing.

Whilst overall evaluations of life satisfaction typically do not vary much from overall evaluations of happiness, subtleties do sometimes emerge. For example, there is more between-country variation in life satisfaction than in evaluative happiness measures, which would impact any judgment of how much happier one country is compared to another (Waldron, 2010). Age affects life satisfaction and evaluations of purpose rather differently too: whereas life satisfaction improves after middle age, evaluations of purpose do not always, and so it would seem that older people are happier than middle aged people according to the life satisfaction data but sometimes not from the data on evaluations of purpose (Blanchflower & Oswald, 2008; Pinquart, 2002; Ryff & Singer, 2008). We are not aware of any studies that would allow a comparison of whether the determinants of how satisfied people feel right now are different to those of experiences of pleasure or purpose right now.

From this discussion, it is evident that it is important for anyone investigating the causes of happiness with only a single measure to be clear that their results may differ if another happiness measure were used. Making general claims about happiness based on analyses of a single measure poses a serious problem to those seeking to understand the causes of happiness because the determinants of happiness differ according to the level and type of happiness measure used. Yet our understanding of the differences between the levels and types of happiness is limited by the fact that we know much less about some aspects of happiness than others, a consideration to which we now turn.

29.3 Accounting for Pleasure and Purpose

Researchers focus more on some dimensions of happiness than others, with the various adjectives of emotion and 'happiness' being the most commonly used terms in the literature to date. This is according to Google Scholar and Web of Knowledge keyword searches of happiness terms. Evaluative happiness and life satisfaction measures are popular in economics and policy (Benjamin, Heffetz, Kimball, & Szembrot, 2014). For example, economic articles often refer to happiness and life satisfaction interchangeably (Easterlin, 2013; Kavetsos & Koutroumpis, 2011; Van Landeghem, 2012), and life satisfaction measures are used for cost benefit analyses by the UK's HM Treasury (Fujiwara, 2010).

Where purpose has been separately referenced, it is typically done so at the evaluation level; that is, whether life overall has meaning or purpose (Huta & Waterman, 2013; Ryff & Keyes, 1995; Shin & Steger, 2014; Huta, Chap. 15, this volume; Steger, Chap. 11, this volume). A common scale used to measure purpose is in fact called "Purpose in Life", with "in life" reflecting the evaluative nature of its items (Ryff & Keyes, 1995). There has been some recognition that experiences of purpose are distinct from evaluations (Krause, 2009, p. 105; Reker & Wong, 1988, pp. 220–221; Steger, 2012, pp. 381–382). White and Dolan (2009) conducted a principal-component exploratory factor analysis of time-use data to determine whether or not positive and negative affect are conceptually distinct from experiences of worthwhileness, meaningfulness, and purposefulness. The results were a two-factor solution where the positive and negative affect items loaded onto the first factor and the purpose items loaded onto the second factor.

The US National Academy of Sciences (2014) report on measuring well-being concluded experiences of purpose are important in addition to experiences of pleasure: "*An important part of people's experiences may be overlooked if concepts associated with purpose and purposelessness are not included alongside hedonic ones like pleasure and pain in measures of [experienced well-being]... People do many things because they are deemed purposeful or worthwhile, even if they are not especially pleasurable* (e.g., *reading the same story over and over again to a child, visiting a sick friend, volunteering*)" (National Academy of Sciences, 2014, p. 43).

There is not yet enough evidence yet to firmly conclude that evaluations and experiences of purpose have different determinants. To add to our understanding of experiences of purpose we have therefore analyzed two major surveys: the 2010 Well-being Module of the American Time Use Survey (ATUS), which is a cross-sectional sample of around 13,000 US residents, and also the German Day Reconstruction Method (DRM), another cross-sectional sample of around 600 German residents (and reported in White & Dolan, 2009). Each survey asks participants to keep a diary of yesterday's activities and rate how they felt during them.

In the ATUS, three activities were selected for affect ratings for a partial DRM, whereas in the German DRM, participants rated the affect they experienced during almost every activity in their diary for a full day. The ATUS is the largest sample of activity diaries that contains affect ratings for a selection of activities, and the German DRM is the largest sample of activity diaries that contains affect ratings on a full day's activities. In the ATUS, the pleasure question was, "From 0 to 6, where a 0 means you were not happy at all and a 6 means you were very happy, how happy did you feel during this time?" and the purpose question was, "From 0 to 6, how meaningful did you consider what you were doing? 0 means it was not meaningful at all to you and a 6 means it was very meaningful to you." In the German DRM, the pleasure question was, "How much happiness did you feel?" and the purpose question was, "I feel the activities in this episode were worthwhile/meaningful", each again rated a 0–6 scale from not at all to very strongly.

We are not aware of any data that would facilitate comparisons between evaluations and experiences of purpose and so here we focus on differences between experiences of pleasure and purpose. These data tell us about three important aspects of experienced purpose that support the notion it manifests itself independently from experienced pleasure. First, as discussed previously and shown in White and Dolan (2009) using the same dataset, the 'pleasure' items load onto different factors than the 'purpose' items. Second, it is evident that some activities are more purposeful than pleasurable (like work) whereas others are more pleasurable than purposeful (like watching TV) in both the ATUS and the German DRM, as can be seen in Figs. 29.1 and 29.2, and was also discovered in another sample of 45 university staff (Christodoulou et al., 2012). Third, the purpose ratings of those aged 15–23 years in the ATUS are lower than the purpose ratings of other age groups as well as their own pleasure ratings, as can be seen in Fig. 29.3.

Although it is possible that selection effects account for the results regarding the second aspect, it is likely that the activity itself does drive some of its effects on pleasure and purpose: someone might feel sad and then start listening to music but eventually the music will impact how that person feels while listening to it. While it would be impossible for age to cause pleasure or purpose, cohort or sampling effects could be responsible for the results regarding the third aspect and future research may help to clarify this. Regardless, these headline results show that if we only looked at people's pleasure scores we would reach different conclusions about how happy the ATUS and the German DRM participants are when engaging in different activities, as well as how happy young people are. Taken together, these findings suggest a distinction between experiences of pleasure and purpose.

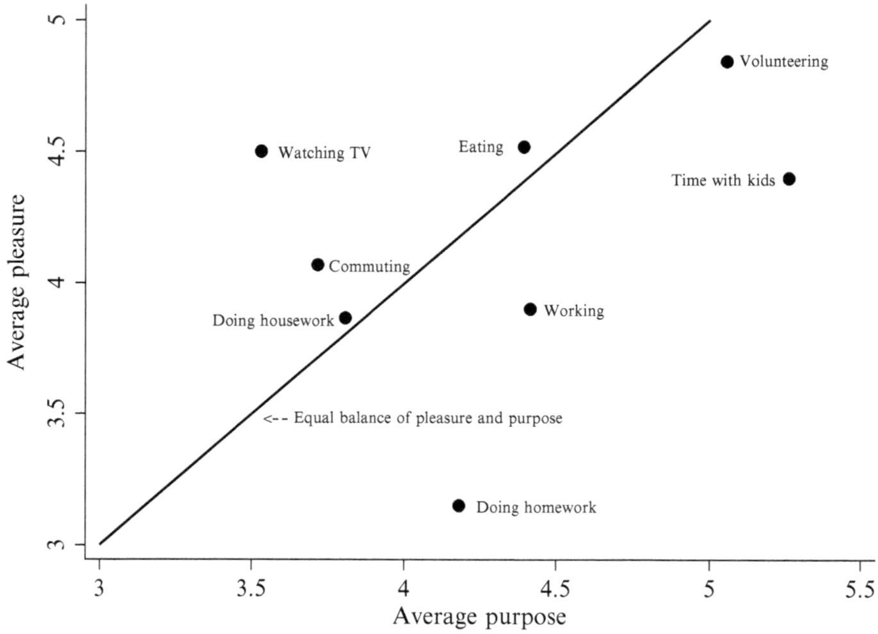

Fig. 29.1 'Pleasure' and 'purpose' ratings by activity in the German DRM

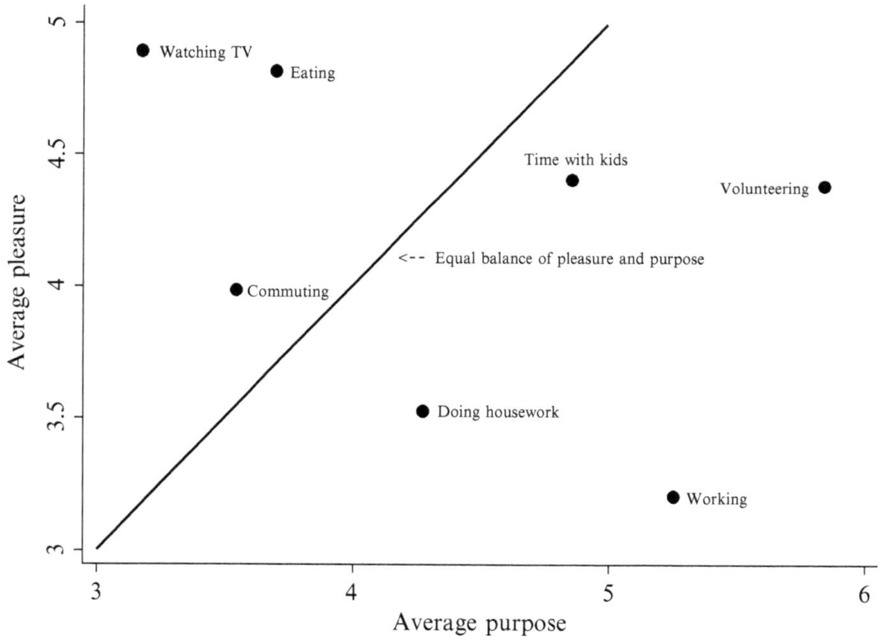

Fig. 29.2 'Pleasure' and 'purpose' ratings by activity in the ATUS

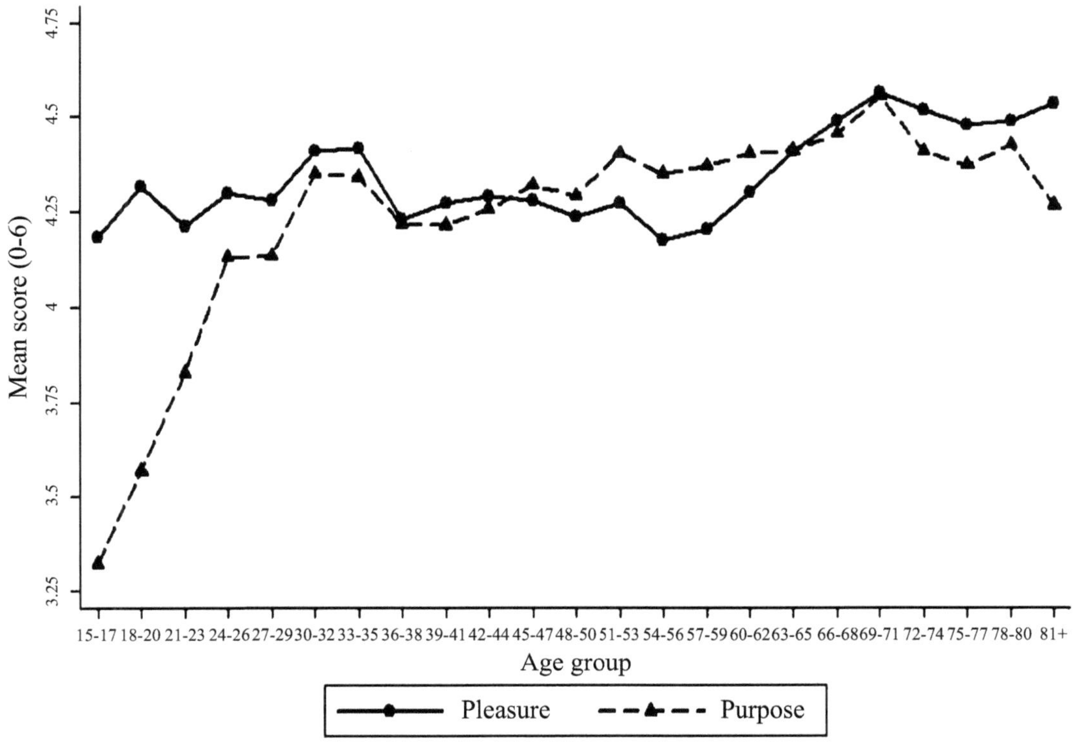

Fig. 29.3 'Pleasure' and 'purpose' ratings by age in the ATUS

29.4 From Evaluation to Experience

We now examine the levels of happiness a little more closely. As discussed in the Introduction, policy-makers around the world are increasingly interested in using measures of happiness to monitor national progress (Diener, Lucas, Schimmack, & Helliwell, 2009; Office for National Statistics, 2013; United Nations, 2012) and to inform resource allocation (Fujiwara, 2010). Most of the policy research to date has been conducted using questions that reflect overall evaluations, such as life satisfaction, and we have already seen that what affects people's evaluations and experiences can be quite different. This means that our conclusions about which countries are doing well and about who should get priority in the race for scarce resources might be different if measures of experience were used instead.

Does this matter? We contend that there are good conceptual and empirical reasons to suppose it does, and that researchers and policy-makers should be paying more serious attention to experience-based measures of happiness than they are currently. This is not an uncontroversial position to take. It is far cheaper and easier for statistical agencies to ask high-level evaluative questions than it is to ask about specific feelings and activities. Still, as we discuss in detail in this section, we believe there are good reasons to favour experiences over evaluations.

Certainly, for researchers especially, the happiness measure does depend on the research question: for questions about experiences of happiness, experiential indicators are more suitable, and for questions about evaluations of happiness, evaluative items are more appropriate. We do not mean to imply that experiential indicators are better for all types of research questions; rather, that the types of questions asked about happiness should more often be about experiential happiness inasmuch as researchers want to understand how well people's lives are going. This is our overarching criterion in this discussion: whether experiential or evaluative indicators better reflect how well people's lives are really going.

It might initially appear as though evaluative questions that ask about life overall are preferable to experiential questions that ask about only a moment in time. "How happy are you feeling right now?" only tells us how well people's lives are going at that moment, whereas "how happy are you with your life overall?" seemingly informs about life as a whole. Unfortunately, it does not appear that people actually aggregate information about their lives as a whole when they answer a question about their life overall. It takes a similar amount of time for people to answer a life satisfaction question as it does a question about their emotions, 4–5 s (Vittersø, Oelmann, & Wang, 2009). This is an issue because the length of time it takes to answer a question can be associated with the depth with which people process that question (Krosnick, 1999; Slovic, Finucane, Peters, & MacGregor, 2002, 2007). Whilst understanding how well people's lives are going overall is a laudable aim, it does not appear that a single question can achieve that aim.

Given that people answer overall questions about their happiness so quickly, is not surprising that people appear to rely on readily available information to construct responses to evaluative happiness questions. For example, being asked about one's political views before being asked about life satisfaction affects reports of satisfaction as much as becoming unemployed does, and life and relationship satisfaction are more highly correlated if the relationship question comes before the life satisfaction question rather than after (Deaton, 2011; Schwarz, Strack, & Mai, 1991). The task of evaluating how well life is going overall is a demanding one and so what is prominent at the time of the assessment will drive responses, similar to the way that people facing the task of recalling how many alcoholic drinks they have had over a period of weeks or months will tend to recall the most prominent drinks, such as regularly having two beers at the bar every Friday (Del Boca & Darkes, 2003). It is also difficult to make an assessment of life overall without making comparisons to other people because the question is so broad, whereas reports of feelings in the moment are arguably more absolute – the pain you feel in your leg is not as affected by the pain others are feeling, although this is an active research area (Meng et al., 2013).

Another reason why we favour experiences to evaluations is that overall evaluations are rarely considered in our daily lives; perhaps they are only ever really triggered in studies that measure them (Feldman, 2004; Haybron, 2008, Chap. 2, this volume; Schwarz & Strack, 1991). People do not often appear to ask themselves how happy or satisfied they are overall, or how much purpose they have in life, and such specific evaluative happiness questions will likely arise more often in the context of a survey interview than in daily life. We need more research into people's thoughts and where their attention is directed, however, to truly know the degree to which people think about whether they are happy or satisfied overall. There are, of course, likely to be individual differences in the extent to which people consider overall evaluations of their lives. Some people may be more prone to think about them than others, such as those who have high trait anxiety, frequently ruminate on the past, or often worry about the future (Watkins, 2008). To understand how well people's lives are going, we maintain that it is preferable to use measures aligned with what people are most likely to consider most often as they go about their lives, rather than momentary snapshots that do not feature as frequently in their considerations.

Moreover, evaluative judgments do not adequately capture the duration of our happiness, which is a problem because our happiness depends on how long our feelings last as well as on their valence and intensity. Someone who reports feeling happy throughout the day is happier than someone who reports feeling happy for only one minute in the day. Recall from earlier that people's evaluations of how they felt on a particular day were more intense than the duration-weighted average of their emotions on the same day (Miron-Shatz et al., 2009; Tadić et al., 2013). Given that the encoding and retrieval of emotional information are largely unconscious processes, it is likely that at least some of the tendency to neglect the duration of an emotional experience in an overall evaluation of it is also unconscious (Robinson & Clore, 2002; Wyer, Clore, & Isbell, 1999). So drawing conscious attention to the difference between evaluation and experience may not fully resolve the issue of duration neglect in the former. Although people who feel more happiness in their experiences report more happiness in their evaluations, capturing experiential variability is important. Consider for instance, those people whose happiness is more susceptible to positive and negative environmental influences (see Pluess, 2015): their happiness is likely to fluctuate more than others' during a period of time, as environments constantly change over time. Yet this experienced variability might not transpire in people's global evaluations, which would then be less informative for policy purposes. Similar issue apply to people with mental health conditions, such as bipolar disorder, which are characterised by extreme fluctuations in mood over time.

There are also concerns with the use of the word 'satisfaction' in many of the evaluative questions. Confusingly, there are several interpretations of satisfaction: it could mean feeling happy in some general sense, or it might indicate the perception of having 'just enough'. For example, a qualitative investigation of how people understood the question, "How satisfied are you with your life nowadays?" revealed that the term 'satisfaction' was interpreted positively by some people and negatively by others, and among those who interpreted it negatively, it was reported that satisfaction was "something not to aim for or that it meant something that was neither good nor bad" (Ralph, Palmer, & Olney, 2011, p. 5). As further evidence of such problems with the comprehension of life satisfaction questions, people who are older, poorer, and less educated are more likely to be provide 'ten out of ten' ratings for their satisfaction with life than those saying 'nine out of ten'. The evidence related to age supports the idea that life satisfaction measures are capturing an endorsement of one's life when approaching the end of life, rather than an actual evaluation of one's life (Dolan, Layard, & Metcalfe, 2011; Oishi, Diener, & Lucas, 2007). We argue that endorsements of life are not good indicators of how well people's lives are really going.

It is also possible that responses to life satisfaction questions capture the degree to which respondents have satisfied their preferences – as opposed to capturing any aspect of their mental state at all. In support of this idea, Akay, Bargain and Jara (2015) show that people's revealed preferences for income-leisure trade-offs closely correspond to their life satisfaction in that as leisure time increases and income decreases, life satisfaction also decreases in a similar manner. Adler (2012) raises legitimate reasons why life satisfaction might not be a good guide to preferences, primarily due to 'scale heterogeneity', whereby two people with similar preference might use the life satisfaction scale differently (King & Wand, 2007; Salomon, Tandon, & Murray, 2004), and 'preference heterogeneity', whereby we cannot infer people's preferences over the ranking of bundles of attributes from a single satisfaction response.

But even if life satisfaction may be an imperfect measure of preference satisfaction, this still leaves open the possibility that the ratings better reflect preferences than they do mental states. Indeed, when considering the high respondent burden associated with the direct reporting of preferences and the high survey costs therein, single-item life satisfaction measures may be a better choice for statistical agencies seeking to capture preferences than people's reports of their preferences (Dolan & Peasgood, 2008).

Experiential happiness is not without its own limitations. It is not clear what the best assessment method is. The experience sampling method (ESM) asks people at random times of day how they are feeling. It is typically considered the gold standard for measuring experiential happiness because it does not allow for the possibility that people inaccurately recall how they were feeling as responses are captured 'in-the-moment' (Kahneman, Krueger, Schkade, & Schwartz, 2004; Scollon, Kim-Prieto, & Diener, 2003). Using the DRM increases the risk of recall bias because it asks people to recall how they felt during various activities over a 24-h period. But a DRM provides information about an entire day's worth of experiences, whereas experience sampling captures only a few points throughout the day to minimise respondent burden. Moreover, the ESM asks people to say how happy they are at the moment they are interrupted from their experiences to report on it. These considerations call into question whether the ESM can really be considered the 'gold standard'. Another issue is that people who report feeling stress do not always show physiological signs of stress (Mauss, Wilhelm, & Gross, 2004). This is surprising because stress is known to be associated with higher heart rate, respiratory rate, and levels of the hormone cortisol. But these findings merely raise the issue of how experiential happiness is best assessed – with the ESM or DRM or other self-reports, or physiological indicators of emotions. It does not call into question whether experiential measures are capturing (the duration of) happiness or another construct such as having 'just enough' or an 'endorsement' of life the same way that the evidence on evaluative measures does. An issue for both evaluations and experiences of happiness is that we do not really know what determines the answer to a survey item about happiness. Cognitive interviews provide some clues but they cannot capture processes people are unaware of (Luhmann, Hawkley, & Cacioppo, 2014).

Another issue with measures of experiences of happiness relate to perceived duration differing from actual duration. Emotional experiences themselves affect the perception of time: when people report experiencing low purpose, such as boredom, time passes slowly, whereas when people report experiencing high pleasure, such as fun, it passes quickly (Droit-Volet & Meck, 2007). Weighting emotional experiences such that they account for perceived rather than actual duration could affect who appears most happy or unhappy. For example, Knabe et al. (2010) found that unemployed people reported feeling sadder than employed people but that their emotional experiences were similar once duration was accounted for. So, the greater intensity of sadness found among unemployed people might occur in periods that are perceived to last longer than their actual duration, and this could bring down the total happiness experienced by unemployed people relative to employed ones.

The implication of taking the position that experiences are more important than evaluations is that the determinants of experiential happiness are more important than those of evaluative happiness. When unemployed people find a new job, they become less satisfied with their lives overall, possibly because they think working again will be better than it actually is (Luhmann et al., 2012). Their experiences of happiness are higher around the time of re-employment than before or after, however, and we believe it is these direct experiences that are more important than evaluative constructions about these experiences.

29.5 Conclusion

This article has provided a simple classification of the various conceptualisations and measures of happiness. Given the evidence that evaluative happiness measures suffer from a range of problems, conceptualising and measuring happiness as an experience appears to better reflect how well our lives are going. By observing the purpose in our experiences of happiness in addition to their pleasure, the criticism that experiential happiness is too limited by only considering experiences of pleasure and pain may be overcome (Aristotle, 2002; Huta & Waterman, 2013; Ryan & Deci, 2001; Ryan and Martela, Chap. 7, this volume). Some activities, like work, might then be afforded a greater contribution to our happiness because they are purposeful even if they are not very pleasurable. That working could contribute to happiness as much as watching television is important for academics, policymakers and the general public to consider when using happiness measures to help improve people's lives.

Given the interpretation of experiences as sentiments, a richer account of experiential happiness would be 'sentimental hedonism', which defines happiness as experiences of pleasure and purpose over time. This is distinct from hedonism, which only recognizes experiences of pleasure. This account of happiness also downplays evaluations of happiness. Again, the aim of this discussion is not to reinvigorate debates about hedonism. Our conceptualization of experiential happiness includes experiences of purpose as well as pleasure and so we recognize some of the limitations of hedonism, especially the criticism that there are things that matter beyond pleasure (Crisp, 2006; Smart et al., 1974; Nozick, 1977).

There are obviously longstanding ethical and philosophical discussions about the extent to which happiness is all that matters (Duncan, 2013). We are inclined to think that it is but we recognize that others will disagree, arguing instead that we might have legitimate desires for things other than happiness, such as morality, freedom, truth, knowledge, aesthetics, or beauty (Bruni, Comim, & Pugno, 2008; Nussbaum & Sen, 1993). We do not seek to add further to this discussion but rather to make the case that, insofar as happiness does matter, it is best measured as experiences of pleasure and purpose over time.

In the future, researchers should be much more explicit about the definition of happiness employed in their work and how it informs the measures they select, ideally according to the distinctions between level and type of happiness that we proposed here, and with a focus on experiences. There is much work to be done in discovering the structure of sentiments and their optimal balance over time. Future work should continue to explore how the determinants of experiences of pleasure and purpose differ, as well as whether experiences of pleasure and purpose can be combined to generate an overall measure of happiness. In general, future work should continue to consider which happiness measures best reflect how happy we all are.

References

Adler, M. D. (2012). Happiness surveys and public policy: What's the use. *Duke LJ, 62*, 1509.

Akay, A., Bargain, O., & Jara. H. X. (2015). *Large-scale comparison of decision versus experienced utility for income-leisure preferences* (Institute for Social and Economic Research, No. 2015-2).

Aknin, L. B., Dunn, E. W., Sandstrom, G. M., & Norton, M. I. (2013). Does social connection turn good deeds into good feelings? On the value of putting the 'social' in prosocial spending. *International Journal of Happiness and Development, 1*(2), 155–171.

Aristotle. (2002). *Nicomachean ethics* (S. Broadie, & C. Rowe, Eds.). Oxford, UK: Oxford University Press.

Baumeister, R. F. (1991). *Meanings of life*. New York: Guilford Press.

Benjamin, D. J., Heffetz, O., Kimball, M. S., & Szembrot, N. (2014). Beyond happiness and satisfaction: Toward well-being indices based on stated preference. *The American Economic Review, 104*(9), 2698–2735.

Bentham, J. (1907). *An introduction to the principles of morals and legislation*. Oxford, UK: Oxford University Press.

Biswas-Diener, R., Kashdan, T. B., & King, L. A. (2009). Two traditions of happiness research, not two distinct types of happiness. *The Journal of Positive Psychology, 4*(3), 208–211.

Blanchflower, D. G., & Oswald, A. J. (2008). Is well-being U-shaped over the life cycle? *Social Science & Medicine, 66*(8), 1733–1749.

Brown, N. J., MacDonald, D. A., Samanta, M. P., Friedman, H. L., & Coyne, J. C. (2014). A critical reanalysis of the relationship between genomics and well-being. *Proceedings of the National Academy of Sciences, 111*(35), 12705–12709.

Bruni, L., Comim, F., & Pugno, M. (2008). *Capabilities and happiness*. Oxford, UK: Oxford University Press.

Bryson, A., Forth, J., & Stokes. L. (2014). *Does worker wellbeing affect workplace performance?* Department for Business Innovation and Skills.

Burton, R. P. D. (1998). Global integrative meaning as a mediating factor in the relationship between social roles and psychological distress. *Journal of Health & Social Behavior, 39*(3), 201–215.

Busseri, M. A., & Sadava, S. W. (2011). A review of the tripartite structure of subjective well-being: Implications for conceptualization, operationalization, analysis, and synthesis. *Personality and Social Psychology Review, 15*(3), 290–314.

Campbell, A., Converse, P. E., & Rodgers, W. L. (1976). *The quality of American life: Perceptions, evaluations, and satisfactions*. New York: Russell Sage Foundation.

Carstensen, L. L., Turan, B., Scheibe, S., Ram, N., Ersner-Hershfield, H., Samanez-Larkin, G. R., … Nesselroade, J. R. (2011). Emotional experience improves with age: Evidence based on over 10 years of experience sampling. *Psychology and Aging, 26*(1), 21–33.

Christodoulou, C., Schneider, S., & Stone, A. A. (2012). Validation of a brief yesterday measure of hedonic well-being and daily activities: Comparison with the day reconstruction method. *Social Indicators Research, 115*, 1–11.

Clarke, P. (2014). *Does worker wellbeing affect workplace performance?* Retrieved from https://app.croner.co.uk/whats-new/does-worker-wellbeing-affect-workplace-performance?topic=3307&product=8

Crisp, R. (2006). Hedonism reconsidered. *Philosophy and Phenomenological Research, 73*(3), 619–645.

Deaton, A. (2011). The financial crisis and the well-being of Americans: 2011 OEP Hicks Lecture. *Oxford Economic Papers, 64*(1), 1–26.

Deeming, C. (2013). Addressing the social determinants of subjective wellbeing: The latest challenge for social policy. *Journal of Social Policy, 42*(3), 541–565.

Del Boca, F. K., & Darkes, J. (2003). The validity of self-reports of alcohol consumption: State of the science and challenges for research. *Addiction, 98*(s2), 1–12.

Diener, E. (2000). Subjective well-being: The science of happiness and a proposal for a national index. *American Psychologist, 55*(1), 34.

Diener, E., Lucas, R., Schimmack, U., & Helliwell, J. (2009). *Well-being for Public Policy*. Oxford, UK: Oxford University Press.

Diener, E., Ng, W., Harter, J., & Arora, R. (2010). Wealth and happiness across the world: Material prosperity predicts life evaluation, whereas psychosocial prosperity predicts positive feeling. *Journal of Personality and Social Psychology, 99*(1), 52.

Dokic, J., & Lemaire, S. (2015). Are emotions evaluative modes? *Dialectica, 69*(3), 271–292.

Dolan, P. (2014). *Happiness by design: Finding pleasure and purpose in everyday life*. London: Penguin.

Dolan, P., Layard, R., & Metcalfe, R. (2011). *Measuring subjective well-being for public policy*. Retrieved from http://eprints.lse.ac.uk/35420/1/measuring-subjective-wellbeing-for-public-policy.pdf

Dolan, P., & Metcalfe, R. (2012). Measuring subjective wellbeing: Recommendations on measures for use by national governments. *Journal of Social Policy, 41*(2), 409–427.

Dolan, P., & Peasgood, T. (2008). Measuring well-being for public policy: Preferences or experiences? *The Journal of Legal Studies, 37*(S2), S5–S31.

Dolan, P., Peasgood, T., & White, M. (2008). Do we really know what makes us happy? A review of the economic literature on the factors associated with subjective well-being. *Journal of Economic Psychology, 29*(1), 94–122.

Droit-Volet, S., & Meck, W. H. (2007). How emotions colour our perception of time. *Trends in Cognitive Sciences, 11*(12), 504–513.

Duncan, G. (2013). Should happiness-maximization be the goal of government? *Journal of Happiness Studies, 11*(2), 163–178.

Easterlin, R. A. (2013). Happiness, growth, and public policy. *Economic Inquiry, 51*(1), 1–15.

Ellyatt, H. (2013, June 6). *Happiness matters, Merkel tells Germany*. CNBC.

Feldman, F. (2004). *Pleasure and the good life: Concerning the nature, varieties, and plausibility of Hedonism*. New York: Oxford University Press.

Fujiwara, D. (2010). *The Department for Work and Pensions Social Cost-Benefit Analysis framework* (Department for Work and Pensions Working Paper Series, 86). London: Department for Work and Pensions.

Hansen, T. (2012). Parenthood and happiness: A review of folk theories versus empirical evidence. *Social Indicators Research, 108*(1), 29–64.

Haybron, D. M. (2008). *The pursuit of unhappiness: The elusive psychology of well-being*. Oxford, UK: Oxford University Press.

Hicks, J. A., Cicero, D. C., Trent, J., Burton, C. M., & King, L. A. (2010). Positive affect, intuition, and feelings of meaning. *Journal of Personality and Social Psychology, 98*(6), 967.

Huta, V., & Waterman, A. S. (2013). Eudaimonia and its distinction from hedonia: Developing a classification and terminology for understanding conceptual and operational definitions. *Journal of Happiness Studies, 14*, 1–32.

Jivraj, S., Nazroo, J., Vanhoutte, B., & Chandola, T. (2014). Aging and subjective well-being in later life. *The Journals of Gerontology Series B: Psychological Sciences and Social Sciences, 69*(6), 930–941.

Kahneman, D., & Deaton, A. (2010). High income improves evaluation of life but not emotional well-being. *Proceedings of the National Academy of Sciences, 107*(38), 16489–16493.

Kahneman, D., & Krueger, A. B. (2006). Developments in the measurement of subjective well-being. *The Journal of Economic Perspectives, 20*(1), 3–24.

Kahneman, D., Krueger, A., Schkade, D., & Schwartz, N. (2004). A survey method for characterizing daily life experience: The day reconstruction method. *Science, 306*(5702), 1776–1780.

Kahneman, D., & Riis, J. (2005). Living, and thinking about it: Two perspectives on life. In A. Hupper, N. Baylis, & B. Keverne (Eds.), *The science of well-being* (pp. 285–304). Oxford, UK: Oxford University Press.

Kavetsos, G., & Koutroumpis, P. (2011). Technological affluence and subjective well-being. *Journal of Economic Psychology, 32*(5), 742–753.

King, G., & Wand, J. (2007). Comparing incomparable survey responses: Evaluating and selecting anchoring vignettes. *Political Analysis, 15*(1), 46–66.

Knabe, A., Rätzel, S., Schöb, R., & Weimann, J. (2010). Dissatisfied with life but having a good day: Time-use and wellbeing of the unemployed. *The Economic Journal, 120*(547), 867–889.

Krause, N. (2009). Deriving a sense of meaning in late life: An overlooked forum for the development of interdisciplinary theory. In M. Silverstein, V. L. Bengtson, & N. M. Putney (Eds). *Handbook of theories of aging, Second Edition* (pp. 101–116). New York: Springer Publishing Company.

Krosnick, J. A. (1999). Survey research. *Annual Review of Psychology, 50*(1), 537–567.

Luhmann, M., Hawkley, L. C., & Cacioppo, J. T. (2014). Thinking about one's subjective wellbeing: Average tends and individual differences. *Journal of Happiness Studies, 15*(4), 757–781.

Luhmann, M., Hofmann, W., Eid, M., & Lucas, R. E. (2012). Subjective well-being and adaptation to life events: A meta-analysis. *Journal of Personality and Social Psychology, 102*(3), 592.

Mauss, I., Wilhelm, F., & Gross, J. (2004). Is there less to social anxiety than meets the eye? Emotion experience, expression, and bodily responding. *Cognition and Emotion, 18*(5), 631–642.

Meng, J., Jackson, T., Chen, H., Hu, L., Yang, Z., Su, Y., et al. (2013). Pain perception in the self and observation of others: An ERP investigation. *NeuroImage, 72*, 164–173.

Miron-Shatz, T., Stone, A., & Kahneman, D. (2009). Memories of yesterday's emotions: Does the valence of experience affect the memory-experience gap? *Emotion, 9*(6), 885.

National Academy of Sciences. (2014). *Subjective well-being: Measuring happiness, suffering, and other dimensions of experience*. National Academies Press. Retrieved from http://www.nap.edu/catalog.php?record_id=18548

Nelson, S. K., Kushlev, K., English, T., Dunn, E. W., & Lyubomirsky, S. (2013). In defense of parenthood: Children are associated with more joy than misery. *Psychological Science, 24*(1), 3–10.

Nozick, R. (1977). *Anarchy, State, and Utopia*. New York: Basic Books.

Nussbaum, M., & Sen, A. (1993). *The quality of life*. Oxford: Oxford University Press.

Office for National Statistics. (2013, July 30). *Personal well-being in the UK, 2012/13. Office for National Statistics*. Retrieved from http://www.ons.gov.uk/ons/rel/wellbeing/measuring-national-well-being/personal-well-being-in-the-uk--2012-13/sb---personal-well-being-in-the-uk--2012-13.html#tab-Sex--age-and-ethnicity

Office of Management and Budget. (2013). 2013 Draft Report to Congress on the Benefits and Costs of Federal Regulations and Agency Compliance with the Unfunded Mandates Reform Act. Retrieved from http://www.whitehouse.gov/sites/default/files/omb/inforeg/2013_cb/draft_2013_cost_benefit_report.pdf

Oishi, S., & Diener, E. (2014). Can and should happiness be a policy goal? *Policy Insights from the Brain and Behavioural Sciences, 1*(1), 195–203.

Oishi, S., Diener, E., & Lucas, R. E. (2007). The optimum level of well-being: Can people be too happy? *Perspectives on Psychological Science, 2*(4), 346–360.

Organisation for Economic Cooperation and Development. (2015). *How's Life? Measuring Wellbeing*. Retrieved from http://www.oecd.org/statistics/how-s-life-23089679.htm

Pavot, W., & Diener, E. (1993). The affective and cognitive context of self-reported measures of subjective well-being. *Social Indicators Research, 28*(1), 1–20.

Pinquart, M. (2002). Creating and maintaining purpose in life in old age: A meta-analysis. *Ageing International, 27*(2), 90–114.

Pluess, M. (2015). Individual differences in environmental sensitivity. *Child Development Perspectives, 9*(3), 138–143.

Ralph, K., Palmer, K., & Olney, J. (2011). *Subjective well-being: A qualitative investigation of subjective wellbeing questions*. London: Office for National Statistics.

Reker, G. T., & Wong, P. T. P. (1988). Aging as an individual process: Toward a theory of personal meaning. In J. E. Birren & V. L. Bengston (Eds.), *Emergent theories of aging* (pp. 214–246). New York: Springer.

Robinson, L. A. (2013). Cost-benefit analysis and well-being analysis. *Duke Law Journal, 62*(8), 1717–1734.

Robinson, M. D., & Clore, G. L. (2002). Belief and feeling: Evidence for an accessibility model of emotional self-report. *Psychological Bulletin, 128*(6), 934.

Ryan, R. M., & Deci, E. L. (2001). On happiness and human potentials: A review of research on hedonic and eudaimonic well-being. *Annual Review of Psychology, 52*(1), 141–166.

Ryff, C. D., & Keyes, C. L. M. (1995). The structure of psychological well-being revisited. *Journal of Personality and Social Psychology, 69*(4), 719–727.

Ryff, C. D., Keyes, C. L., & Hughes, D. L. (2003). Status inequalities, perceived discrimination, and eudaimonic well-being: Do the challenges of minority life hone purpose and growth? *Journal of Health and Social Behavior, 44*, 275–291.

Ryff, C. D., & Singer, B. H. (2008). Know thyself and become what you are: A eudaimonic approach to psychological well-being. *Journal of Happiness Studies, 9*(1), 13–39.

Salomon, J. A., Tandon, A., & Murray, C. J. (2004). Comparability of self rated health: Cross sectional multi-country survey using anchoring vignettes. *British Medical Journal, 328*(7434), 258.

Schwarz, N., & Strack, F. (1991). Evaluating one's life: A judgment model of subjective well-being. *Subjective Well-Being: An Interdisciplinary Perspective, 21*, 27–47.

Schwarz, N., Strack, F., & Mai, H. P. (1991). Assimilation and contrast effects in part-whole question sequences: A conversational logic analysis. *The Public Opinion Quarterly, 55*(1), 3–23.

Scollon, C. N., Kim-Prieto, C., & Diener, E. (2003). Experience sampling: Promises and pitfalls, strengths and weaknesses. *Journal of Happiness Studies, 4*(1), 5–34.

Shin, J. Y., & Steger, M. F. (2014). Promoting meaning and purpose in life. In S. Schueller (Ed.), *The Wiley-Blackwell handbook of positive psychological interventions* (pp. 90–111). Malden: Wiley.

Slovic, P., Finucane, M., Peters, E., & MacGregor, D. G. (2002). Rational actors or rational fools: Implications of the affect heuristic for behavioral economics. *The Journal of Socio-Economics, 31*(4), 329–342.

Slovic, P., Finucane, M. L., Peters, E., & MacGregor, D. G. (2007). The affect heuristic. *European Journal of Operational Research, 177*(3), 1333–1352.

Smart, J., Quinton, A., & Williams, B. (1974). Utilitarianism; for and against. *Philosophical Quarterly, 24*(96), 279.

Son, J., & Wilson, J. (2012). Volunteer work and hedonic, eudemonic, and social well-being. *Sociological Forum, 27*, 658–681.

Steger, M. F. (2012). Making meaning in life. *Psychological Inquiry, 23*(4), 381–385.
Steger, M. F., Kashdan, T. B., & Oishi, S. (2008). Being good by doing good: Daily eudaimonic activity and well-being. *Journal of Research in Personality, 42*(1), 22–42.
Stiglitz, J. et al. (2009) *Report by the Commission on the Measurement of Economic Performance and Social Progress*. Retrieved from: http://www.stiglitz-sen-fitoussi.fr/en/index.htm
Tadić, M., Braam, H., Van Vliet, K., & Veenhoven, R. (2013). Memory-experience gap in early adolescents' happiness reports. *Child Indicators Research, 7*, 1–20.
United Nations. (2012). *Defining a new economic paradigm: The report of the high-level meeting on wellbeing and happiness*. Thimbu: The Permanent Mission of the Kingdom of Bhutan to the United Nations.
Van Landeghem, B. (2012). A test for the convexity of human well-being over the life cycle: Longitudinal evidence from a 20-year panel. *Journal of Economic Behavior & Organization, 81*(2), 571–582.
Vittersø, J., Oelmann, H. I., & Wang, A. L. (2009). Life satisfaction is not a balanced estimator of the good life: Evidence from reaction time measures and self-reported emotions. *Journal of Happiness Studies, 10*(1), 1–17.
Waldron, S. (2010). *Measuring subjective wellbeing in the UK*. London: Office for National Statistics.
Watkins, E. R. (2008). Constructive and unconstructive repetitive thought. *Psychological Bulletin, 134*(2), 163–206.
Watson, D., & Tellegen, A. (1985). Toward a consensual structure of mood. *Psychological Bulletin, 98*(2), 219.
Weiss, H. M. (2002). Deconstructing job satisfaction: Separating evaluations, beliefs and affective experiences. *Human Resource Management Review, 12*(2), 173–194.
White, M. P., & Dolan, P. (2009). Accounting for the richness of daily activities. *Psychological Science, 20*(8), 1000–1008.
Wyer, R. S., Jr., Clore, G. L., & Isbell, L. M. (1999). Affect and information processing. *Advances in Experimental Social Psychology, 31*, 1–77.

The Eudemonics of Education 30

Hans Henrik Knoop

30.1 Introduction

For more than two centuries, the world has built educational systems on principles of mass production and industry. In many ways this has been a successful endeavor, as still more people have learned to read, write, count, and have been introduced to scientific, artistic and moral understandings of the world, far beyond what their home surroundings would allow for. Yet, it has also become increasingly clear that education comes with a price, not only as concerns the financial budget but also immaterially, personally, and socially. For as education has grown more and more powerful in selecting young people for different paths in life, the risks of young people losing self-confidence, direction and ultimately hope has increased too. To be sure, competition between people can be great fun, be educational, and be very productive as we see in sports, gaming, and all kinds of voluntary activity in which people immerse themselves in tough challenges (thereby "competing with the challenge"). But there are delicate limits to be respected if to avoid fun turning into to anxiety, and learning turning into desperation. The limits may be difficult to determine, but the assumption that they are real should be uncontroversial. It could be limits regarding the kind and amount of experiencing meaninglessness a person can sustain before taking lasting damage. It may be limits to mere levels of challenge: as the level of challenge increases, the fun and excitements does too, until a certain point that is, where fun morphs to fear, where learning changes to self-defense, and where phobia and similar auto-immune reactions begin to flourish, rather than the person hosting them. A third variant could be limits regarding social belonging and the complex problem of accelerating change in the world potentially compromising every human relation depending on continuity, trust and long-term perspectives.

To be sure, there are countless other such limits to human capacity to be recognized, yet these few examples should suffice to exemplify what may be perceived as psychological tipping-points of crucial educational importance. Indeed, the relevance of tipping-points as regards human flourishing becomes clear by merely recognizing how all living organisms come into the world with all the motivation for life one could ever wish for, and in principle this motivation to live may remain intact until the last day, if only the sense of life being worth living is not corrupted along the way. So whenever the pursuit of flourishing is corrupted, that is: whenever a person start losing interest in life, there is danger. And should this happen in formal learning conceived

H.H. Knoop (✉)
Department of Education, University of Aarhus, Niels Juels Gade 84, building 2110, room 139, 8200 Aarhus N, Denmark
e-mail: knoop@edu.au.dk

J. Vittersø (ed.), *Handbook of Eudaimonic Well-Being*, International Handbooks of Quality-of-Life,
DOI 10.1007/978-3-319-42445-3_30

and promoted to stimulate the exact opposite: human flourishing above all, we are clearly in serious trouble. Which unfortunately seems to be the case: a paramount problem in education, perhaps the one above them all, is the grim fact that millions, if not billions, of learners don't really want to learn in settings and ways provided by traditional, educational institutions, boldly evidenced by the fact that so many learners prefer staying home on an ordinary school day rather than showing up if given the choice. Another way of framing this is to assume that the tipping-points, the "psychological thresholds of bearability" so to speak, by definition must have been transgressed, since so many lose motivation. In any case, we have massive evidence of how children and adolescents are learning about the world in ways they'd rather avoid if possible without punishment. However good reasons for education are proposed, they cannot stand against evidence about learners losing interest in learning by being educated. It simply makes no sense, as being psychologically completely unsustainable.

An often heard response to this is that life is hard, and that children have to learn to work hard if they are to make it in this world, and certainly this point has some validity as the capacity to delay gratification has benefits (e.g. Mischel, Shoda, & Rodriguez, 1989) and effortful perseverance is key to much academic, and personal, achievement (Baumeister & Tierney, 2012; Duckworth, Peterson, Matthews, & Kelly, 2007). Yet, excess delay of say water supply kills a person, and, while not quite as dramatic, delaying educational rewards may indeed tax a person quite severely also. Indeed, losing interest in learning broadly equals nothing less than loss of adaptability and thus viability. No small matter, evolutionarily, or even culturally, speaking.

One of the most interesting, general, and often over-looked, features of educational policy is that there is really no provision for hurting learners. Indeed, the Danish Ministry of Education has recently gone as far as to directly declare well-being a right of all pupils and it has decided to measure well-being among all pupils annually in order to see this flourishing happen (Danish Ministry of Education, 2015). In effect, building on scientific knowledge of learning and well-being, this means that every learner is entitled to enjoy educational life sufficiently for it to be worth living in itself, since an uninspired life generally predicts failure in all aspects and walks of life. Thriving is not provided by simply succeeding at the end of a school-term but rather a broad measure of how life feels while underway. Moreover, when applying the fuller spectrum of well-being, implying for instance self-determination (e.g. Deci & Ryan, 2000; Ryan and Martela, Chap. 7, this volume), self-efficacy (e.g. Bandura, 1994), willpower (e.g. Baumeister & Tierney, 2012; Duckworth, 2007), health (e.g. Zachariae, 2011), positive emotions (i.e. Fredrickson, 2009, Chap. 12, this volume), engagement (e.g. Csikszentmihalyi, 1990), meaning (e.g. Damon, 2008), social relatedness (e.g. Deci & Ryan, 2000) to learning, success is almost invariably predicted (e.g. Knoop, 2011, 2013). In short: just as a healthy mind-body generally predicts success in handling daily challenges so does it as regards educational success, defined as personal growth.

So neither by political intention or scientific evidence may we accept educational processes doing damage to learners. A main reason explaining why it is nevertheless happening, may be that it has simply been difficult be prove whether a given learner has actually been hurt mentally by others, and difficult to determine how much of the cause rests within the learner him- or herself. Psychological damage is less tangible than a broken leg. Yet, the better we understand the threshold between the tolerable and the intolerable pressures, the better the chances for improving education will clearly be. And the better we understand that the (eudemonic) joy of learning requires considerable effort when learning abstract content, such as acquiring written language, theory and most academic content of which educational curricula mostly consist, the more important it becomes to discern the pathways to thriving (e.g. Baumeister & Tierney, 2012; Gardner, 1999; Hattie & Yates, 2014; Kahneman, 2011; Knoop, 2011; Waters, 2011).

The following is an overview of some of the most important scientific contributions to be employed in this endeavor.

30.2 Early Psychological Findings of Particular Educational Importance

Some of the first direct humanistic psychological strides towards what eventually became Positive Psychology (PP) were made through acknowledging how people are not born as blank slates but quite to the contrary with unique genetic and mental dispositions, occurring in the form of basic individual needs to be played out in unique contexts every second of a person's life (e.g. Deci & Ryan, 2000; Maslow, 1954; Pinker, 2002). Abraham Maslow, maybe stronger than anyone else, paved the way for this understanding by arguing for a third type of psychology, a humanistic psychology based on evidence of well-functioning individuals, broadly living an intrinsically motivated life worth living. Indeed, Maslow even coined the term "positive psychology" half a century before its formal induction a scientific field of study, as something close to being a synonym to humanistic psychology, focusing on human strengths rather than the weaknesses, as it was predominantly the case within the up until then highly influential behavioristic and psychoanalytic paradigms of psychology. Many of Maslow's basic observations remain valid and much of what is known as "progressive" and "creative" in education has been strongly informed and inspired by humanistic thought of this kind, as has much of the so-called "human relation/resource management" in work-life. Akin, the growth-directed psycho-therapeutical approach of Carl Rogers (1961, 1969) remains of premiere influence among therapists to this day and is but another example of how humanistic psychology continues to inform culture and progress. Indeed, shortly after the inception of humanistic psychology Rogers expressed a humanistic approach to education as forcefully as anyone:

> *If we value independence, if we are disturbed by the growing conformity of knowledge, of values, of attitudes, which our present system induces, then we may wish to set up conditions of learning which make for uniqueness, for self-direction, and for self-initiated learning* (Rogers, 1961, p. 24)

- thereby echoing progressive educational ideas of John Dewey (2009) half a century earlier.

On the shoulders of Maslow and peers, an equally important theoretical contribution, yet with a much stronger empirical base, has come from Ed Deci and Richard Ryan's (2000) work on self-determination. Over more than 40 years they have developed a robust theory of human motivation elaborating and corroborating humanistic psychology, especially by convincingly showing how human beings are well understood as biological organisms that depend on an organismic understanding of themselves, strongly in line with Maslow, but also acknowledging how these organisms are very sophisticated mammals, capable of, indeed fundamentally requiring, communication, social relatedness, learning, creativity and autonomous action at a level unparalleled by any other known species on the planet.

Self-determination theory obviously has strong implications for education as, in the words of Niemiec and Ryan (2009, p. 133), it

> *…assumes that inherent in human nature is the propensity to be curious about one's environment and interested in learning and developing one's knowledge. All too often, however, educators introduce external controls into learning climates, which can undermine the sense of relatedness between teachers and students, and stifle the natural, volitional processes involved in high-quality learning…A large corpus of empirical evidence based on SDT suggests that both intrinsic motivation and autonomous types of extrinsic motivation are conducive to engagement and optimal learning in educational contexts. In addition, evidence suggests that teachers' support of students' basic psychological needs for autonomy, competence, and relatedness facilitates students' autonomous self-regulation for learning, academic performance, and well-being.*

Of particular educational importance here are numerous findings showing how individual and social flourishing in all age groups depends directly on the personal experience of autonomous motivation. In other words, self-determination theory argues forcefully for giving priority to autonomous motivation in almost any kind of learning environment, if the particular type of learning is to be effective and joyful enough to be self-reinforcing (Deci & Ryan, 2000). Many other findings from biology, evolutionary psychology, and systems science are in line with this research, and have produced insights congruent, or indirectly corroborating self-determination theory (e.g., Camazine et al., 2001; Csikszentmihalyi, 1993, 1996; Kauffman, 2000; Pinker, 2002).

Almost "synergistically" with self-determination theory stands Albert Bandura's (1994) equally robust theory of the development of individual self-efficacy. Self-efficacy is "the belief in one's capabilities to organize and execute the courses of action required to manage prospective situations" (Bandura, 1995, p. 2). In other words, self-efficacy is a belief in one's own ability to meet important challenges successfully. The degree of self-efficacy has been shown highly predictive of individuals' performances in many different settings, for better or worse, and Henry Ford's conviction that "Whether you think you can, or you can't – you're right", holds considerable truth, potentially directly related to the mechanisms known as placebo effects. Learner's self-efficacy thus being the learner's expectation regarding own performance can meaningfully be understood as complementary to the teachers' expectation towards the learners, yielding the so-called Pygmalion-effect (when positive) and Golem-effect (when negative), originally studied by Robert Rosenthal, where teachers' expectation of pupil outcomes are almost eerily predictive: Low expectations predict low achievement, high expectations the opposite (Rosenthal & Jacobson, 1992). Also Bandura's work (e.g. 1977, 1994) has fundamental implications for education, where most pupils have first-hand experience of insurmountable failure as they found themselves stalling, gradually being sorted into classes, categories, levels of status, as they saw their more competent, or otherwise privileged, peers proceed and advance into the distance. The predictive value of self-efficacy, and its precise and rather easily manageable measures, compared to related but more vague concepts such as self-confidence, have made it popular not only in psychology but also in many bordering areas of study such as stress-research and preventive medicine (e.g. Zachariae, 2011). Maybe the most important educational implication of the research on self-efficacy is that it provides an irrefutable argument for ensuring that all students experience school learning as an overall successful venture because self-efficacy grows from own experience of success, that is: for a learner, to a considerable degree, success requires previous success. This is another reason why rigidly standardized teaching, learning and testing is bound to discourage a large percentage of pupils as they come to see learning as a no-win-game. In support of this point, Robert Rosenthal offers his only conclusion of prescriptive nature from his decades of research:

> *Superb teachers can teach the "unteachable"; we know that. So, what I think this research shows is that there's a moral obligation for a teacher: if the teacher knows that certain students can't learn, that teacher should get out of that classroom* (Rhem, 1999, p. 4).

Contrasting, yet also almost complementing, both self-determination theory and self-efficacy theory, is the theory of learned helplessness (Seligman & Maier, 1967; Overmier & Seligman, 1967). This theory explains how it is possible to brutalize animal, and humans, into complete passivity and apathy by removing their sense of control over their own (unpleasant and meaningless) situation. Also this theory, though obviously running counter to any defendable educational endeavor, has important explanatory power in the cases of young people burning out in school due to continuous failure to succeed meaningfully. Yet, maybe equally important was the follow-up finding to the studies of learned helplessness indicating that learned helplessness is much less likely to occur if preceded by experiences of success in overcoming challenges similar to the given (Seligman & Maier, 1967), exactly as predicted by self-efficacy-theory (Bandura, 1994). Extrapolating, the latter finding is also congruent with the massive evidence of the importance of early childhood experiences for later life as regards harmonious physical, emotional, cognitive, and social development all predicting resilience (O'Dougherty et al., 2013).

Of maybe unparalleled theoretical importance in expanding humanistic psychology towards the positive psychology movement, are the contributions of Mihaly Csikszentmihalyi (e.g. 1990, 1993, 1996). Csikszentmihalyi's work is best known though the concept of "flow", which is a construct developed to frame the optimal experience in which an engaged person is completely immersed in activity to a degree that the activity becomes autotelic, a goal in itself, ultimately completely intrinsically motivating, worth doing for its own sake (Csikszentmihalyi, 1990). A glimpse of how deep this theory goes, not the least in the context of education, may be given by a simple reflection on time and life-quality. Thus, when considering what one finds really worth doing in life, it becomes clear that almost nothing done in a state of haste qualifies. By and large, hurrying things through simply does not provide worthwhile experiences – at least not for those who do it (others may cynically benefit from it for a period of time, of course).[1] Indeed, the point generalizes: being asked to recall great moments, almost no one recalls being aware of the time at these moments. Moreover, flow-theory is embedded in a much deeper appreciation of complexity theory elaborated in the magnum opus *The Evolving Self: A psychology for the third millennium* (Csikszentmihalyi, 1993). The groundbreaking understanding of flow and complexity has had profound influence in many fields, but arguably most directly in education as the concept of flow serves as an almost perfect description of play in academic terms, with play being the preferred state of consciousness for children during their early years, as indeed it remains to be throughout life if the concept of flow is elaborated a bit to encompass also the play-like state people find themselves in when employing hobbies, curiously studying and shaping their worlds. There is massive evidence of the effectiveness of play and flow on learning, with the research of Csikszentmihalyi and colleagues specifically demonstrating that the more intrinsically motivated learners are, the more they enjoy learning, the more they will learn, the more inclined they will be to learn more, and the more inclined they will be to contribute to the greater good (e.g. Anderson, Manoogian, & Reznick, 1976; Csikszentmihalyi & Rathunde, 1993; Csikszentmihalyi, Abuhamdeh, & Nakamura, 2005; Deci & Ryan, 2000; Fredrickson, 2009; Gray, 2013; Harter, 1978; Knoop, 2011; Ryan, 1995; Shernoff & Hoogstra, 2001). Indeed, flow is almost the perfect description of the processual aspects of eudemonia, inherent in Aristotle's ideal of joyfully striving towards virtuous excellence and perfection. Thus, if the content is right, virtuous, in essence flow may be understood as a near-optimal processual vehicle for educational, indeed more generally personal, flourishing.

Needless to say, many other lines of psychological inquiry contribute to the foundation of humanistic psychology and PP, but the findings mentioned above have proven so influential and robust that it will be rather unsurprising should they prove themselves universal, and consequently of universal importance to educators also. As such, they provide a firm and congruent basis of understanding, which cannot be neglected if education is to promote learning in ethically defendable ways. On a further note, the scholars mentioned above seem to share an ambition of going beyond the "ism-game", gradually leaving the battle of psychological paradigms behind, aiming to synthesize psychological science at a higher level, employing all relevant methodologies and perspectives. To be sure, this has not protected for instance PP against itself being perceived as a new paradigm by many even so, but, echoing Gregory Bateson, rather than reducing the experience through paradigmatic blinders it should be a noble aim to employ a holistic approach to understanding academic disciplines

[1] Obviously, this is not the place for a detailed investigation of the philosophy of time, but the implications of this as regards an educational system being run by digital time-frames for over two centuries should be fairly clear even so. Almost none of what makes life worth living is about getting it over with and in the vernacular this boldly means that very little quality of life is to be expected by trying to get from A to B as quickly as possible.

and domains as merely different ways of looking at the world, at life, and at being human, all of which may inform and inspire, and none of which may reduce or dominate unjustly. And indeed, as regards eudemonia, an influential attempt at such a more holistic view of well-being, drawing broadly on previous psychological theories has been made by Carol Ryff (1989, 2014, Chap. 6, this volume) and subsequently expanded in collaborations (Ryff & Keyes, 1995; Ryff & Singer, 1998; Keyes, Shmotkin, & Ryff, 2002) by development of the construct "psychological well-being", which is an operationalized understanding/interpretation of eudemonia as multidimensional construct consisting of six distinct components of psychological functioning found in earlier key contributions to psychology: a positive attitude toward oneself and one's past life (self-acceptance); high quality, satisfying relationships with others (positive relations with others); a sense of self-determination and freedom from norms (autonomy); having life goals and a belief that one's life is meaningful (purpose in life); the ability to manage life and one's surroundings (environmental mastery); and being open to new experiences and making use of one's personal talents and potential (personal growth). As complementing the construct of subjective well-being (Diener, 1984) measuring primarily hedonic components (high positive affect, low negative affect, and satisfaction with life), Ryff et al.'s model has been important in promoting research on eudemonia, and clearly every one of the six component bear relevance for education also. In recent years however, the sharp distinction between the hedonic and eudemonic well-being has been contested, in part on the grounds that a very high correlation ($r=0.96$) between hedonia and eudemonia (Disabato et al., 2015). As such there seems to be fair agreement that the distinction between hedonia and eudemonia needs further clarification and empirical investigation, in order to approach full scientific fruition itself. Indeed, an attempt at such clarification is already provided by Huta and Waterman (2014) and Huta (Chap. 15, this volume) arguing for clarity as regards operationalizations, clarity in core and close-to-core elements of definitions, and clarity in level of measurement (state/trait). However, this is very much work in progress and for all educational purposes, every proposed element of both hedonia and eudemonia remains indispensable. Thus one may ask: On ethical and/or developmental grounds, which learner could be left neglected as concerns growth, meaning, authenticity, excellence, virtue, relatedness, competence, engagement, awareness, acceptance/self-acceptance, effort, physical health or subjective well-being – the core definitions of eudemonia used in the literature as summarized by Huta and Waterman (2014)? And, turning to the summarized definitions of hedonia from the same review: Which learner may be restrained from pleasure, enjoyment, satisfaction, happiness, low distress, an appropriately evaluative mindset, pursuit of homeostasis?

Based on these findings, and as elaborated below in chapters below, I submit that for the time being our best options for eudemonic education lie in a more or less unified approach to education, acknowledging the value of both hedonic and eudemonic well-being without losing anything thereby. It may even make sense to coin two complementary constructs with slightly different loading: "pleasurable meaning" and "meaningful pleasure" to allow for the distinctions without losing the unity. And as for education, the term "edutainment" may indeed be an already well-known special case of this complementarity.

30.3 More Recent Findings in Positive Psychology of Particular Educational Importance

More recent psychological evidence, of course still standing on the shoulders of those who went before, include the authoritative mapping the negativity-bias – a tendency to experience bad (negative) aspects of life stronger than good ones, relating to almost every aspect of live (Baumeister, Bratslavsky, Finkenauer, & Vohs, 2001; Rozin & Royzman, 2001). By all likelihood, nature selected our ancestors primarily for fitness of survival and propagation, and only indirectly for well-being apart from basic health and fitness. According to this understanding, it has always been more important to be good at feeling acutely stressed than to be good at savoring the riches of life, even if positive emotions do seem to provide survival advantages too as detailed below. This broad finding is so important that it may be viewed as PP's deepest single *raison d'etre*. It directly or indirectly influences almost every aspect of human life and interaction, and explains, maybe stronger than any other single factor, why it is necessary to give special attention to, and foster, the brighter sides of life, if we wish to see them for ourselves. Understanding the negativity-bias has both hidden and overt implications for education in that a good-enough educational experience, i.e. one promoting flourishing, appears to generally require positivity quantitatively overwhelming negativity in individuals, groups, and cultures. Thus, directly related to the pivotal challenge of keeping negativity within limits, while certainly not disregarding the importance of being able to employ a full emotional spectrum, are two ground-breaking findings by Barbara Fredrickson and colleagues regarding positivity. First, the discovery of the link between positive emotions and learning though the Broaden-and-Build theory (Fredrickson, 2009, 2013) stands out. While already Thorndike's "law of effects" (1927) was an attempt to understand the basic role of emotions in learning, the broaden-and-Build theory clarifies how humans react to positive emotions in ways that broaden their capacity to learn and consequently tend to make them better at learning (building). Secondly, the exposure of a "positivity ratio", stating that a person needs considerably more positive than negative emotions) in order to flourish, is important (Fredrickson, 2013b).[2] It is hard to find better arguments than these two connected theories for ensuring the individual experience of positive emotions as an essential part of any educational experience and they signal almost the exact opposite of the burning-platform-message so often promoted in order to make people more "willing to change", echoing the laboratory where frightened rats tend not to explore the maze.

A further major contribution to PP regards the mapping and advanced employment of individual strengths. To be sure, within general psychology individual strengths have long been studied as traits, intelligences, styles, interest and values, but data from millions of users of online surveys such as the Clifton Strengths Finder, the Values-in-Action – Inventory of Strengths (VIA-IS) measuring character strengths, and the Realise2[3] are catalyzing inspiring theoretical developments and applications. In education these strength-approaches are crossing the traditional divisions of disciplines lighting up a host of human qualities (strengths) that have hitherto been difficult to identify because the sciences, arts, and crafts often do not readily reveal them. Thus, for instance the strength of perseverance may obviously be of great use in any domain but typically not a strength that is given particular attention, let alone one that is tested in education (though it certainly contributes to performances that are tested).

The VIA Classification (Peterson & Seligman, 2004) and VIA-IS are used by researchers and practitioners around the world (Niemiec, 2012), making it one of the most substantial initiatives to emerge from the burgeoning science of PP to date. Research on the VIA Classification is flourishing and like other practitioners, educators are working to find ways to apply the research to their practices. Research on character strengths across "educational" disciplines, is seen in positive psychotherapy (Seligman, Rashid, & Parks, 2006); in various forms of coaching, ranging from executive to life, health, and parent coaching; use with children, adolescents, teachers, and school systems (Eades, 2008; Park & Peterson, 2009; Proctor & Fox Eades, 2011); in positive education (e.g. Geelong Grammar School and St Peters College in Australia; a significant number of schools in Denmark (Andersen, 2013; Knoop,

[2] The precise ratio is still contested but that a ratio exists is rather consensual, as negative events almost invariably affect us more than positive ones (Baumeister et al., 2001; Rozin & Royzman, 2001).

[3] See: www.strengthsfinder.com, www.viacharacter.org, www.cappeu.com

2011); Penn Resiliency Program)[4]; positive institutions, business, and Appreciative Inquiry (Cooperrider, 2009; Cooperrider & Whitney, 2005); and faculty development and teaching (McGovern & Miller, 2008).

In reviewing educational applications of strengths broadly, Lopez and Louis (2009) find that there are generally five recommendable principles of strengths-based education: measurement, individualization, networking, deliberate application, and intentional development. Lopez and Louis argue that through a parallel process, educators practice the principles of strengths-based education when advising and teaching while students learn to put their strengths to work in learning and social situations. These recommendations are clearly in line with the central elements of self-determination theory, that show how individuals function at optimal levels and are most authentically motivated when three psychological needs are met: competence, autonomy, and relatedness (Deci & Ryan, 2000). Lopez and Louis highlight how helping students understand the connection between their strengths and their personal goals, and offering guidance in the application of their strengths in the most effective ways, may elicit feelings of competence. Further, providing students with choices and opportunities for self-direction can support their need for autonomy: "When educators establish a learning culture where students view themselves and others through 'strengths-colored glasses'" (Clifton, Anderson, & Schreiner, 2006, p. 73), they help to foster appreciation for differences, highlight the value of collaboration and teamwork, and establish a powerful sense of relatedness" (Lopez & Louis, 2009).

Related to the work on character strengths are also studies of grit showing how effort explains up to two thirds of academic performance while talent only accounts for one third for normally gifted and above (Duckworth et al., 2007). This further relates to the work of Carol Dweck (2006) showing how there are important differences in pupil's mindsets explaining both their well-being and their performance, specifically differences accounted for by the so-called "fixed mindset" (the belief that one cannot become a better learner) versus the growth mindset (the belief than one does become a better learner by learning). And in line with all this, the recent inception of the International Positive Psychology Network (IPEN) must be mentioned, as it constitutes an international initiative whereby academic training and character formation are promoted as equally important as academic skills in modern education, and where flourishing skills are taught to teachers and learners with the aim of making education a better experience hedonically as well as eudemonically, promoting learning through thriving and preventing mental illness such as depression (e.g. O'Shaughnessy, Larson, & Seligman, 2014). IPEN may be seen as a subdivision of IPPA, the International Positive Psychology Association.

30.4 How Educational Research on Effectiveness Aligns with Science of Well-Being

Looking more directly at educational research, the meta-studies of John Hattie and colleagues (e.g. Hattie, 2008; Hattie & Yates, 2014) have been very influential in recent years. While controversial, and to psychologists sometimes even bordering on triviality, John Hattie and Gregory Yates have tried to map cognitive learning theory that may explain earlier findings from hugely influential meta-studies of educational effectiveness, which is relevant in this context. The meta-study of meta-studies provides a thorough, if critiqued, review of quantitative studies, so far representing close to half a billion learners, and Hattie and colleagues hold the high ground in many countries struggling to get educational policy and practice to work. This is not the place for a thorough review of this work, rather just a brief investigation of whether the principles of learning summarized by Hattie and Yates as undergirding their educational recommendations are congruent with recommendations based on science of well-being such as outlined above. If

[4] See: www.ggs.vic.edu.au; www.stpeters.sa.edu.au; www.ppc.sas.upenn.edu/prpsum.htm

so, we may have yet another reason for applying science of well-being to education. Hence, in the following, Hattie and Yates's "nine principles of learning" are cited verbatim with a brief commentary by this author. The nine principles are written in italic and my commentary in normal typeface:

1. *Explanations of human learning in terms of native ability, talent, or intelligence are severely constrained by one consistent and persistent finding: that substantial investments of time, energy, structured tuition, and personal effort are all required in order to develop mastery in all knowledge domains investigated. Notions such as talent, ability, and intelligence exist as useful descriptive terms. But they are not sufficient to explain learning or achievement.* This principle is completely in line "eudemonic" findings e.g. showing how passion (Vallerand et al., 2007; Vallerand, Chap. 13, this volume), effort (Duckworth et al., 2007), perseverance and willpower (Baumeister & Tierney, 2012), and mindset (Dweck, 2006) are all important variables in explaining educational success.
2. *We naturally learn from exposure to information detected by our senses. But to increase our knowledge base, this information has to possess a level of organization which matches how our minds are structured and organized—and our minds change in how we structure and organize as we age.* This conforms with psychological insights showing how effective teaching employs characteristics/strengths of the individual learner rather than just pressing the learning into a standardized curricular form (e.g. Donaldson, Dollwet, & Rao, 2015; Dunn, 2009; Knoop, 2011; Peterson, & Seligman, 2004); O'Shaughnessy & Watson, 2015).
3. *Our mind has severe and inherent limitations, as built-in characteristics. When these limitations are reached, through experiences or depletion, deep and meaningful processing becomes impossible, and only shallow learning will occur from that point.* This again relates to the characteristics/strengths of the individual learner, to studies of willpower, inhibition and ego-depletion (Baumeister, 2014), cognitive limitations of "system 2" in processing abstract information (Kahneman, 2011), and studies of deep attentional immersion and flow-states of mind (Csikszentmihalyi & Knoop, 2008). An important exception from the ego-depletion tendency has been noted by Deci and Ryan (2008) arguing that in cases of autonomously motivated activity during ego-depletion tends not to occur.
4. *Human learners benefit enormously from social examples, from directed instruction, and from corrective feedback. Learning from exposure to the information provided by other people represents a fundamental aspect underpinning human adjustment and evolution; the more expert these 'other people' are in understanding the progression of learning, the more effective is the learning.* From a well-being scientific perspective almost every sub-branch of research informs the educator and learner on how learning can be understood as uninterruptedly affected by the physical and mental states of the learner – that is the level of well-being in all its forms (e.g. Knoop, 2011). Social examples and model are powerful but people learn enormously from non-other-directed, self-determined activity also, which Hattie and Yates tend to downplay here.
5. *We will exert strong efforts to perform at a high level, calling upon hidden and guarded reserves of effort, once we become confident that worthwhile goals are achievable in the short term.* This is directly related to, maybe even derived from, flow-research (e.g. Csikszentmihalyi's collected works, and indirectly with the broader body of knowledge regarding self-efficacy (Bandura, 1994). Indirectly it also underscores the importance of affect, pleasure, in the pursuit of meaningful virtue.
6. *Short-term goals are highly motivating. But they may exist in conflict with other long-term values we harbor. Hence, one of the key aspects of personal development and happiness involving learning and activating strategies that enable us to control impulses and*

delay gratification. From a positive psychology perspective this again relates directly to studies of willpower, inhibition, ego-depletion, and the intimate relation between the hedonic and eudemonic (e.g. Baumeister, 2014; Mischel et al. 1989, though the argument for keeping them distinct is indirectly being made).

7. *Learners possess human traits requiring a consistent level of maintenance. These include ego esteem needs, as well as the need to synchronize actions with other people within the immediate social context.* This matches broadly findings regarding individual strength profiles (e.g. Donaldson et al., 2015), regarding the basic need for relatedness (e.g. Deci & Ryan, 2000), and regarding the need of experiencing success on an ongoing basis in order to be able to perceive self-discipline as meaningful (e.g. Bandura, 1994; Knoop, 2013).
8. *Neurologically, we possess a remarkably social brain. This evolved organ becomes a tool enabling us to react to the physical presence of others, to learn from information they dispense, and to become familiar with the characteristics of up to 150 individuals within our wider social world.* This is but another good reason to make sure the social relations are not compromised during formal learning as this predicts negative emotional and virtuous effect on all learning. Moreover, this mirrors findings on the basic need for social relatedness throughout life (e.g. Deci & Ryan, 2000; Peterson, 2006).
9. *Within both public and professional domains, fallacious ideas of human learning continue to be promoted despite being contradicted by available scientific opinion and evidence. Many such fallacies are potentially destructive and driven by false promises, pecuniary interests, or an overreliance on anecdotes.* This is parallel to problems regarding premature application of for instance PP but it also, conversely, relates to premature and ill-informed application of grand-scale meta-research whereby smaller-scale, successful intervention may be obscured in statistical noise (e.g. Dunn, 2009; Gardner, 1999; Knoop, 2011; Wilson et al., 2012).

Again, this is not the place for a proper review of this educational effect research. Yet, it should suffice for the aim of showing how these influential educational findings are quite congruent with essential psychological research on well-being and strengths. Thus, it seems quite possible to form coherent understandings of learning based on educational and psychological research.

As for eudemonia, Hattie and Yates appear to be all for it. What this author finds missing is particularly the appreciation of self-determined and self-regulated educational activity. To be sure, Hattie (2008) has argued forcefully for "visible learning", implying both that learners see themselves as teachers and that teachers view their teaching through the eyes of the learners, but the frame in which this is most often to take place according to Hattie may likely lead to educational micro management, i.e. be extremely detail-controlled by the professional teacher with very little real freedom for the learner. Indeed, one serious criticism against Hattie's methodology is that he produces anachronistic results by looking at what works in traditional schools and finding that traditional teaching does – ignoring how much "better pedagogy" is more or less impossible in the traditional frames (e.g. Sjøberg, 2015). In the final chapter below this potential problem is further discussed.

30.5 Towards a Coherent Understanding of Human Flourishing

It is a plain truth about human life, shared with all other life-forms, that we are propelled by a pervasive tendency to stay alive, from the moment of fertilization to the very end. This tendency can be observed *directly* in two specific and intertwined processes: *self-regulated growth processes* and *self-regulated balancing processes*, and *indirectly* in attempts to avoid getting "stuck" in unpleasant and/or meaningless situations. Through these processes, adaptation to distinct life circumstances becomes possible (e.g. Forrester, 1994). For instance, self-regulating growth processes at the cellular level are seen in cell division and in the brain by forming and strengthening neural connections. Learning can in part be understood as differentiation and integration of neural connections whereby and individual becomes able to understand differences where before there were only similarities, and understand similarities where before there were only differences. Thus, an individual's world view and competence grows – and barriers against the experience of growth, that are de facto threats of stagnation or actual stagnation, will be experienced as unpleasant and/or meaningless. Complementary, self-regulating balancing processes in living organisms can be appreciated at all levels aimed at adaptation by adjustment of the internal state of the body's sugar levels, pulse, speed of breath, temperature, of emotions, of decisions and behavior. And in cases where these self-regulating processes are barred, problems almost certainly occur.

Thus, assuming that self-regulated growth and self-regulated balancing are foundational processes for all forms of well-being, learning processes and creative processes, by deduction the general prediction that *well-being, learning, and creativity*, i.e. *educational processes, will be promoted or inhibited through promotion or inhibition of the learner's ability to self-regulate hedonically as well as eudemonically*, can be made. As such, human autonomy in this foundational sense, within any given frame of constraints, is generally indispensable in the pursuit of quality education.

Model 30.1 offers an illustration of this systems approach as a key to a flourishing life in education and beyond.

The model illustrates how the basic motivation for self-regulated growth and self-regulated balancing are foundational processes for all forms of well-being, and for learning processes and creative processes. The basic motivation is equally relevant for hedonic and eudemonic components, which supports the hypothesis that hedonia and eudemonia works synergistically, and that the employment of individual strengths may be understood as equally foundational if genetic dispositions, personality traits and behavioral preferences are included as "strengths". Importantly, every component in the model can be promoted and inhibited by the individual as well as by the environment/authorities, thus providing an argument for combining psychological and sociological perspectives. Graphically, it may be noted that as a systems model of the body and psyche, double arrows could be applied throughout, but for the present purpose of illustration how multiple forms of well-being are crucial predictors of harmonious educational/personal growth processes, single arrows are mostly preferred here.

The basic systems theory of the model is developed by Jay Forrester (1994) and congruent with the organismic theory of self-determination by Deci and Ryan (2000). Theories on the importance of employing human strengths and virtues is dating back to Greek philosophy, but is now being refined and elaborated by modern scientific theory and inquiry (e.g. Donaldson et al., 2015; Linley, 2008; Niemiec, 2013; Peterson & Seligman, 2004). Model 30.1 also includes all the components of the PERMA model developed by Martin Seligman (2010) – the components being positive emotion, engagement, relations, meaning and achievement – yet as it figures, with these embedded in a more comprehensive frame of human growth including also basic motivations, physical health, learning, creativity and key environmental conditions promoting each component.

Indeed, expanding the perspective, Model 30.1 further allows for an integrative perspective on just about every proposed element of eudemonia and hedonia summarized by Huta and Waterman (2014), assumed to represent the most important components of well-being found in the current literature:

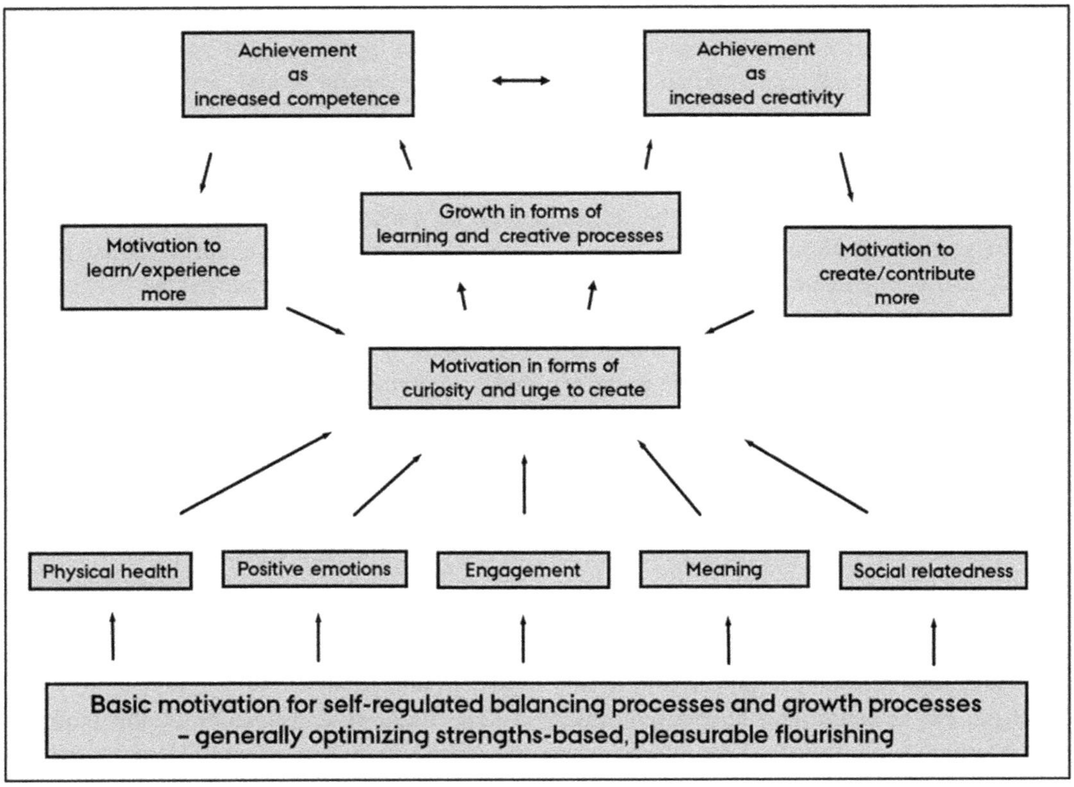

Model 30.1 Systems model of human flourishing: how well-being predicts learning and creativity, which in turn predicts well-being

Summarized Definitions of Eudemonia

- Growth/self-realization/self-actualization/development of potentials/full functioning/maturity
- Meaning/purpose/long-term perspective/caring about and contributing to the broader context
- Authenticity/identity/personal expressiveness/autonomy/constitutive goals/integrity
- Excellence/virtue/using the best in oneself/reaching a high standard/signature strengths
- Relatedness/positive relationships/social well-being
- Competence/environmental mastery
- Engagement/interest/flow
- Awareness/contemplation/mindfulness
- Acceptance/self-acceptance
- Effort/engaging with challenge
- Physical health
- Subjective well-being

Summarized Definitions of Hedonia

- Pleasure/enjoyment/life satisfaction/happiness
- Low distress/comfort/relaxation
- Evaluative mindset
- Pursuit of homeostasis

As stated earlier, none of these "life-qualities" may meaningfully be disregarded in modern education, as they clearly each carry importance for the well-being of every person, human diversity notwithstanding. Moreover, life-qualities (traits and/or states) like self-efficacy and resilience are likewise predicted by well-being and harmonious growth through learning and creativity. Thus, assuming that the model is correct, two kinds of research questions emerge in addition to those addressing the relations between the components: (*1*) *questions regarding lower and upper thresholds/limits/tipping-points/cut-off points of each component*, and (2) *questions regarding how to support and inhibit for optimal flourishing*. In other words: what are the outer limits of the "zone predicting flourishing" for each component of well-being and how may we best ensure staying within the zones? An example of a specific question could be: How and when do low levels of engagement turn into apathy – and how do we effectively avoid this happening? Another example: At what point does meaninglessness turn into self-destruction – and how does one effectively avoid this happening? And yet another: What is the minimal happiness-set-point necessary for flourishing?

When attempting to answer such questions, and specifically as regards "eudemonic education", I submit that Model 30.1 represents a mapping of key components of well-being and the relations between these and the growths-processes inherent in all educational endeavors. From the perspective of this author the model thus offers a rather precise account of, what today may be understood by the eudemonic ambition of joyfully and virtuously striving for our potential, as Aristotle argued, though now also informed by testable empirical evidence. It also reminds us, how every component of well-being can actually be cared for and trained by the individual and be promoted by the surrounding culture and leadership. And how the opposite is equally true: that one may indeed damage oneself by neglect of own potential just as a culture or a specific type of leadership may damage employees and citizens. Obviously, processes thus infused with pleasure, engagement and meaning, and even leading to a positive outcome will be self-reinforcing and as such psychological sustainability/flourishing is predicted at both the component level (well-being being intrinsically motivating) and at the systems level (learning and creative processes being successful will function rewardingly), thus not stressing, depressing, or burning out learners.[5]

30.6 Practical Predictors of Well-Being

Examples of what may be done by the individual or the surroundings to promote wellbeing are exemplified in Model 30.2. The examples are just that, and by no means exhaustive, yet aligned with scientific evidence (e.g. Knoop, 2011). Thus *physical health* (reflecting dynamic order in the body)[6] is strongly predicted by proper nutrition, physical exercise, appropriate sleep and hygiene, all of which tend to have psychological benefits as well. *Positive emotions* (reflecting dynamically ordered understanding) are predicted by a good social atmosphere, by aesthetic experiences and by functionality that make moment-to-moment progress possible. *Engagement* (reflecting dynamic order in consciousness) is predicted by the so-called flow-conditions, implying situations that allow a person to take and maintain initiative and control; that have concrete, energizing goals; that are governed by manageable, non-bureaucratic rules; that are characterized by clear, non-humiliating information about moment-to-moment performance; that allows appropriate levels of challenges matched to the skills; and that make it possible to remove distracting factors thereby to concentrate. *Meaning* (reflecting dynamic existential order) is predicted by usability and convincing justification / good reasons that further predict particularly motivation and

[5] To be noted, of course, every person is sensing some level and kind of well-being at any time awake and will be learning and acting one way or the other at any particular moment, so it may be argued that it is difficult, maybe at times even impossible, to determine, whether one aspect of a mood (e.g. curiosity), or and action (e.g. reading), comes before the other. But keeping that in mind, for analytical purposes, it may still make sense to outline, how indeed mental states predict one another, how certain acts predict certain states, and how states may predict certain actions. Indeed, without this assumption, we probably would not have psychological science at all.

Also, to be noted, well-being in all forms are intrinsically motivated, which means that a completely functioning system will be highly, psychologically sustainable, unless overdone as when, for instance, purpose becomes so overwhelming as to become obsessive, or some type of pleasure becomes to dominating as to be addictive and thereby undermining self-determination.

[6] In other texts, I have used the systems theoretical term of "dynamic order" to describe general aspects of well-being on different levels (Knoop, 2013). See also Csikszentmihalyi and Knoop (2008).

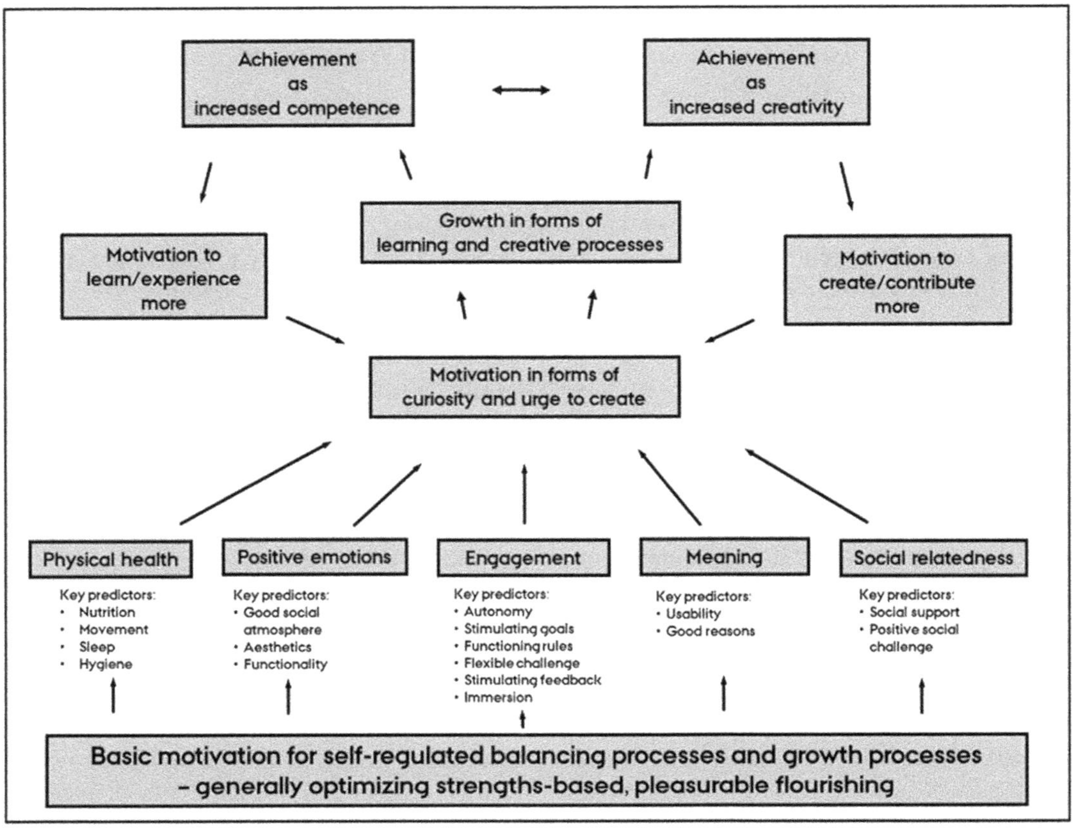

Model 30.2 Systems model of human flourishing with key predictors of well-being

resilience. *Social relatedness* (reflecting dynamic social order) is predicted by social support providing safety and positive social challenge providing interesting encounters.

Again, these predictors are but examples but they are all well documented as being important for human flourishing and thus to be respected and promoted just as human rights for physical safety and shelter are. Thus, the science of well-being increasingly assumes a critical role in the formation of future society – in both meanings of the word. Indeed, as science of well-being provides ever more knowledge about the requirements for human flourishing it obviously becomes increasingly difficult to ignore it from a moral philosophical perspective also. To be sure, we might not derive *ought* from *is*, as David Hume taught us – that is, we may not imply moral justifications for genocide, because genocide appears to have been virtually routine throughout most of our natural history (Wrangham & Peterson, 1997). Yet, as we know more and more about human well-being, we may turn the argument around as well, and state that we may not organize human life in ways that are scientifically proven to be harmful.

30.7 Flourishing in Greater Ecologies

We should measure what matters because what we measure matters.

So far, education has had mainly three functions: qualifying young people for life's challenges, socializing young people into cultural traditions, and selection of young people for different working positions available in society. It is strongly debatable how well education has succeeded in overcoming, or better, living up to these tasks. Indeed, one may (un-)comfortably argue that only the last function has been fulfilled, if ever so unjust. That is: only the selective function has fully worked insofar people have been divided horizontally into domains and fields, and vertically into stratified, unequally privileged, layers of society. To be sure, it is difficult to imagine a modern society where some kind of horizontal and vertical division of labor is not in place, but importantly in this context is to note how scientific understandings of well-being evidences the justification of combatting any form of inequality barring sufficient social appreciation, positive experiences, and future perspective necessary for making life worth living. Certainly, science of well-being is no more than knowledge to be used for better or worse, but knowledge nevertheless to be employed wisely by the able and willing. Of course, it may be cynically ignored for political reason, yet it may be heartwarming to realize that the more we learn about human well-being, and the clearer the findings are communicated to the public, the harder it becomes to disregard this knowledge in forming moral philosophies or policies, unless one is willing to openly employ hypocrisy.

Still, while the science and the application hereof does hold great promises, the challenges of overcoming basic *structural* limitations affecting learners' well-being and thriving in traditional educational settings remain overwhelming. As a particularly harsh critic of traditional schooling Peter Gray (2013) offers a dark summary of what educators, in his view, are up against:

> *...The unfortunate fact is that one of our most cherished institutions is, by its very nature, failing our children and our society. School is a place where children are compelled to be, and where their freedom is greatly restricted — far more restricted than most adults would tolerate in their workplaces. In recent decades, we have been compelling our children to spend ever more time in this kind of setting, and there is strong evidence (summarized in my recent book) that this is causing serious psychological damage to many of them. Moreover, the more scientists have learned about how children naturally learn, the more we have come to realize that children learn most deeply and fully, and with greatest enthusiasm, in conditions that are almost opposite to those of school...*

Gray summarizes the seven structural problems of what he calls coercive education as denial of liberty without due cause and due process; interference with the development of personal responsibility and self-direction; undermining of intrinsic motivation to learn; judging students in ways that foster shame, hubris, cynicism, and cheating; interference with the development of cooperation and promotion of bullying; inhibition of critical thinking; and reduction in diversity of skills and knowledge (Gray, 2013a). In David Sloan Wilson's words after reviewing Gray (ibid.):

> *The modern educational system is like a wish made in a folk tale gone horribly wrong. Peter Gray's Free to Learn leads us out of the maze of unforeseen consequences to a more natural way of letting children educate themselves. Gray's message might seem too good to be true, but it rests upon a strong scientific foundation...*

Thus, what Gray is basically arguing is that the very institution to teach and prepare young people for a flourishing life is often doing the exact opposite by denying them the necessary possibility of self-determined, responsible learning, in effect making eudemonic education impossible, if correct. While this is not the place for a detailed account on the pros and cons of traditional educational structures it does bear mention how the educational world – being the millions of educators with ideals and practices guiding their thoughts and actions – are violently challenged by changes in modern society.

Today the educational world finds itself in constant tension between, on one side the ambition of being foundational in preserving and furthering society and culture – and on the other side being one of society's most threatened institutions. Internally, deep ideological conflicts combined with widespread failure to thrive in both learners and educators abound. From the outside, political dissatisfaction and distrust is aired almost daily, while ever more challenging competition from informal "learning environments" – real as well as virtual/digital – continues to emerge at accelerating speed and often even with higher quality of content and higher impact (that is: de facto stronger educational potential(!))

How can any school library match online resources like Google books? And who has ever heard of a student getting addicted to school the way they get addicted to gaming and other "learning" through the Internet? Connected to the Internet, today "education" can take place anywhere, and good autodidacts will be those best set to employ these new possibilities. The general, virtually free, access to knowledge thus provided may almost be regarded as an educational bypass operation if not properly employed by the educational system itself. And, in this context especially relevant: if not providing individualized, strengths-based, differentiated learning in non-humiliating form.

Doubtlessly, any educator today will be aware of the importance of embracing information technology if appropriate, yet much technology driven learning nevertheless takes place completely without formal education being part of the equation. This is not to do away with formal education but if the future of humanity is to be more flourishing, education certainly needs to provide therefore by teaching the skills necessary and by providing experiences of flourishing through the structuring of daily life from kindergarten to university. In short, education must be seriously interesting, even fun, to be worth its name. Being in a depressing school not only makes academic achievement unlikely, it does not even socialize appropriately as the norms inculcated in a depressive setting will be associated with unpleasantness and thus de facto taught as something to be avoided. A depressive school is an anti-socializing school. For instance, if reading a book is unpleasant the desire to read more books is automatically diminished, squarely against all educational ideals. Thus, such experiences are simply to be avoided, and especially so in cultural and societal foundational institutions. Yet, as we have seen, too often they are not. For instance, the first national survey of well-being of pupils in Danish schools shows, that only about one in five pupils in fourth to ninth grade feel that the can do something for making learning more exciting in case they are bored (Danish Ministry of Education, 2015). The rest are taught to accept boredom as part of learning, obviously. This is a national problem, to say the least. Four out of five young citizens are thus taught to accept meaningless passivity, apparently. To be sure, on other measures Danish pupil seem to thrive, but the devil is in the detail and by looking at items like aforementioned we may get a fairly good idea of what is going on in detail. If asking about root causes for the alarming numbers of stress and depression reported among young people, here should be a good candidate, easy to understand. And not only is it depressing to be stuck in unpleasant conditions – it also implies pupils learning less than they could and, as mentioned, that they lose motivation for further learning and improvement, all lacking any positive perspective.

This is not the place for a detailed account on these complex and complicated issues but we have to recognize that educational institutions today act alongside private vendors who offer high quality information and learning for, in principle, all of humanity, and a host of leading universities following up with so called Massive Online Open Courses (MOOCS) to engage from your home whenever you prefer. Again, this happens while the administration of educational institutions and professionals continues to disengage many, completely opposing what is needed. What can be recommended in this situation that jeopardizes people, academic authority or social responsibility in one sweep? What is the role of education? And how can educational work be done in ways that are psychologically sustainable, that is: ways that do not burn out its practitioners in the process? By definition eudemonic education worth the name, promoting flourishing amongst all involved will have answers to offer. And by all likelihood, the answers will not imply the demise of educational institutions, for how may a culture or a society prevail without foundational institutions? Neither does the present Global Educational Reform Movement (GERM) (Sahlberg, 2014), built on standardization, testing, and nulsum-competition (at best) between learners as well as institutions seem likely to continue in its current form because the unintended side-effects of massive demotivation in learners and professionals simply cannot be sustained. And maybe, anecdotally speaking, because a country like Finland exemplifies the likelihood of success by *not* accepting the premises of GERM (Sahlberg, 2014).

Thus, it seems that whatever solution is sought, it must take into account what we know of human flourishing, learning and creativity. And it must employ knowledge both about how individuals may approach own and others flourishing, and how organizations and societies can be structured as to promote this happening. Today, eudemonic education, optimizing self-regulated, strength-based growth for all, should be considered a Human Right. Scientifically justified, socially legitimate, and what every parent wants for their child.

References

Andersen, F. Ø. (2013). *Drengeakademiet*. København: Løkkefonden.

Anderson, R., Manoogian, S. T., & Reznick, J. S. (1976). The undermining and enhancing of intrinsic motivation in preschool children. *Journal of Personalitv and Social Psychology, 34*, 915–922.

Bandura, A. (1977). Self-efficacy: Toward a unifying theory of behavioral change. *Psychological Review, 84*, 191–215.

Bandura, A. (1994). Self-efficacy. In V. S. Ramachandran (Ed.), *Encyclopedia of human behavior* (4th ed., pp. 71–81). New York: Academic.

Bandura, A. (1995). *Self-efficacy in changing societies*. Cambridge, MA: Cambridge University Press.

Baumeister, R. F. (2014). Self-regulation, ego depletion, and inhibition. *Neuropsychologia, 65*, 313–319.

Baumeister, R. F., Bratslavsky, E., Finkenauer, C., & Vohs, K. D. (2001). Bad is stronger than good. *Review of General Psychology, 5*, 323–370.

Baumeister, R. F., & Tierney, J. (2012). *Willpower: Rediscovering the greatest human strength*. New York: Penguin Books.

Camazine, S., Deneubourg, J. L., Franks, N. R., Sneyd, J., Theraulaz, G., & Bonabeau, E. (2001). *Self-organization in biological systems*. Princeton, NJ: Princeton University Press.

Clifton, D. O., Anderson, C. E., & Schreiner, L. A. (2006). *StrengthsQuest: Discover and develop your strengths in academics, career, and beyond* (2nd ed.). New York: Gallup Press.

Cooperrider, D. (2009). *The discovery and design of positive institutions*. Presentation at the International Positive Psychology Association conference on June 20.

Cooperrider, D., & Whitney, D. (2005). *Appreciative inquiry: A positive revolution in change*. San Francisco: Berrett-Koehler.

Csikszentmihalyi, M. (1990). *Flow – The psychology of optimal experience*. New York: Harper & Row Publishers.

Csikszentmihalyi, M. (1993). *The evolving self*. New York: HarperCollinsPublishers.

Csikszentmihalyi, M. (1996). *Creativity – Flow and the psychology of discovery and invention*. New York City: HarperCollins Publishers.

Csikszentmihalyi, M., Abuhamdeh, S., & Nakamura, J. (2005). Flow. In A. J. Elliot & C. S. Dweck (Eds.), *Handbook of competence and motivation*. New York: The Guilford Press.

Csikszentmihalyi, M., & Knoop, H. H. (2008). Kompleksitet: universelt ideal og global trussel. I J. Lyhne, & H. H. Knoop (red.), *Positiv psykologi: positiv pædagogik* (1 udg., s. 243–263). Kbh: Dansk Psykologisk Forlag.

Csikszentmihalyi, M., & Rathunde, K. (1993). The measurement of flow in everyday life: Towards a theory of emergent motivation. In J. E. Jacobs (Ed.), *Developmental perspectives on motivation. Nebraska symposium on motivation*. Lincoln, UK: University of Nebraska Press.

Damon, W. (2008). *The path to purpose*. New York: Free Press.

Danish Ministry of Education. (2015). *Trivselsmåling*. Retrieved February 25, 2016, from https://www.uvm.dk/Uddannelser/Folkeskolen/Elevplaner-nationale-test-og-trivselsmaaling/Trivselsmaaling

Deci, E. L., & Ryan, R. M. (2000). The 'what' and 'why' of goal pursuits: Human needs and the selfdetermination of behaviour. *Psychological Inquiry, 11*(4), 227–268.

Deci, E., & Ryan, R. (2008). Self-determination theory: A macrotheory of human motivation, development, and health. *Canadian Psychology, 49*(3), 182–185.

Dewey, J. (2009). *Democracy and education: An introduction to the philosophy of education*. New York: WLC Books (Originally published in 1916).

Diener, E. (1984). Subjective well-being. *Psychological Bulletin, 95*, 542–575.

Disabato, et al. (2015). Different types of well-being? A cross-cultural examination of hedonic and eudaimonic well-being. *Psychological assessment*. Washington, DC: American Psychological Association.

Donaldson, S. I., Dollwet, M., & Rao, M. A. (2015). Happiness, excellence, and optimal human functioning revisited: Examining the peer-reviewed literature linked to positive psychology. *The Journal of Positive Psychology, 10*, 185–195.

Duckworth, A. L., Peterson, C., Matthews, M. D., & Kelly, D. R. (2007). Grit: Perseverance andpassion for long-term goals. *Journal of Personality and Social Psychology, 92*(6), 1087–1101.

Dunn, R. (2009). *Answer to Mr Jensen*. New York: St John's University.

Dweck, C. S. (2006). *Growth mindset: The new psychology of success*. New York: Random House Publishing.

Eades, J. (2008). *Celebrating strengths: Building strengths-based schools*. Warwick: CAPP Press.

Forrester, J. (1994). System dynamics, systems thinking, and soft OR. *System Dynamics Review, 10*(2–3), 245–256.

Fredrickson, B. L. (2009). *Positivity: Groundbreaking research reveals how to embrace the hidden strength of positive emotions, overcome negativity, and thrive*. New York: Crown.

Fredrickson, B. L. (2013). Updated Thinking on Positivity Ratios. *American Psychologist*. Advance online publication. doi:10.1037/a0033584.

Gardner, H. (1999). *The disciplined mind: Beyond facts and standardized tests, the K-12 education that every child deserves*. New York: Basic Books.

Gray, P. (2013). Retrieved online: http://www.salon.com/2013/08/26/school_is_a_prison_and_damaging_our_kids/

Harter, S. (1978). Effectance motivation reconsidered: Toward a developmental model. *Human Development, 1*, 661–669.

Hattie, J. (2008). *Visible learning: A synthesis of over 800 meta-analyses relating to achievement* (1st ed.). New York: Routledge.

Hattie, J., & Yates, G. C. R. (2014). *Visible learning and the science of how we learn*. London: Routledge.

Huta, V., & Waterman, A. S. (2014). Eudaimonia and its distinction from Hedonia: Developing a classification and terminology for understanding conceptual and operational definitions. *Journal of Happiness Studies, 15*, 1425–1456.

Kahneman, D. (2011). *Thinking, fast and slow*. New York: Penguin.

Kauffman, S. A. (2000). *Investigations*. New York: Oxford University Press.

Keyes, Shmotkin, & Ryff. (2002). Optimizing well-being: The empirical encounter of two traditions. *Journal Personality and Social Psycholy, 82*(6), 1007–1022.

Knoop, H. H. (2011). Education in 2025: How positive psychology can revitalize education. In S. I. Donaldson, S. I. M. Csikszentmihalyi, J. Nakamura (Eds.), *Applied positive psychology: Improving everyday life, health, schools, work, and society*. London: Routledge Academic.

Knoop, H. H. (2013). Positive education, or just education. In C. Proctor & P. A. Linley (Eds.), *Research, application, and interventions for children and adolescents – A positive psychology perspective*. Dordrecht, The Netherlands: Springer. Chapter 9.

Linley, A. (2008). *Average to A+ – Realising strengths in yourself and others*. Warwick, UK: CAPP Press.

Lopez, S. J., & Louis, M. C. (2009, April). The principles of strengths-based education. *Journal of College & Character X*(4), 1–8.

Maslow, A. (1954). *Motivation and personality*. New York: Harper.

McGovern, T. V., & Miller, S. L. (2008). Integrating teacher behaviors with character strengths and virtues for faculty development. *Teaching of Psychology, 35*(4), 278–285.

Mischel, W., Shoda, Y., & Rodriguez, M. L. (1989). Delay of gratification in children. *Science, 244*, 933–938.

Niemiec, R. (2012). VIA character strengths – Research and practice: The first 10 years. In H. H. Knoop & A. Delle Fave (Eds.), *Well-being and cultures: Perspectives from positive psychology (cross-cultural advancements in positive psychology)*. Dordrecht, The Netherlands: Springer.

Niemiec, R. (2013). VIA character strengths - research and practice: The first 10 years. In H. H. Knoop & F. Delle (Eds.), *Well-being and cultures: Perspectives from positive psychology*. Dordrecht: Springer.

Niemiec, C. P., & Ryan, R. M. (2009). Autonomy, competence, and relatedness in the classroom: Applying self-determination theory to educational practice. *Theory and Research in Education, 7*, 133–144.

O'Dougherty Wright, M., Masten, A. S., & Narayan, A. J. (2013). Resilience processes in development: Four waves of research on positive adaptation in the context of adversity. In S. Goldstein & R. B. Brooks (Eds.), *Handbook of resilience in children* (pp. 15–37). New York, NY: Springer.

O'Shaughnessy & Watson. (2015). Online article at: http://www.ipositive-education.net/

O'Shaughnessy, J., Larson, E., & Seligman, M. (2014). Online article at: http://www.ipositive-education.net/

Overmier, J. B., & Seligman, M. E. P. (1967). Effects of inescapable shock upon subsequent escape and avoidance responding. *Journal of Comparative and Physiological Psychology, 63*, 28–33.

Park, N., & Peterson, C. (2009). Strengths of character in schools. In R. Gilman, E. S. Huebner, & M. J. Furlong (Eds.), *Handbook of positive psychology in schools* (pp. 65–76). New York: Routledge.

Peterson, C. (2006). *A primer in positive psychology*. Oxford: Oxford University Press.

Peterson, C., & Seligman, M. E. P. (Eds.). (2004). *Character strengths and virtues – A handbook and classification*. New York: Oxford University Press.

Pinker, S. (2002). *The blank slate – The modern denial of human nature*. London: BCA.

Proctor, C., & Fox Eades, J. (2011). *Strengths gym: Build and exercise your strengths!* St Peter Port, Guernsey: PPRC.

Rhem, J. (1999, February). Pygmalion in the classroom. *The National Teaching & Learning Forum. 8*(2), 1–4.

Rogers, C. (1961). *On becoming a person: A therapist's view of psychotherapy*. London: Constable.

Rogers, C. (1969). *Freedom to learn: A view of what education might become* (1st ed.). Columbus, OH: Charles Merill.

Rosenthal, R., & Jacobson, L. (1992). *Pygmalion in the classroom* (Expandedth ed.). New York: Irvington.

Rozin, P., & Royzman, E. B. (2001). Negativity bias, negativity dominance, and contagion. *Personality and Social Psychology Review, 5*(4), 296–320.

Ryan, R. M. (1995). Psychological needs and the facilitation of integrative processes. *Journal of Personality, 63*, 397–427.

Ryff, C. D. (1989). Happiness is everything, or is it? Explorations on the meaning of psychological wellbeing. *Journal of Personality and Social Psychology, 57*, 1069–1081.

Ryff, C. D. (2014). Psychological well-being revisited: Advances in the science and practice of eudaimonia. *Psychotherapy and Psychosomatics, 83*, 10–28.

Ryff, C. D., & Keyes, C. L. M. (1995). The structure of psychological well-being revisited. *Journal of Personality and Social Psychology, 69*, 719–727.

Ryff, C. D., & Singer, B. H. (1998). The contours of positive human health. *Psychological Inquiry, 9*, 1–28.

Sahlberg, P. (2014). Global educational reform movement and its impact on schooling. In K. Mundy, A. Green, R. Lingard, & A. Verger (Eds.), *The handbook of global policy and policy-making in education*. West Sussex, UK: Wiley-Blackwell.

Seligman, M. E. P. (2010). *Flourish – A visionary new understanding of happiness and well-being*. New York: Free Press.

Seligman, M. E. P., & Maier, S. F. (1967). Failure to escape traumatic shock. *Journal of Experimental Psychology, 74*, 1–9.

Seligman, M. E. P., Rashid, T., & Parks, A. (2006). Positive psychotherapy. *American Psychologist, 61*, 774–778.

Shernoff, D. J., & Hoogstra, L. (2001). Continuing motivation beyond the high school classroom. *New Directions in Child and Adolescent Development, 93*, 73–87.

Sjøberg, S. (2015). Skoleforskning som børs og katedral. Kronik i *Aftenposten*, Oslo, May 4th.

Vallerand, R. J., Salvy, S. J., Mageau, G. A., Elliot, A. J., Denis, P., Grouzet, F. M. E., et al. (2007). On the role of passion in performance. *Journal of Personality, 75*, 505–533.

Waters, L. (2011). A review of school-based positive psychology intervention. *The Australian Educational and Developmental Psychologist, 28*(2), 75–90.

Wrangham, R., & Peterson, D. (1997). *Demonic males: Apes and the origins of human violence*. New York: Mariner Books.

Zachariae, R. (2011, December 8). Unpublished lecture on positive psychology, health and stress, Aarhus University.

31 Developing Well-Being and Capabilities as a Goal of Higher Education: A Thought-Piece on Educating the Whole Student

Eranda Jayawickreme and Sara E. Dahill-Brown

The role of well-being in higher education has received increased attention from both researchers and practitioners in recent years (Dahill-Brown & Jayawickreme, 2016; Seligman, Ernst, Gillham, Reivich, & Linkins, 2009). Here we argue that (a) the multiplicity of approaches notwithstanding (Jayawickreme, Forgeard, & Seligman, 2012), a eudaemonic approach to well-being represents an important lens through which to examine well-being in the educational context; (b) such an approach is consistent with the progressive school of thought in educational theory and learner-centered approaches to education; (c) multiple educational curricula consistent with eudaemonic principles already exist in the U.S. context, and (d) an educational system that has as its goal the expansion of eudaemonic well-being—*depending on how well-being is defined*—can contribute to a more just society and world. Centering education around the promotion of eudaimonic ends, as well as promoting a healthy discussion of what those ends are, engenders a broader discourse about what best practices in education should be, rather than the narrow ones that seem to be favored at present.

E. Jayawickreme (✉)
Department of Psychology, Wake Forest University, Winston-Salem, NC, USA
e-mail: jayawide@wfu.edu

S.E. Dahill-Brown
Department of Politics and International Affairs, Wake Forest University, Winston-Salem, NC, USA
e-mail: dahillse@wfu.edu

31.1 What Is "Well-Being" in Education?

Given Aristotle's (1998) emphasis on the lifelong pursuit of eudaemonia (defined as the highest good achievable by human activity), it is not surprising that he has views on how it should be facilitated through education. However, it is instructive to note that even during his time, controversy prevailed over the appropriate goals of education:

> [F]or there are no generally accepted assumptions about what the young should learn, either for virtue or for the best life; nor yet is it clear whether their education ought to be conducted with more concern for the intellect than for the character of the soul. The problem has been complicated by the education we see actually given; and it is by no means certain whether training should be directed at things useful in life, or at those conducive to virtue, or at exceptional accomplishment. (Aristotle, Poetics, VIII, ii, 1337a33)

This tension that Aristotle highlights remains just as relevant today, and Thomas (2013) notes that the core focus of education—the development of the intellect, "virtue" or accomplishment? —remains just as unclear today as it did millennia ago. The tension between formal and

J. Vittersø (ed.), *Handbook of Eudaimonic Well-Being*, International Handbooks of Quality-of-Life,
DOI 10.1007/978-3-319-42445-3_31

progressive educational traditions captures much of this tension. The progressive educational tradition emphasizes "development from within" as opposed to "formation from without" (Dewey, 1938). The focus here is on activity, freedom and the personal growth of the student, with a focus on both group and individual work, and with teachers and students operating in a mentor-apprentice relationship, as opposed to the teacher operating purely in an instructional capacity. Such growth-focused goals are broadly concordant with eudaemonic approaches, yet the question of which "virtues" should be developed remains unclear.

Indeed, a wide range of traits, skills and abilities that arguably count as eudaemonic youth outcomes have been identified as important "non-academic" youth outcomes. These constructs have been variously termed skills that promote or constitute "character", "character virtue development", "social emotional learning", "pro-social behavior", "positive youth development", "learning mindsets and skills", "capacity for accomplishment", "thriving", "non-cognitive skills" and "personal success skills". As Berkowitz and Bier (2004) note when discussing definitions of research-based character education, "service learning, social-emotional learning, and prevention programs all share significant features with character education and could be considered forms of character education" (p. 74).

Given that eudaemonic notions of well-being and character may be defined, presented, and encouraged differently for different student populations, part of the challenge is thus to understand whether a conceptualization of eudaemonic well-being can be specified that successfully promotes the education of the whole student while helping to ensure that no single aspect of well-being or character are lost in the shuffle or subverted to other ends, such as social control (e.g. Davies, 2015). Eudaemonic well-being, however, with its emphasis on character, morality, meaning and spiritual concerns, defies simple definition.

31.2 The Multiplicity of Eudaemonic Approaches in Psychology

The empirical study of eudaemonic approaches to well-being, while at least as ancient as Socrates, has made a comeback in the wake of the advent of positive psychology. While meaning was a central topic in the humanistic psychology tradition (Frankl, 1985; Maslow, 1968; Rogers 1961), the anti-empirical stance of the field led the topic to be largely abandoned after the 1960s (Yalom, 1980). However, the notion that meaning is a valid component of well-being has become established in psychology during the last 20 years (Baumeister, 1992; Deci & Ryan, 2000; Kasser & Ryan, 1993; King & Hicks, 2007; Ryff, 1989, Chap. 6, this volume; Seligman, 2002). In particular, happiness and meaning have come to be seen as two different concepts. As Baumeister has noted, having children may decrease happiness among parents, but contributes very significantly to their levels of meaning. Nussbaum (2008) presents the examples of the happy warrior going into battle and the misanthropic David Trimble, who shared the 1998 Nobel Peace Prize, as models of meaning-rich lives that are not necessarily "happy" ones.

31.2.1 Self-Determination Theory

One eudaemonic approach that is sympathetic to many of the core assumptions in the progressive education traditions is self-determination theory (SDT). The SDT perspective is founded on the notion of *intrinsic motivation*—the pursuit of an activity for its own sake, interest and rewards, which is contrasted with extrinsic motivation, which refers to the pursuit of activities for instrumental ends (Deci & Ryan, 1980; Ryan and Martela, Chap. 7, this volume). A second focus concerned the process through which extrinsic goals come to be assimilated and accommodated, or *internalized* (Deci & Ryan, 1985). This study of goal pursuit and its determinants and consequences, has uncovered a distinction between goals based on their content. Kasser and Ryan (1996) found that life goals could be differentiated into those relating to *intrinsic aspirations* (including growth, affiliation, community contributions and health) and those relating to *extrinsic aspirations* (wealth, fame, image, etc.). Building on this foundation, Deci and Ryan (2000) posited three basic psychological needs as foundational to personal growth, integrity and well-being: autonomy, relatedness, and competence. The need for autonomy points to a feeling of choice and volition in the regulation of behavior. Relatedness refers to the importance of feeling a close connection to and being cared for by others. The need for competence refers to the sense of efficacy that one has with regards to internal and external environments (Ryan, Huta, & Deci, 2008). One distinctive claim they make is that these needs are related to intrinsic values that are an essential part of human nature, although they are careful to point out that this short list is not exhaustive. However, these three needs are essential for the development of intrinsic aspirations and psychological well-being (Kasser & Ryan, 1996). Moreover, the theory hypothesizes that attaining intrinsic goals will lead to the satisfaction of these needs, and that attaining such goals would increase well-being: that is, need satisfaction would mediate the relationship between intrinsic goal attainment and well-being (Ryan et al., 2008).

In addition to positing a relationship between the content of (intrinsic and extrinsic) goals, the SDT perspective also stresses the importance of the reason *why* individuals pursue important goals (Deci & Ryan, 2000). Organismic integration theory (OIT, a sub-theory of SDT: Deci & Ryan, 1985) distinguishes between intrinsic motivation (the most autonomous form of regulation), amotivation (the state of lacking the intention to act) and different forms of extrinsic motivation, which assess the extent to which regulation is autonomous. The theory specifies a continuum of extrinsically motivated behaviors that resembles Aristotle's discussion of the range of virtuous behavior (which spans virtuous, continent, incontinent and vicious behavior). On this account, the most heteronomous form of regulation is *external regulation*. An example of such regulation would be an individual acting to avoid pain or gain a reward. A second form of external motivation is *introjected regulation*. This involves accepting a motivation but not completely seeing it as one's own; that is, it still has an externally perceived locus of causality, although the motivation may be internally driven. In this form of regulation, actions are taken for the purpose of avoiding feelings of guilt or anxiety or to attain feelings of pride or self-esteem.

A significantly more self-determined form of extrinsic motivation is *identified motivation*, which involves the conscious and explicit valuing of a behavioral goal or regulation, leading to that goal being seen as personally important. The most autonomous form of extrinsic motivation is *integrated motivation*, where identified regulations are fully assimilated and brought into congruence with an individual's other values.

While it is important to note that intrinsic goals tend to be subject more frequently to autonomous regulation, the relative autonomy of a goal has effects independent of the content of the goal on well-being (Sheldon, Ryan, Deci, & Kasser, 2004). Of relevance to the present discussion, identified regulation was related to higher levels of interest and enjoyment among school children, as well as greater levels of effort at school, and more positive coping styles (Ryan & Connell, 1989). Subsequently, a series of studies have linked more autonomous extrinsic motivation with better health behaviors (Williams, Rodin, Ryan, Grolnick, & Deci, 1998), physical exercise (Chatzisarantis, Biddle, & Meek, 1997), political activity (Koestner, Losier, Vallerand, & Carducci, 1996), greater behavioral effectiveness, greater volitional persistence, higher levels of SWB and improved assimilation of the individual within the social group (Ryan, Kuhl, & Deci, 1997). Additionally, students who were securely connected to and cared for by their teachers and parents reported a greater sense of control, autonomy, and engagement in school (Ryan, Stiller, &

Lynch, 1994). Thus, these needs are seen to play an important role in the successful regulation and integration of behavior. Such findings are consistent with views in the progressive education tradition on intrinsic motivation—young learners are only motivated to complete tasks that intrinsically interest them (Thomas, 2013).

31.2.2 The Psychological Well-Being Tradition

A second approach more directly rooted in Aristotelian notions of eudaemonia is the psychological well-being tradition (PWB: Ryff, 1989, 1995; Ryff & Keyes, 1995; Ryff & Singer, 1998), which arose as a complementary approach to the happiness or subjective well-being (SWB) perspective. While the subjective well-being perspective does not specify a single conception of well-being—preferring instead to leave such matters to the individual—the PWB perspective adopts a more theory-guided approach to well-being, and argues that focusing solely on affect and life satisfaction neglects important aspects of positive psychological functioning (Ryff, 1989).

Ryff's (1989) definition of psychological well-being combines insight from three domains of psychological theory that emphasize character development. *Personal growth models* include Jung's (1933) notion of individuation, Allport's (1961) conception of maturity, Rogers (1962) theory of the fully functioning individual and Maslow's (1968) notion of self-actualization. *Life-span development perspectives* include Buhler's (1935) basic life tendencies towards life-fulfillment, Erikson's (1959) psychosocial stage model, and Neugarten's (1968, 1973) perspectives on personality change in adulthood and old age. Finally, Jahoda's (1958) *positive metal health* model provides a detailed description of what constitutes psychological health. Such models are consistent with PWB being understood as a character-based model of well-being (Peterson & Seligman, 2004).

One of the main goals of the PWB perspective is to provide a parsimonious and empirically robust conception of well-being derived from the theoretical perspectives noted above. This conception contains six dimensions (Ryff, 1989):

1. Self-acceptance: Holding positive attitudes towards oneself and one's past life
2. Positive relations with others: Having warm, trusting inter-personal relationships
3. Autonomy: Possessing qualities such as self-determination, independence, self-regulation of behavior, and an internal locus of evaluation
4. Environmental mastery: Having the ability to choose and/or create environments suitable to his/her psychic condition
5. Purpose in life: Having beliefs that give the individual the feeling that there is purpose in and meaning to life
6. Personal growth: Developing one's potential, and growing and expanding as a person

Ryff (2014) has noted that over 350 publications in 150 different scientific journals have examined the PWB construct. This output has focused on examining PWB in the context of development and aging; personality correlates of PWB; the impact of family experiences; work and other engagements; health and biological research; and clinical and intervention studies. For example, two PWB dimensions, personal growth (PG) and environmental mastery (EM), have been used to identify three paths of adult development among women— Achievers (high on PG and EM), Conservers (high on EM, low on PG), and Seekers (high on PG, low on EM; Helson & Srivastava, 2001). Ryff and Singer (1996) have also found that while mastery and autonomy showed incremental patterns from young adulthood to midlife, personal growth and purpose in life presented a decremental pattern from mid-life to old age. Positive relations and self-acceptance, on the other hand, did not show significant changes across the three domains. Keyes, Shmotkin, and Ryff (2002) have argued that while the PWB and SWB constructs are related to each other, they are empirically distinct, and while this view ties in with lay conceptions of happiness and meaning as separate components of the good life (King & Napa, 1998, but see Ward and King, Chap. 35, this volume, for a different view), other empirical work seems to suggest substantial empirical overlap between the two constructs (Disabato, Goodman, Kashdan, Short, & Jarden, 2015).

In recent work directly examining the link between eudaemonic well-being and academic outcomes, Yeager and colleagues (2014) have examined how purpose in life can contribute to self-regulation in academic settings. They found that promoting a pro-social, self-transcendent purpose for working hard in school in general promoted greater self-regulation among students even in the absence of a compelling reason to engage in a specific task in a specific class. In other words, providing students with a morally-motivated, eudaemonically-sourced "why" for learning motivated them to persevere on boring tasks, which would arguably assist them with later knowledge acquisition.

31.2.3 Seligman's Well-Being Theory

A more recent theoretical approach that also arguably lies within the eudaemonic tradition is Seligman's (2011) Well-Being theory. Well-Being theory is a revision of Seligman's (2002) Authentic Happiness (AH) theory, which proposed to "decompose" well-being into three more scientifically manageable components: *positive emotion* (*the pleasant life*), *engagement* (*the engaged life*), *and meaning* (*the meaningful life*). This original trichotomy was not claimed to be exclusive or exhaustive at this point, but rather a first approximation toward a scientifically useable unpacking of the lay term "happiness." The original theory relied on a set of empirical and analytic methods for moving the trichotomy toward becoming more exclusive and exhaustive (Peterson & Seligman, 2004). This approach is described as a "first cousin" to the "Subjective Well Being" approach (Jayawickreme, Pawelski, & Seligman, 2008), and on this account "happiness" was therefore achievable by pursuing one or more of these facets. As a result, individuals low in one aspect could still be "happy" if they nurtured other components. Individuals low in positive emotions could, for instance, flourish by being highly engaged in their lives, or by cultivating a rich sense of meaning in their lives.

Seligman (2011) subsequently revised AH theory by adding two facets to his original account: positive relationships and accomplishment. In addition, Seligman redefined the endpoint of his theory as "well-being" rather than "happiness" in order to stress the multifaceted nature of human flourishing over simple positive affect. Well-Being theory posits that well-being consists of the nurturing of one or more of the five following elements that are the best approximation of what humans pursue *for their own sake*: Positive emotion, Engagement, Relationships, Meaning, and Accomplishment (abbreviated as the acronym PERMA). According to Well-Being theory, while individuals may sometimes pursue of these elements for other ends (e.g., they may for instance think that accomplishment will bring positive emotion), many choose to do so because these elements are themselves intrinsically motivating. Of note, four of the five elements Seligman proposes as important elements of well-being constitute psychological facets of eudaemonic well-being. One important question that awaits clarification with Well-Being theory is whether, and if so how the various facets of well-being should be weighted if researchers want to be able to come up with a single summary measure of well-being (Forgeard, Jayawickreme, Kern, & Seligman, 2011).

31.3 The Multiplicity of Eudaemonic Approaches in Political Theory

The PWB approach represents the most direct approach to assessing the psychological facets of eudaemonic well-being (Forgeard et al., 2011). However, defining the good or full life has also been a project of political philosophers and human development researchers, and multiple accounts have been advocated over the last

60 years (Ranis, Stewart, & Samman, 2006). Alkire (2002) has noted 39 different attempts at defining what makes for a good or flourishing life between 1938 and 2000. While a detailed review of this literature will not be attempted here, we follow Ranis and colleagues (2006) in summarizing a number of accounts that each adopts a different conceptual approach and justification:

- Rawls (1999) identifies a set of primary goods that "are in general necessary for the framing and execution of a rational plan of life" (p. 359). He identifies these goods through a process of deliberative rationality, which he defines as "a careful consideration of the relevant facts and after a careful consideration of the consequences" (p. 380).
- Finnis (1980) and colleagues (Finnis, Boyle, & Grisez, 1987) use a similar approach to Rawls in defining a list of goods, but unlike Rawls' approach, which sees primary goods as necessary requirements for the good life, Finnis sees his goods as constitutive elements of a flourishing existence.
- The *Human Development Index* (UNDP, 1990), which emphasizes three important factors that enable individuals to increase their life choices: leading a long and healthy life, receiving an adequate education and maintaining a decent standard of living. This perspective is derived from Sen's (1993) capability approach.
- Doyal and Gough's (1991) *Basic Needs Approach* is founded on the principle "do no harm", where harm is defined as factors that prevent individuals from realizing activities central to their life plan.
- Nussbaum's (2000) account, which will be discussed in substantial detail later in this piece.
- Narayan-Parket's (2000) *Voices of the Poor* analysis lists the needs identified by the poor, which have been collected through focus groups with poor people in the developing world.
- Camfield's (2005) ESRC Research Group of Well-Being in Developing Countries attempts to collect information of how individuals perceive well-being in four separate countries.

Of these perspectives, the capabilities approach has arguably gained the most traction (Jayawickreme & Pawelski, 2013), and is one of the most prominent eudaemonic theories to have cut across human development studies, political theory and theories of education (Robeyns, 2006).

31.3.1 The Capabilities Approach

Sen (1999) argued that while income analysis presents the best starting point for assessing development, it is misguided to limit one's attention to income alone. He claimed that any meaningful analysis of the relationship between income and well-being requires a consideration of other relevant informational spaces. This argument for the necessity for considering factors in addition to income is in part based on Adam Smith's analysis of "necessities" (1776, quoted in Sen, 1999, pp. 73–74), and political philosopher John Rawls' argument on the importance of primary goods (1971/1999, quoted in Sen, 1999, p. 72) and "self-respect" (1971, quoted in Sen, 1992, p. 8).

Sen builds on these accounts by claiming that what is important are the "substantive freedoms" that individuals enjoy. Income is only important insofar as helps us achieve these freedoms. Sen quotes Aristotle's maxim that wealth is "merely useful and for the sake of something else" (Sen, 1999, p. 14), and it should be noted that in general he acknowledges strong conceptual similarities between his approach and the Aristotelian conception of *eudemonia* or optimal human functioning (Sen, 1993, p. 46, 1999, p. 73), although his account does not rely on Aristotle as heavily as Nussbaum's (Jayawickreme & Pawelski, 2013).

For Sen, what is required is a framework that focuses on the extent to which individuals can function successfully with the goods that they have at hand. In setting up this framework, Sen distinguishes between functionings, capabilities, functioning vectors and capability sets (Sen, 1999, p. 75). Functionings—the core notion in his account— refer to the various activities that an individual may value doing or being, while that individual's capability refers to "the alternative combinations of functionings that are feasible for her to achieve" (p. 75). Capability is therefore a form of freedom, as it affords the opportunity to achieve multiple functioning combinations. A functioning vector can be said to describe the combinations of these "doings and beings" that she enjoys at a particular point in life, while the capability set describes the set of possible or attainable functioning vectors that an individual can achieve. In this sense, capability can be defined as a *set* of functionings n-tuples, representing the various alternative combinations of beings and doings any one combination of which an individual can choose. The concept of capability is thus defined *in the space* of functionings. The focus of the capability approach can be either on the realized functionings (what the individual has achieved) or on the capability set of alternatives she has (p. 75). While Sen has (perhaps deliberately) kept the concept of capability vague, Gasper (1997, 2002, 2007) has distinguished between three types of capabilities:

- Potential-Capabilities (P-capabilities), which are inborn potentials
- Skill-Capabilities (S-capabilities), which refer to trained potentials that constitute skills, abilities and aptitudes
- Option- or Opportunity Capabilities (O-capabilities), attainable outcomes that are the joint implications of environmental opportunities and a person's abilities

It should be noted that while most people would see capabilities as S-capabilities, Sen seems to endorse an O-capabilities perspective (Gasper, 2007), especially when he describes capabilities as "opportunity freedom" (Sen, 1999).

One advantages of Sen's approach is that it is "inescapably pluralistic" (p. 76). Sen does not identify his approach with a single list of functionings, and as a result his approach is amenable to development and adaptation in a number of different ways and contexts (Clark, 2006). Moreover, Sen acknowledges that his approach does not provide an exhaustive theory of justice or development and that other principles must be taken into consideration. Sen sees this non-exhaustive flexibility as a strength: "To insist that there should only be one homogeneous magnitude that we value is to reduce drastically the range of our evaluative reasoning" (1999, p. 77).

While Sen's emphasis on human freedom and capability has been widely regarded as groundbreaking, it has also been criticized as being vague on the extent to which capability, well-being and freedom are spelled out (Gasper, 2004). Nussbaum (2003) has been critical of Sen's approach on this account, and her *capabilities* approach (to be distinguished from Sen's *capability* approach) seeks to rectify this shortcoming by offering a substantive set of human capabilities which, while non-exhaustive, are non-negotiable in their equal worth, as they are together constitutive of what it means to live a truly human existence.

Nussbaum's account draws heavily from Aristotelian notions of flourishing: "The basic intuitive idea of my version of the capabilities approach is that we begin with a conception of the dignity of the human being, and of a life that is worthy of that dignity" (Nussbaum, 2006, p. 74). In particular, her early work (1990, 1992) draws explicitly from the writings of Aristotle, and in many ways represent a development of his ideas concerning optimal human functioning. Writing of Aristotle's conception of happiness as eudaimonia, she notes:

> By (Aristotle's) account, pleasure is just not the right thing to focus on in a normative account of the good life for a human being. Some pleasures are bad; evil people take pleasure in their evil behavior. Happiness, by contrast, is a normative notion: since it is constitutive of what we understand as "the human good life," or "a flourishing life for a human being," we cannot include evil pleasures in it. (Nussbaum, 2004, p. 62)

Her account offers a view of "happiness" as "a thick vague theory of the good" that is both empirical and normative (Nussbaum, 1992, pp. 214–215) and "aims to be as universal as possible" (p. 215). The capabilities are presented as an "internal-essentialist account" that reveals "what the most central features of our common humanity are" (p. 215). Her current list (2006) of the ten Central Human Capabilities is as follows:

1. Living a normal life span;
2. Bodily health, including rights to adequate nourishment and shelter;
3. Bodily integrity (including freedom of movement and security against assault, as well as freedom of choice in reproduction and in matters of sexual satisfaction);
4. Being able to use the senses, the imagination, and thought (including freedom of expression and religious exercise, and adequate education), and being able to have pleasurable experiences;
5. Experiencing normal human emotions, including longing, grief, anger, etc., and having emotional attachments to others (i.e., love, friendships, and the normal range of affective emotions);
6. Development of one's capacities for practical reason, including the capacity of critical reflection upon one's good or plan of life (protected by liberty of conscience and religious freedom, among other rights);
7. Capabilities for affiliation (including both having the capacities to care for and commiserate with others, and having social bases of self-respect and non-humiliation (with rights to nondiscrimination on the basis of race, sex, sexual orientation, ethnicity, caste, religion, and national origin));
8. Living with other species;
9. Play, including the ability to enjoy recreational activities;
10. Control over one's environment (including rights to political participation, freedom of association, and having property rights on an equal basis with others and equal opportunities)
(Nussbaum, 2006, pp. 76–78)

Nussbaum has utilized various methods over the years to justify her list of capabilities (Jayawickreme & Pawelski, 2013). Her early work on capabilities (1990, 1992) derived a list of capabilities from Aristotle, and represented a development of his ideas concerning optimal human functioning. Nussbaum is strongly dismissive of relativist accounts, seeing them as ultimately confused and reactionary (Jaggar, 2006; see Nussbaum, 1999, for an extended discussion). Nussbaum's later accounts, captured in *Women and Human Development* (2000) and *Frontiers of Justice* (2006) are more open to claims of open-endedness and revision, although little such revision has in fact occurred (Jayawickreme & Pawelski, 2013). She however claims that the list is vague enough to be open to a multiplicity of interpretations, stands as a "partial moral conception" without being grounded in any metaphysical tradition, and—in line with Sen—focuses on protecting people's capabilities as opposed to functionings. The list also includes liberties that protect plurality, and Nussbaum sees her account as primarily offering a basis for persuasion, not intervention (pp. 78–80).

31.4 How Should "Well-Being" Be Defined in Education? An Integrative Note

We have provided a brief overview of selected theories of eudaimonic well-being in psychology and political theory. Building on this overview, we provide some integrative suggestions that fall directly out of these perspectives. We should note at the outset that we are not being bold enough to offer a model of eudaimonic well-being for use in education—we are simply offering some thoughts that we believe should be kept in mind by those interested in promoting well-being in the educational context:

1. A eudaemonic model of well-being in the education context needs to be sensitive to the distinction between O-capabilities and S-capabilities (Gasper, 2007). O-capabilities

refer to opportunities in the environment that afford the achievement of an individual's flourishing and functioning, while S-capabilities refer to skills, abilities and aptitudes that are traditionally the target of educational and psychological interventions. We note that one of the most persistent criticisms of certain education programs that fall within the rubric of well-being and character is that they both define character in very narrow terms (in many cases in terms of self-regulatory behavior) and are targeted at students from low-income and marginalized populations (e.g. Strauss, 2012).

2. With regards to addressing the different backgrounds of students and the impact this has for their long-term life prospects, a thorough and complete model of eudaemonic well-being in the educational context should confront and integrate environmental factors such as poverty and class and marginalization and their role in inhibiting flourishing, since such factors are vital in determining how individuals can converts their potential and skills into actual flourishing lives. We also posit that a thorough and complete model of eudaemonic well-being should confront and integrate environmental factors and that in addition to recognizing legitimate barriers to flourishing, an additional consequence of a wholistic approach might be to provoke greater recognition of the strengths and skills that students from low-income backgrounds have, helping educators and scholars to move away from the damaging 'deficit mindset' which attributes student failure to factors within the student as opposed to examining how schools are structured to prevent underprivileged students from learning (Valencia, 2010).
3. Educators should be encouraged to consider well-being in a holistic manner that ensures that the education of the whole student is promoted without prioritizing one aspect of well-being and character above others. The emphasis of certain character education programs on traits such as grit and self-control, and on values such as individual achievement call into question the ultimate value of such programs (Snyder, 2014). Such programs should however be tailored to be culturally sensitive to the target population (see point 6 below).
4. In this context, one helpful model of eudaemonic well-being that may be sufficiently holistic to capture the vital dimensions relevant in an educational context is Seider's (2012) distinction between moral character ("character of a good neighbor," including traits such as compassion, trust and kindness), civil character ("character of a good citizen," including traits such as tolerance, respect and civic-mindedness), and performance character ("achievement traits," including traits such as conscientiousness and grit) as promoted in three Boston-area charter schools. In reviewing this tripartite distinction, Baehr (2015) suggested the addition of the fourth category of intellectual character (traits that foster life-long learning like critical thinking and open-mindedness). These four dimensions arguably represent a model of eudaemonic well-being that captures all the important dimensions without prioritizing one dimension (such as traits associated with performance character, for example) over another.
5. We believe that engaging educators in discussions of these dimensions can assist with the development of a comprehensive model of well-being for education that can both educate the "whole student" and be sensitive to the development of O-capabilities (opportunities not afforded to all students due to differences in opportunity and other background conditions) and S-capabilities (for example, the capabilities Nussbaum argues are essential to flourishing and are frequently denied equal expression for reasons including gender inequality or poverty). For example, the validity of Ryff's (1989) PWB model or Seligman's (2011) PERMA model for education can be ascertained in part by evaluating such models against the comprehensive dimensions listed above (e.g. does the PWB or PERMA model promote intellectual character, as defined by Baehr

6. We also note one significant question relevant to education that eudaimonic theories are largely silent on; none of these theories discuss in any significant detail *cultural differences* in notions of well-being or in emphasis on and prioritization of different traits relevant to flourishing. This is in part because of the universalist nature of eudaimonic theories themselves, which focus on common characteristics across gender, religions, cultures and philosophical traditions. For example, philosophers advocating universalist approaches such as Nussbaum have appealed to these commonalities to argue that all individuals must have at least some minimum rights necessary for human functioning (Nussbaum, 1993). We acknowledge however that such approaches fail to account for the fact that certain significant differences among communities cannot simply be reconciled by pointing to commonalities among cultures. We believe that culture is an important factor at play in education, as the challenge of addressing cultural differences is one driver of the tendency to focus narrowly on academic outcomes when teaching children from diverse backgrounds. We note that careful attention needs to be paid to ensure that educational programming based on character education principles or other eudaimonic perspectives be tailored to be culturally appropriate to the target population.

As we noted at the beginning of this thought piece, eudaemonic notions of well-being and character are often defined, presented, and encouraged differently for different populations of students. Educators interested in promoting well-being as a goal of education should be mindful of the skills, capacities and traits they want to promote as part of that goal. A serious consideration of the role of well-being in higher education should ideally incorporate a conceptualization of eudaemonic well-being that successfully promotes the education of the whole student while ensuring that no single aspect of well-being and character is subverted to other ends. Such a conceptualization of well-being has the potential to play a significant role in shaping thinking about education in the future, particularly in ensuring that as many individuals as possible enjoy the "substantive freedoms" that Sen and other eudaemonic theorists argue should be the ultimate goal of policy.

References

Alkire, S. (2002). Dimensions of development. *World Development, 30*(2), 181–205.

Allport, G. (1961). *Pattern and growth in personality*. New York: Holt, Rinehart, & Winston.

Aristotle. (350BC/1998). *Nichomachean ethics*. New York: Oxford University Press.

Baehr, J. (2015). Appendix A: Varieties of character: Moral, civic, performance, and intellectual. In *Cultivating good minds: A philosophical and practical resource guide for educating for intellectual virtues*. Available at: http://intellectualvirtues.org

Baumeister, R. F. (1992). *Meanings in life*. Hillsdale, NJ: Erlbaum.

Berkowitz, M. W., & Bier, M. C. (2004). Research-based character education. *The Annals of the American Academy of Political and Social Science, 591*(1), 72–85.

Buhler, C. (1935). The curve of life as studied in biographies. *Journal of Applied Psychology, 43*, 653–673.

Camfield, L. (2005). Researching quality of life in developing countries. *ESRC Research Group on Well-Being in Developing Countries Newsletter*, p. 3.

Chatzisarantis, N. L., Biddle, S. J., & Meek, G. A. (1997). A self-determination theory approach to the study of intentions and the intention–behaviour relationship in children's physical activity. *British Journal of Health Psychology, 2*(4), 343–360.

Clark, D. A. (2006). The capability approach: Its development, critiques and recent advances. In D. A. Clark (Ed.), *The Elgar companion to development studies* (pp. 1–18). Cheltenham, UK: Edward Elgar.

Dahill-Brown, S. E., & Jayawickreme, E. (2016). What constitutes indices of well-being among college students? In D. Harward (Ed.), *Well-being and higher education: A strategy for change and the realization of education's greater purposes*. New York City: Endeavor Foundation.

Davies, W. (2015). *The happiness industry: How the government and big business sold us well-being*. London: Verso Books.

Deci, E. L., & Ryan, R. M. (1980). Self-determination theory: When mind mediates behavior. *Journal of Mind and Behavior, 1*, 33–43.

Deci, E. L., & Ryan, R. M. (1985). *Intrinsic motivation and self-determination in human behavior*. New York: Taylor & Francis.

Deci, E. L., & Ryan, R. M. (2000). The "what" and "why" of goal pursuits: Human needs and the self-determination of behavior. *Psychological Inquiry, 11*(4), 227–268.

Dewey, J. (1938). *Education and experience*. New York: Simon & Schuster.
Disabato, D. J., Goodman, F. R., Kashdan, T. B., Short, J. L., & Jarden, A. (2015). Different types of well-being? A cross-cultural examination of hedonic and eudaimonic well-being. *Psychological Assessment*. Washington, DC: American Psychological Association.
Doyal, L., & Gough, I. (1991). *A theory of human need*. London: Macmillan.
Erikson, E. H. (1959). Identity and the life cycle: Selected papers. *Psychological Issues, 1*, 1–171.
Finnis, J. (1980). *Natural law and natural rights*. Oxford, UK: Clarendon.
Finnis, J., Boyle, J. M., & Grisez, G. (1987). *Nuclear deterrence, morality and realism*. Oxford, UK: Clarendon.
Forgeard, M. J. C., Jayawickreme, E., Kern, M. L., & Seligman, M. E. P. (2011). Doing the right thing: Measuring wellbeing for public policy. *International Journal of Wellbeing, 1*(1), 79–106.
Frankl, V. E. (1985). *Man's search for meaning*. New York: Simon and Schuster.
Gasper, D. (1997). Sen's capability approach and Nussbaum's capability ethics. *Journal of International Development, 9*, 281–302.
Gasper, D. (2002). Is Sen's capability approach an adequate basis for considering human development? *Review of Political Economy, 14*, 435–461.
Gasper, D. (2004). *The ethics of development*. Edinburgh, UK: Edinburgh University Press.
Gasper, D. (2007). What is the capability approach? Its core, rationale, partners and dangers. *Journal of Socio-Economics, 36*, 335–359.
Helson, R., & Srivastava, S. (2001). Three paths of adult development: Conservers, seekers, and achievers. *Journal of Personality and Social Psychology, 80*(6), 995.
Jaggar, A. M. (2006). Reasoning about well-being: Nussbaum's methods of justifying the capabilities. *Journal of Political Philosophy, 14*(3), 301–322.
Jahoda, M. (1958). *Current concepts of positive mental health*. New York: Basic Books.
Jayawickreme, E., Forgeard, M. J. C., & Seligman, M. E. P. (2012). The engine of well-being. *Review of General Psychology, 16*(4), 327–342.
Jayawickreme, E., & Pawelski, J. O. (2013). Positivity and the capabilities approach. *Philosophical Psychology, 26*(3), 383–400.
Jayawickreme, E., Pawelski, J., & Seligman, M. E. P. (2008). *Happiness: Positive psychology and Nussbaum's capabilities approach. Library of living philosophers: The philosophy of Martha Nussbaum*. Chicago: Open Court.
Jung, C. G. (1933). *Modern man in search of a soul*. New York: Harcourt.
Kasser, T., & Ryan, R. M. (1993). A dark side of the American dream: Correlates of financial success as a central life aspiration. *Journal of Personality and Social Psychology, 65*(2), 410.
Kasser, T., & Ryan, R. M. (1996). Further examining the American dream: Differential correlates of intrinsic and extrinsic goals. *Personality and Social Psychology Bulletin, 22*, 280–287.
Keyes, C. L. M., Shmotkin, D., & Ryff, C. D. (2002). Optimizing well-being: The empirical encounter of two traditions. *Journal of Personality and Social Psychology, 82*(6), 1007.
King, L. A., & Hicks, J. A. (2007). Whatever happened to "What might have been"? Regrets, happiness, and maturity. *American Psychologist, 62*(7), 625.
King, L. A., & Napa, C. K. (1998). What makes a life good? *Journal of Personality and Social Psychology, 75*(1), 156.
Koestner, R., Losier, G. F., Vallerand, R. J., & Carducci, D. (1996). Identified and introjected forms of political internalization: Extending self-determination theory. *Journal of Personality and Social Psychology, 70*(5), 1025.
Maslow, A. (1968). Some educational implications of the humanistic psychologies. *Harvard Educational Review, 38*(4), 685–696.
Narayan-Parker, D. (2000). *Crying out for change: Voices of the poor*. Oxford, UK: Oxford University Press for the World Bank.
Neugarten, B. L. (1968). The awareness of middle age. In B. L. Neugarten (Ed.), *Middle age and aging* (pp. 93–98). Chicago: University of Chicago Press.
Neugarten, B. L. (1973). Personality change in late life: A developmental perspective. In C. Eisodorfer & M. P. Lawton (Eds.), *The psychology of adult development and aging* (pp. 311–335). Washington, DC: American Psychological Association.
Nussbaum, M. C. (1990). Aristotelian social democracy. In R. Bruce Douglass, G. Mara, & H. Richardson (Eds.), *Liberalism and the good*. New York: Routledge.
Nussbaum, M. C. (1992). Human functioning and social justice in defense of Aristotelian essentialism. *Political Theory, 20*(2), 202–246.
Nussbaum, M. C. (1999). *Sex and social justice*. New York: Oxford University Press.
Nussbaum, M. C. (2000). *Women and human development*. Cambridge, UK: Cambridge University Press.
Nussbaum, M. C. (2003). Capabilities as fundamental entitlements: Sen and social justice. *Feminist Economics, 9*(2–3), 33–59.
Nussbaum, M. C. (2004). Mill between Aristotle & Bentham. *Daedalus, 133*(2), 60–68.
Nussbaum, M. C. (2006). *Frontiers of justice: Disability, nationality, species*. Cambridge, MA: Belknap.
Nussbaum, M. C. (2008). Who is the happy warrior? Philosophy poses questions to psychology. *The Journal of Legal Studies, 37*(S2), S81–S113.
Peterson, C., & Seligman, M. E. P. (2004). *Character strengths and virtues: A classification*. Oxford, UK: Oxford University Press.

Ranis, G., Stewart, F., & Samman, E. (2006). Human development: Beyond the human development index. *Journal of Human Development, 7*, 323–358.

Rawls, J. (1999). *A theory of justice*. Oxford, UK: Oxford University Press.

Robeyns, I. (2006). Three models of education rights, capabilities and human capital. *Theory and Research in Education, 4*(1), 69–84.

Rogers, C. (1961). *A therapist's view of psychotherapy: On becoming a person*. London: Constable.

Rogers, C. R. (1962). The process equation of psychotherapy. *American Journal of Psychotherapy, 15*, 27–45.

Ryan, R. M., & Connell, J. P. (1989). Perceived locus of causality and internalization: Examining reasons for acting in two domains. *Journal of Personality and Social Psychology, 57*(5), 749.

Ryan, R. M., Huta, V., & Deci, E. L. (2008). Living well: A self-determination theory perspective on eudaimonia. *Journal of Happiness Studies, 9*, 139–170.

Ryan, R. M., Kuhl, J., & Deci, E. L. (1997). Nature and autonomy: An organizational view of social and neurobiological aspects of self-regulation in behavior and development. *Development and Psychopathology, 9*(04), 701–728.

Ryan, R. M., Stiller, J. D., & Lynch, J. H. (1994). Representations of relationships to teachers, parents, and friends as predictors of academic motivation and self-esteem. *The Journal of Early Adolescence, 14*(2), 226–249.

Ryff, C. D. (1989). Happiness is everything, or is it? Explorations on the meaning of psychological well-being. *Journal of Personality and Social Psychology, 57*(6), 1069.

Ryff, C. D. (1995). Psychological well-being in adult life. *Current Directions in Psychological Science, 4*, 99–104.

Ryff, C. D. (2014). Psychological well-being revisited: Advances in the science and practice of eudaimonia. *Psychotherapy and Psychosomatics, 83*(1), 10–28.

Ryff, C. D., & Keyes, C. L. M. (1995). The structure of psychological well-being revisited. *Journal of Personality and Social Psychology, 69*(4), 719.

Ryff, C. D., & Singer, B. (1996). Psychological well-being: Meaning, measurement, and implications for psychotherapy research. *Psychotherapy and Psychosomatics, 65*(1), 14–23.

Ryff, C. D., & Singer, B. (1998). The contours of positive human health. *Psychological Inquiry, 9*(1), 1–28.

Seider, S. (2012). *Character compass: How powerful school culture can point students towards success*. Cambridge, MA: Harvard Education Press.

Seligman, M. E. P. (2002). Positive psychology, positive prevention, and positive therapy. *Handbook of Positive Psychology, 2*, 3–12.

Seligman, M. E. P. (2011). *Flourish*. New York: The Free Press.

Seligman, M. E., P., Ernst, R. M., Gillham, J., Reivich, K., & Linkins, M. (2009). Positive education: Positive psychology and classroom interventions. *Oxford Review of Education, 35*(3), 293–311.

Sen, A. (1992). *Inequality reexamined*. Oxford: Clarendon Press.

Sen, A. K. (1993). Capability and well-being. In M. C. Nussbaum & A. K. Sen (Eds.), *The quality of life*. Oxford, UK: Clarendon.

Sen, A. K. (1999). *Development as freedom*. Oxford, UK: Oxford University Press.

Sheldon, K. M., Ryan, R. M., Deci, E. L., & Kasser, T. (2004). The independent effects of goal contents and motives on well-being: It's both what you pursue and why you pursue it. *Personality and Social Psychology Bulletin, 30*(4), 475–486.

Snyder, J. A. (2014, May 6). Teaching kids 'Grit' is all the rage. Here's What's wrong with it. *The New Republic*.

Strauss, V. (2012, October 3). Sick of "grit" already. *The Washington Post*.

Thomas, G. (2013). *Education: A very short introduction*. Oxford, UK: Oxford University Press.

United Nations Development Program. (1990). *Human development report 1990*. New York: Oxford University Press.

Valencia, R. R. (2010). *Dismantling contemporary deficit thinking: Educational thought and practice*. New York: Routledge.

Williams, G. C., Rodin, G. C., Ryan, R. M., Grolnick, W. S., & Deci, E. L. (1998). Autonomous regulation and long-term medication adherence in adult outpatients. *Health Psychology, 17*(3), 269.

Yalom, I. D. (1980). *Existential psychotherapy*. New York: Basic Books.

Yeager, D. S., Henderson, M. D., Paunesku, D., Walton, G. M., D'Mello, S., Spitzer, B. J., et al. (2014). Boring but important: A self-transcendent purpose for learning fosters academic self-regulation. *Journal of Personality and Social Psychology, 107*(4), 559.

32 Developing a Eudaimonia Research Agenda in Travel and Tourism

M. Joseph Sirgy and Muzaffer Uysal

32.1 Introduction

The field of travel and tourism has achieved a significant amount of academic success and recognition for the past 40 years or so. The accumulation of knowledge as reflected in journals and other publication outlets support this. The scope of travel and tourism research has covered a broad range of issues such as antecedents of travel behaviour, satisfaction, motivation, benefits received, social-cultural and environmental impacts of tourism activities, host and guest interactions, tourism planning and development, and economic significance of tourism in destinations where travel and tourism activities take place. Similarly, the research tools and approaches used to examine these issues also reveal a high degree of methodological sophistication and theoretical underpinnings that help us understand the production and consumption of tourism experiences and services. A most recent research trend also reveals that while acknowledging economic significance, the value of tourism activities has transitioned to focus more on non-economic measures such as quality of life (QOL) of stakeholders, satisfaction, wellness, an increased focus on abstract forms of value such as perceived quality of life, sense of well-being and sustainable business practices. More specifically, there has been a notable increase in the amount of research that has focused on QOL and well-being of tourism stakeholders in the past 15 years or so. In this vein, the goal of this chapter is to contribute to this growing body of knowledge by developing a eudaimonia research agenda in travel and tourism. The chapter has three main sections. The first section introduces the term of eudaimonia and its conceptual foundations. The second section, which is the main focus of the chapter, introduces to the reader selected eudaimonia theories and show how these theories can guide future research in travel and tourism. The chapter ends with a conclusion section.

32.2 Eudaimonia: Conceptual Foundations

The first author of this chapter made a clear distinction among three programs of research in quality-of-life studies and well-being research (Sirgy, 2012). These three programs of research are essentially referred to as hedonic well-being, life satisfaction, and eudaimonia. Three distinct programs of research were identified based on Haybron's (2000, 2008) distinction among three philosophical concepts of happiness:

M.J. Sirgy (✉) • M. Uysal
Pamplin College of Business, Virginia Polytechnic Institute & State University, Blacksburg, VA, USA
e-mail: sirgy@vt.edu; samil@vt.edu

J. Vittersø (ed.), *Handbook of Eudaimonic Well-Being*, International Handbooks of Quality-of-Life,
DOI 10.1007/978-3-319-42445-3_32

psychological happiness (philosophical basis for much of the research in hedonic well-being), prudential happiness (philosophical basis for much of the research in life satisfaction), and perfectionist happiness (philosophical basis for much of the research in eudaimonia). Dan Haybron is a happiness philosopher.

32.2.1 Psychological Happiness: Hedonic Well-Being

Psychological happiness is essentially hedonic or emotional well-being. According to Haybron (2000, 2008, Chap. 2, this volume), *psychological happiness* is indeed a state of mind involving feelings of joy, serenity, and affection. Psychological happiness is the experience of positive emotions over time. David Phillips (2006), a philosopher of happiness, clearly distinguishes between two approaches to happiness: hedonic and eudaimonic. He argues that the hedonic tradition highlights the individual and assumes that the individual is motivated to enhance personal freedom, self-preservation, and self-enhancement. Thus, the focus is on the integrity of the individual and his own judgment about what makes him happy. In contrast, the eudaimonic tradition derives from the Aristotelian conception of the good life, prudence, reason, and justice. The goal is to have people flourish or to function to meet their full potential, to contribute to society, and achieve the highest standards of morality. Thus, hedonic well-being is clearly distinguished from eudaimonia.

To help the reader better appreciate the concept of hedonic well-being, let us review some research that have operationalized this concept. Specifically, the affective dimension of subjective well-being is customarily measured by two types of affect, positive and negative, and then summing up the scores to derive an index of subjective well-being (e.g., Diener & Emmons, 1984; Diener, Smith, & Fujita, 1995; Lucas, Diener, & Suh, 1996). That is, a person who has a high level of subjective well-being is one who has a preponderance of positive affect (such as joy, contentment, or pleasure) over negative affect (such as sadness, depression, anxiety, or anger). The concepts of positive and negative affect capture what some well-being researchers also call emotional well-being. For example, Simsek (2009) has argued that the traditional measures capturing psychological happiness in terms of positive and negative affect (e.g., the PANAS measure) do not make reference to "life."

Daniel Kahneman, a Nobel Laureate and a leading scholar in the psychology of well-being research, has conceptualized happiness as sensations that are associated with real-time feelings of happiness (Kahneman, 1999). He calls this happiness as "objective happiness." To measure this concept of happiness, he employs an experiential sampling method. Subjects are contacted at set time intervals during the day and are asked to report their positive and negative feelings they experienced now (or during the last hour or so).

At a much more micro level, one can argue that psychological happiness or hedonic well-being can be viewed at a molecular level in terms of neuronal activity related to the release of dopamine (and possibly other neurochemicals) in the brain. For example, Warburton (1996) argues that happiness is a pleasant, physiological sensation caused by neurochemical responses in the dopamine system in response to external stimuli that have rewarding properties (e.g., food, drugs, sex, and music). Therefore, people have a natural proclivity to increase their happiness by experiencing stimuli that triggers the release of dopamine in the brain—the reward system.

32.2.2 Prudential Happiness = Life Satisfaction

In contrast with psychological happiness, prudential happiness refers to a different state of well-being. Psychological happiness may be a necessary but not sufficient condition of prudential happiness. Prudential happiness is achieved when a person achieves a high state of well-being, both mentally and physically. Prudential happiness is leading a good life. It involves both the feelings of happiness and the action that generates personal growth.

In the context of Seligman's (2002) distinction among the pleasant life, the engaged life, and the meaningful life, psychological happiness seems to represent the pleasant life, whereas prudential happiness seems most consistent with the engaged life. Seligman's meaningful life is what we think is eudaimonia. Peterson, Park, and Seligman (2005) developed a measure based on Seligman's theory of authentic happiness. The measure seems to capture the three major dimensions of happiness—hedonic well-being, life satisfaction, and eudaimonia. Examples of items capturing hedonic well-being (or what they call the "pleasant life") include: "life is too short to postpone the pleasures it can provide," "I go out of my way to feel euphoric," and "in choosing what I do, I always take into account whether it will be pleasurable." Example items for the life satisfaction dimension (or what they call "the engaged life") include "regardless of what I am doing, time passes very quickly," "I seek out situations that challenge my skills and abilities," and "I am always absorbed in what I do." Example items for the eudaimonia dimension (or what they call "the meaningful life") include: "my life serves a higher purpose," "in choosing what I do, I always take into account whether it will benefit other people," and "I have a responsibility to make the world a better place." The scale used to capture responses is a 5-point rating scale varying from 1 ("Very Much Unlike Me") to 5 ("very Much Like Me").

Haybron (2000, 2008) illustrates the state of prudential happiness by describing a brain in a container. That brain may experience perfect bliss (psychological happiness), but physically it is not leading a good life as a person (prudential happiness). In other words, happiness is more than feelings of joy. It necessitates engagement in life to realize one's potentiality. It is what people do in life to achieve personal fulfilment. It is leading the good life.

A great majority of well-being researchers view life satisfaction as self-avowals of happiness (see Diener, 1984; Veenhoven, 1984a, 1984b; Veenhoven et al., 1994 for literature reviews). Life satisfaction is viewed as a "cognitive" conceptualization of happiness or subjective well-being. It may involve judgments of fulfilment of one's needs, goals, and wishes. This view is essentially based by seminal studies of the founding fathers of the life satisfaction research movement: Andrews and Withey (1976), Campbell, Converse, and Rodgers (1976), Cantril (1965), Diener (1984), and Michalos (1985). Diener, Emmons, Larsen, and Griffin (1985) defined life satisfaction as "a cognitive judgmental process dependent upon a comparison of one's circumstances with what is thought to be an appropriate standard" (p. 71); thus, the lower the discrepancy between the perception of life achievements and some standard the higher the life satisfaction.

32.2.3 Perfectionist Happiness = Eudaimonia

In contrast to psychological and prudential happiness, perfectionist happiness refers to a life that is good in all respects, including the moral life. It is a life that is desirable without qualification, both enviable and admirable. Perfectionist happiness is achieved when a person achieves a state of well-being plus leading a moral life (Haybron, 2000, 2008). Haybron illustrates the concept of perfectionist happiness by describing an evil person. This person may be psychologically happy (high on psychological happiness), is highly engaged in life (high on prudential happiness), but is a parasite to society (low on perfectionist happiness).

Political psychologist, Paul Lane, defined QOL as the relation between a person's subjective and objective sets of circumstances (Lane, 2001). The *subjective* set of a person reflecting a high quality of life involves nine elements: (1) capacity for enjoying life, (2) cognitive complexity, (3) a sense of autonomy and effectiveness, (4) self-knowledge, (5) self-esteem, (6) ease of interpersonal relations, (7) an ethical orientation, (8) personality integration, and (9) a productivity orientation. Lane believes that these nine elements describing the psychological makeup of a person are the hallmark of mental health and social responsibility. These elements combined are responsible for a sense of subjective well-being and moral development. This subjective set makes up what Lane calls the "quality of the person," or what we call "eudaimonia."

32.3 Eudomania Theories to Guide Future Research in Travel and Tourism

In recent years a number of psychological theories of eudoaimonia have been developed: self-determination theory, the broaden-and-build theory of positive emotions, the theory of human flourishing, meaning and purpose in life theory, theory of positive mental health, need hierarchy theory, and eudaimonstic identity theory. We will discuss these theories and we'll suggest ideas that should help travel/tourism scholars apply these theories to help explain eudaimonia as experienced through travel and tourism activities and programs.

32.3.1 Self-Determination Theory

With respect to self-determination theory, Ryan and Deci (2000) suggest that human beings can be proactive and engaged in life. They have the potential to determine their own destiny and the destiny of others. Those who are proactive and engaged in life tend to be intrinsically motivated. Intrinsic motivation is directly related to three innate psychological needs, namely the need for *competence*, *relatedness*, and *autonomy*. People who are proactive and engaged in life are likely to have these three psychological needs met to a large extent. Meeting these psychological needs constitute human flourishing (i.e., eudaimonia). Much research in tourism has shown that individuals engage in leisure and tourism activities for intrinsic as well extrinsic reasons in their travel experiences (e.g., Iso-Ahola, 1980; Driver, Brown, & Peterson, 1991; Snepenger, King, Marshall, & Uysal, 2006; Jackson, 2008; Prebensen, Woo, & Uysal, 2013). Furthermore, there is a plethora of research in tourism that have focused on motivation with its variants as antecedent to travel, involvement, and emotional and physical engagement in creating and consuming tourism experiences in different settings (e.g., Filep, 2008; Hills, Argyle, & Reeves, 2000; Nawijn, 2011, Nawijn, Mitas, Lin, & Kerstetter, 2013; Prebensen et al., 2013; Prebensen, Chen, & Uysal, 2014).

With respect to the specific three dimensions of self-determination theory (competence, relatedness, and autonomy), we do have research that has focused on the development of competency and mastery in skills and levels of knowledge in travel behaviour. Such competency and mastery have been shown to contribute to enjoyment, happiness, and subjective well-being of participants (e.g., Dolnicar, Yanamandram, & Cliff, 2012; Gilbert & Abdullah, 2004). Furthermore, some studies have documented the fact that tourism activities and experiences tend to be relational and social in nature, meeting social needs. Given the preceding discussion, one can argue that tourist activities that have elements of competence, relatedness, and autonomy are likely to contribute significantly to tourists' eudaimonia. Future research could test this theoretical proposition explicitly in various travel/tourism settings for different tourist groups.

32.3.2 Broaden-and-Build Theory of Positive Emotions

Further, Fredrickson's (2001, Chap. 12, this volume) *broaden-and-build theory of positive emotions* suggests that cultivating positive emotions (e.g., joy, interest, contentment, and love) is useful in several ways. First, the experience of positive emotions broadens an individual's thought-action repertoire in different ways. Examples may include a positive emotion such as joy sparking the urge to play; interest may spark the urge to explore; contentment may spark the urge to savour and integrate; and love may spark reinforce the urge to play, explore, savour, and integrate within safe and close relationships. In contrast, negative emotions (e.g., anger, anxiety, fear, depression, jealousy, envy, hate, and disgust) function to narrow one's mind set. The consequences of having a broadened mind set include creativity and discovery and the reinforcement of social bonds. These outcomes, in essence, serve to build personal resources for the individual—physical, intellectual, social, and psychological resources. These resources serve to enhance future coping behaviour and survival given adversity (Prebensen & Foss, 2011). Hence, positive emotions not only serve to optimize health, well-being, and eudaimonia.

In a travel/tourism context, Nawijn et al. (2013) conducted a study tracking daily the emotions of 39 American and Dutch travelers during their vacation using a diary. The study showed that although fluctuations in emotions are related to length of vacation, vacationers on an 8- to 13-day trip experienced significant changes in the balance of their emotions over the course of their trip. In general, they felt good; but positive feelings declined towards the end of the vacation. Future research could be conducted to test the notion that tourists experiencing a large dose of positive emotions on their vacation are likely to gain in eudaimonia compared to those who do not experience much positive emotions.

32.3.3 Theory of Human Flourishing

The *theory of human flourishing* by Carol Ryff (1989, Chap. 6, this volume) focuses on defining and measuring human flourishing in terms of psychological well-being. This construct involves five dimensions: autonomy (e.g., "I am not afraid to voice my opinions even when they are in opposition to the opinions of most people), positive relations with others (e.g., "most people see me as loving and affectionate"), environmental mastery (e.g., "I am quite good at managing the responsibilities of my daily life"), and personal growth (e.g., "I think it is important to have new experiences that challenge how I think about the world") (cf. Burns & Machin, 2009; Ryff; Ryff & Keyes, 1995; Ryff & Singer, 1996, 1998; Van Dierendonck, Diaz, Rodriguez-Carvajal, Blanco, & Moreno-Jimenez, 2008).

A more recent attempt to capture human flourishing is the *Flourishing Scale* (Diener et al., 2010). This is a brief eight-item summary measure of the respondent's self-perceived success in important areas such as relationships (e.g., "my social relationships are supportive and rewarding"), self-esteem (e.g., "I am a good person and live a good life"), purpose (e.g., "I lead a purposeful and meaningful life"), and optimism (e.g., "I am optimistic about my future").

A number of studies that have focused on such leisure activities as dancing (e.g., flamenco), mountain climbing, scuba diving and skiing in tourism destinations reported "flourishing" through participating in activities. For example, Kler and Tribe (2012) found that scuba divers as their study participants gained meaning and fulfilment from the acts of learning and personal growth as a result of scuba diving experience. Another study by Tsan, Yen, and Hsiao reported similar results from a study that examined the relationships among transcended, experience, flow and happiness from a group of 339 Taiwanese mountain claimers. The study indicated that transcendent experience positively affects flow and happiness. Similarly, Matteucci (2013) conducted a study demonstrating that learning to dance Flamenco over an extended period of time can be a spiritual tourist journey. Participants were observed to experience flourishing and growth, derived a sense of accomplishment and happiness, from the act of intense engagement and social interactions. Future research could help identify specific tourist activities that are most eudaimonic. Furthermore, future research can decompose the specific dimensions of specific tourist activities as a direct function of the various dimensions of flourishing such as self-acceptance, positive relations with others, personal growth, purpose in life, environmental mastery, and autonomy. Specific programs can be designed and tested to induce specific aspects of flourishing (e.g., a golf excursion can be designed and tested to enhance tourists' sense of environmental mastery).

32.3.4 Meaning and Purpose in Life Theory

Well-being researchers have shown that the concept of purpose and meaning in life plays a very important role in eudaimonia. They make reference to ideas developed by Victor Frankl (1963, 1967) and the panoply of subsequent writings (e.g. Steger, Frazier, Oishi, & Kaler, 2006; Steger, Chap. 11, this volume). Much of these writings support the notion that purpose and meaning are beneficial to individual and social functioning. People who are conscientiously embrace social values and live their lives consistently with those values are characterized as high in eudaimonia.

Examples of eudaimonia measures based on the concept of purpose and meaning in life include the *Meaning in Life Questionnaire-Presence Subscale* (MLQ-P; Steger et al., 2006). The MLQ-P measure captures the degree to which people feel their lives are meaningful through five items (e.g., "I have a good sense of what makes my life meaningful"). Responses to each item are captured on a 7-point rating scale varying from "1=absolutely untrue" to "7=absolutely true."

More recently, Schulenberg and Melton (2010) have provided some evidence of construct validity in relation to the *Purpose-in-Life* (PIL) measure (Chamberlain & Zika, 1988; Dyck, 1987; Hicks & King, 2007; Melton & Schulenberg, 2008; Morgan & Farsides, 2009). Respondents express the extent to which they feel enthusiasm in living, whether they feel life is exciting, if they have clear life goals, whether the life they live has been worthwhile, whether they have a reason for being alive, whether the world is meaningful, and whether they feel they have a life purpose (cf. Schulenberg, Schnetzer, & Buchanan, 2011).

In the context of tourism, there is enough published evidence to infer that through tourism activities some tourists make travel a life quest. These travellers make the constructive use of their travel time as central to their lifestyle (Neulinger, 1981). That is, activities such as travel, learning about different cultures, meeting new people and visiting places create experiential values, excitement, and provide meaning to their lives. One can hypothesize that the desire for exploration through travel is inherent in most youth and young adults. That young people find meaning through travel to not only explore new places but also to seek meaning in their own lives and to come to understand themselves. There may be gender differences too in that this inherent motive is likely to be stronger among male than female travellers. People who are single and romantically unattached to others may be more involved in travel and exploration, compared to those who have established relationships and family roles.

32.3.5 Theory of Positive Mental Health

Corey Keyes, a social psychologist from a sociology tradition, has made quite an impact in well-being research by advocating a mental health concept of eudaimonia. Specifically, he equates eudaimonia with positive mental health, which involves feeling good and functioning well (Keyes, 1998). He argues that the presence of mental health is flourishing in life, and the absence of mental health is languishing in life. *Mental health* is thus a syndrome of symptoms of both positive feelings and positive functioning in life. Keyes (2002) identified 13 dimensions of positive mental health: (1) positive emotions; (2) avowed satisfaction with life; (3) making a contribution to society; (4) social integration, (5) social growth and potential; (6) acceptance of others; (7) social interest and coherence; (8) self-acceptance; (9) environmental mastery (control); (10) positive relations with others; (11) personal growth; (12) autonomy, and (13) having purpose in life. A measure of positive mental health was positively related to several personality traits such as extraversion, conscientiousness, agreeableness, and negatively related to neuroticism (Joshanloo & Nostrabadi, 2009) — a pattern of findings consistent with much of the research on personality and subjective well-being (cf. Keyes, 2006a, 2006b).

There is some evidence in the tourism literature that travel and tourism contribute to physical and mental well-being through leisure (e.g., Hobson & Dietrich, 1994; Nawijn, 2011; Chen, Fu, & Lehto, 2014). If so, future research could flesh out the mediating mechanism using the theory of positive mental health. In other words, future research can test the hypothesis that engagement in leisure activities contribute to mental well-being through the 13 dimensions of positive mental health, namely positive emotions; avowed satisfaction with life; etc.

32.3.6 Need Hierarchy Theory

Based on humanistic psychology, perfectionist happiness can be construed as the kind of need satisfaction related to the full spectrum of human development needs. One popular humanistic approach is Maslow's *hierarchy of needs* (Maslow, 1954/1970). The idea here is that eudaimonia reflects a state of being in which the individual experiences satisfaction with basic needs (e.g., biological needs, safety needs, and economic needs), as well as growth needs (e.g., social, esteem, self-actualization, knowledge, and aesthetic needs) (cf. Sirgy & Wu, 2009).

The first author of this chapter and colleagues (Kosenko, Sirgy, & Efraty, 1990; Sirgy et al., 1995) developed a measure of eudaimonia based on Maslow's need hierarchy theory. Four need categories were used: survival needs (e.g., "the feeling of having been secure"), social needs (e.g., "the feeling of having developed close friendships"), ego needs (e.g., the feeling of prestige or reputation one person has about oneself"), and self-actualization needs (e.g., "the feeling of having experienced personal growth and development").[1]

Guided by need hierarchy theory, new eudaimonia constructs and measures were formulated to capture work well-being (e.g., Sirgy, Efraty, Siegel, & Lee, 2001) and consumer well-being (Sirgy, Lee, & Kressmann, 2006). Consider the case of work well-being. Sirgy and his colleagues conceptualized and measured quality of work life by the extent to which the workplace (specifically job requirements, the work environment, supervisory behaviour, and other ancillary programs) serve to meet employees human development needs (both basic and growth needs). Seven major needs were identified and measured: (1) health and safety needs (protection from ill health and injury at work and outside of work, and enhancement of good health), (2) economic and family needs (pay, job security, and other family needs), (3) social needs (collegiality at work and leisure time off work), (4) esteem needs (recognition and appreciation of work within the organization and outside the organization), (5) actualization needs (realization of one's potential within the organization and as a professional), (6) knowledge needs (learning to enhance job and professional skills), and (7) aesthetic needs (creativity at work as well as personal creativity and general aesthetics). This construct was found to be a significant predictor of organizational and employee well-being outcomes. Similar constructs and measures were developed in relation to the marketplace. For example, Sirgy et al. (2006) developed a consumer well-being measure to capture the extent to which personal transportation contributes to the overall health and well-being of the consumer. The idea that if an automobile (and its supporting services) can contribute significantly to individual and social well-being by meeting the full spectrum of the human development needs.

In the context of tourism, Lee, Kruger, Whang, Uysal, and Sirgy (2014) conducted a study to validate a consumer well-being index related to natural wildlife tourism. The index was formulated based on need hierarchy theory. The index

[1]The following scales are used to record responses for each measurement items:

How much is there now?	Minimum 1 2 3 4 5 6 7 Maximum
How much should there be?	Minimum 1 2 3 4 5 6 7 Maximum

The overall score of life satisfaction of a particular respondent is computed by taking the absolute difference score (between "how much is there now" and "how much should there be") for each item and deriving an average score. The lower the resultant average score, the higher the overall life satisfaction.

was successful in predicting travel outcomes such as length of stay, number of visits, and total amount of money spent at the park. The study was based on four waves of surveys of customers (overnight visitors) intercepted at a natural wildlife park in South Africa in a 2-year period. Future research could test the hypothesis that most tourist attractions can be designed to meet a larger spectrum of basic and growth needs—the more an attraction meets more needs (both basic and growth needs) the more likely that the attraction would contribute significantly to tourists' eudaimonic experiences.

32.3.7 Eudaimonistic Identity Theory

According to eudaimonistic identity theory (Waterman, 1993, 2005; Waterman et al., 2003; Waterman, Schwartz, & Conti, 2008), human activities have two need components in terms of the individual's intrinsic motivation: self-expressiveness and hedonic enjoyment (McMahan & Estes, 2011; Voigt, Howata, & Browna, 2010). Self-expressiveness associated with an activity refers to the extent to which the activity helps the individual identify his or her potential and moves the individual toward realizing that potential. People are likely to engage in an activity when that activity contributes to self-expressiveness (exercise to realize one's ideal self-image). For example, research has demonstrated that self-expressiveness with physical exercise has a positive and enduring impact on one's health (e.g., Huta & Ryan, 2006; Lee, Sirgy, Yu, & Chalamon, 2015; Ryan and Martela, Chap. 7, this volume; Huta, Chap. 15, this volume).

Bosnjak, Brown, Lee, Yu, and Sirgy (2014) conducted a study to test a self-expressiveness model in sport tourism. Self-expressiveness in a sport activity experienced by a tourist was successfully predicted by the activity's perceived difficulty, perceived effort, perceived importance, and potential for self-realization. Furthermore, tourist's self-expressiveness in a sport activity was found to contribute subjective well-being. The study was based on two surveys involving 1251 travelers who participated in a dance festival (study 1) and ski activities (study 2) during their vacations. Future research can extend this line of research by testing the self-expressiveness hypothesis in relation to non-sport tourist activities such visiting tourist attractions. If so, what under what conditions (situational, personality, and cultural conditions) tourists may experience self-expressiveness with the non-sport activity? Such information can be very beneficial in guiding tourists' programs designed to induce feelings of self-expressiveness.

32.4 Conclusion

The broader concept of eudaimonia embodies the elements of psychological happiness (hedonic well-being, emotional well-being, and subjective well-being), prudential happiness (life satisfaction), and perfectionist happiness (mental health, self-actualization, psychological well-being and flourishing). It is important to note that these concepts of eudaimonia are not necessarily mutually exclusive but they are rather complementary in nature depending on research settings and context. The theories that fall under the domain of eudaimonia research agenda independently or collectively help us understand and explain the concept of well-being as it relates to tourism experiences and activities.

As tourism plays a central role in lives of many people across the globe, its expected benefits would include not only economic measures but also non-economic value of tourism measures such as quality of life (QOL) and well-being of participants at different levels of units of analysis. The chapter presents that tourism activities have the inherent potential to contribute to hedonic and emotional well-being as well mental and physical well-being of individuals as consumers of tourism goods and services.

Although we have seen a number of recent studies that have examined the link between the concept of eudaimonia and tourism activities, there is still ample opportunity to conduct research in this area with different targets, goals, and units of analysis in mind. We wholeheartedly encourage tourism researchers to further contribute to this growing body knowledge by developing and applying appropriate measures of eudaimonia in different tourism settings. From the perspective of providers, tourism professionals and practitioners should design their experience settings in a way that would be conducive to enhancing and facilitating experiential value of what is being consumed. Benefits provided should also relate to growth needs of participants regardless of target, context, or gaols. As there is more demand for extraordinary tourism experiences, people as travellers partake more in creating and consuming tourism experiences, and make travel as part of their lifestyle. As such we should increase our research to closely examine the connection between tourism activities and their contribution to eudaimonia.

References

Andrews, F. M., & Withey, S. B. (1976). *Social indicators of well-being: America's perception of life quality*. New York: Plenum Press.

Bosnjak, M., Brown, C. A., Lee, D-J., Yu, G. B., & Sirgy, M. J. (2014). Self-expressiveness in sports tourism: Determinants and consequences. *Journal of Travel Research*. Published online; doi:10.1177/0047287514535845).

Burns, R. A., & Machin, M. A. (2009). Investigating the structural validity of Ryff's psychological well-being scales across two samples. *Social Indicators Research, 93*, 359–375.

Campbell, A., Converse, P. E., & Rodgers, W. L. (1976). *The quality of American life: Perceptions, evaluations, and satisfactions*. New York: Russell Sage.

Cantril, H. (1965). *The pattern of human concerns*. New Brunswick, NJ: Rutgers University Press.

Chamberlain, K., & Zika, S. (1988). Measuring meaning in life: An examination of three scales. *Personality and Individual Differences, 9*, 589–596.

Chen, Y., Fu, X., & Lehto, X.Y. (2014). Chinese tourist vacation satisfaction and subjective well-being. *Applied Research Quality Life*. doi:10.1007/s11482-014-9354-y.

Diener, E. (1984). Subjective well-being. *Psychological Bulletin, 75*, 542–575.

Diener, E., & Emmons, R. A. (1984). The independence of positive and negative affect. *Journal of Personality and Social Psychology, 47*, 1105–1117.

Diener, E., Emmons, R. A., Larsen, R. J., & Griffin, S. (1985). The satisfaction with life scale. *Journal of Personality Assessment, 49*, 71–75.

Diener, E., Smith, H., & Fujita, F. (1995). The personality structure of affect. *Journal of Personality and Social Psychology, 69*, 130–141.

Diener, E., Wirtz, D., Tov, W., Kim-Prieto, C., Choi, D., Oishi, S., et al. (2010). New well-being measures: Short scales to assess flourishing and positive and negative feelings. *Social Indicators Research, 97*, 143–156.

Dolnicar, S., Yanamandram, V., & Cliff, K. (2012). The contribution of vacations to quality of life. *Annals of Tourism Research, 39*(1), 59–83.

Driver, B. L., Brown, P. J., & Peterson, G. L. (1991). *Benefits of leisure*. State College, PA: Venture Publishing.

Dyck, M. J. (1987). Assessing logotherapeutic constructs: Conceptual and psychometric status of the purpose in life and seeking of noetic goals tests. *Clinical Psychology Review, 7*, 439–447.

Filep, S. (2008). Applying the dimensions of flow to explore visitor engagement and satisfaction. *Visitor Studies, 11*(1), 90–108.

Frankl, V. (1963). *Man's search for meaning* (Revisedth ed.). London: Hodder & Stoughton.

Frankl, V. (1967). *Psychotherapy and existentialism*. New York: Simon & Schuster.

Fredrickson, B. L. (2001). The role of positive emotions in positive psychology: The broaden-and-build theory of positive emotions. *American Psychologist, 56*, 219–226.

Gilbert, D., & Abdullah, J. (2004). Holidaytaking and the sense of well-being. *Annals of Tourism Research, 31*(1), 103–121.

Hayborn, D. M. (2008). *The pursuit of unhappiness*. Oxford, UK: Oxford University Press.

Haybron, D. M. (2000). Two philosophical problems in the study of happiness. *Journal of Happiness Studies, 1*, 207–225.

Hicks, J. A., & King, L. A. (2007). Meaning in life and seeing the big picture: Positive affect and global focus. *Cognition and Emotion, 21*, 1577–1584.

Hills, P., Argyle, M., & Reeves, R. (2000). Individual differences in leisure satisfactions: An investigation of four theories of leisure motivation. *Personality and Individual Differences, 28*(4), 763–779.

Hobson, J. S. P., & Dietrich. (1994). Tourism health and quality of life: Challenging the responsibility of using the traditional tenets of sun, sea, sand and sex in tourism marketing. *Journal of Travel and Tourism Marketing, 3*(4), 21–38.

Iso-Ahola, S. E. (1980). *Social psychological perspectives on leisure and recreation*. Springfield, Ill: Charles C. Thomas.

Jackson, L. T. (2008). Leisure activities and quality of life. *Activities, Adaptation, & Aging, 23*(4), 19–24.

Joshanloo, M., & Nostrabadi, N. (2009). Levels of mental health continuum and mental health traits. *Social Indicators Research, 90*, 211–224.

Kahneman, D. (1999). Objective happiness. In D. Kahneman, E. Diener, & N. Schwartz (Eds.), *Well-being: The foundations of hedonic psychology* (pp. 3–25). New York: Russell Sage.

Keyes, C. L. M. (1998). Social well-being. *Social Psychology Quarterly, 61*, 121–140.

Keyes, C. L. M. (2002). The mental health continuum: From languishing to flourishing in life. *Journal of Health and Social Behavior, 43*, 207–222.
Keyes, C. L. M. (2006a). Subjective well-being in mental health and human development research worldwide: An introduction. *Social Indicators Research, 77*, 1–10.
Keyes, C. L. M. (2006b). Mental health in adolescence: Is America's youth flourishing? *The American Journal of Orthopsychiatry, 76*, 395–402.
Kler, B. V. K., & Tribe, J. (2012). Flourishing through scuba: Understating the pursuit of dive experiences. *Tourism in Marine Environments, 8*(1/2), 19–32.
Kosenko, R., Sirgy, M. J., & Efraty, D. (1990). A life satisfaction measure based on need hierarchy theory. In H. L. Meadow & M. J. Sirgy (Eds.), *Quality-of-life studies in marketing and management* (pp. 657–667). Blacksburg, VA: Virginia Tech, Center for Strategy and Marketing Studies.
Lane, R. E. (2001). *The loss of happiness in market democracies*. New Haven, CT: Yale University Press.
Lee, D.-J., Kruger, S., Whang, M.-J., Uysal, M., & Sirgy, M. J. (2014). Validating a consumer well-being index related to natural wildlife tourism. *Tourism Management, 45*, 171–180.
Lee, D.-J., Sirgy, M. J., Yu, G. B., & Chalamon, I. (2015). The well-being effects of self-expressiveness and hedonic enjoyment associated with physical exercise. *Applied Research in Quality of Life, 10*, 141–159.
Lucas, R. E., Diener, E., & Suh, E. (1996). Discriminant validity of well-being measures. *Journal of Personality and Social Psychology, 71*, 616–628.
Maslow, A. H. (1954, 1970). *Motivation and personality*. New York: Harper.
Matteucci, X. (2013). Experiencing flamenco: An examination of a spiritual journey. In S. Fliep & P. Pearce (Eds.), *Tourist experience and fulfilment: Insights from positive psychology*. New York: Routledge.
McMahan, E. A., & Estes, D. (2011). Hedonic versus eudaimonic conceptions of well-being: Evidence of differential associations with self-reported well-being. *Social Indicators Research, 103*, 93–108.
Melton, A. M. A., & Schulenberg, S. E. (2008). On the measurement of meaning: Logotherapy's empirical contributions to humanistic psychology. *Humanistic Psychologist, 36*, 31–44.
Michalos, A. C. (1985). Multiple discrepancies theory (MDT). *Social Indicators Research, 16*, 347–413.
Morgan, J., & Farsides, T. (2009). Measuring meaning in life. *Journal of Happiness Studies, 10*, 197–214.
Nawijn, J. (2011). Determinants of daily happiness on vacation. *Journal of Travel Research, 50*(5), 559–566.
Nawijn, J., Mitas, O., Lin, Y., & Kerstetter, D. (2013). How do we feel on vacation? A closer look at how emotions change over the course of a trip. *Journal of Travel Research, 52*(2), 265–274.
Neulinger, J. (1981). *To leisure – an introduction: A psychological approach to leisure and its relationships to the quality of life*. Boston: Allyn and Bacon.
Peterson, C., Park, N., & Seligman, M. E. P. (2005). Orientations to happiness and life satisfaction: The full life versus the empty life. *Journal of Happiness Studies, 6*, 24–41.
Phillips, D. (2006). *Quality of life: Concept, policy and practice*. London: Routledge.
Prebensen, N., Woo, E., & Uysal, M. (2013). Experience value: Antecedents and consequences. *Current Issues in Tourism, 16*(7–8), 1–15.
Prebensen, N., Chen, J., & Uysal, M. (Eds.). (2014). *Creating experience value in tourism*. Oxfordshire, UK: CABI Publishing. 288 pages.
Prebensen, N., & Foss, L. (2011). Coping and co-creating in tourist experiences. *International Journal of Tourism Research, 13*, 54–67.
Ryan, R. M., & Deci, E. L. (2000). Self-determination theory and the facilitation of intrinsic motivation, social development, and well-being. *American Psychologist, 55*, 68–78.
Ryff, C. D. (1989). Happiness is everything, or is it? Explorations on the meaning of psychological well-being. *Journal of Personality and Social Psychology, 57*, 1069–1081.
Ryff, C. D., & Keyes, C. L. M. (1995). The structure of psychological well-being revisited. *Journal of Personality and Social Psychology, 69*, 719–727.
Ryff, C. D., & Singer, B. (1996). Psychological well-being: Meaning, measurement, and implications for psychotherapy research. *Psychotherapy and Psychosomatics, 65*, 14–23.
Ryff, C. D., & Singer, B. (1998). The contours of positive human health. *Psychological Inquiry, 9*, 1–28.
Schulenberg, S. E., & Melton, A. M. A. (2010). A confirmatory factor-analytic evaluation of the purpose in life test: Preliminary psychometric support for a replicable two-factor model. *Journal of Happiness Studies, 11*, 95–111.
Schulenberg, S. E., Schnetzer, L. W., & Buchanan, E. M. (2011). The purpose in life test-short form: Development and psychometric support. *Journal of Happiness Studies, 12*, 861–876.
Seligman, M. E. P. (2002). *Authentic happiness: Using the new positive psychology to realize your potential for lasting fulfillment*. New York: The Free Press.
Simsek, O. F. (2009). Happiness revisited: Ontological well-being as a theory-based construct of subjective well-being. *Journal of Happiness Studies, 10*, 505–522.
Sirgy, M. J., Cole, D., Kosenko, R., Meadow, H. L., Rahtz, D., Cicic, M., et al. (1995). Developing a life satisfaction measure based on need hierarchy theory. In M. J. Sirgy & A. C. Samli (Eds.), *New dimensions of marketing and quality of life* (pp. 3–26). Westport, CT: Greenwood Press.
Sirgy, M. J., Efraty, D., Siegel, P., & Lee, D.-J. (2001). A new measure of quality-of-work life (QWL) based on need satisfaction and spillover theories. *Social Indicators Research, 55*, 241–302.
Sirgy, M. J., Lee, D.-J., & Kressmann, F. (2006). A need-based measure of consumer well-being (CWB) in relation to personal transportation: Nomological validation. *Social Indicators Research, 79*, 337–367.

Sirgy, M. J., & Wu, J. (2009). The pleasant life, the engaged life, and the meaningful life: What about the balanced life? *Journal of Happiness Studies, 10*, 183–196.

Sirgy, M. J. (2012). *The psychology of quality of life: Hedonic well-being, life satisfaction, and eudaimonia*. Dordrecht, The Netherlands: Springer.

Snepenger, D., King, J., Marshall, E., & Uysal, M. (2006). Modeling Iso-Ahola's motivation theory in the tourism context. *Journal of Travel Research, 45*(2), 140–149.

Steger, M. F., Frazier, P., Oishi, S., & Kaler, M. (2006). The meaning in life questionnaire: Assessing the presence and search for meaning in life. *Journal of Counseling Psychology, 53*, 80–93.

Van Dierendonck, D., Diaz, D., Rodriguez-Carvajal, R., Blanco, A., & Moreno-Jimenez, B. (2008). Ryff's six-factor model of psychological well-being: A Spanish exploration. *Social Indicators Research, 87*, 473–479.

Veenhoven, R. (1984a). *Conditions of happiness*. Boston: Reidel.

Veenhoven, R. (1984b). *Data book on happiness*. Boston: Reidel.

Veenhoven, R., et al. (1994). *World database of happiness: Correlates of happiness*. Rotterdam, The Netherlands: Erasmus University.

Voigt, C., Howata, G., & Browna, G. (2010). Hedonic and eudaimonic experiences among wellness tourists: An exploratory enquiry. *Annals of Leisure Research, 13*, 541–562.

Warburton, D. (1996). The functions of pleasure. In D. Warburton & N. Sherwood (Eds.), *Pleasure and quality of life*. Chichester, UK: Wiley.

Waterman, A. S. (1993). Two conceptions of happiness: Contrasts of personal expressiveness (eudaimonia) and hedonic enjoyment. *Journal of Personality and Social Psychology, 64*, 678–691.

Waterman, A. S. (2005). When effort is enjoyed: Two studies of intrinsic motivation for personally salient activities. *Motivation and Emotion, 29*, 165–188.

Waterman, A. S., Schwartz, S. J., Goldbacher, E., Green, H., Miller, C., & Philip, S. (2003). Predicting the subjective experience of intrinsic motivation: The roles of self-determination, the balance of challenges and skills, and self-realization values. *Personality and Social Psychology Bulletin, 29*, 1447–1458.

Waterman, A. S., Schwartz, S. J., & Conti, R. (2008). The implications of two conceptions of happiness (hedonic enjoyment and eudaimonia) for the understanding of intrinsic motivation. *Journal of Happiness Studies, 9*, 41–79.

Hedonism, Eudaimonia, and the Serious Leisure Perspective

33

Robert A. Stebbins

33.1 Introduction

Alan Waterman (1993), in a review of some of the modern literature on eudaimonism, describes it as an "ethical theory." Its practical message is that people should recognize and live in accordance with the *daimon*, or their true self (Norton, 1976). The theory is ancient, with roots at least as far back as classical Hellenic philosophy. There Aristotle, in his *Nicomachean Ethics*, weighed in extensively on the subject. Waterman's discussion shows clearly the import of eudaimonism for the serious leisure perspective (SLP):

> The *daimon* refers to those potentialities of each person, the realization of which represents the greatest fulfillment in living of which each is capable. These include both the potentialities that are shared by all humans by virtue of our common specieshood and those unique potentials that distinguish each individual from all others. The daimon is an ideal in the sense of being an excellence, a perfection toward which one strives and, hence, it can give meaning and direction to one's life. Efforts to live in accordance with the daimon, to realize those potentials (self-realization), give rise to a condition termed *eudaimonia*. Such efforts can be said to be personally expressive of the individual. (Waterman, 1993, p. 678)

It is during their serious pursuits that leisure participants are eudaimonic, are living according to the daimon. The casual leisure activities, which are hedonic (hedonism is the doctrine in which the proper pursuit is that of pleasure), have a dramatically different appeal. The third form constituting the SLP – project-based leisure – is also eudaimonic but significantly more weakly so than the serious pursuits.

We consider first the SLP, showing in the process how eudaimonism and hedonism are experienced in modern leisure. A treatment of the relationship of the SLP to well-being rounds out the chapter. Here I use the concept of optimal leisure lifestyle to show how all three forms of the Perspective can contribute to personal well-being. That is, both eudaimonism and hedonism are important ingredients in the recipe for a life of lasting happiness.

33.2 The Serious Leisure Perspective

The serious leisure perspective (SLP) is a theoretic framework that synthesizes three main forms of leisure, showing, at once, their distinctive features, similarities, and interrelationships (Stebbins, 2007/2015). The forms are the serious pursuits (Stebbins, 2012) and casual and project-based leisure, briefly defined as follows:

R.A. Stebbins (✉)
University of Calgary, Calgary, Canada
e-mail: stebbins@ucalgary.ca

J. Vittersø (ed.), *Handbook of Eudaimonic Well-Being*, International Handbooks of Quality-of-Life,
DOI 10.1007/978-3-319-42445-3_33

- **Serious Pursuits**
  - *Serious leisure* is the systematic pursuit of an amateur, hobbyist, or volunteer activity sufficiently substantial, interesting, and fulfilling for the participant to find a (leisure) career there acquiring and expressing a combination of its special skills, knowledge, and experience.
  - *Devotee work* is activity in which participants feel a powerful devotion, or strong, positive attachment, to a form of self-enhancing work. In such work the sense of achievement is high and the core activity endowed with such intense appeal that the line between this work and leisure is virtually erased (Stebbins, 2004b/2014).
- **Casual leisure** is immediately intrinsically rewarding, relatively short-lived pleasurable activity requiring little or no special training to enjoy it. It is fundamentally hedonic, pursued for its significant level of pure enjoyment, or pleasure.
- **Project-based leisure** is a short-term, reasonably complicated, one-off or occasional, though infrequent, innovative undertaking carried out in free time, or time free of disagreeable obligation. Such leisure requires considerable planning, effort, and sometimes skill or knowledge, but is for all that neither serious leisure nor intended to develop into such (Stebbins, 2005a).

The SLP offers a classification and explanation of all presently-known leisure activity and experience, as these two are framed in the social, psychological, social, cultural, and historical contexts in which the activity and experience take place (a diagram of the SLP is available at www.seriousleisure.net/SLP Diagram).

33.2.1 Serious Leisure

Let us now add to the foregoing definition, by noting that amateurs are distinguished from hobbyists by the fact that the first, who are found in art, science, sport, and entertainment, have a professional counterpart, whereas the second do not. Hobbyists, some of whom have commercial counterparts, fall into five types: collectors; makers of, or tinkerers with, things; participants in activities (e.g., silo ice climbing, wall climbing, indoor mountain biking); players of sports and games (they lack professional counterparts); and the liberal arts hobbies (self-education in an area of life or literature). Serious leisure volunteers offer un-coerced, altruistic help either formally or informally with no or, at most, token pay and done for the benefit of both other people (beyond the volunteer's family) and the volunteer.

Serious leisure is further defined by six distinguishing qualities (Stebbins, 2007, pp. 11–13), qualities found among amateurs, hobbyists, and volunteers alike. One is the occasional need to *persevere*, such as in learning how to be an effective museum guide. Yet, it is clear that positive feelings about the activity come, to some extent, from sticking with it through thick and thin, from conquering adversity. A second quality is that of finding a *career* in the serious leisure role, shaped as it is by its own special contingencies, turning points and stages of achievement or involvement. Careers in serious leisure commonly rest on a third quality: significant personal *effort* based on specially acquired *knowledge*, *training*, *experience*, or *skill*, and, indeed, all four at times. Fourth, several *durable benefits*, or broad outcomes, of serious leisure have so far been identified, mostly through research on amateurs. They are self-development, self-enrichment, self-expression, regeneration or renewal of self, feelings of accomplishment, enhancement of self-image, social interaction and belongingness, and lasting physical products of the activity (e.g., a painting, scientific paper, piece of furniture). Self-gratification, or the combination of superficial enjoyment and deep fulfilment, is a further benefit and also one of the main benefits of casual leisure, where however, the enjoyment part dominates. Of these benefits, self-fulfillment – realizing, or the fact of having realized, to the fullest one's gifts and character, one's potential – is the most powerful of all.

A fifth quality of serious leisure is the *unique ethos* that grows up around each instance of it, a central component of which is a special social world where participants can pursue their free-time interests. Unruh (1980) developed the following definition:

> A *social world* must be seen as a unit of social organization which is diffuse and amorphous in character. Generally larger than groups or organizations, social worlds are not necessarily defined by formal boundaries, membership lists, or spatial territory. . . . A social world must be seen as an internally recognizable constellation of actors, organizations, events, and practices which have coalesced into a perceived sphere of interest and involvement for participants. Characteristically, a social world lacks a powerful centralized authority structure and is delimited by . . . effective communication and not territory nor formal group membership.

The sixth quality revolves around the preceding five: participants in serious leisure tend to *identify* strongly with their chosen pursuits. In contrast, casual leisure, although hardly humiliating or despicable, is nonetheless too fleeting, mundane, and commonplace for most people to find a distinctive identity there.

33.2.2 Rewards, Costs, and Flow

The rewards of a serious leisure pursuit are the more or less routine values that attract and hold its enthusiasts. Every serious leisure career both frames and is framed by the continuous search for these rewards, a search that takes months, and in some fields years, before the participant consistently finds deep satisfaction in his or her amateur, hobbyist, or volunteer role. Ten rewards have so far emerged in the course of the various exploratory studies of amateurs, hobbyists, and career volunteers. As the following list shows, the rewards are predominantly personal.

Personal rewards

1. Personal enrichment (cherished experiences)
2. Self-actualization (developing skills, abilities, knowledge)
3. Self-expression (expressing skills, abilities, knowledge already developed)
4. Self-image (known to others as a particular kind of serious leisure participant)
5. Self-gratification (combination of superficial enjoyment and deep fulfillment)
6. Re-creation (regeneration) of oneself through serious leisure after a day's work
7. Financial return (from a serious leisure activity)

Social rewards

8. Social attraction (associating with other serious leisure participants, with clients as a volunteer, participating in the social world of the activity)
9. Group accomplishment (group effort in accomplishing a serious leisure project; senses of helping, being needed, being altruistic)
10. Contribution to the maintenance and development of the group (including senses of helping, being needed, being altruistic in making the contribution)

Further, every serious leisure activity contains its own costs – a distinctive combination of tensions, dislikes and disappointments – which each participant confronts in his or her special way. Tensions and dislikes develop within the activity or through its imperfect mesh with work, family, and other leisure interests. Put more precisely, the goal of gaining fulfillment in the serious pursuits is the drive to experience the rewards of a given leisure activity, such that its costs are seen by the participant as more or less insignificant by comparison. This is at once the meaning of the activity for the participant and that person's motivation for engaging in it. It is this motivational sense of the concept of reward that distinguishes it from the idea of durable benefit set out earlier, an idea that emphasizes outcomes rather than antecedent conditions.

Nonetheless, the two ideas constitute two sides of the same social psychological coin. Thus, a golfer anticipates the reward of playing well on a particular day on the links (self-expression) but has there instead a bad day such that the outcome is not seen as a benefit. Moreover, this brief discussion shows that some positive psychological states may be founded, to some extent, on particular negative, often noteworthy, conditions (e.g., tennis elbow, frostbite [cross-country skiing], stage fright, frustration [in acquiring a collectable, learning a part in theater]). Such conditions can make the senses of achievement and self-fulfillment even more pronounced as the enthusiast manages to conquer adversity.

Thrills are part of this reward structure. *Thrills*, or high points, are the sharply exciting events and occasions that stand out in the minds of those who pursue a kind of serious leisure or devotee work. In general, they tend to be associated with the rewards of self-enrichment and, to a lesser extent, those of self-actualization and self-expression. That is, thrills in serious leisure and devotee work may be seen as situated manifestations of certain more abstract rewards; they are what participants in some fields seek as concrete expressions of the rewards they find there. They are important, in substantial part, because they motivate the participant to stick with the pursuit in hope of finding similar experiences again and again and because they demonstrate that diligence and commitment may pay off. Because thrills, as defined here, are based on a certain level of mastery of a core activity, they know no equivalent in casual leisure. The thrill of a roller coaster ride is qualitatively different from a successful descent in a kayak down a roaring rapids, where the boater has the experience, knowledge, and skill to accomplish this.

These thrills are exceptional instances of the *flow* experience, a concept that originated with the work of Mihalyi Csikszentmihalyi (1990). The intensity with which some participants approach their leisure suggests that in it they may at times be in psychological flow. Flow, a form of optimal experience, is possibly the most widely discussed and studied generic intrinsic reward in the psychology of work and leisure. Although many types of work and leisure generate little or no flow for their participants, those that do are found primarily in the "devotee occupations" (discussed in the next section) and serious leisure. Still, it appears that each work and leisure activity capable of producing flow does so in terms unique to it. And it follows that each of these activities, especially their core activities, must be carefully studied to discover the properties contributing to the distinctive flow experience it offers.

33.2.3 Devotee Work

Devotee work and the attitude occupational devotion conceptualize the fact that occupational devotees feel a powerful devotion – a strong, positive attachment – to a form of self-enhancing work. In such work the sense of achievement is high and the core activity endowed with such intense appeal that the line between this work and leisure is virtually erased. Further, it is by way of the core activity of their work that devotees realize a unique combination of, what are for them, strongly seated cultural values (Williams, 2000, p. 146): success, achievement, freedom of action, individual personality, and activity (being involved in something). Other categories of workers may also be animated by some, even all, of these values, but fail for various reasons to realize them in gainful employment.

Occupational devotees turn up chiefly, though not exclusively, in four areas of the economy, providing their work there is, at most, only lightly bureaucratized: certain small businesses, the skilled trades, the consulting and counseling occupations, and the public- and client-centered professions. Public-centered professions are found in the arts, sports, scientific, and entertainment fields, while those that are client-centered abound in such fields as law, teaching, accounting, and medicine (Stebbins, 1992, p. 22). It is assumed in all this that the work and its core activity to which people become devoted carries with it a respectable personal and social identity within their reference groups, since it would be difficult, if not impossible, to be devoted to work that those groups regarded with scorn. Still, positive identification with the job is not a defining condition of occupational devotion, since such identification can develop for other reasons, including high salary, prestigious employer, and advanced educational qualifications.

The fact of devotee work for some people and its possibility for others signals that work, as one of life's domains, may be highly positive. Granted, most workers are not fortunate enough to find such work. For those who do find it, the work meets six criteria (Stebbins, 2004a, p. 9). To generate occupational devotion:

1. The valued core activity must be profound; to perform it acceptability requires substantial skill, knowledge, or experience or a combination of two or three of these.
2. The core must offer significant variety.
3. The core must also offer significant opportunity for creative or innovative work, as a valued expression of individual personality. The adjectives 'creative' and 'innovative' stress that the undertaking results in something new or different, showing imagination and application of routine skill or knowledge. That is, boredom is likely to develop only after the onset of fatigue experienced from long hours on the job, a point at which significant creativity and innovation are no longer possible.
4. The would-be devotee must have reasonable control over the amount and disposition of time put into the occupation (the value of freedom of action), such that he can prevent it from becoming a burden. Medium and large bureaucracies have tended to subvert this criterion. For, in interest of the survival and development of their organization, managers have felt they must deny their nonunionized employees this freedom, and force them to accept stiff deadlines and heavy workloads. But no activity, be it leisure or work, is so appealing that it invites unlimited participation during all waking hours.
5. The would-be devotee must have both an aptitude and a taste for the work in question. This is, in part, a case of one man's meat being another man's poison. John finds great fulfillment in being a physician, an occupation that holds little appeal for Jane who, instead, adores being a lawyer (work John finds unappealing).
6. The devotees must work in a physical and social milieu that encourages them to pursue often and without significant constraint the core activity. This includes avoidance of excessive paperwork, caseloads, class sizes, market demands, and the like.

Sounds ideal, if not idealistic, but in fact occupations and work roles exist that meet these criteria. In today's climate of occupational deskilling, over-bureaucratization, and similar impediments to fulfilling core activity at work, many people find it difficult to locate or arrange devotee employment. The six criteria just listed also characterize serious leisure, giving further substance to the claim put forward here that such leisure and devotee work occupy a great deal of common ground. Together they constitute one class of the eudaimonic leisure pursuits. The other class is that of project-based leisure, to be discussed shortly.

33.3 Casual Leisure

So far we have been able to identify eight types of casual leisure, which is the classificatory home of the creature pleasures and hedonism:

- Play (including dabbling, dilettantism, fiddling)
- Relaxation (e.g., sitting, napping, strolling)
- Passive entertainment (e.g., through TV, books, recorded music)
- Active entertainment (e.g., games of chance, party games)
- Sociable conversation (e.g. gossip, "idle chatter," banter)
- Sensory stimulation (e.g., sex, eating, drinking, sight-seeing)
- Casual volunteering (e.g., handing out leaflets, stuffing envelopes, pouring coffee)
- Pleasurable aerobic activity

The last and newest addition to this typology – pleasurable aerobic activity (Stebbins, 2004a) – refers to physical activities that require effort sufficient to cause marked increase in respiration and heart rate. Here I am referring to "aerobic activity" in the broad sense, to all activity that calls for such effort, which to be sure, includes the routines pursued collectively in (narrowly conceived of) aerobics classes and those pursued individually by way of televised or video-taped programs of aerobics. Yet, as with its passive and active cousins in entertainment, pleasurable aerobic activity is, at bottom, casual leisure. That is, to do such activity requires little more than minimal skill, knowledge, or experience.

33.4 Project-Based Leisure

Whereas systematic exploration may reveal others, two types of project-based leisure have been identified to date: one-off projects and occasional projects. As noted already, these relatively short undertakings are eudaimonic, but only weakly so compared with the much more involved and long-lived serious pursuits.

33.4.1 One-Off Projects

In all these projects people generally use the talents and knowledge they have at hand, even though for some projects they may seek certain instructions beforehand, including reading a book or taking a short course. And some projects resembling hobbyist activity participation may require a modicum of preliminary conditioning. Always, the goal is to undertake successfully the one-off project and nothing more, and sometimes a small amount of background preparation is necessary for this. It is possible that a survey would show that most project-based leisure is hobbyist in character and next most common, a kind of volunteering. First, the following hobbyist-like projects have so far been identified:

- Making and tinkering:
  - Interlacing, interlocking, and knot-making from kits
  - Other kit assembly projects (e.g., stereo tuner, craft store projects)
  - Do-it-yourself projects done primarily for fulfillment, some of which may even be undertaken with minimal skill and knowledge (e.g., build a rock wall or a fence, finish a room in the basement, plant a special garden). This could turn into an irregular series of such projects, spread over many years, possibly even transforming the participant into a hobbyist.
- Liberal arts:
  - Genealogy (not as ongoing hobby)
  - Tourism: special trip, not as part of an extensive personal tour program, to visit different parts of a region, a continent, or much of the world
- Activity participation: long backpacking trip, canoe trip; one-off mountain ascent (e.g., Fuji, Rainier, Kilimanjaro)

One-off volunteering projects are also common, though possibly somewhat less so than hobbyist-like projects. And less common than either are the amateur-like projects, which seem to concentrate in the sphere of theater.

- Volunteering
  - Volunteer at a convention or conference, whether local, national, or international in scope.
  - Volunteer at a sporting competition, whether local, national, or international in scope.
  - Volunteer at an arts festival or special exhibition mounted in a museum.
  - Volunteer to help restore human life or wildlife after a natural or human-made disaster caused by, for instance, a hurricane, earthquake, oil spill, or industrial accident.
- Arts projects:
  - Entertainment theatre: produce a skit or one-off community pageant; prepare a home film, video or set of photos.
  - Public speaking: prepare a talk for a reunion, an after-dinner speech, an oral position statement on an issue to be discussed at a community meeting.
  - Memoirs: therapeutic audio, visual and written productions by the elderly; life histories and autobiographies (all ages); accounts of personal events (all ages).

33.4.2 Occasional Projects

The occasional projects seem more likely to originate in or be motivated by agreeable obligation than their one-off cousins. Examples of occasional projects include the sum of the culinary, decorative, or other creative activities undertaken, for example, at home or at work for a religious occasion or someone's birthday. Likewise, national holidays and similar celebrations sometimes inspire individuals to mount occasional projects consisting of an ensemble of inventive elements.

33.5 Optimal Leisure Lifestyle

According to eudaimonic theory people, to realize their potentials, should recognize and live in accordance with the *daimon*, or their true self. The SLP, backed by its extensive foundation of contemporary theoretical and empirical work (listed in www.seriousleisure.net/Bibliography), encourages such recognition while also setting out the merits of other kinds of free-time activities. For example, well-being is one of the several benefits that can flow from participating in certain types of casual leisure. Relaxation is another.

Nevertheless, it can be argued that the greatest sense of well-being is achieved when a person develops an *optimal leisure lifestyle*. Such a lifestyle is "the deeply satisfying pursuit during free time of one or more substantial, absorbing forms of serious leisure, complemented by a judicious amount of casual leisure" (Stebbins, 2007/2015). People find optimal leisure lifestyles by partaking of leisure activities that individually and in combination realize human potential and enhance quality of life and well-being. Project-based leisure can also enhance a person's leisure lifestyle (see below). The study of kayakers, snowboarders, and mountain and ice climbers (Stebbins, 2005b) revealed that the vast majority of the three samples used various forms of casual leisure to optimally round out their use of free time. For them their serious leisure was a central life interest. Yet, their casual leisure also contributed to their overall well-being. It allowed for relaxation, regeneration, sociability, entertainment, and other activities less intense than their serious activities.

Be that as it may, well-being experienced during free time is more than this. For casual leisure, say Hutchinson and Kleiber (2005), can contribute to self-protection, as by buffering stress and sustaining coping efforts. Such leisure can also preserve or restore a sense of self. This was sometimes achieved in their samples when their respondents rediscovered in casual leisure fundamental personal or familial values or a view of themselves as caring people.

Project-based leisure fits into leisure lifestyle in its own peculiar way as interstitial activity. In this it resembles some casual leisure but not most serious leisure. Project-based leisure can therefore help shape a person's optimal leisure lifestyle. For instance, it can often be pursued at times convenient for the participant. It follows that project-based leisure is nicely suited to people who, out of proclivity or extensive non-leisure obligations or both, reject serious leisure and, yet, who also have no appetite for a steady diet of casual leisure. Among the candidates for project-based leisure are people with heavy workloads; homemakers, mothers, and fathers with extensive domestic responsibilities; unemployed individuals who, though looking for work, still have time at the moment for (I suspect, mostly one-shot) projects; and avid serious leisure enthusiasts who want a temporary change in their leisure lifestyle. Retired people who often do have time for discretionary activity may find project-based leisure attractive as a way of adding spice and variety to their lifestyles. Beyond these special categories of participant, project-based leisure offers a form of substantial leisure to all adults, adolescents, and even children looking for something interesting and exciting to do in free time that is neither short-term as casual leisure is or long-term as the serious pursuits are.

33.6 The Serious Pursuits and Well-Being

The first question to pose in this section is whether an activity, even though freely chosen, can engender well-being when encumbered with significant costs and a marginal status *vis-à-vis* the social institutions of work, leisure, and the family (see Stebbins, 1979). The answer is that it can. For, to the extent that well-being is fostered by enjoyment of and satisfaction with the activities of everyday life, research evidence suggests that it is an important by-product of serious leisure (Haworth, 1986; Haworth & Hill, 1992; Mannell, 1993). Furthermore, when interviewed, the respondents in the many studies of the serious pursuits (Stebbins, 2007/2015, ch. 2) invariably described in detail and with great enthusiasm the fulfillment they get from their amateur, hobbyist, and career volunteer activities.

All this evidence, however, is correlational. No one has yet carried out a study expressly designed to ascertain whether long-term involvement in a form of serious leisure leads to significant enduring increases in feelings of well-being. The extent to which serious leisure can generate major interpersonal role conflict for some practitioners – it led to two divorces among the 25 respondents in the theatre study (Stebbins, 1979, pp. 81–83) – should be sufficient warning to avoid postulating an automatic link between this kind of leisure and well-being. I also have anecdotal evidence that serious leisure activities can generate intrapersonal conflict, such as when people fail to establish priorities among their many and varied leisure interests. Even an approach-approach conflict between two cherished leisure activities can possibly affect well-being unfavorably. Hamilton-Smith (1995, pp. 6–7) says our lack of knowledge about the link between serious leisure and well-being is a major lacuna in contemporary leisure research.

Finally, are we being realistic when we argue that the serious pursuits are a primary source of personal well-being in life? There is probably no sphere in life where well-being can take root and grow in pure, undiluted form. In other words, I suspect that when we are filled with feelings of well-being, whether at work, during leisure or while performing non-work obligations, we are, in effect, experiencing those feelings as a significant profit of rewards against costs. Moreover, what is noteworthy about the theoretical link between any kind of leisure and well-being is that, in commonsense, we seldom expect costs in the former, whereas we routinely expect them at work and during the execution of obligatory tasks. That we expect to find pure enjoyment everywhere in our leisure, however unrealistic, may be shown some day to have a powerful effect on how much we enjoy, or are satisfied with or happy about, the serious leisure we pursue. And when a sense of well-being does emerge here – as it surely will – this expectation will influence the level of intensity with which the well-being is felt. Certainly, we can be mildly *or* highly satisfied with a serious pursuit or activity, enjoy it somewhat *or* enjoy it immensely, find it highly fulfilling or mildly fulfilling. The serious pursuits and well-being would seem to make a perfect couple, but their relationship appears destined to be far more complicated than current levels of theory and research would suggest.

33.7 Conclusions

If, as noted at the start of this chapter, people should recognize and live in accordance with the *daimon*, or their true self, how do they do this? Self-efficacy and personal agency are two critical processes that generate eudaimonia. Psychologist Albert Bandura pioneered the concept of *self-efficacy*, defining it as "people's beliefs in their capabilities to produce desired effects by their own actions" (Bandura, 1997, p. vii). He argued that people develop "efficacy expectations" bearing on particular goals they hope to realize and on what they must do to achieve this. These expectations are based on the capabilities individuals believe they have to accomplish the goals they are pursuing in a particular setting. Bandura says that efficacy expectations constitute the cognitive state immediately preceding goal-directed actions. Additionally efficacy is enhanced to the extent that people's *locus of control* is high; in other words they sense that their activities result from their own efforts rather than from such impersonal forces as fate, luck, and chance (Rotter, 1990).

The main belief here is in one's own self-efficacy to pursue in a fulfilling way particular activities in serious leisure or devotee work. This belief in oneself is born of the numerous routine successes that accumulate with the enduring, systematic pursuit of an activity and of the encouragement from positive others who also partake of it or who are otherwise close associates of the participant.

In leisure studies personal agency is both a social arrangement for enabling and a personal capacity for putting into effect what an individual intends to do. The individual thus enabled (not constrained) by society can become his own agent in producing the intended outcome. Here agency refers to seizing the initiative to reach a goal, short- or long-term. It includes figuring out how to reach the goal, which includes organizing to this end oneself and such relevant other entities as individuals, organizations, groups, and social networks. Agency rests on the participant's sense of self-efficacy in planning, organizing, working with others, and so on. Thus, a concert violinist can only perform her concerto when accompanied by an orchestra guided by its conductor, a quarterback in American football cannot express his agency as a passer unless there is a teammate downfield trying to catch the ball that person is passing. Agency is also at work when a participant arranges for necessary resources.

It is through particular activities that people, propelled by their own agency and belief in their own efficacy, find positive things in life, which they blend and balance with the negative, or disagreeably obligatory, things they must also deal with. Un-coerced, people in leisure believe they are doing something they are not pushed to do, something they are not disagreeably obliged to do. In this definition emphasis is *ipso facto* on the acting individual and on his self-direction through personal agency.

A key condition nurturing eudaimonia is for participants to gain control over any tendency to pursue selfishly the leisure that generates it. The failure to do so can give rise in close relationships to conflict capable of substantially reducing the positiveness of the activity for both members of the dyad. I have discussed this matter elsewhere in detail (Stebbins, 1995, 2009, pp. 115–117).

Selfishness is the act of a self-seeker judged as selfish by the victim of that act. When we define an act as selfish, we make an imputation. This imputation is most commonly hurled at perceived self-seekers by their victims, where the self-seekers are felt to demonstrate a concern for their own welfare or advantage at the expense of or in disregard for those victims. The central thread running through the fabric of selfishness is exploitative unfairness – a kind of personal favoritism infecting the everyday affairs of many people in modern society.

In comparing the three forms, it is evident that serious leisure is nearly always the most complicated and enduring of them and, for this reason, often takes up much more of a participant's time. It is therefore much more likely to give rise to charges of selfishness. For instance, some types of the serious pursuits and even some project-based leisure can only be pursued according to a rigid schedule (e.g., amateur theatrical rehearsals, volunteer guiding at a zoo, volunteer ticket selling at an arts festival), which unlike most casual leisure, allows little room for compromise or maneuver. Thus imputations of selfishness are considerably more likely to emerge with reference to the first two, and if the activity is to be pursued at all, behavior definable as selfish may be difficult to avoid.

In short, it is all well and good to encourage the search for eudaimonia by way of the SLP, but through therapy and education, we must also inform leisure enthusiasts about how selfishness can undermine that search.

References

Bandura, A. (1997). *Self-efficacy: The exercise of control*. New York: Freeman.

Csikszentmihalyi, M. (1990). *Flow: The psychology of optimal experience*. New York: Harper & Row.

Hamilton-Smith, E. (1995, March 4–9). The connexions of scholarship. *Newsletter* (Official newsletter of RC13 of the International Sociological Association).

Haworth, J. T. (1986). Meaningful activity and psychological models of non-employment. *Leisure Studies, 5*, 281–297.

Haworth, J. T., & Hill, S. (1992). Work, leisure, and psychological well-being in a sample of young adults. *Journal of Community & Applied Social Psychology, 2*, 147–160.

Hutchinson, S. L., & Kleiber, D. A. (2005). Gifts of the ordinary: Casual leisure's contributions to health and well-being. *World Leisure Journal, 47*(3), 2–16.

Mannell, R. C. (1993). High investment activity and life satisfaction among older adults: Overcoming psychological inertia through committed, serious leisure, and flow activites. In J. R. Kelly (Ed.), *Activity and aging: Staying involved in later life* (pp. 125–145). Newbury Park, CA: Sage.

Norton, D. L. (1976). *Personal destinies*. Princeton, NJ: Princeton University Press.

Rotter, J. B. (1990). Internal versus external locus of control of reinforcement: A case history of a variable. *American Psychologist, 45*(4), 489–493.

Stebbins, R. A. (1979). *Amateurs: On the margin between work and leisure*. Beverly Hills, CA: Sage. Also freely available in the Digital Library, www.seriousleisure.net

Stebbins, R. A. (1992). *Amateurs, professionals, and serious leisure*. Montreal, QC: McGill-Queen's University Press.

Stebbins, R. A. (1995). Leisure and selfishness: An exploration. In G. S. Fain (Ed.), *Reflections on the philosophy of leisure* (Leisure and ethics, Vol. II, pp. 292–303). Reston, VA: American Alliance for Health, Physical Education, Recreation, and Dance.

Stebbins, R. A. (2004a). Pleasurable aerobic activity: A type of casual leisure with salubrious implications. *World Leisure Journal, 46*(4), 55–58.

Stebbins, R. A. (2004b/2014). *Between work and leisure: The common ground of two separate worlds*. New Brunswick, NJ: Transaction. (Published in paperback in 2014 with new Preface).

Stebbins, R. A. (2005a). Project-based leisure: Theoretical neglect of a common use of free time. *Leisure Studies, 24*, 1–11.

Stebbins, R. A. (2005b). *Challenging mountain nature: Risk, motive, and lifestyle in three hobbyist sports*. Calgary, AB: Detselig. Also freely available in the Digital Library, www.seriousleisure.net

Stebbins, R. A. (2007/2015). *Serious leisure: A perspective for our time*. New Brunswick, NJ: Transaction. (Published in paperback in 2015 with new Preface).

Stebbins, R. A. (2009). *Personal decisions in the public square: Beyond problem solving into a positive sociology*. New Brunswick, NJ: Transaction.

Stebbins, R. A. (2012). *The idea of leisure: First principles*. New Brunswick, NJ: Transaction.

Unruh, D. R. (1980). The nature of social worlds. *Pacific Sociological Review, 23*, 271–296.

Waterman, A. S. (1993). Two conceptions of happiness: Contrasts of personal expressiveness (eudaimonia) and hedonic enjoyment. *Journal of Personality and Social Psychology, 64*, 678–691.

Williams, R. M., Jr. (2000). American society. In E. F. Borgatta & R. J. V. Montgomery (Eds.), *Encyclopedia of sociology* (2nd ed., Vol. 1, pp. 140–148). New York: Macmillan.

34 Eudaimonia and 'Species Being': A Marxist Perspective

Hartley Dean

34.1 Introduction

The object of this chapter is to observe the influence of the concept, *eudaimonia*, on the concept, 'species being', as advanced by Karl Marx (1818–1883), and to discuss the combined relevance of both concepts to current contestation around the meanings of 'welfare' and 'well-being'. As such, it is a contribution to key debates in the multi- and interdisciplinary academic subject, known as Social Policy (Dean, 2012). To that end the chapter will first discuss the ostensibly paradoxical contribution by Aristotle (384–322 BCE), a defender of slavery and misogyny, to the thinking of Marx, the ultimate opponent of all human exploitation. We shall also mention an equally paradoxical contribution to our understanding of species being subsequently made by Hannah Arendt (1906–1975), notwithstanding that she was a savage critic of Marx. Each of these discussions offers a reframing of the idea of *eudaimonia*. The chapter then seeks to draw out four elements of human species being as identified by a contemporary Marxist philosopher, György Márkus (2014); those elements which are *essentially* constitutive of humanity – namely, consciousness, work, sociality and historical development. These are presented as a basis for a model of eudaimonic well-being. Finally, the chapter will consider the implications of that model for the substantive development of social policies and the articulation of human need through social rights.

34.2 Reframing Eudaimonia

Previous chapters in the volume have discussed the distinction between hedonic and eudaimonic components of well-being (e.g., the chapters by Besser (Chap. 3); Haybron (Chap. 2); Fowers (Chap. 4); Ryan and Martela (Chap. 7); Huta (Chap. 15); Proctor and Tweed (Chap. 18); and Vittersø (Chap. 17)). Broadly understood it is a distinction between, on the one hand, human beings' struggle for survival and their pursuit of pleasure and, on the other, their search for human fulfilment. The hedonic and eudaimonic components of well-being are equally necessary to well-being: one cannot achieve fulfilment if one does not survive. But, is survival a means or another end? What beyond the enjoyment of pleasure might human fulfilment or *eudaimonia* entail?

H. Dean (✉)
Department of Social Policy, London School of Economics, London, UK
e-mail: h.dean@lse.ac.uk

J. Vittersø (ed.), *Handbook of Eudaimonic Well-Being*, International Handbooks of Quality-of-Life,
DOI 10.1007/978-3-319-42445-3_34

34.2.1 Aristotle and Good Spirit

Any account of *eudaimonia* as a concept begins with Aristotle and classical Greek philosophy.[1] An approximate literal interpretation of the word, *eudaimonia*, is 'good spirit'. The prefix 'eu-' can allude both to 'wellness' and to 'goodness' and may be taken to imply that – for human beings – well-being and virtue are coterminous. The word 'daimon' originally referred to what might be regarded as a person's soul or essence; or to what Kant would later describe as the 'noumenal self'. (It is, incidentally, only later derivatives of the word – *daemon* or *demon* – that allude to notions of supernatural spirits, whether good or bad, that might possess or inhabit a person's being.) For Aristotle, therefore, *eudaimonia* described the realisation of a 'good' or ethical life; of Man's natural purpose.

Aristotle's teleological conceptualisation of 'natural' purpose was premised on a categorical distinction between humans and other animals; but a distinction also between, on the one hand, free men and, on the other, women and slaves, whose capabilities and potential he deemed to be 'naturally' constrained. Nevertheless, he offered what might be regarded as a theory of personhood: a theory concerning that which characterises the human species and, to an either greater or lesser extent, sets its members apart *within* nature; a theory that defines what is constitutively necessary for human well-being (Aristotle, c. 350 BCE; Russell, 1961). Like other animals, human beings require material resources in order to survive, and beyond mere survival, it is natural that they should seek pleasure in life. But the fulfilment of personhood entails:

- The maximum and unimpeded realisation of human capabilities. Human beings are removed from mere animal existence by their ability through their activity consciously to shape and control the world around them.
- The exercise of intelligence. Such capabilities require intelligence, a distinctive capacity for thinking that must be progressively developed and applied.
- The exercise of deliberation and choice. Effective thinking requires, in turn, the capacity for reason and the freedom thereby to shape one's own life through deliberation and choice. The idea of self-determined rational activity was captured in the Aristotelian concept of 'praxis' and in his acknowledgment that the human being is a 'political animal', whose existence is predicated on social intercourse.
- The expression of good character. In choosing how to behave or to act a person must choose what she judges for herself to be right. Virtue stems not from obedience to rules that are imposed, but from the good that is chosen for its own sake; from a balancing of personal pleasure and civic duty in a manner that achieves a harmonious 'Golden mean'.
- The enjoyment of friendship. Friendship, or *philia*, in this sense extends to the love, care and companionship experienced between intimates, family members, neighbours and fellow-citizens and is an essential and constitutive feature of human society.

Aristotelian thought has influenced a variety of contradictory philosophies, which may, for example, be seen contemporarily, on the one hand, in the liberal-individualist capability approach (Nussbaum, 2000; Sen, 1982, 1999) and, on the other, in communitarian interpretations, most explicitly that informed by virtue ethics (MacIntyre, 2007). The historical evolution of such influences is arcanely complex, but the specific influence that is of concern in this chapter, is the influence on Marxist theory. For such purposes it is necessary, however, first to mention Hegel's response to the dominance following the so called European Enlightenment of materialist philosophising and mind-body dualism, in which he sought to recapture a more holistic and essential understanding of the place of the individual both in human society and in the cosmos (Depew, 1992; Hegel, 1805–1806, 1821; Smith, 1992).

[1] My treatment here of Aristotle will be brief and thinly referenced, since his work is extensively discussed elsewhere in this volume.

Significantly, Hegel combined the introduction of dialectical philosophical method with a claim that the ultimate mover in the dialectical unfolding of human history is 'absolute spirit' (or 'absolute mind', since the German word for spirit, *geist*, also means mind). The notion of absolute spirit may in one sense be seen to reflect the fullest possible expression of *eudaimonia*, as both an idea and an ideal.

34.2.2 Marx and the Essence of Humanity

While the influence of Hegel on Marx is widely recognised, the extent to which Marx drew, both in his early and later writings, directly on Aristotle is frequently overlooked (McCarthy, 1992). Marx's epic critique of capitalism may be understood as an analysis of the way that capitalism systemically denies the majority of people the requirements of a 'good life', as identified by Aristotle (Miller, 1992). Put another way, Marx's claim was that capitalism was anti-eudaimonic:

- It impaired the realisation of human capabilities. Human beings who were dependent for their survival on the performance of wage labour were removed barely if at all from mere animal existence, having little or no opportunity consciously to shape and control the world around them and being alienated from the fruits of their own labour.
- Though industrial capitalism harnessed the latest scientific knowledge, for the majority of workers it restricted the exercise of intelligence or creativity, condemning them to routinised, mindless activity.
- The lives of workers and their families under capitalism were governed by alien forces that restricted the exercise of deliberation and choice and curtailed their freedom to shape their own future. The scope for self-determined rational activity was systematically constrained.
- The narrowing of life's compass to the sale of labour power as a means to obtain life's necessities and the subjection of the wage labourer to the discipline of the factory and to regulation by the capitalist state undermined the expression of good character. Such conditions attenuated the opportunity to behave or to act as one might judge for oneself to be right.
- The capacity of free-market capitalism to generate social relationships between things and material relationships between persons, threatened the enjoyment of friendship. Commodification and competition were inimical to social connectedness and mutual caring.

But underpinning this critique of capitalism lay new historical insights regarding the essence of humanity; insights that were 'eudaimonist' in inspiration (Gilbert, 1992), albeit that in connecting the natural and social context of human existence these insights, unlike Aristotle's, encompassed *all* humanity, regardless of gender or status. Here, Marx borrowed the term *gattungswesen* – meaning 'species essence' or 'species being' – from Hegel. However, whereas Hegel equated such essence in an idealist sense with absolute spirit, Marx equated it with the materiality of history. In doing so he was alluding not merely to the objective materiality of nature, but the materiality of human, and therefore social, action; of 'revolutionary, or practical-critical activity' (Marx, 1845: 82). As Fromm (1961: 26) interprets this, 'History is the history of man's self-realization; it is nothing but the self-creation of man'. This view of human activity constituted Marx's alternative concept of 'praxis', which differed from that of Aristotle, who had regarded the human essence to be invariant and inherent to the individual, rather than dynamic and constitutive of the human species (Margolis, 1992).

Marx's writings, generated over a period of some 40 years (between 1841 and 1883), are as complex as they are voluminous. They have been subject to a great deal of misunderstanding or, some would claim, 'falsification' (Fromm, 1961: ch. 1). In part this is attributable to problems entailed by the translation and editing of his work; to popularised conceptual misunderstandings; to distorted interpretations on the part of Marxian followers; and to the adverse outcomes of various socialist/communist revolutions, most notably the totalitarian nature of the former Soviet Union. There is also dispute among Marxist scholars as to whether there was a point of discontinuity – an 'epistemological break' (Althusser, 1971) – between Marx's earlier humanistic philosophical work and his later economistic work, in which he applied the method of dialectical materialism in order to develop the labour theory of value. Alternatively, it is suggested, the normative and cognitive elements of his work are essentially complementary (Soper, 1981) and represent two interdependent accounts: one concerning the 'humanisation of nature' occasioned by the self-creation of the human species, the other with the need to 'naturalise humanity' by realising materially its eudaimonic essence (Benton, 1988; Márkus, 2014). The argument to be developed below is broadly consistent with this last conclusion.

34.2.3 Arendt and Living Well

Before doing so, however, we shall briefly consider the thinking of a third philosopher, Hannah Arendt, whose reflections upon the horrors of the Second World War and the consequences of totalitarianism led to new insights into the essence of the human condition. Unfortunately, Arendt was amongst those critics who associated Marx's original thinking with its totalitarian misapplications. Yet in a recent study, Tama Weisman (2014: 1–2) has commented that 'Arendt criticizes Marx with one stroke of her pen while in the next she appropriates his thought without acknowledgement'. Arendt's peculiarly partial reading of Marx's work elided any explicit engagement on her part with the concept of species being (Weisman, 2014: 72), yet there remains a sense in which she has in various ways clarified what might be meant by 'species being'.

Whereas Marx's critique was directed against the capitalist form of modernity, Arendt's was directed against modernity itself and its inherent totalitarian social tendencies. Her complaint was that 'today we consider both history and nature alien to the essence of man' (Arendt, 1951: 435). Western modernity, she contended, was eroding the human condition, reducing humanity to an abstract quality vested in essentially individuated beings, rather than a quality that arises through effective membership of a concrete political community. Arendt sought to re-express the Aristotelian ideal of *eudaimonia* as the *raison d'être* of human action: 'The ultimate end of human acts is *eudaimonia*, happiness in the sense of living well, which all men desire; all acts are but different means chosen to arrive at it.' (Arendt, 1968: 61). Neither labour nor work, but 'acts' constitute the most definitive component of what Arendt called the *vita activa*. And human acts depend axiomatically for their meaning on common engagement between human beings, without which human beings cannot live well (see Parekh, 2008: 31). In seeking to define the different 'realms' in which human activity occurs, Arendt drew distinctions between those realms in which human conduct is governed by *necessity* and those in which it is fashioned by *free will*. The former she refers to as the private and the social realms, which are driven by biological and instrumental motives and constraints. The latter she refers to as the public and the political, which are concerned with acts undertaken for their own sake. Elements of these definitions remain problematic, but the underlying distinction between, on the one hand, the things people do for utilitarian purposes and the idea, on the other, that living well entails engagement in acts 'for their own sake' is important; especially in the context of Arendt's insistence that human beings are shaped not by their nature, but by their condition; by the world they inhabit in common with others. Such insistence implies particular consequences for the meaning of 'eu' in eudaimonia; for 'wellness' and what is 'good'. To live well one must be free not in the sense of a freedom that is negatively defined in terms of constraints upon interference *by* others, but in the radical sense of a positive freedom to act *with* others.

34.3 Constitutive Species Characteristics

In his attempt to distil from Marx's concept of 'species being' an anthropological account of human essence, György Márkus contends that

Table 34.1 The eudaimonic character of our human species being

Essential species characteristics	Which define …	Are realised through …	Are 'good' when …
Consciousness	Who we are	Our search for meaning	We exercise critical reason
Work	What we do	Our activity	We express human creativity
Sociality	How we relate to one another	Our mutual interdependence	We sustain love, solidarity and rights
Historical development	What we might accomplish	Our part in human history	We contribute to human 'betterment'

'For Marx "human essence" lies precisely in the "essence" or inner unity of the total social development of humanity' (2014: 63). What characterises the human species and it's mode of existence according to Márkus' reading of Marx is human consciousness, work and sociality. And to these three interconnected characteristics should be added the universality and freedom that 'mark the general direction of the historical progress of humanity' (2014: 61): this fourth and last characteristic I shall, for the sake of brevity, refer to as 'historical development'. These then are the characteristics that are constitutive of humanity and define the human species in relation to other species and in relation to the natural world. These characteristics also define each member of that species as a generic being. We shall consider each in turn, but a highly reductive version of the account that follows is offered in Table 34.1.

34.3.1 Consciousness

The consciousness that characterises the human species is something beyond mere sentience. What we now refer to as *the* human species, is *homo sapiens*, which has existed on this planet for around 150,000 years. There had been other species of genus *homo*, some of whom developed the use of tools and of fire, and the oldest of which may have first appeared some 2.5 million years ago. Some of these species (such as *homo erectus* and *homo neanderthalensis*) coexisted and may to a limited extent have interbred with *homo sapiens* until as recently as 12,000 years ago. The *homo sapiens* brain was twice as large as that of the earliest hominid species, but what set it apart was a process characterised by Harari (2011) as a 'Cognitive Revolution', which unfolded between 70,000 and 30,000 years ago as our species began to colonise the world, travelling in boats, hunting with bows and arrows, sewing with needles, etc.; but more importantly evolving elaborated forms of language and communication, and developing artistic and symbolic modes of representation. This entailed thinking: a form of consciousness that made uniquely human action possible in the sense that it is action that has purpose and meaning to the actor; and an intersubjective awareness on the part of members of the species as to their selfhood and identity in relation the natural world and to each other.

Descartes, the seventeenth century philosopher, insisted upon a dualistic distinction between body and mind. The human capacity for conscious thinking, he contended, was essentially independent of bodily functions. This fuelled a debate that continues to divide scientists and philosophers concerning the 'mystery of consciousness' (Searle, 1997). Is thinking and awareness of our own existence no more than a neurological activity unique to the human brain, or does it entail something more essential about a human being compared with a highly trained and emotionally intelligent dog on the one hand or a highly sophisticated and artificially intelligent robot on the other?

Marx's answer was that 'Thought and being are indeed distinct, but they also form a unity', insofar as an individual human's species being 'confirms itself in species consciousness' (Marx, 1844: 351). Species consciousness was more than the capacity for passive contemplation, but the capacity for 'sense activity' (Marx, 1845: 82); it was not about the capacity for reason alone, but the capacity for 'praxis', in the sense discussed above. For Marx consciousness was the dynamic relationship between thinking and being that characterises human action and therefore human history. This was the meaning of human essence: a phenomenon that is neither distinctively biological nor spiritual, but precisely human. The essence of *homo sapiens* lies in the process of human history that, according to recent supposition, was 'kick-started' (Harari, 2011: 3) by the Cognitive Revolution some 70,000 years ago. According to Harari's much attenuated history of humankind the cognitive revolution was followed much later by an Agricultural Revolution (12,000 years ago) and more recently by a Scientific Revolution (just 500 years ago). Marx's understanding of those revolutions was focused on the unfolding of the 'human essence of Nature and the natural essence of Man' (Marx, 1844: 355). It is in the process of harnessing Nature for the purposes of Man that human beings have begun to realise their species being, albeit in ways that have been in many instances suboptimal, self-destructive and unsustainable. His contention was that – specifically under industrial capitalism – the greater part of humanity was self-alienated; the full potential of its species being was denied. But central to humanity's species being is the consciousness that allows us to act.

Notwithstanding her concern that the revolutionary actions that Marx supposedly inspired proved themselves inimical to free thinking, Arendt's understanding of the relationship between thought and action would seem to chime precisely with that of Marx. Her enigmatic statement that 'There are no dangerous thoughts; thinking itself is dangerous' (1978: 176) reflected her conclusion that there were tendencies portended by modernity that denied or coercively inhibited human beings' capacity to think; that the most monstrous excesses of totalitarianism resulted not, after all, from radically evil thinking, but from 'thoughtlessness'; in the sense of a total absence of moral reasoning, or 'thought-defying banality'. She argues, that 'only the good has depth and can be radical' (1978: 250–251). Arendt draws upon a distinction between, on the one hand, the intellectual quest for evidence-based truth and, on the other, critical reason, which is itself the most essential of human capacities; a capacity not reserved exclusively for philosophers, but which defines what it takes for any human being to be good and to live well (Parekh, 2008: ch. 6; Yarbrough & Stern, 1981).

Consciousness, therefore, is the means by which a human, as a species being, has a personal and an inter-subjective awareness of her identity; seeks meaning in the world around her and in her relationships to others; can critically engage with that world in conjunction with others.

34.3.2 Work

It follows that conscious human activity, or what we might call 'work', is equally definitive of human essence. Aristotle, Marx and Arendt each applied a concept of praxis in relation to the idea of work, but they did so differently.

For Aristotle, praxis as active and fulfilling engagement with public life and political discourse – the activity valued by the patrician elite of ancient Athens, was to be distinguished from necessary physical labour, performed by slaves, who were not recognised as fully human. The rise of industrial capitalism, it might be supposed, portended the final end of slavery and of feudal serfdom, since productive labour power became a commodity to be voluntarily bought and sold under free market conditions. The dominant form of 'work' – both physical and intellectual – began to assume the form of wage labour. For Marx, all forms of work – whether materially productive or socially reproductive – entail human self-realisation, and the essence of work lies not in its exchange value, but in its dynamic capacity to fulfil the radical needs of the human species (Heller, 1974). Under capitalist social relations, however, work tends to be an alienated rather than a self-affirming activity. Arendt, eschewing (or ignoring) the holistic character of Marx's conception of work and human need (Weisman, 2014) conceives of praxis through her notion of the *vita activa*, the components of which she distinguishes as 'labour' (for the fulfilment of biological need), 'work' (for the fulfilment of socially constructed need) and 'action' (for freely willed engagement with others). For Arendt, modernity marginalises our capacity for *action*, which, like Aristotle, she prized above labour and work. Nonetheless, the term *vita activa* chimes with, and perhaps enhances, Marx's encompassing conception of 'work' as a constitutive element of our species being.

For Marx, work encompasses the uniqueness of the human species' metabolism with Nature; the species' symbiotic appropriation of natural resources and manipulation of natural forces. He wrote specifically of *stoffvechsel* (a term best translated as 'social-ecological metabolism') as a fundamental condition of human existence (Marx, 1887: 183–4), but also warned of the 'metabolic rift' occasioned by capitalism (see Foster, 1999). Through the wage relation, capitalism estranges human beings from their metabolism with Nature and, through the commodity form, it reduces their species being to an 'alien essence' (Chitty, 2009), or else in the late modern era the managerial ethos associated with even the best-rewarded employment can be corrosive of the human character (Sennett, 1998). Where paid employment is organised informally, on the margins of, or outwith, formally regulated labour markets it is chronically precarious (Standing, 2011).

But the manner of human beings' metabolism with Nature is that it is socially, not naturally, organised and reproduced. We shall return to the subject of human sociality in a moment, but if we expand our understanding of work as human activity that lies beyond wage labour, it extends to the entire arena of social and cultural reproduction as well as to the realm of political engagement. It encompasses: care work – including care for children and for frail, sick or disabled adults; creative endeavour – including artistic expression, sporting and recreational activity undertaken for its own sake; all forms of study, learning and scholarly activity; engagement in voluntary and community activities as well as engagement in formal politics. Work as activity is what a human being does; it is the realisation of her species being and, whether or not it is *materially* productive, it is, potentially and in essence, the expression of her human creativity.

34.3.3 Sociality

Aristotle defined the human being as a *zöon politikon*, a term usually translated as 'political animal', though, in historical and etymological context, it might also translate as 'social animal'. Importantly, however, Aristotle was distinguishing the human form of sociality – the most refined (and exclusive) version of which was to be found in the Athenian *agora* – from animalistic herd or pack behaviours. Marx observed that 'the human being is in the most literal sense a *zöon politikon*, not merely a gregarious animal, but an animal that can only individuate itself in the midst of society (Marx, 1857: 84). The concept of sociality elicited from Marx's writing by Márkus (2014: 32–35) has two interconnected components, *Gemeinwesen* (alluding to the communal character of human life) and *Gattungsleben* (alluding to the generic socio-historic shaping of human life).

Human life has a communal character in the sense that the human individual is not, and cannot wholly be, the isolated irreducible atom of liberal social contract theory: she is an inherently vulnerable, interdependent creature (Dean, 2000; Turner, 2006). It is not mere ingenuity, but socially organised care and collaboration that have allowed human beings to survive and flourish despite their limited stature and strength relative to other more physically powerful species and often in spite of adverse natural and climatic conditions. Human beings' sociality is founded on a loyalty to one another, 'clinging together against the dark' (Rorty, 1982: 166). But human beings are also generically social in the sense that 'clinging together' is made possible through shared language, customs, institutions, knowledge and beliefs – all of which are dynamically socio-historically constructed and contested; and which, through social or 'interpsychological' processes, shape the personal development of every human being (Vygotsky, 1978).

We have already observed Arendt's contention that a life not lived among other humans is not a human life. It is a contention premised on a concept of intersubjectivity not necessarily dissimilar to Vygotsky's concept of 'interpsychological' process (Parekh: ch. 3). Arendt insisted that respect for other human beings required that they be *recognised* 'as builders of worlds or co-builders of a common world' (1951: 458). The common world to which Arendt refers is, in her own peculiar terminology, to be found in the realm of public and political, rather than the private or the social, since it is concerned not with the specific 'world alienating' conditions of modernity, but a radical intersubjective understanding of a better world. Arendt shares with Marx the idea that humanity is alienated from the essence of its species being, but she shares with Aristotle an ambiguous and abstracted understanding of *zöon politikon*. Certainly, she did not share Marx's understanding of sociality. Nevertheless, her call upon the idea of recognition demonstrates a common connection with Hegelian philosophy. In clinging together against the dark, one of humanity's struggles has been the struggle for the mutual recognition upon which sociality depends. A recent and influential contribution to the philosophy of recognition debate has been provided by Axel Honneth (1995; and see Smyth, 2012), who discusses three modes of recognition upon which a good life (i.e. *eudaimonia*) depends:

- Love. Being oneself in and through an intimate relationship with another is an axiomatic requirement of self-identity.
- Solidarity. Participation and engagement with others in a community or social group establishes who one is and what one can do, affording shared collective identity and fostering self-esteem.
- Rights. Exercising rights and respecting others' rights provides the foundation on which mutually to recognise the claims that strangers or distant others may make upon one that that one may make upon them.

Sociality is a constitutive characteristic of an individual's human species being in the sense that she is shaped through, and depends for her identity upon her immediate and historical social context; it is realised though her mutual interdependence with other human beings; it may be sustained through love, solidarity and rights.

34.3.4 Historical Development

According to Márkus, what Marx primarily meant by the 'human essence' of our species being was '... those characteristics of the real historical existence of mankind which made it possible to comprehend history as a continuous and unified process that has a developmental tendency'. Humanity's conscious social being and engagement in material productive self-activity provided the constitutive dimensions of 'a total developmental process, on the basis of which [this] historical tendency unfolds and in the spheres of which it becomes manifest' (2014: 61). This is an understanding quite different, on the one hand, from Aristotle's idea that human nature was immutable and fixed and, on the other, from Arendt's idealised notion of a common world. When Marx asserted that 'Philosophers have hitherto only interpreted the world; the point is to change it' (1857: 84) his appeal was to a *eudaimonia* that was not some latent potential of a *zöon politikon*, but to the gritty everyday reality of human beings' continuing and ever-evolving struggle for a *better* life, for self-fulfilment, for moral progress (Gilbert, 1992) or emancipation.

As a species being a human being is defined and constrained not merely by nature, but by her historical context; her actions have meaning not only because they contribute to species survival, but because they are a contribution to an historical process and, notwithstanding the constraints of history, they might potentially contribute to the betterment of that process. It is in the context of historical development that matters of social policy and social development come into focus and it is to these that we now turn.

34.4 Towards a Eudaimonic Social Policy

I shall attempt here tentatively to consider how to reframe our understanding of the purpose of social policy as the ongoing historical realisation of our human species being. To do so I shall first briefly re-visit the idea of social rights and the role of rights in human sociality and historical development. Secondly, I shall draw on Marx's theory of human need in order to outline the basis for a 'life-first' ethic of social policy; an approach that prioritises the realisation of species being.

34.4.1 Social Rights and Social Development

Social rights may be understood as 'expressions of sociality' and, specifically, as 'articulations of human need' (Dean, 2015). The earliest human societies, as associations of interdependent beings, will, through the negotiation of claims made one upon another, have established customary rules by which to govern the processes by which they ensured not only their collective survival (Sahlins, 1974), but their shared well-being. Whereas Neanderthals, the archaeological evidence would suggest, may have ensured the survival of certain sick and infirm members of their species (Harari, 2011: 15), human beings (i.e. *homo sapiens*), with the benefit of language and cognitive reasoning, in their struggle for survival and fulfilment have clearly come not merely to care for one another's needs, but to articulate the ethical premises by which to recognise or, indeed, to refute the needs and claims of others. We have seen that the classical 'civilisation' of ancient Athens refuted the needs and claims of slaves and women. The agricultural and industrial revolutions transformed the means by which, and the extent to which, human beings materially provide for one another. But they also imposed particular social relations of power and exclusion; social relations that systemically refuted or failed fully to recognise the evolving needs and claims of the greater part of humanity.

It has been argued that in the later stages of industrial capitalism, the advent in the global North of modern welfare states provided a mechanism by which human altruism could be expressed not primarily through individual gift giving – as might have been possible in earlier, less complex social formations – but collectively through tax-funded state provision for social security, healthcare, education and housing (Titmuss, 1970). Other commentators saw the modern welfare state not as a mechanism for collective gift giving, but as the realisation of a new social form of citizenship (Marshall, 1950); an advanced form of citizenship that encompassed not only hard-won civil and political freedoms, but rights to basic minimum social standards.

In practice, the social rights of citizenship in advanced capitalist nations can be 'fine-tuned' so as to be more or less inclusive (Lockwood, 1996). And the origins of modern social policy and capitalist welfare states have been fuelled by competing demands, reflecting different approaches to human well-being (Esping-Andersen, 1990). Though it is not possible to draw clear lines of distinction between hedonic and eudaimonic forms of social policy, it is possible to draw a closely related distinction between utilitarian and solidaristic forms of social provision. Contemporary social policy may exhibit on the one hand, an approach with roots in utilitarian social assistance principles; and on the other, a more solidaristic approach founded either pragmatically on risk-sharing social insurance, or else inclusively on principles of universalism. Actual welfare states incorporate a mixture of these competing principles so far as provision for social protection, health care and other social services is concerned and it is possible to situate different welfare states on a continuum depending on the balance they strike between a hedonic understanding of well-being implied by a selective social assistance approach and more or less eudaimonic understanding implied by various types of solidaristic approach.

Social rights of citizenship are creatures of welfare state capitalism and do not have the same purchase in the global South, where concepts of social rights have been driven to a greater extent by the human rights agenda and the UN's Universal Declaration of Human Rights of 1948. In the wake of two world wars, the declaration gave expression to a loose and uneasy international consensus (Davy, 2013) and expressly incorporated a new generation of 'economic, social and cultural rights' (an expression for which the term 'social rights' is widely regarded as a synonymous contraction), including rights to work, social security, health, education and adequate housing. The International Covenant that eventually gave effect to social rights required not that they be immediately implemented, but only their 'progressive realisation'. Several countries of the global South went on to incorporate social rights into national constitutions or regional charters, but the capacity progressively to realise such rights was invariably constrained. Such constraint fed demands for a right to social development; a right that should be underwritten by the international community as a whole. The demand was conceded through the UN's Declaration of the Right to Development of 1986, which was supposed finally to afford not just a right to live, but 'the right to live better' (M'Baye, 1972). The emphasis was on social, not economic, development and what might be regarded as a quintessentially eudaimonic aspiration.

The impact of that aspiration, which would later find expression in the setting of the Millennium Development Goals (United Nations General Assembly, 2000), has been significantly diluted by two factors: by the hegemonic effects of a global neo-liberal consensus; and by a certain degree of resistance within the global South to the imposition of the cultural values of the global North. What came to be known in the 1980s as the Washington Consensus (Williamson, 1990) favoured trade liberalisation – including trade in human services – low public spending and selective social safety nets (i.e. conditional relief for the poorest). This prescription resulted initially in 'structural adjustment' programmes, which signally failed to assist social development in the world's poorest countries. But despite a subsequent shift in emphasis on the part of key institutions such as the World Bank (2001), the underlying logic of the Washington Consensus endures (Deacon, 2007). At the same time, attempts to establish 'Global Social Policy Principles' (Ferguson, 1999) have foundered in the face of charges against the global North of hypocrisy and cultural imperialism, made by some poorer nations, who fear, for example, that the imposition of labour regulation standards could in practice result in the further impoverishment of some of the world's most vulnerable people (e.g. Kabeer, 2004).

Debates in social and public policy have lately been preoccupied with new ways of assessing human progress, including the measurement of 'happiness', or subjective well-being (Dolan & Metcalfe, 2012; Layard, 2005; Stiglitz, Sen, & Fitoussi, 2009); Dolan and Kudrna, Chap. 29, this volume) a metric that implies a primarily hedonic understanding of human well-being and a utilitarian approach to human welfare. The immanent concern, it may be argued, is not so much with human fulfilment, as popular satisfaction; with the capacity of the global economy to adjust or accommodate, rather than overcome systemic inequality and social disadvantage. Such trends, arguably, have been further driven by the post-2008 global financial crisis and associated calls for greater austerity in social provision (Farnsworth & Irving, 2015).

34.4.2 Radical Need and a Life-First Ethic

The trend towards a hedonic understanding of human well-being has been, or might be, countered in a variety of ways by positions favouring more holistic understandings of human welfare:

- One of these is the social quality movement (see www.socialquality.org), which began life in 1997 as the European Foundation on Social Quality, but has since developed into the International Association on Social Quality (Beck, Van der Maesen, & Walker, 1997; van der Maesen & Walker, 2014). The IASQ define social quality as 'the extent to which people are able to participate in social relationships under conditions which enhance their well-being, capacity and individual potential', placing specific emphasis on the objective, the subjective and the normative conditions of life. It represents a broadly social democratic, academically driven, riposte to neo-liberal hegemony.

- A more loosely framed conceptual perspective, dubbed by Woodiwiss (2005: 134) the 'minor tradition' within human rights discourse, is that which regards the individual bearer of rights as fundamentally vulnerable and interdependent, rather than free-born and autonomous and frames its understanding of social rights as a system of mutual protection (Turner, 2006; Twine, 1994).
- There are related perspectives focused not so much on rights, as specifically on care: calls by feminists for an alternative 'ethic of care' (e.g. Sevenhuijsen, 1998; Tronto, 1994) and by the global Left commentator, De Sousa Santos (2006) for an of 'axiology of care'. These calls accord priority to the centrality within human lives of caring relationships and the meaning and value of care for human well-being.
- De Sousa Santos also alludes to the existence in the global South of alternative epistemologies; ways of understanding quite different to those which inform market capitalism and liberal democracy. Some of these, it must be said, entail ostensibly conservative religiously-framed principles, which offer nevertheless notions of well-being that are clearly more solidaristic than utilitarian and may be said to be quite clearly eudaimonic in character. For example, the Confucian idea of *Rén*, which translates as a state of ultimate human-ness (Chan, 1999); the ancient pan-African belief system, *Ubuntu*, captured by the aphorism 'a person is only a person through other persons' (Ramose, 2003); and the Islamic principle of *Zakat*, a central pillar of faith requiring all Muslims to share wealth with needier members of the community (Dean & Khan, 1997).
- Within academic Social Policy there has of late been something of a turn in the direction of psycho-social approaches (Stenner & Taylor, 2008) focusing on the role that social policies can play not simply in relieving individual stress and promoting individual coping, but in addressing social harm or 'social suffering' (cf. Bourdieu, 1999); in promoting the social conditions for eudaimonic well-being.
- Another Social Policy commentator, Bill Jordan (2008), argues for a definition of well-being as the realisation of 'social value', a term that captures, perhaps, a less ambiguous meaning than that of 'social quality' (see above), since it is premised explicitly on a rejection of utilitarian conceptions of value.

Jordan's discussion of social value as a social policy principle resonates, but is not coterminous, with Marx's concept of 'radical need' (see Heller, 1974). Marx defined human need in relation to the 'species characteristics' outlined earlier in this chapter, these being the constitutive features of humanity and the axiomatic requirements of a human's species being. Marx's vision was of a social order that would succeed from capitalism; an order in which the measure of things would flow from the recognition and fulfilment of needs, rather than fetishised conceptions of market value. Though Hannah Arendt deplored the reality of communism, her claim that that which is good in life is 'radical' echoes the sense in which Marx claimed that human needs – the things we need to be fully human – are dynamic and radical. The historical failure of the communist experiment need in no way detract from the significance of Marx's re-conceptualisation of *eudaimonia* and a 'good life' in terms of the radical essence of a human's species being. Nor did that failure signal the end of history (*pace* Fukuyama, 1992) or in any way a conclusion to the process of historical development that is a constitutive characteristic of the human species.

It is in this context that I argue for a eudaimonic social policy, premised on what might be called a 'life-first' ethic (Dean, 2014, 2015). The term originated in an attempt to frame an alternative to aggressive 'work-first' labour market activation policies and a more meaningful framing of 'work-life balance' policies in the UK. Its significance, however, may be extended to encompass the idea that eudaimonic well-being is a social right – the right to live well; and that axiomatically the realisation of that right is a collectively shared responsibility. It is a flexible and potentially unifying idea, that is to some extent commensurate, or can at least communicate, with some or all the six positions outlined above. Its simple meaning is that human life is about more than individual utility and that this provides a foundation for social policy making. A life-first ethic, by implication is, on the one hand, concerned with the species being of specific human individuals: it is essentially compassionate and caring. On the other hand, it is concerned with the condition of the human species as a whole: it is cosmopolitan and solidaristic.

Social policy, clearly, is something unique to the human species, but its formulation entails the negotiation of social rights; a struggle over needs (Fraser, 1989, ch. 8), which entails the 'publicising' or politicisation of strictly hedonic needs experienced in what Arendt dismissively referred to as the private sphere. The recognition of everyday needs, especially the exacerbated needs of subordinated social groups, into the public sphere – a process referred to by Fraser as a 'politics of needs interpretation' – transforms their significance. The process of social development and the considered purpose of social policy are, or ought to be, essentially eudaimonic: they are, or ought to be, the personal and historical fulfilment of human species being. This chapter is not the place to extol a manifesto for eudaimonic social policy, since the struggle over needs is an ever evolving struggle. Fundamentally, however, we can see that publicly framed policy for the fulfilment of species being would:

- Nourish human **consciousness** through forms of education that might, for example, expressly promote a process that Friere (1972) described as 'conscientization'; a process by which every human person may discover 'an ontological vocation'.
- Recognise and facilitate all forms of **work**. Not only such work as may be specified by the International Labour Organisation as 'decent' (1999), but all purposeful human activity, whether materially productive, socially reproductive, culturally creative or politically constructive.
- Extend and fully support the realisation of human **sociality** through inclusive social security mechanisms; and the collective provision of, and/or effective democratic control over, universal human services, including health, social care and housing.
- Enable a sustainable process of **historical development** capable of fulfilling the radical character of human needs.

34.5 Summary/Conclusion

This chapter has reviewed the concept of *eudaimonia*, which constituted – for Aristotle, the natural purpose of a privileged minority of humanity; for Marx, the historical and developmental purpose of an entire species radically characterised by its specific forms of consciousness, work and sociality; for Arendt, what it means for a human being to live well in common with others. Seizing on the idea that in the contemporary era social policy and social development are, or ought to be, concerned not only with living well, but living better, the chapter has returned to Marx's particular concept of species being as the basis for a life-first ethic: an ethic that seeks consensually to define and prioritise human fulfilment and that which is *essentially* 'good'.

References

Althusser, L. (1971). *Lenin and philosophy and other essays* (B. Brewster, Trans.). London: New Left Books.

Arendt, H. (1951). *The burden of our time*. London: Secker & Warburg.

Arendt, H. (1968). *Life of mind: Vol. 2 willing*. London: Secker & Warburg.

Arendt, H. (1978). *Life of mind: Vol. 1 thinking*. London: Secker & Warburg.

Aristotle. (c. 350 BCE). *Eudemian ethics – Books I. II and VIII* (1982 edn. M. Woods, Tran.). Oxford, UK: Clarendon Press.

Beck, W., Van der Maesen, L., & Walker, A. (Eds.). (1997). *The social quality of Europe*. Bristol, UK: The Policy Press.

Benton, T. (1988). Humanism = specieism: Marx on humans and animals. *Radical Philosophy, 50*, 4–18.
Bourdieu, P. (1999). *The weight of the world: Social suffering in contemporary society*. Cambridge, UK: Polity.
Chan, J. (1999). A Confucian perspective on human rights for contemporary China. In J. Bauer & D. Bell (Eds.), *The east Asian challenge for human rights*. Cambridge, UK: Cambridge University Press.
Chitty, A. (2009). Species-being and capital. In A. Chitty & M. McIvor (Eds.), *Karl Marx and contemporary philosophy*. Basingstoke, UK: Palgrave Macmillan.
Davy, U. (2013). Social citizenship going international: Changes in the reading of UN-sponsored economic and social rights. *International Journal of Social Welfare, 22*(Supplement 1), S15–S31.
De Sousa Santos, B. (2006). *The rise of the global left: The world social forum and beyond*. London: Zed Books.
Deacon, B. (2007). *Global social policy and governance*. London: Sage.
Dean, H. (2000). Towards an embodied account of welfare. In K. Ellis & H. Dean (Eds.), *Social policy and the body: Transitions in corporeal discourse*. Basingstoke, UK: Macmillan.
Dean, H. (2012). *Social policy* (2nd ed.). Cambridge, UK: Polity.
Dean, H. (2014). Life first welfare, the need/right to work and the scope for a 'eudemonic ethic' of social security. In M. Keune & A. Serrano (Eds.), *Deconstructing flexicurity and developing alternative approaches: Towards new concepts and approaches for employment and social policy*. London: Routledge.
Dean, H. (2015). *Social rights and human welfare*. Abingdon, UK: Routledge.
Dean, H., & Khan, Z. (1997). Muslim perspectives on welfare. *Journal of Social Policy, 26*(2).
Depew, D. (1992). The polis transfigured: Aristotle's politics and Marx's critique of Hegel's philosophy of right. In G. McCarthy (Ed.), *Marx and Aristotle: Nineteenth century German social theory and classical antiquity*. Annapolis, MD: Rowman & Littlefield.
Dolan, P., & Metcalfe, P. (2012). Measuring subjective wellbeing: Recommendations for use by national governments. *Journal of Social Policy, 41*(2), 409–427.
Esping-Andersen, G. (1990). *The three worlds of welfare capitalism*. Cambridge, UK: Polity Press.
Farnsworth, K., & Irving, Z. (Eds.). (2015). *Social policy in times of austerity*. Bristol, UK: The Policy Press.
Ferguson, C. (1999). *Global social policy: Human rights and social justice*. London: Department for International Development.
Foster, J. (1999). Marx's theory of metabolic rift: Classical foundations for environmental sociology. *American Journal of Sociology, 105*(2), 366.
Fraser, N. (1989). *Unruly practices: Power, discourse and gender in contemporary social theory*. Minneapolis, MN: University of Minnesota Press.
Friere, P. (1972). *Pedagogy of the oppressed*. Harmondsworth, UK: Penguin.
Fromm, E. (1961). *Marx's concept of man*. New York: Frederick Unger Publishing.
Fukuyama, F. (1992). *The end of history and the last man*. New York: Basic Books.
Gilbert, A. (1992). Marx's moral realism: Eudaimonism and moral progress. In G. McCarthy (Ed.), *Marx and Aristotle: Nineteenth century German social theory and classical antiquity*. Annapolis, MD: Rowman & Littlefield.
Harari, Y. (2011). *Sapiens: A brief history of humankind*. London: Vintage.
Hegel, G. (1805–1806). Jena lectures on the philosophy of spirit. In L. Rauch (Ed.), *Hegel and the human spirit (1983)*. Dettroit, MI: Wayne State University Press.
Hegel, G. (1821). In A. Wood (Ed.), *Elements of the philosophy of rights* (1991st ed.). Cambridge, UK: Cambridge University Press.
Heller, A. (1974). *The theory of need in Marx*. London: Alison & Busby.
Honneth, A. (1995). *The struggle for recognition: The moral grammar of social conflicts*. Cambridge, UK: Polity.
International Labour Organisation (ILO). (1999). *Report of ILO Director-General: Decent work, international labour conference, 87th session*. Geneva, Switzerland: ILO.
Jordan, B. (2008). *Welfare and well-being: Social value in public policy*. Bristol, UK: The Policy Press.
Kabeer, N. (2004). Globalization, labor standards, and women's rights: Dilemmas of collective (in)action in an interdependent world. *Feminist Economics, 10*(1), 3–35.
Layard, R. (2005). *Happiness: Lessons from a new science*. New York: Penguin.
Lockwood, D. (1996). Civic integration and class formation. *British Journal of Sociology, 47*(3), 531–550.
M'Baye, K. (1972). Le Droit au Développement comme un droit de l'Homme. *Revue des Droits de l'Homme, 5*, 503–505.
MacIntyre, A. (2007). *After virtue* (3rd ed.). Notre Dame, IN: Notre Dame Press.
Margolis, J. (1992). Praxis and meaning: Marx's species being and Aristotle's political animal. In G. McCarthy (Ed.), *Marx and Aristotle: Nineteenth century German social theory and classical antiquity*. Annapolis, MD: Rowman & Littlefield.
Márkus, G. (2014). *Marxism & anthropology: The concept of 'human essence' in the philosophy of Marx* (special, ed.). Sydney, Australia: Modem-Verlag.
Marshall, T. H. (1950). Citizenship and social class. In T. Marshall & T. Bottomore (Eds.), *Citizenship and social class* (1992nd ed.). London: Pluto.
Marx, K. (1844). Economic and philosophical manuscripts. In L. Colletti (Ed.), *Early writings* (1975th ed.). Harmondsworth, UK: Penguin.

Marx, K. (1845). Theses from Fuerbach (extract from). In T. Bottomore & M. Rubel (Eds.), *Karl Marx: Selected writings in sociology and social philosophy*. Harmondsworth, UK: Penguin.
Marx, K. (1857). *Grundrisse* (1973rd ed.). London: Penguin.
Marx, K. (1887). *Capital* (1970th ed., Vol. I). London: Lawrence & Wishart.
McCarthy, G. (Ed.). (1992). *Marx and Aristotle: Nineteenth century German social theory and classical antiquity*. Annapolis, MD: Rowman & Littlefield.
Miller, R. (1992). Marx and Aristotle: A kind of consequentialism. In G. McCarthy (Ed.), *Marx and Aristotle: Nineteenth century German social theory and classical antiquity*. Annapolis, MD: Rowman & Littlefield.
Nussbaum, M. (2000). *Women and human development: The capabilities approach*. Cambridge, MA: Cambridge University Press.
Parekh, S. (2008). *Hannah Arendt and the challenge of modernity*. Abingdon, UK: Routledge.
Ramose, M. (2003). Globalisation and ubuntu. In P. Coetzee & A. Roux (Eds.), *The African philosophy reader*. London: Routledge.
Rorty, R. (1982). *Consequences of pragmatism*. Minnesota, MD: University of Minnesota.
Russell, B. (1961). *History of western philosophy* (2nd ed.). London: Routledge.
Sahlins, M. (1974). *Stone age economics*. Chicago: Aldine.
Searle, J. (1997). *The mystery of consciousness*. London: Granta.
Sen, A. (1982). Equality of what? In A. Sen (Ed.), *Choice, welfare and measurement*. Oxford: Blackwell.
Sen, A. (1999). *Development as freedom*. Oxford, UK: Oxford University Press.
Sennett, R. (1998). *The corrosion of character: The personal consequences of work in the new capitalism*. New York: Norton.
Sevenhuijsen, S. (1998). *Citizenship and the ethics of care*. London: Routledge.
Smith, S. (1992). The origins of the dialectic: Hegel's appropriation of the ancient skeptics. In G. McCarthy (Ed.), *Marx and Aristotle: Nineteenth century German social theory and classical antiquity*. Annapolis, MD: Rowman & Littlefield.
Smyth, B. (2012). Review of Zurn, F. and Schmidt Am Busch, H-C (Eds.) The philosophy of recognition. *Marx & Philosophy Review of Books*. Retrieved December 2, 2015, from, http://marxandphilosophy.org.uk/reviewofbooks/reviews/2012/632
Soper, K. (1981). *On human needs*. Brighton, UK: Harvester.
Standing, G. (2011). *The Precariat: The new dangerous class*. London: Bloomsbury.
Stenner, P., & Taylor, D. (2008). Psychosocial welfare: Reflections on an emerging field. *Critical Social Policy, 28*(4), 415–437.
Stiglitz, J., Sen, A., & Fitoussi, J.-P. (2009). *Report by the commission on the measurement of economic performance and social progress*. See www.stiglitz-sen-firoussi.fr
Titmuss, R. (1970). *The gift relationship*. London: Allen and Unwin.
Tronto, J. (1994). *Moral boundaries: A political argument for an ethic of care*. New York: Routledge.
Turner, B. (2006). *Vulnerability and human rights*. Harrisburg, PA: Pennsylvania State University.
Twine, F. (1994). *Citizenship and social rights: The interdependence of self and society*. London: Sage.
United Nations General Assembly. (2000). *United nations millennium declaration (resolution 2 session 55)*. New York: UN.
van der Maesen, L., & Walker, A. (2014). *The development of social quality between 1994 and 2014* (Working Paper Series nr. 13). Amsterdam: IASQ. www.socialquality.org
Vygotsky, L. (1978). *Mind and society: The development of higher mental processes*. Cambridge, MA: Harvard University Press.
Weisman, T. (2014). *Hannah Arendt and Karl Marx*. Annapolis, MD: Lexington Books.
Williamson, J. (1990). What Washington means by policy reform. In J. Williamson (Ed.), *Latin American adjustment: How much has happened?* Washington, DC: Institute for International Economics.
Woodiwiss, A. (2005). *Human rights*. London: Routledge.
World Bank. (2001). *World development report 2000/2001*. Retrieved from Oxford.
Yarbrough, J., & Stern, P. (1981). Vita activa and vita contemplativa: Reflections on Hannah Arendt's political thought in life of mind. *The Review of Politics, 43*(3), 323–354.

Part V

Against Eudaimonia

35 Socrates' Dissatisfaction, a Happiness Arms Race, and the Trouble with Eudaimonic Well-Being

Sarah J. Ward and Laura A. King

Classically, eudaimonia represents the highest human good. It implies a concern for character, ethics, morality, and a code of conduct. For Aristotle (3 BCE/1986), living true to one's *daimon*, pursuing virtue in accord with reason, is the key to a life well lived. Of course, for Aristotle only some members of society were likely to possess a daimon at all and eudaimonia was quite unlikely for a person lacking in good birth, good children, beauty, external resources, and sophisticated reasoning skills. The inherent elitism of its origins notwithstanding, it would seem that only the most unreasonable curmudgeon would find serious fault with the current psychological take on the concept of eudaimonia. All that is required of us is to allow the *daimon* to be a natural birthright, a built-in tendency toward self-expression, growth, and actualization. At once, a more pleasing, democratic promise of eudaimonia emerges: If you live a life of authenticity, follow your calling, use proper reasoning to guide you to your best outcomes, value intrinsic over extrinsic ends, realize your potentials, and dedicate yourself to virtue and excellence, then you will have made serious progress toward a Good Life.

Some might quibble with these ideas and certainly about how much they jibe at all with Aristotle's ideas, but eudaimonia would seem here to represent a straightforward humanistic approach to human nature and motivation. It would make a fine philosophy of life or code of conduct. What it would not make, in our view, is a kind of well-being. And indeed, contemporary psychologists do not only espouse eudaimonia as merely a philosophy of life or code of conduct. They assert that eudaimonia is an approach to or kind of well-being (see reviews in Huta & Waterman, 2014; Ryan & Deci, 2001; Huta, Chap. 15, this volume; Ryan and Martela, Chap. 7, this volume). Although there are certainly numerous approaches to eudaimonia, they share some central ideas. Most importantly, *eudaimonic well-being* is promulgated as an alternative to run-of-the-mill hedonic well-being (i.e., how a person feels). Although it too is typically measured using self-report, eudaimonic well-being is considered more objective than simple happiness and to involve something above and beyond happiness.

In this essay, we describe some of the problems with the notion of eudaimonic *well-being*. We suggest that although scholars have taken pains to separate eudaimonic functioning from experienced happiness or positive affect conceptually and theoretically, the term eudaimonic well-being and its typical use in the literature have very clear implications for the subjective experience of happiness. This reflexive linking of eudaimonic activities and motivations with well-being has led to a happiness arms race with one

S.J. Ward • L.A. King (✉)
University of Missouri, Columbia, MO, USA
e-mail: kingla@missouri.edu

J. Vittersø (ed.), *Handbook of Eudaimonic Well-Being*, International Handbooks of Quality-of-Life,
DOI 10.1007/978-3-319-42445-3_35

type of well-being presented as *better* (qualitatively, quantitatively, morally) than the other. The idea of eudaimonic well-being and its superiority to hedonic well-being has blurred the lines between predictors and outcomes and has had negative consequences for research on human functioning. We maintain that such an approach does a disservice to eudaimonia, a philosophy of life or code of conduct. Eudaimonia should best be considered separate from well-being. It may predict well-being. It may be predicted by well-being. But it is not a kind of well-being.

To begin, we first consider a construct that appears to be lacking in the eudaimonia literature, Socrates' dissatisfaction. For inasmuch as eudaimonic approaches disavow the centrality of hedonic happiness to a Good Life, in practice, such happiness continues to occupy a vital place even in the science of eudaimonia.

35.1 Socrates' Dissatisfaction

Discussions of the eudaimonic-hedonic distinction sometimes include reference to Mill's (1863/2001, p. 13) famous assertion, "It is better to be a human being dissatisfied than a pig satisfied; better to be Socrates dissatisfied than a fool satisfied." In the context of the eudaimonic-hedonic well-being distinction (and with no disrespect meant for either side), it is clear who is the implied Socrates and who are the implied pigs and fools. Mills' quotation captures well the eudaimonic ideal about the place of pleasure in a Good Life. Satisfaction is a good but it is certainly not the highest good nor the only one. What is interesting, though, is what is shockingly *missing* from contemporary approaches to eudaimonic well-being, namely, Socrates' *dissatisfaction*. Within contemporary eudaimonic approaches, the eudaimonic person, Socrates, is not only *not* dissatisfied, he is quite satisfied. Indeed, he enjoys a satisfaction that is not only greater in quantity than the pigs' and the fools', it is, in fact, qualitatively superior, and potentially immune to the kinds of processes that reduce hedonic enjoyment over time (Waterman, 2007; 2013). Eudaimonia carries no risk of loss to personal happiness. Instead, it is portrayed as a route to ever greater levels of fulfillment.

The concept of eudaimonic well-being requires that we revisit the promise of eudaimonia reviewed above: If you live a life of authenticity, follow your calling, use proper reasoning to guide you to your best outcomes, value intrinsic over extrinsic ends, realize your potentials, and dedicate yourself to virtue and excellence, then *you will be happy*. You will not simply be happy but happi*er* than those who pursue happiness itself. Eudaimonists contend that happiness, pleasure, or positive emotion is merely a byproduct of eudaimonic pursuits and not an end in itself. However, the associations between eudaimonic pursuits and subjective happiness provide the key form of validity for the construct of eudaimonia. Within psychology, eudaimonic constructs have been exalted *because* they relate to subjective reports of happiness, despite being conceptualized as somehow distinct from them.

In this sense, the promise of eudaimonic well-being is a kind of psychological prosperity gospel: If you do well, you will feel well. As if, within this world of upward spirals of delight, not only bad things but also bad *feelings* never happen to good people. Such a perspective not only reveals naïve just world thinking, it overlooks the numerous good lives that are lived in sometimes less than optimal circumstances. It misses precisely the person who might most embody the eudaimonic ideal: One who legitimately sacrifices personal happiness, not for the promise of even greater joy later, but for the good of another person or in the name of principle. Eudaimonic approaches to well-being were introduced to represent something other than happiness, to demonstrate that happiness was not, actually everything (Ryff, 1989, Chap. 6, this volume; Ryff & Singer, 1998). Yet, in the intervening years, the portrait of eudaimonia that has emerged, from many eudaimonic scholars, is almost entirely a portrait of a happy person. Is it still possible for someone to do the right thing and *not* be happy about it? Is such a person, the dyspeptic (even dysphoric) but morally excellent person not living a good life?

Consider, as an example, the life of Mother Teresa, a woman who is often trotted out as an example when psychologists search for a contemporary exemplar of a good person. During her young adulthood as a nun living a typical life in a convent surrounded by her sisters, she was happy, possessed of a daily joy and, for her, the strong and constant felt presence of God. Once she received her calling, however, and embarked on the work with the poorest of the poor in Calcutta, she never felt that happiness again. The titles of the books authored in her name (which often included the word joy) notwithstanding, her private letters reveal that her days in service to the poor, those works for which she is best known and most recognized as a self-actualizer and moral exemplar, were not happy times (Mother Teresa, 2007). They were times of doubt, sorrow, loneliness, and questioning (Zaleski, 2003). These were the times when she felt the most disconnected from God.

Considering Mother Teresa's hidden unhappiness, we would likely conclude that the works themselves are what ought to matter, not how the person feels while or after doing it. That sentence would seem to reflect a eudaimonic sentiment. Works that are for the greater good are more important than subjective feelings. Yet, consider how eudaimonic well-being is portrayed in the literature and how it is studied and it is easy to see that eudaimonia is not considered valuable in and of itself. If it were, eudaimonic behaviors would be the end or outcome not the predictor of something else. And that something else would not so very often be subjective well-being. If eudaimonia is an end in itself, and it may well be, why must happiness so often appear in the role of carrot?

Just how absent is the unhappy eudaimonic person in the literature? Consider the results of a recent study examining the prevalence of flourishing in a representative sample of over 5,000 individuals in the Netherlands (Schotanus-Dijkstra, et al., 2015). Like most studies of eudaimonic well-being it (along with hedonic well-being) was assessed using self-reports. The investigators measured both eudaimonic well-being and hedonic well-being in order to divide the sample into quadrants: languishing (low on both) and flourishing (high on both per Keyes, 2002); as well as individuals falling into the low/high groups (i.e., high on eudaimonic/low on hedonic and vice versa). Although the study was focused on languishing (about 20 % of the sample) vs. flourishing (about 37 % of the sample), an examination of the mismatched groups is revealing. Over 40 % of the participants were categorized as "not high" on eudaimonic well-being but high on hedonic well-being. In contrast, *less than 2 %* of the sample scored high on eudaimonic well-being without also being high on hedonic well-being. Where, again, is Socrates dissatisfied? Where is Mother Teresa, dedicated to a difficult sometimes joyless but morally correct life?

The absence of individuals who pursue eudaimonic ends despite the cost of this pursuit to personal happiness suggests a serious problem in either the conceptualization or the operationalization of eudaimonia. It would also seem to be disingenuous to claim that subjective feelings of happiness are irrelevant to eudaimonia when the unhappy appear quite unlikely to pursue eudaimonic ends. Perhaps these results suggest just how likely it is that eudaimonic activities lead to positive affect. They might also indicate that positive affect lays a foundation for the experience of eudaimonic well-being (including, for instance, meaning in life, King et al., 2006). Whatever the causal direction between positive emotion and eudaimonic activities, these results show that in modern measures of eudaimonic well-being, happiness is hardly beside the point.

As noted already, eudaimonic experiences are thought to lead, not simply to pleasure but to *a better, more virtuous and more durable, form of pleasure*. These perspectives assume that one's pleasure or happiness is guided by a sort of moral or self-actualizing compass, with beneficial or virtuous pursuits boosting happiness and negative or unethical actions diminishing it. Although surely virtuous actions can promote positive affect, so too can unethical behaviors, such as cheating (e.g., Ruedy, Moore, Gino, & Schweitzer, 2013). The association between virtuous aims and subjective happiness is more tenuous than eudaimonists claim. Not only is the assumption that people's affective states are closely tied to lofty, abstract considerations inaccurate, but it is also potentially damaging, as it may cause scholars to ignore the host of prosaic circumstances that do stimulate subjective happiness as well as experiences thought to be eudaimonic (e.g., meaning in life, King et al., 2006). Not only is the eudaimonic ideal—the person who achieves virtue and perfection with no concern for personal happiness—a rarity among actual people, but there is no evidence that this paragon would even have a qualitatively superior form of well-being.

35.2 Happiness Arms Race and Its Consequences

Although eudaimonic functioning has traditionally been considered more "objective" than hedonic well-being, it is important to bear in mind that both of these aspects of well-being are generally assessed with self-reports. Despite the inherently subjective nature of self-reports, eudaimonist thinkers have suggested that eudaimonia is not a subjective state but a set of motivations and behaviors representing "the best within us" (Huta & Waterman, 2014; p. 1427). Positive feelings that emerge from success at eudaimonic pursuits are not viewed as goals, but rather as byproducts of attaining virtue or excellence. These ideas downplay the extraordinarily strong association between eudaimonic and hedonic well-being. This very strong relationship has been understated to the detriment of science. Arguments in this vein have been proffered elsewhere (see Biswas-Diener, Kashdan, & King, 2009; Kashdan, Biswas-Diener, & King, 2008). Briefly, there is no evidence that the happiness that emerges from eudaimonic endeavors differs, *qualitatively*, from the happiness that comes from other activities. Importantly, instead, reports of eudaimonic well-being are very strongly related to reports of hedonic well-being.

Research has continued to strongly support the possibility that there is only one general well-being that covaries with the pursuit of eudaimonic motivations. Even when researchers take pains to include measures of eudaimonic and hedonic well-being, these variables tend to share correlations suggestive of reliabilities. For example, a recent cross-cultural assessment of eudaimonic and hedonic well-being in nearly 8000 people (Disabato, Goodman, Kashdan, Short & Jarden, 2015) found relationships ranging from .78 to .92, ultimately estimating *92%* of the shared variance between the latent factors.

Of course, it is not uncommon in psychology to have the same construct be given two different names and then have scientists make great hay out of miniscule distinctions between them. Does it really matter if the same occurs in the realm of well-being? Yes it does. Perhaps because the *conceptual* distinction between eudaimonic and hedonic well-being has become so entrenched and reified, scholars have ignored their very strong empirical association unwisely. The illusion of a very strong distinction has led otherwise excellent scholars to take variables that are extremely highly correlated (e.g., $r=.79$; Fredrickson et al., 2013; r's = .63, .70; Baumeister, Vohs, Aaker, & Garbinsky, 2013) and predict outcomes from one while controlling for the other. Assuming that there are two qualitatively different kinds of well-being leads to conclusions that are very likely multicollinearity (see, Brown et al., 2014). Importantly, it is unlikely that anyone would even think of splitting the hairs of the good life in this way if this distinction did not exist.

Additionally, consider the message such research sends to people struggling to live a good life. Interested parties should know that the happiness they experience must be of the right kind, experienced for the right reasons. Moreover, those who find living the morally good life at all problematic, who struggle and sacrifice personal happiness for some greater end, must be doing something wrong.

The proliferation of new eudaimonic constructs may portray well-being as challenging to achieve and even, perhaps, rare. Notions of eudaimonia necessitate personal virtues to produce well-being, leading to the conclusion that well-being may be uncommon or only achievable by the lucky few. Yet both subjective happiness and even more eudaimonic forms of well-being (e.g., meaning in life) are actually quite prevalent across the world, even in difficult circumstances (e.g., Diener & Diener, 1996; Heintzelman & King, 2014). It does not appear that well-being is only available to a select few who exude virtue and personal excellence.

35.3 Beyond Well-Being and Toward Eudaimonia

In some ways, attaching eudaimonia to well-being has led to an unfortunate dearth of information about eudaimonia as a code of conduct or philosophy of life. We know very little about the antecedents and consequences of eudaimonic motivation that do not involve subjective well-being. Eudaimonic well-being is defined, to some extent, by its antecedents. The happiness of a person has just volunteered for a day with Habitat for Humanity is eudaimonic; the happiness of a person who just got off an awesome roller coaster is not. But it seems that the many differences between these people might be a better place to look for defining features of eudaimonia. If happiness is merely a byproduct of eudaimonic activity and is not synonymous with it, then researchers and theorists ought to begin to study eudaimonia apart from subjective happiness (King & Hicks, 2007). What else might it do besides (sometimes) make people happy?

A fascinating possibility is that eudaimonic pursuits may offer wider social benefits due to their outward, rather than personal, focus. For example, Huta and colleagues (2012) found that respondents' self-reported eudaimonic, but not hedonic, motivation was associated with higher well-being in their close friends or relatives, gathered from peer-reports. These findings are important because they demonstrate that eudaimonic motivation may offer unique social benefits that are distinct from a hedonic motivation and potentially irrelevant to personal happiness.

Disabato and colleagues (2015) suggested that eudaimonic and hedonic well-being may differ in their motivational content. For instance, some people may endeavor to avoid unpleasant circumstances and opportunities altogether, focusing primarily on maintaining positive affective states, whereas other people may be willing to endure unpleasant circumstances if they have the potential to promote growth or further one's goals. Huta and Ryan (2010) found that motives for hedonic pursuits promoted positive affect, whereas motives for eudaimonic pursuits related to enhanced meaning. (Though we stress, yet again, that positive affect and meaning share a very strong robust relationship).

One important caveat about the utility of this motivational approach is that people's motives for either hedonic or eudaimonic aims may overlap with other personality traits (e.g., eudaimonic aims reflecting conscientiousness). Studies that aim to differentiate between hedonic and eudaimonic motives should include additional measures of personality in order to address whether these motivations are unique. Moreover, we caution that reliance on self-reports in the assessment of behaviors and motives may reflect more about how people construe behaviors rather than the benefits of eudaimonic behaviors, per se.

Another important avenue for research is investigating how various life circumstances and personality factors influence whether people emphasize eudaimonic goals or conceive of their behavior as eudaimonic. For example, Lucas and Diener (2015) suggest that eudaimonic activities may themselves be a product of traits such as conscientiousness and other characteristics such as education, income, marital status, and so forth. It is possible that some people, for instance, those with low education or socioeconomic status, may potentially be less prone to endorse notions of eudaimonic well-being, having not been as entrenched in the variegated notions of well-being that are perhaps more common in wealthy, intellectual communities. Understanding how demographic factors, culture, and personality traits influence the manner in which people strive towards well-being, as well as the aspects of well-being they prioritize, remains an important area for research.

In a similar vein, it may be valuable to examine whether eudaimonic constructs and motivations influence societal or occupational functioning, ideally using measures of these outcomes *besides self-report*. Although eudaimonia has generally been considered more objectively beneficial than hedonia, there is scant empirical evidence for this claim. Perhaps eudaimonic constructs or motivations do provide objective benefits, such as increased prosocial behavior or dedication at work, that hedonic well-being does not offer. Moving eudaimonic constructs into a broader social and societal realm, and away from the domain of individual well-being, will allow a better understanding of their function and utility.

The current state of eudaimonic well-being gives the impression that those who sacrifice to do the right thing will be rewarded with greater happiness. That is simply not reliably true nor universal. It may be that eudaimonia is best captured when personal happiness is *sacrificed for* and not enhanced by moral, ethical, or virtuous action. When a person gives up their own happiness for the good of another or for the sake of principle, such a person need not be viewed as "happier in the end" or less likely to experience regret in the long run. Personal unhappiness can also be a consequence of living a virtuous life. The emphasis on eudaimonia as an aspect of individual well-being, rather than as virtues or qualities that are useful to hone for their own sake, has obfuscated the broader importance of these motivations and behaviors. For a life of virtue, happiness should be beside the point.

References

Aristotle. (1986). *Nicomachean ethics*. New York: Macmillan (Original work published 4th Century BCE).

Baumeister, R. F., Vohs, K. D., Aaker, J. L., & Garbinsky, E. N. (2013). Some key differences between a happy life and a meaningful life. *The Journal of Positive Psychology, 8*(6), 505–516. doi:10.1080/17439760.2013.830764.

Biswas-Diener, R., Kashdan, T., & King, L. A. (2009). Two traditions of happiness research, not two distinct types of happiness. *Journal of Positive Psychology, 4*, 208–211. doi:10.1080/17439760902844400.

Brown, N. L., MacDonald, D. A., Samanta, M. P., Friedman, H. L., & Coyne, J. C. (2014). A critical reanalysis of the relationship between genomics and well-being. *PNAS Proceedings of the National Academy of Sciences of the United States of America, 111*(35), 12705–12709. doi:10.1073/pnas.1407057111.

Diener, E., & Diener, C. (1996). Most people are happy. *Psychological Science, 7*(3), 181–185.

Disabato, D. J., Goodman, F. R., Kashdan, T. B., Short, J. L., & Jarden, A. (2015). Different types of well-being? A cross-cultural examination of hedonic and eudaimnic well-being. *Psychological Assessment* (in press).

Fredrickson, B. L., Grewen, K. M., Coffey, K. A., Algoe, S. B., Firestine, A. M., Arevalo, J. G., & ... Cole, S. W. (2013). A functional genomic perspective on human well-being. *PNAS Proceedings of the National Academy of Sciences of the United States of America, 110*(33), 13684–13689.

Heintzelman, S. J., & King, L. A. (2014). Life is pretty meaningful. *American Psychologist, 69*(6), 561–574. doi:10.1037/a0035049.

Huta, V., Pelletier, L., Baxter, D., & Thompson, A. (2012). How eudaimonic and hedonic motives relate to the well-being of close others. *Journal of Positive Psychology, 7*, 399–404.

Huta, V., & Ryan, R. M. (2010). Pursuing pleasure or virtue: The differential and overlapping well-being benefits of hedonic and eudaimonic motives. *Journal of Happiness Studies, 11*, 735–762.

Huta, V., & Waterman, A. S. (2014). Eudaimonia and its distinction from hedonia: Developing a classification and terminology for understanding conceptual and operational definitions. *Journal of Happiness Studies, 15*, 1425–1456.

Kashdan, T. B., Biswas-Diener, R., & King, L. A. (2008). Reconsidering happiness: The costs of distinguishing between hedonics and eudaimonia. *Journal of Positive Psychology, 8*, 219–233.

Keyes, C. L. M. (2002). The mental health continuum: From languishing to flourishing in life. *Journal of Health and Social Research, 43*, 207–222.

King, L. A., & Hicks, J. A. (2007). Whatever happened to" What might have been"? Regrets, happiness, and maturity. *American Psychologist, 62*(7), 625.

King, L. A., Hicks, J. A., Krull, J. L., & Del Gaiso, A. K. (2006). Positive affect and the experience of meaning in life. *Journal of Personality and Social Psychology, 90*(1), 179–196. doi:10.1037/0022-3514.90.1.179.

Lucas, R. E., & Diener, E. (2015). Personality and subjective well-being: Current issues and controversies. In M. Mikulincer, P. R. Shaver, M. L. Cooper, & R. J. Larsen (Eds.), *APA handbook of personality and social psychology, volume 4: Personality processes and individual differences* (pp. 577–599). Washington, DC: American Psychological Association. doi:10.1037/14343-026.

Mill, J. S. (1863/2001). *Utilitarianism*. Kitchener, ON: Batoche Books.

Mother, T. (2007). In B. Kolodiejchuk (Ed.), *Mother Teresa: Come be my light: The private writings of the saint of Calcutta*. New York: Random House.

Ruedy, N. E., Moore, C., Gino, F., & Schweitzer, M. E. (2013). The cheater's high: The unexpected affective benefits of unethical behavior. *Journal of Personality and Social Psychology, 105*(4), 531–548. doi:10.1037/a0034231.

Ryan, R. M., & Deci, E. L. (2001). On happiness and human potentials: A review of research on hedonic and eudaimonic well-being. *Annual Review of Psychology, 52*, 141–166.

Ryff, C. D. (1989). Happiness is everything, or is it? Explorations on the meaning of psychological well-being. *Journal of Personality And Social Psychology, 57*(6), 1069–1081. doi:10.1037/0022-3514.57.6.1069.

Ryff, C. D., & Singer, B. (1998). The contours of positive human health. *Psychological Inquiry, 9*(1), 1–28.

Schotanus-Dijkstra, M., Pieterse, M. E., Drossaert, C. H. C., Westerhof, G. J., de Graaf, R., ten Have, M. et al. (2015). What factors are associated with flourishing? Results from a large representative national sample. *Journal of Happiness Studies* (in press).

Waterman, A. S. (2007). On the importance of distinguishing hedonia and eudaimonia when contemplating the hedonic treadmill. *American Psychologist, 62*(6), 612–613. doi:10.1037/0003-066X62.6.612.

Waterman, A. S. (Ed.). (2013). *The best within us: Positive psychology perspectives on eudaimonia*. Washington, DC: American Psychological Association. 10.1037/14092-000.

Zaleski, C. (2003, May). The dark night of Mother Teresa. *First Things*. http://www.firstthings.com/article/2003/05/the-dark-night-of-mother-teresa downloaded 10/9/2015.

Putting Eudaimonia in Its Place

On the Predictor, Not the Outcome, Side of the Equation

36

Kennon M. Sheldon

36.1 Introduction

"Putting eudaemonia in its place" is, intentionally, a provocative title. There have been positive benefits to the emergence of eudaimonia as a research topic during the last 20 years: mainly, that it has helped bring greater empirical attention to the important question of how people can maximally fulfill and develop themselves. However in my view, the eudaimonia concept has been more confusing than edifying for the field, more harmful to the cause of scientifically-backed positive psychology than helpful (Kashdan, Biswas-Diener, & King, 2008; King, 2009; Sheldon, 2013). There has been a rush to climb aboard the eudaimonia bandwagon, just as there was a rush to join the positive psychology bandwagon, without full consideration of what tune the bandwagon was playing. As a result, the bandwagon has grown to contain a jarring discordance of different melodies and themes, with the different musicians sometimes pounding (or blaring) away without really listening to each other. Also, some musicians continue to play melodies or themes that are unnecessary or even irrelevant to the full ensemble!

Thus, in this chapter I will begin with a critique of the eudaimonia concept – but only in one way. I will argue that ***eudaimonia goes wrong when it is conceptualized as a form of well-being, whose measures are proposed to supplement, or even supplant, traditional well-being measures.*** The Psychological Well-Being scales (Ryff & Keyes, 1995; Ryff, Chap. 6, this volume), which assess experiences of autonomy, mastery, positive relationships, purpose, personal growth, and self-acceptance, exemplify this tendency. Ryff and Keyes suggested that these are six additional forms of well-being which should be measured and considered, in addition to conventional mood and satisfaction-based well-being measures, in order to understand the fully thriving human being. And indeed, the six Psychological Well-Being scales seemed to fill a gap in the literature, explaining their immediate resonance and popularity. Surely there is more to a truly meaningful life than mere "good mood and satisfaction?"

While I agree that the topics contained within the PWB measure (self-acceptance, autonomy, mastery, personal growth, positive relations, and purpose) are all important topics, I do NOT agree that what is being measured is alternate forms of

---

This article was prepared within the framework of a subsidy granted to the HSE by the Government of the Russian Federation for the implementation of the Global Competitiveness Program.

K.M. Sheldon (✉)
University of Missouri, Columbia, MO, USA

International Laboratory of Positive Psychology of Personality and Motivation, National Research University Higher School of Economics, Moscow, Russia
e-mail: SheldonK@missouri.edu

J. Vittersø (ed.), *Handbook of Eudaimonic Well-Being*, International Handbooks of Quality-of-Life,
DOI 10.1007/978-3-319-42445-3_36

well-being. These are all potential experiential *causes* of well-being, which should be empirically tested as such, rather than just assumed a priori to be aspects of well-being. Sheldon (2013) discussed at length the problems the a priori approach creates. Among them was the fact that one researcher's list of the multiple facets of eudaimonic well-being may not concur with another researcher's list. For example, Ryff's sixfold PWB model (Ryff & Keyes, 1995) does not line up with Seligman's fourfold PARMA model (Seligman, 2011), which does not line up with Huppert and So's (2009) ninefold Flourishing model. It becomes a matter of mere argumentation, not science, as to which list is more accurate or useful. Relatedly, it is difficult to get an item from an a priori list *off* of the list, once it is *on* the list, if there is no emphasis on empirically comparing and testing the various list elements (cf. Sheldon, Elliot, Kim, & Kasser, 2001). Proliferation of these kinds of theories could cause the list of proposed characteristics of the good life to get longer and longer, with none of the winnowing that is also beneficial for science. The "corral" of eudaimonic constructs could grow larger and larger, until it has almost caught up in size to the larger corral of positive psychology constructs.

In contrast, ***eudaimonia "goes right" when it focuses on understanding the nature of virtuous activity, with a goal of finding out which activities are demonstrably best for people.*** Eudaimonia is to be found in the things that people *do,* not in the ways that they *feel*. Regarded in this way, the scientific enterprise of eudaimonia involves trying to determine *which* activities, done in *which* ways by *which* people, are most productive of well-being and development – both in the individual and in his/her community and culture. I will argue that eudaimonia should almost always be kept on the predictor, not the outcome, side of the equation, and that on the outcome side we should keep things simple, by relying on subjective well-being (SWB), i.e., the combination of high positive mood, high life-satisfaction, and low negative mood. I will also show that SWB is fully sufficient to use as a criterion variable for comparing and distinguishing between "lower" and "higher" candidate measures of eudaimonic activity and living. In particular, SWB should not be conceptualized or presented as a measure of "mere hedonic well-being," defined as well-being based on mere pleasure and self-indulgence.

In the second part of the chapter I will argue that the organismic philosophical perspective is most fruitful for conceptualizing and categorizing the various candidate eudaimonic activities. This perspective views each human being as a living system, which in the optimal case grows and evolves throughout its life-time, continually enhancing its own skills and capacities while achieving ever-greater levels of personal complexity and social integration. The organismic perspective provides a way of refuting Nussbaum's (2008) proposal that feelings of satisfaction are a sign that one is only a "dumb animal," smug in its abandonment of growth and development. From the organismic perspective (and a proper eudaimonic perspective), feelings of satisfaction are precisely the rewards that we should expect for jobs well done, tasks well completed, and developmental stages well negotiated. I will tie this view to the decades-long research program of Self-determination theory, focusing on the vital role of intrinsic motivation, with its concomitant feelings of enjoyment and satisfaction, in peoples' growth and development.

I will conclude the chapter with a discussion of my own theory of "self-concordance," which reframes important SDT concepts within a personal goal striving context. The self-concordance model provides a way to conceptualize optimal self-initiated activity, and also provides a way to approach the eudaimonic concept of "the daimon." The self-concordance model asserts that the ignorant conscious self, whose function is (in part) to select and endorse life-goals to pursue, often selects wrongly. Peer pressures, advertising messages, incorrect self-images, immaturity, and inability to process emotional information, can all lead people to select personally inappropriate goals – goals that do not express a person's daimon, i.e., his or her actual developmental potentials. The self-concordance model is a well-validated eudaimonic theory of well-being, specifying the most effective kinds of goal contents and goal motivations for enhancing happiness and well-being. Also, it is a model validated almost entirely with respect to the effects of self-concordance on "mere" garden-variety SWB. In the context of this chapter, the self-concordance research serves as a case example of how (I believe) a eudaimonic theory should be constructed and tested.

36.2 The True Meaning of Eudaimonia

To burrow deeper into this topic, we need only turn to the Encyclopedia Brittanica (http://www.britannica.com/EBchecked/topic/194960/eudaemonism):

> ***Eudaimonism: in ethics, a self-realization theory that makes happiness or personal well-being the chief good for man. The Greek word eudaimonia means literally "the state of having a good indwelling spirit, a good genius"; and "happiness" is not at all an adequate translation of this word. Happiness, indeed, is usually thought of as a state of mind that results from or accompanies some actions. But Aristotle's answers to the question "What is eudaimonia?" (namely, that which is "activity in accordance with virtue"; or that which is "contemplation") show that for him eudaimonia was not a state of mind consequent on or accompanying certain activities but is a name for these activities themselves. "What is eudaimonia?" is then the same question as "What are the best activities of which man is capable?"***

I am in agreement with every facet of this definition, because it precisely describes the focus of most of my research activity during my career! Below, I will first discuss each sentence within this definition. Then, I will explain how many different strains of my past research program have followed from this definition, approaching it from a variety of different angles. Then I will conclude the section by describing a very current research example.

"Happiness or well-being is the chief good for man." This sentence suggests that well-being, properly conceived, is an important good, the desired end of all of our personal and economic activity. This statement is tremendously useful, because it makes very clear how we can evaluate all behavioral prescriptions, interventions, practices, and beliefs: do they (or do they not) improve the well-being of those who engage in them? In the same way that "the health of the patient" is the primary criterion to use in judging whether a medical treatment is efficacious, the "well-being of the person" is the primary criterion to use in judging whether a psychological (or other) intervention is efficacious. Of course, there are other potential targets for psychological interventions besides well-being or happiness, such as stress management skills, critical thinking skills, optimistic reframing skills, and so on. I am merely suggesting that when the target of the intervention is peoples' overall positive state of mind, then SWB should be the primary outcome measure. Of course, it would be dubious to insist that "no activity can have value unless it brings SWB." There are many bases for valuation besides "whether it makes me happy." It would probably be more accurate to say that "if an activity harms SWB, its value is questionable."

In my own research I use the terms "Well-being" and "Happiness" interchangeably, just as does the first sentence of the Brittanica definition. Empirically, I use Diener's (1984, 1994) conception of Subjective Well Being (SWB), which is operationalized as the combination of high positive mood, high life-satisfaction, and low negative mood. Busseri and Sadava (2011) showed that these three measures form a single latent construct (upon which negative affect loads negatively), justifying the creation of a single combination variable, although of course the component measures can be examined separately for some purposes.

SWB is a desirable criterion measure not only because it is singular, but also, because it is relatively content-free: It references biologically-based emotions with straightforward translations into nearly every language, and makes no content-based assumptions about the causes or sources of mood (be they physiological, cognitive, circumstantial, or cultural), and it references general life-satisfaction, making no assumptions about the causes or sources of satisfaction (be

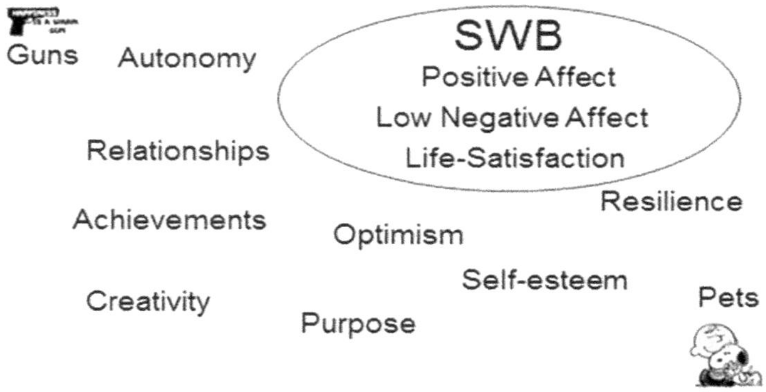

Fig. 36.1 Restricting the empirical the empirical definition of happiness to SWB

they biological, cognitive, circumstantial, or cultural). Defining happiness in this way keeps "psychosocial content" (Sheldon, 2013) out of the criterion measure, putting content only on the predictor side, so that the effects of each type of content (or activity, or practice, or attitude) can be evaluated against a consistent, unbiased standard. Figure 36.1 graphically depicts my proposal, showing that the entities "on the inside of the well-being circle" should be strictly limited, rather than being expanded to include the many additional qualities or characteristics of experience that might tempt researchers. In this same vein, Kashdan and Steger (2011) discussed "bracket creep," in which more and more constructs become encompassed within an ever-expanding conception of well-being.

Keeping psychosocial content on the predictor side allows us to avoid the potential pitfalls of confusing the causes of happiness with the outcome of happiness. Remember the saying: "Happiness is a warm puppy." Wrong! Happiness may be *caused* by a warm puppy (or by a warm gun, or by a warm friend), but a warm puppy is not happiness itself! Happiness itself is SWB. Consistent with this assertion, the philosopher Daniel Haybron argues: "to be happy is roughly for one's emotional condition to be broadly positive with only minor negatives, embodying a stance of psychic affirmation" (Haybron, 2008; p. 182). Again, this is SWB.

But doesn't the SWB measure miss the finer, more virtuous aspects of a life well lived? In point of fact, it does *not* miss them. SWB *suffices* to distinguish "higher" from "lower" forms of activity. Twenty years of research have now shown us that activities or goals that are overly hedonistic, narcissistic, self-centered, anti-social, self-indulgent, materialistic, and so on, are detrimental to, not helpful for, SWB (Crocker & Canevello, 2012; Kasser, 2002; Sheldon, 2014). Non-eudaimonic happiness strategies (i.e., being selfish, self-indulgent, or addicted) do not pay off, even though we may secretly believe that they do! (I call this "the myth of the happy hedonist") In short, we do not need to posit alternative forms of well-being beyond simple SWB, in order to find out what makes for a good life; SWB is itself sufficient to empirically distinguish between mere happiness *pretenders* and *actual* producers of happiness. To put it somewhat poetically, when there is eudaimonic (or organismically congruent) living, there is a "fire burning brightly." Feelings of well-being, the natural reward for a life well lived, predominate within such living systems (Sheldon, 2013). What's more, they have demonstrable strong positive effects on a myriad of life outcomes (Lyubomirsky, King, & Diener, 2005).

The Greek word eudaimonia means literally "the state of having a good indwelling spirit, a good genius"; and "happiness" is not at all an adequate translation of this word. The thrust of this second definitional sentence is that we must define eudaimonia not as a feeling, but as a way of living (Ryan, Huta, & Deci, 2013; Huta, Chap. 15, this volume; Ryan and Martela, Chap. 7, this volume). Although the first sentence of the definition suggests that happiness (a feeling) is the ultimate good, this second sentence indicates that eudaimonia itself is NOT this ultimate good; instead, eudaimonia involves enhancing or augmenting the manifestation of "a good indwelling spirit." In my own research, such spirit is best represented by the state of "self-concordance," in which a person has managed to select personal goals that properly represent his or her growth and happiness potentials (i.e. his/her daimon). When a person's goals are in harmony with his or her enduring values, talents, and interests, then that person is able to act in a way that is more effective, connective, and happiness-producing. These ideas will be considered in greater detail at the end of the chapter.

Happiness, indeed, is usually thought of as a state of mind that results from or accompanies some actions. But Aristotle's answers to the question "What is eudaimonia?" (Namely, that which is "activity in accordance with virtue"; or that which is "contemplation") show that for him eudaimonia was not a state of mind consequent on or accompanying certain activities but is a name for these activities themselves. The third sentence can be read as criticizing the unfortunate tendency of some eudaimonia researchers to think of eudaimonia as an outcome – as a state of mind that results from activity. Arguably, the very title of this book makes this mistake, by referring to "Eudaimonic well-being!" Again, I am advocating keeping eudaimonia only on the "predictor" side. The fourth sentence reinforces this argument with the assertion that eudaimonia is NOT a state of mind consequent upon doing certain activities, rather, it is the activities themselves. Hence, the problem of eudaimonic living becomes, for all of us: "What activities should I choose, and how should I pursue them?" Good answers to these questions, I believe, are the answers (activities) that bring us greater SWB.

"What is eudaimonia?" is then the same question as "What are the best activities of which man is capable?" This final sentence precisely summarizes the main point of this part of the chapter. Eudaimonia is not a diverse set of well-being outcomes (feelings or states of mind), which must somehow all be approached and optimized simultaneously. Rather, it is "right living," i.e. living that is in accordance with one's own strengths and developmental potentials. Right living brings its own reward, namely, SWB.

36.3 A Current Empirical Example

In sum, I advocate a research approach in which various candidate measures of eudaimonic living (i.e. whatever constructs that the researchers hypothesize might be virtuous, praise-worthy, or pursuit-worthy) are simultaneously compared as predictors of SWB. This allows a clear determination of which constructs actually work, or work better, at least for the purposes of bringing psychological well-being. I have taken this approach to examine which "candidate psychological needs" are actually needed (Sheldon et al., 2001); which measures of optimal functioning at which levels of personality are most conducive to well-being (Sheldon & Tan, 2007; Sheldon, Cheng, & Hilpert, 2011); which type of goals, once attained, best enhance people's well-being (Sheldon & Elliot, 1999, Sheldon & Kasser, 1998); which measure of balanced time-use best predicts well-being (Sheldon, Cummins, & Khamble, 2010); which type of personality integration best predicts well-being (Sheldon & Kasser, 1995); which type of law job better predicts well-being, money or service (Sheldon & Krieger, 2014); whether material affluence or time affluence best predicts well-being (Kasser & Sheldon, 2009); and so on (Sheldon & Elliot, 2000; Sheldon & Lyubomirsky, 2012).

Most recently, Sheldon, Jose, Kashdan, and Jarden (2015) explored the concept of "personality strengths" using a large longitudinal data-set ($N = 755$). They compared ten personality strengths that have emerged within recent positive psychology research (Grit, Gratitude, Curiosity, Savoring, Control beliefs, Meaning in Life-Presence, Strength-Use, Engagement Orientation, Pleasure Orientation, and Meaning Orientation), in two different regards: (1) as variables that might predict enhanced goal attainment, 6 months later; and (2) as variables that might amplify (moderate) the effects of enhanced goal attainment upon enhanced SWB. That is, each of the candidate strengths was comparatively evaluated as a baseline personality characteristic that might (a) boost people's ability to achieve their goals, and (b) enable them to derive proportionally greater well-being boosts from their goal attainments. To evaluate the robustness of the findings, we adopted an internal replication criterion. Specifically, we only interpreted effects that emerged twice: both during a T1-T2 period (a 6-month interval) and during a T2-T3 period (a second 6-month interval).

As hypothesized, the analyses revealed that initial Grit was the personality strength (out of ten strengths) that was most relevant for boosting peoples' goal-attainment, a finding which was replicated during both time periods. This made sense because Grit is defined as an attitude of perseverance in the face of any and all obstacles; Grit involves dogged persistence no matter what (Duckworth). Also as hypothesized, initial Curiosity (Kashdan) was the only personality strength (again, out of ten strengths) that significantly moderated the effects of increased goal-attainment upon increased SWB, in both time periods. This made sense because Curiosity is close in meaning to Intrinsic motivation, which has previously been shown to amplify goal-attainment effects upon well-being (Sheldon & Elliot, 1999; Sheldon & Kasser, 1998). When one acts to satisfy one's curiosity, one learns, develops, and becomes happier through one's attainments. This latter finding is very relevant to my arguments in the next section of this chapter.

The significance of Sheldon et al. (2015) study of personality strengths is that it: (a) winnows rather than expands the number of constructs researchers need to consider, at least within the particular domain of personal goal strivings, inviting studies of the finer details of the identified constructs; (b) models an important general strategy for testing and comparing competing theories and measures of optimal functioning, via their demonstrated effects upon SWB; and (c) shows which personality strengths are worthy of strengthening, if we want to boost peoples' goal-functioning (namely, their curiosity and their grit). Should the other eight personality strengths that we examined be abandoned or de-valued? Not necessarily – they may have positive effects on SWB via other routes or mechanisms besides goal-striving. For example, gratitude may boost SWB via positive interpersonal processes, processes which were not studied by Sheldon et al. Gratitude could be tested, at the same time that forgiveness, empathy, intimacy, and altruism are also tested, as interpersonal personality strengths that can boost peoples' SWB. The field is ripe for such studies.

The main point of describing this study was to show the usefulness of keeping happiness, and its potential predictors, within separate categories. SWB can thus be used as a sword, to cut through the thickets of positive psychology and eudaimonic psychology. Arguably, positive psychology has engendered a bewildering proliferation of strengths and constructs (Sheldon, 2011), with few ways to decide what they're really good for. In the Sheldon et al. (2015) study, were were instead left with a more parsimonious number of strengths (two of the ten initial candidate strengths), a pair now shown to be most salubrious in this particular context, of longitudinal goal-strivings. I believe that most eudaimonia research should be similarly organized.

36.4 The Role of Satisfaction in Optimal Functioning

One focus of this edited volume is Nussbaum's (2008) philosophical analysis of happiness, and her critique of the way that some psychologists use (or mis-use) the term. I confess to lacking the background to fully understand and appreciate Nussbaum's analysis, as is often the case when I read the philosophical literature on happiness. Some of the distinctions seem like unnecessary relics from entrenched or outmoded conceptual systems, or seem of questionable relevance to current psychological theories and research findings. However, in this section of the chapter I would like to address one of Nussbaum's statements in particular. On p. 82 she writes, concerning her personal attitude towards happiness: "So, if I ever notice myself feeling feelings of satisfaction, I blame myself and think that, insofar as I have those feelings, I am like Mill's 'pig satisfied' or Aristotle's 'dumb grazing animals,' and thus, reflectively, I report dissatisfaction with my life as a whole." I think that Nussbaum is attempting to characterize feelings of satisfaction (such as might be reported in response to the Satisfaction with Life Scale, an aspect of SWB; Diener, Emmons, Larsen, & Griffin, 1985) as antithetical to growth and development – suggesting that satisfaction is *not* an appropriate criterion variable for evaluating the eudaimonic quality of the life being lived. Satisfaction functions, Nussbaum implies, as a "Stop" rule that halts and de-energizes activity – and we should not succumb to it.

But what if feelings of satisfaction actually function more like a "Go" rule than a "Stop" rule? Consider – when Nussbaum finished writing her essay, she likely had some feeling of satisfaction, a job well-done. Perhaps she felt that this is a good direction of inquiry for her, one that is interesting and likely to be a fruitful avenue for further development. If so, I would argue that she *deserved* to have and to enjoy this experience. Positive feelings of satisfaction and enjoyment are precisely the rewards and reinforcements that we are given for pursuing interests, meeting challenges, rising to occasions, and so on. When we experience satisfaction, we do not then back away from further engagement in the arena in which it was felt; instead, we are likely to push further into that arena (after a period of rest), in search of further satisfactions.

In the language of Self-determination theory (Deci & Ryan, 1985; Ryan & Deci, 2008), "intrinsic motivation" is behavior that is undertaken for its own sake, i.e. because one is curious, intrigued, fascinated, or simply enjoys the journey. The concept of intrinsic motivation was once radical (Deci & Ryan, 1985) because it did not fit with formerly dominant drive-based or biological deficit-reduction accounts of motivation. Now, however, it is widely accepted that intrinsic motivation is vital for cognitive development. Humans need to engage in much self-initiated, self-directed activity to get the stimulation needed to develop their brains to their full potential. Intrinsic motivation is one of the most important ways in which this happens.

In this view, feelings of satisfaction are not antithetical to growth – rather, they are essential for growth! Feelings of satisfaction are precisely the sign that tells one that one is pointed in the right direction (Sheldon, 2011). Nussbaum's statements only make sense *if* one assumes that satisfaction is a lower, merely "hedonic" form of well-being, a form that is based ultimately in animal laziness or self-indulgence. But again, I believe it would be a huge mistake to define SWB as mere "hedonic" well-being, a lower order or quality well-being than eudaimonic well-being. Instead, SWB is perhaps our best, most unbiased metric for evaluating and comparing the eudaimonic quality of various styles or approaches to life. Which eudaimonic candidates for "living well" produce "the supreme good," namely, SWB?

36.5 The Organismic Perspective

My arguments are based in organismic or living systems approaches to conceptualizing human nature. According to Deci and Ryan (2000), humans have a natural growth instinct or propensity, that is, a desire to become more differentiated and integrated, to create and consolidate new psychic structures, and to become more deeply embedded within relationships and their communities. This instinct unfolds in a dialectical process in which the environment (at times) resists the agency and self-authorship of developing individuals, posing challenges that must be overcome. Growth and development are not a given; they must be actively pursued, within (ideally) a supportive environment. Again, however, environments often fail to support peoples' intrinsic motivations and growth impulses, instead coercing, bribing, or controlling people to act in ways that do not serve their growth and well-being. Personality development is in large part a quest for greater ego autonomy in the face of such impediments so as to become more self-determining and self-regulating over time.

In this view, the main "eudaimonic problem" that many people face is *not* that they are *too* satisfied; instead, it is that they have been induced to take up goals or pursuits that are too *un*-satisfying, which do not represent their growth impulses, and which even actively impede their growth and development. Sheldon (2014) discussed the case of "Anna," an unhappy 30 year old lawyer whose main goal in life was to escape her terrible job by becoming wealthy and retiring in "only" 15 years, at the age of 45. Although Anna was fictional, her case is prototypical in many ways. Somewhere along the way Anna lost the ideals that originally brought her to law school, becoming corrupted by her success to take the highest-paying job offered to her (e.g., within a very large private law firm). Knowing that "making partner" was the standard of success within this context, and knowing that this would make her wealthy, Anna subscribed to a miserable life involving extremely long hours, intensive competition and back-biting, and the degrading process of padding her billable hours. Anna's long-time friends talk about the negative changes the job has caused within Anna. However, Anna herself seems oblivious (a fact that is itself a symptom of her condition). Is she really going to tolerate 15 more years of misery, before she can finally retire and escape? Would she have any remaining capacity to enjoy life, at that point?

One day at work, the image of an old college friend ("Sarah") flashed across Anna's mind, and not for the first time. Although Anna did not know it, this image was actually a growth impulse, bubbling up from her unconscious. This time Anna googled Sarah, and discovered that she is still active in the environmental interests that she and Anna once shared. A reconnection was made, and Anna soon found herself spending much time doing volunteer work for Sarah's current organization. It felt so good, so right! After a few months, Anna was finally able to make the break: she resigned her high pressure, money-focused job, to take a position with an environmental law firm at less than half the salary, leading a team of younger lawyers working on an array of environmental initiatives. Half the money, but twice the SWB – and she hopes to keep working until she is 75, not 45! In this example, notice that the feelings of satisfaction deriving from trying out the new volunteer activity were precisely the "Go" rule that supported Anna's attempt to re-make her life, not a "Stop" rule limiting her to animal-like contentedness, as suggested by Nussbaum's (2008) analysis.

It is also worth noting that there was no certainty that Anna *would* be able to escape her plight; many people in her position do not, instead choosing "the money" (or financial entanglements) over intrinsic motivation and fulfillment. Consistent with the dialectical process posited by organismic perspective, development is never certain; it depends on the person's ability to find and express a sense of agency within their lives, to become an origin rather than a pawn within their own lives (deCharms, 1968). In some cases, positive movement and change could be stalled for years, for decades, or even permanently.

36.6 The Self-Concordance Model

My Self-concordance model (Sheldon & Elliot 1999; Sheldon, 2004; Sheldon, 2014) focuses on the idiographic, self-generated life-goals that people select for themselves. The model assumes that conscious processes are strongly involved in goal selection, as consciousness is required to "cross the Rubicon" from deliberation to implementation (Gollwitzer, 2012), and to begin to process of regulating the action system in accordance with the selected goals (Carver & Scheier, 1981; Sheldon, 2014). However, the model also assumes that consciousness has only a tenuous connection to the personality as a whole. The conscious self serves as a "representative" of the personality, a kind of self-simulation being enacted in real-time (Sheldon, 2004). Also, consciousness (or system 2 thinking; Kahneman, 2011) is easily swayed by various biases, including self-enhancing biases, the impact bias, and the focalism bias, and by various salient concepts and messages that have been promoted or primed by the person's environment. Also, consciousness is seriously limited in how much information it can consider at once, and in its access to the information derivable from emotional experience. As a result, people can have serious problems "knowing what to want." What's more, the nature of the goal striving system is such that people have serious difficulty even *knowing* that they do not know what to want! Without adequate information or reflection, we lurch towards targets that seized our attention in the past, resisting all of our friends' attempts to get us to "hit the re-set button." We are myopic and single-minded as we "stumble towards happiness" (Gilbert, 2006).

Anna is a case in point. Earlier in her life she had virtuous (eudaimonic) ideals, revolving around using the study of the law to advance meaningful causes in the world. However she lost touch with those ideals, getting swept up in the heady sense of being a hot-shot law student who edits the Law Review and gets interviews with all the biggest and "best" firms (Sheldon & Krieger, 2014). Now at age 30, despite much outward success, she seems to be spiraling downward, emotionally, with no idea how to correct the problem (the best she can come up with is sticking it out for another 15 years, when she can finally retire early!). Her current goals ("get wealthy and retire by age 45") are clearly "non-concordant" with her best developmental and happiness potentials. What happened?

What happened was this: at some point, Anna stopped paying attention to what was satisfying and what wasn't. When she thought about it at all, satisfaction had become a "matter for the future" or "a problem that would be resolved after the next promotion." The only way back for her (and people like her) is to start trying different kinds of activities, and to rely on the satisfactions these bring (or don't bring) to guide them. Fortunately, in Anna's case, she was able to begin this process and see it through, ultimately creating a much more fulfilling and rewarding career, even though it only paid half as much. She was able to select, and dedicate her life to, a more self-concordant set of goals (e.g. "clear the way for green energy initiatives in my state," "mentor my team so they grow personally as well as professionally"). This helps her to chart a course towards becoming the wise and generative leader she could possibly become. Anna's new job affords her a precious opportunity: to actualize her growth potentials, to move towards and finally become one with her own "daimon."

Importantly, I do not view "the daimon" as a mystical entity, as a soul, or as a pre-determined destiny. Instead, the daimon is simply individual human potential (or stated differently, potential humanness!) – the most skilled, compassionate, wise, and altruistic person that each of us has the capacity to become, if all goes well. Of course, we may never know about some or even many of these potentials, unless we find a way to develop them. Furthermore, potential is not just a one way street: for example, Anna might have been a skilled outreach counselor or a skilled systems engineer, rather than a skilled environmental lawyer. However, I do believe that each human living system tends to have a "best solution" or "small set of best solutions" to the problem of "what should I do with myself in life?," solutions which best solve the massive parallel constraint-satisfaction problem that we all face as we consider our options in light of our evolving interests, talents, and commitments. For example, although "stay-at-home mother" may be a perfectly self-concordant dominant activity for some or many women, Anna's high need for achievement and highly logical mind made it unlikely that this activity alone would have expressed and channeled her potential. Indeed, "environmental lawyer" may in fact be the best Anna could have done, given her values and talents. She got herself halfway to this eudaimonic occupation by getting a law degree, and was finally able to get herself the rest of the way there, with encouragement from her friend Sarah and with considerable personal courage.

This concludes a conceptual consideration of the self-concordance construct. Normally in a chapter of this kind I would review the multifaceted longitudinal research that supports the premises of the model, but instead I will refer the reader to my recent review article on self-concordance ("Becoming oneself: The important role of self-concordant goal striving;" Sheldon, 2014). Now, I will extend the primary argument of this chapter one step further.

36.7 SWB as a National Indicator

Joining with Diener and others (Diener & Seligman, 2004, Diener, 2006), I believe that *the world needs to agree on a single indicator of well-being, and that every country needs to use that measure as it tracks the effects of various policy initiatives*. Simply getting politicians to agree that their job security and approval requires them to maximize the subjective well-being of their constituents would be a huge step forward. Unfortunately, we are still stuck in a "halfway zone" in which (a) Gross National Product (GNP) is still the predominantly used indicator of national thriving, and (b) Gross National Happiness (GNH) is still too often ignored, or measured by a fractured variety of different indicators which make cross-national comparisons impossible. Again, I advocate using SWB for this GNH index, i.e., some combination of negative mood, positive mood, and life-satisfaction. However, it is not essential that the measures be the ones I use (the SWLS and the PANAS); SWB can probably be measured reasonably well with many fewer items, which might come from the SWLS or the PANAS, or from other satisfaction or mood measures. The important thing is to *agree on what SWB is, and agree on a consistent set of items to measure it*.

Unfortunately, the concept of "Eudaimonic well-being" (EWB; the very topic of this book!), and continuing research under the aegis of the term "EWB", is likely to forestall agreement on a standard conception and measure of well-being. I believe that EWB confuses things because it conflates the causes of well-being with well-being itself and makes the concept of happiness seem ever more broad and diffuse. Happiness is NOT a warm puppy, nor a warm friend, nor a warm gun: Happiness is SWB. Puppies, guns, and friends all need to be tested as potential causes of SWB, not assumed to be part of SWB themselves. "Living well" (Ryan et al., 2013) brings happiness (SWB), and "living poorly" does not. Hedonic, materialistic, selfish, and narcissistic ways of being and living do *not* suffice to bring SWB: the "myth of the happy hedonist" is false!

If the field would agree to my proposal to define happiness as SWB, and to locate all of the constructs that eudaimonic researchers study within a different category (i.e., the category of activities/behaviors, or the category of psychosocial experiences resulting from those activities), then we could present a unified front to the governments and surveying organizations of the world when they look to psychology for guidance on how to assess the elusive state of individual thriving. Let's keep it simple (SWB), thereby opening up the field for rapid advancement in understanding the causes of happiness!

References

Busseri, M. A., & Sadava, S. W. (2011). A review of the tripartite structure of subjective well-being: Implications for conceptualization, operationalization, analysis, andsynthesis. *Personality and Social Psychology Review, 15*(3), 290–314. doi:10.1177/1088868310391271.

Carver, C. S., & Scheier, M. F. (1981). *Attention and self-regulation*. New York: Springer.

Crocker, J., & Canevello, A. (2012). Consequences of self-image and compassionate goals. In P. Devine, A. Plant, P. Devine, & A. Plant (Eds.), *Advances in experimental social psychology, Vol 45* (pp. 229–277). San Diego, CA: Academic.

deCharms, R. (1968). *Personal causation*. New York: Academic.

Deci, E. L., & Ryan, R. M. (1985). *Intrinsic motivation and self-determination in human behavior*. New York: Plenum.

Deci, E. L., & Ryan, R. M. (2000). The "what" and "why" of goal pursuits: Human needs and the self-determination of behavior. *Psychological Inquiry, 11*, 227–268.

Diener, E. (1984). Subjective well-being. *Psychological Bulletin, 95*, 542–575.

Diener, E. (1994). Assessing subjective well-being: Progress and opportunities. *Social Indicators Research, 31*, 103–157.

Diener, E. (2006). Guidelines for national indicators of subjective well-being and ill-being. *Journal of Happiness Studies, 7*, 397–404.

Diener, E., Emmons, R., Larsen, R., & Griffin, S. (1985). The satisfaction with life scale. *Journal of Personality Assessment, 47*, 1105–1117.

Diener, E., & Seligman, M. P. (2004). Beyond money: Toward an economy of well-being. *Psychological Science in the Public Interest, 5*(1), 1–31. doi:10.1111/j.0963-7214.2004.00501001.

Gilbert, D. (2006). *Stumbling on happiness*. New York: Alfred A. Knopf.

Gollwitzer, P. M. (2012). Mindset theory of action phases. In P. M. Van Lange, A. W. Kruglanski, E. T. Higgins, P. M. Van Lange, A. W. Kruglanski, & E. T. Higgins (Eds.), *Handbook of theories of social psychology (Vol 1)* (pp. 526–545). Thousand Oaks, CA: Sage.

Haybron, D. (2008). *The pursuit of unhappiness*. Oxford: Oxford University Press.

Huppert, F., & So, T. (2009). Retrieved March 21, 2011, from http://www.isqols2009.istitutodeglinnocenti.it/Content_en/Huppert.pdf

Kahneman, D. (2011). *Thinking, fast and slow*. New York: Farrar, Straus and Giroux.

Kashdan, T. B., Biswas-Diener, R., & King, L. A. (2008). Reconsidering happiness: The costs of distinguishing between hedonics and eudaimonia. *Journal of Positive Psychology, 3*, 219–233.

Kashdan, T. B., & Steger, M. F. (2011). Challenges, pitfalls, and aspirations for positive psychology. In K. M. Sheldon, T. B. Kashdan, & M. F. Steger (Eds.), *Designing positive psychology: Taking stock and moving forward* (pp. 9–24). New York: Oxford University Press.

Kasser, T. (2002). *The high price of materialism*. Cambridge, MA: MIT Press.

Kasser, T., & Sheldon, K. M. (2009). Material and time affluence as predictors of subjective well-being. *Journal of Business Ethics, 84*, 243–255.

King, L. A. (2009). Are we there yet? What happened on the way to the demise of positive psychology. In K. Sheldon, T. Kashdan, & M. Steger (Eds.), *Designing positive psychology: Taking stock and moving forward* (pp. 439–446). New York: Oxford University Press.

Lyubomirsky, S., King, L. A., & Diener, E. (2005). The benefits of frequent positive affect: Does happiness lead to success? *Psychological Bulletin, 131*, 803–855.

Nussbaum, M. (2008). Who is the happy warrior? *The Journal of Legal Studies, 37*, xx.

Ryan, R. M., & Deci, E. L. (2008). Self-determination theory and the role of basic psychological needs in personality and the organization of behavior. In O. P. John, R. W. Robins, L. A. Pervin, O. P. John, R. W. Robins, & L. A. Pervin (Eds.), *Handbook of personality: Theory and research* (3rd ed., pp. 654–678). New York: Guilford Press.

Ryan, R. M., Huta, V., & Deci, E. L. (2013). Living well: A self-determination theory perspective on eudaimonia. In A. Delle Fave & A. Delle Fave (Eds.), *The exploration of happiness: Present and future perspectives* (pp. 117–139). New York: Springer.

Ryff, C. D., & Keyes, C. L. M. (1995). The structure of psychological well-being revisited. *Journal of Personality & Social Psychology, 69*, 719–727.

Seligman, M. E. P. (2011). *Flourish: A visionary new understanding of happiness and well-being*. New York: Free Press.

Sheldon, K. M. (2004). *Optimal human being: An integrated multi-level perspective*. Mahwah, NJ: Erlbaum.

Sheldon, K. M. (2011). What's positive about positive psychology? Reducing value-bias and enhancing integration within the field. In K. M. Sheldon, T. Kashdan, & M. Steger (Eds.), *Designing the future of positive psychology: Taking stock and moving forward* (pp. 421–429). Oxford: Oxford Press.

Sheldon, K. M. (2013). Individual daimon, universal needs, and subjective well-being: Happiness as the natural consequence of a life well lived. In A. Waterman (Ed.), *The best within us: Positive psychology perspectives on eudaimonic functioning* (pp. 119–137). Washington, DC: American Psychological Association.

Sheldon, K. M. (2014). Becoming oneself: The central role of self-concordant goal selection. *Personality and Social Psychology Review, 18*, 349–365.

Sheldon, K. M., Cheng, C., & Hilpert, J. (2011). Understanding well-being and optimal functioning: Applying the Multilevel Personality in Context (MPIC) model. *Psychological Inquiry, 22*, 1–16.

Sheldon, K. M., Cummins, R., & Khamble, S. (2010). Life-balance and well-being: Testing a two-pronged conceptual and measurement approach. *Journal of Personality, 78*, 1093–1134.

Sheldon, K. M., & Elliot, A. J. (1999). Goal striving, need-satisfaction, and longitudinal well-being: The self-concordance model. *Journal of Personality and Social Psychology, 76*, 482–497.

Sheldon, K. M., & Elliot, A. J. (2000). Personal goals in social roles: Divergences and convergences across roles and levels of analysis. *Journal of Personality, 68*, 51–84.

Sheldon, K. M., Elliot, A. J., Kim, Y., & Kasser, T. (2001). What's satisfying about satisfying events? Comparing ten candidate psychological needs. *Journal of Personality and Social Psychology, 80*, 325–339.

Sheldon, K. M., Jose, P. E., Kashdan, T. B., & Jarden, A. (2015). Personality, effective goal-striving, and enhanced well-being: Comparing 10 candidate personality strengths. *Personality and Social Psychology Bulletin, 4*, 575–585.

Sheldon, K. M., & Kasser, T. (1995). Coherence and congruence: Two aspects of personality integration. *Journal of Personality and Social Psychology, 68*, 531–543.

Sheldon, K. M., & Kasser, T. (1998). Pursuing personal goals: Skills enable progress, but not all progress is beneficial. *Personality and Social Psychology Bulletin, 24*, 1319–1331.

Sheldon, K. M., & Krieger, L. (2014). Service job lawyers are happier than money job lawyers, despite their lower income. *Journal of Positive Psychology, 9*, 219–226.

Sheldon, K. M., & Lyubomirsky, S. (2012). The challenge of staying happier: Testing the hedonic adaptation prevention (HAP) model. *Personality and Social Psychology Bulletin, 38*, 670–680.

Sheldon, K. M., & Tan, H. (2007). The multiple determination of well-being: Independent effects of positive needs, traits, goals, selves, social supports, and cultural contexts. *Journal of Happiness Studies, 8*, 565–592.

Social Planning Without Bentham or Aristotle: Towards Dignified and Socially Engaged Well-being

37

Neil Thin

37.1 Introduction

As well-being research matures into a new phase of active public engagement, we must consider the user-friendliness and effectiveness of our analytical language. In public discourse, obscure jargon is unwelcome and unhelpful unless it is demonstrably better than everyday speech in some way. Either it has to be more precise, or else it must inspire new ways of talking and thinking. I will argue here that the first of these justifications certainly doesn't apply to 'eudaimonia', which is far too diverse in its referents to serve as an analytical term (as previously pointed out by Kashdan, Biswas-Diener, & King, 2008). If we must use an ancient Greek term for well-being, its justification is more likely to come rather indirectly from its ability to stoke interesting enquiries and productive arguments.

But can't we just discuss the goodness of life in plain English terms that are more readily understood, more specific, and less confusing? 'Happiness' is a familiar term that has served well as a bridge between everyday conversations and academic research on many aspects of well-being, including a limitless variety of kinds of pleasures, motivations, personal growth, satisfactions, and overall flourishing. But happiness evidently isn't any one definable or measurable thing, and the common tendency to reduce its meaning to mental pleasures and satisfactions may justify the introduction of other terms that point towards greater sophistication. 'Well-being' serves this function if you want to talk about the good life in general, or 'functional well-being' (Vittersø, 2013, Chap. 17, this volume) if you want to make a general insistence on actively living well, or 'autonomy' or 'sense of coherence' and so on if you want to identify more specific dimensions. As well as pointing towards the need for specification, we can use a variety of terms to inspire people by reminding them that 'happiness isn't everything' (Ryff, 1989). We don't need a hard-to-pronounce and often confusing term like 'eudaimonia' to make progress in conversations about well-being.

Implicitly recognizing that the term has to offer something else, users seem to want to make eudaimonia fit their particular purposes, many of which have questionable relevance to the ways in which, for example, Aristotle used the term. Two striking examples are its new roles as a general term for the 'nonhedonic' aspects of well-being, or for approaches to learning about well-being that de-emphasise emotional experiences and subjective evaluations. These are perplexing, given that Aristotle clearly associated eudaimonia with pleasure and with subjective exploration of what it means to live well. Psychological eudaimonists have fought hard to justify the

N. Thin (✉)
University of Edinburgh, Edinburgh, Scotland
e-mail: n.thin@ed.ac.uk

J. Vittersø (ed.), *Handbook of Eudaimonic Well-Being*, International Handbooks of Quality-of-Life,
DOI 10.1007/978-3-319-42445-3_37

belief in distinctive nonhedonic mental goods, but their supporting evidence is mixed (Coyne, 2013; Disabato, Goodman, Kashdan, Short, & Jarden, 2015; Joshanloo, 2016). Eudaimonism has become embroiled.in forced polemics associated with snobbish moral disparagement of pleasure, with suspicious attitudes towards subjective experiences and self-reports, and with overheated enthusiasm for the relentless pursuit of 'authentic' and perfectionist forms of personal growth that may be associated with unnecessary psychological distress. When they sidestep such adversarialisms, most scholars and planners alike can quickly agree that we want people to live well and not only to feel good (Henderson & Knight, 2012). But you don't need to declare yourself a 'eudaimonist' or an Aristotelian to agree on that.

I would like to propose here a simple analytical approach to identifying what eudaimonism is all about, with a view to thinking more clearly about how well-being concepts add value in scholarship, policy and practice. Eudaimonism is, first and foremost, a 'positivity' discourse about how to live well. But it is also a particular kind of positivity discourse that casts suspicion on some other kinds of positivity (let's call this 'positivity minus') while also insisting on specifying characteristics of really good positivity ('positivity plus'). By outlining what these three aspects of eudaimonism have to offer, I will explore here some of the ways in which eudaimonism debates may have been generative, while also recognizing that busy social planners may justifiably choose to move on without feeling they ought to identify themselves with any particular camp. I will mainly focus on the various ways in which arguments, ideas, and concepts associated with eudaimonia manifest in discourses relating fairly directly to policy and practice in the promotion of well-being.

37.2 Positivity and Positivity Minus: What Is Eudaimonism Better Than?

There's a lunch place near my office which has a fine notice with one arrow pointing inside to 'soup' and another pointing away to 'not soup'. If only moral decisions could be that simple. Should I join the 'eudaimonist' camp or the non-eudaimonist? Have I any idea what these options mean? Those who argue that there are 'two traditions' in well-being scholarship, one organized around the concept of 'eudaimonia' and the other not (Deci & Ryan, 2008; Nussbaum, 2008/2012), seem to expect scholars and planners alike to choose one or the other as if this were an important and fairly clear choice. Is the eudaimonia option about truth (choosing 'real happiness' versus 'fake happiness'), or objectivity (subjective self-evaluations versus observations by others), or sophistication ('noble well-being' versus 'ignoble well-being'), or is it just about 'well-being' versus 'not well-being'?

A recent publication of a nine-point wishlist for 'eudaimonic' socio-economic policies seems to be based on the belief that eudaimonism makes important differences to planning (Crespo & Mesurado, 2015). Yet for all the meticulous examination of many debates between neo-Aristotelian moral philosophers and contemporary positive psychologists, the authors seem only to have come up with a general plea for 'egalitarian' policies, plus a mix of reminders that governments need to ensure provision of citizens' basic needs plus education and rule of law. This all looks like basic decent governance, but none of it looks distinctively 'eudaimonic', nor even interestingly well-being-focused. The core function of eudaimonism is simply that it draws our attention to well-being, but this positivity mainly becomes interesting through exploration of what it is different from, and what particular values it adds to public well-being discourse.

Let's have a look at some of the alternative worldviews or approaches that eudaimonist scholars and planners might say they are transcending. First, let's remind ourselves of three kinds of worldview that all well-being researchers and promoters urge us to transcend:

- **Pathological learning strategies**: the belief that researchers can learn about the human good mainly by looking at what goes wrong.
- **Negative utilitarianism and remedialist practices**: the principle that planners' priority (or only duty) should be to minimise or mitigate harms, not promote goods.

- **Instrumentalism**: the default practice of planners and researchers who emphasise goods that have instrumental rather than intrinsic value – e.g. economic activity rather than quality of life; medical services rather than health; or academic test scores rather than wisdom.

Eudaimonists and hedonists have far more in common with one another than they do with any of these three worldviews. They are interested in positivity, and in conversations about ultimate values and how to promote them. They foster appreciative learning strategies and aspirational policies and practices aimed at facilitating really good lives not just minimally adequate living conditions. Appreciative scholars want to learn about what goes right in people's lives. Aspirational planners want to actively facilitate opportunities for flourishing, not merely deal with problems and facilitate economic growth. Positive psychology announced itself by transcending the dominance of pathology and remedialist, deficit-oriented clinical practice. Among happiness survey researchers, 'beyond money' is a common call, steering our attention from means to ends (e.g. Diener & Seligman, 2004). In social planning, 'beyond GDP [Gross Domestic Product]' is the usual slogan (Fleurbaey & Blanchet, 2013). Tired of the naïve economic instrumentalism and more-is-betterism that tends to dominate public political discourse, social well-being promoters invite people to think instead about what really matters. As labels for these moves, 'well-being' or 'flourishing' are readily understood (Keyes and Haidt, 2002; Seligman, 2011), and even 'happiness' serves fine as a general rubric provided that you make it clear you aren't confining it to the narrow psychological senses of enjoyment and satisfaction.

But eudaimonists aren't satisfied with mere positivity. They insist that we take an interest in and promote the right kinds of positivity – those that amount to better living, not merely more enjoyment or more positive self-regard. So they distance themselves from two further sets of attitudes:

- **Hedonism**: the claim that the goodness of life is all about pleasure.
- **Subjectivism**: belief that individuals are the best judges of how much pleasure they experience, and of which kinds of pleasure are valuable to them.

It is, however, highly debatable whether either of these two polemical antagonisms is plausible if you want to promote better living. A sophisticated hedonist has no trouble explaining that so-called 'eudaimonic' goods (such as active virtue and self-actualisation) offer different kinds of pleasure, and that the good life is one in which a rich diversity or interesting balance of pleasures is enjoyed. Similarly, subjectivists can respond to eudaimonist challenges by simply pointing out that eudaimonism is about ultimate values, and that the process of valuation is unavoidably subjective. In other words, if 'beyond pleasure' and 'beyond subjectivism' are the value supposedly added by eudaimonism, this doesn't seem to justify the jargon. If someone is being naïve about the pursuit of simple pleasures or unduly respectful of particular subjective self-reports, you can simply say so, without trying to elevate your objections to the status of a principled objection to hedonism or subjectivism.

Eudaimonists often seem to become drawn into a position that seems polemically opposed to 'hedonic' conceptions of well-being (e.g. Huta & Waterman, 2014), so that 'eudaimonic' indicators, for example, are often explicitly addressed to 'nonhedonic' issues as if the possibility of pleasurable associations with the goods concerned were a form of contamination. This is counterintuitive to anyone who doesn't reduce 'pleasure' to some ignoble category of simple, short-lived, harmful or ignoble temptations. This function also risks tempting people into snobbish disparagement of simple pleasures as if they had no legitimate place in the good life. Instead of pitting pleasure against good living, we need to persuade people to find, for them, an optimal balance between pursuits that are mainly about pleasure and those that are mainly for the sake of other goods that are valuable in themselves

(Bates, 2013). The idea of 'nonsubjective' assessment of well-being seems more plausible, but someone still needs to choose the criteria, and the goods being assessed still largely depend for their value on mental processing, i.e. on subjectivity. In any case, those who assess subjective indicators aren't normally in the habit of claiming that these tell you all you need to know about well-being.

There is one further thing that eudaimonic objections tend to point us away from:

- **Quantitative reductionism**: the belief that well-being, complex though it is, can be effectively represented with a simple numerical report on a scale from bad to good.

Despite their adoption of the term 'statistics' (which used to mean 'descriptive facts about external realities' but nowadays generally just means 'numbers'), few quantitative well-being scholars would actually defend the idea that the numbers tell us all we need to know about well-being. Nonetheless, when survey-based numbers are reported as 'The Danes *are* happier than the French,' there is an implicit slippage from numerical indicator to a belief that this is the reality it is meant to represent. At this point, eudaimonist objectors have a very strong argument for insisting that we look beyond the numbers to explore those aspects of well-being that tend not to be well represented in numerical self-reports. Once again, however, the term 'eudaimonism' isn't needed to make this objection, and it seems better to insist, positively, on specific better alternatives to quantitative reductionism, such as biographical, qualitative, and interpretive studies of how well people live.

To summarise this section, the two attitudes that eudaimonists make their most objections to, hedonism and subjectivism, are both important approaches to understanding how people live well. It's good to learn about and promote pleasures, and in doing so it's essential to listen to people's own views on how they experience and value various aspects of their lives. There are four other categories of attitudes that eudaimonists ought to have more important quarrels with: pathologism, remedialism, instrumentalism, and quantitative reductionism. But these quarrels are ones that all well-being scholars and promoters ought to pick. The concept of 'eudaimonia' doesn't itself seem to add significant value to the conversations.

In short, it is possible to have sophisticated discussions about well-being in social planning without engaging in a battle between 'eudaimonist' followers of Aristotle and 'hedonist' followers of Bentham (or Epicurus, for example). Trying to do so may feel a little bit like trying to talk politics without resorting to 'left versus right', or to discuss culture and evolution without resorting to 'nature versus nurture'. But by refusing to play the game, you may avoid some pointlessly caricatured positions. You won't, of course, avoid discussions of value and morality, but the important question is whether you can have a good-enough grasp of the implicit evaluations and moral implications of your decisions without becoming a seasoned debater of ancient Hellenistic ethics and its modern versions.

37.3 Positivity Plus: What Goods Do Eudaimonists Specify?

The most overt function of the term eudaimonia is to recommend that people familiarise themselves with ancient Greek moral discourse as a source of enlightenment. The lecture notes put together by Aristotle's students are of course intriguing and inspiring, and worth exploring (along with philosophical texts from many other cultures and periods) for those that have the time to engage in crosscultural moral philosophy. Unsurprisingly, however, since they come from scraps of papyrus thousands of years old, they are extremely diverse, incomplete and hence lacking in overall coherence. Aristotle's views on well-being and value are subject to many interpretations that have perplexed many generations of moral philosophers. If you accept the gist of his argument and try to enrich your understanding of ultimate value by carefully thinking through your hierarchy of motives, you'll probably thank him for the overall approach but not want to follow him on all details such as his specific interpretation of human nature, his 'divine' model for good conduct, or his disparagement of slaves and women.

Because academic moralisers have all the time in the world, lists of the key features of eudaimonist theorising and of specific features of eudaimonia identified by Aristotle and others can expand almost indefinitely. Probably the most parsimonious list of common features would come down to a 'big four' list of very general categories of ethical qualification: *truth*; *active virtue*; *excellence*; and *intrinsic goodness*. These seem to constitute the bulk of Aristotelian and neo-Aristotelian thinking. Adjectivally, the qualities of well-being that we are looking for are that it should be: *reflective and objectively authenticated*; *actively functional* and representative of the best uniquely human dispositions and capabilities; *worthy*, based on a longterm challenging process of personal growth; and *intrinsically good* for particular agents, based on careful scrutiny of the relationships between ends and means. The corresponding verbs for living well would be: *verifying* (working towards accurate awareness of self and situations); *engaging* (actively practising virtues); *striving* (pursuing and encouraging personal growth in interestingly challenging ways); and *evaluating* (thinking about how goals interact in hierarchical ways leading from resources and instrumental goods towards intrinsic goods).

There are many more specific and very important Aristotelian themes, most of which can be fitted into these four clusters in some way. Relational goods or social qualities are important parts of distinctively human functioning or excellence. Social engagement is one of various forms of self-transcendence that seem important for the engaged life and for avoidance of undignified selfishness, others being engagement with the natural environment or with elusive senses of a 'spiritual' environment or cosmos. The gradual, goal-directed pursuit of excellence can entail recognition of the importance of biographical narrativity. Recognizing the multiplicity of goals can lead to awareness of the importance of moderation in all intentional behaviour, and of the virtues of a harmonious diversity of life pursuits.

37.3.1 Truth: Reflective, Deliberate, Authentic Well-being

Cautious and deliberative reality checks, especially of the long-term philosophical kind, are the hallmark of eudaimonism. Socrates gave us the memorable challenge that 'the examined life is not worth living,' and Aristotle strongly endorsed this somewhat egocentric and snobbish idea that the philosopher's life is best and noblest. In more modern times Thoreau gave this a practical twist when he wrote about the benefits and virtues of 'living deliberately' in his short-lived experiment with semi-rural simplicity. Robert Nozick's thought-experiment 'the experience machine' is a diatribe against 'fake' forms of happiness, and his later essay collection *The Examined Life* (1989) is a key text for those who promote neo-Aristotelian objections to forms of happiness that lack real-world authentication. Another philosopher, Martha Nussbaum, argues that 'the omission of this reflective element in happiness is one of the most disturbing aspects of the conceptual breeziness of contemporary subjective-state psychology, insofar as it is laying the groundwork for normative recommendations' (2008/2012: 344).

In our pursuit of well-being, we must recognize that some states, traits, or pleasures may seem like well-being but are actually bad for the individual concerned (as distinct from being antisocial). Subjective experience may clash with objective reality, if someone misconstrues how well they are living. In this regard, eudaimonism is sometimes understood as an 'objectivist' critique of 'subjective well-being'. However, a lot of the truth-checking promoted by eudaimonists is better understood as promoting more careful and sophisticated forms of intentional subjectivity, and as a critique of inadequately reflective or downright self-delusive subjectivity.

In one of the most influential diagrams ever drawn, the humanist psychologist Maslow (1943) put 'self-actualisation' at the pinnacle of his hierarchy of needs. But what kind of self is it good to actualise, and how do we know that we are actualising the right kind of self? Eudaimonists invite us to check whether people are pursuing false hopes, or displaying inauthentic emotions or identities. In self-help industries and in positive psychology, we are often urged to think about 'authentic happiness' or 'true happiness' or to search for our 'real self' and to avoid 'fake' promises of happiness or 'inauthentic' or 'extrinsic' motives (York, 2015). 'Authenticity' discourse is particularly troubling but rife in self-help discourse. It can serve as a casual reminder of the need to think critically about our own characters. But the idea that we can discover our 'true self' (Schlegel, Hirsch, & Smith, 2013; Schlegel, Hicks, & Christy, Chap. 14, this volume) is a fantasy, and it is highly questionable to claim that some kinds of happiness are 'false' or 'inauthentic' (Seligman, 2003). Related to the idea of distinguishing true from false selves and true from false well-being is the idea that by default, motivations and pathways towards well-being that are autonomously selected or 'self-determined' stand a better chance of being authentic, sustainable, and successful than those dictated by or acquired from other people. There is little or no discussion of these matters in Aristotle's work, but it is included as a 'eudaimonic well-being' theme because the authors of 'self-determination theory', Richard Ryan and Edward Deci, also happen to be key instigators of positive psychology's interest in eudaimonia (Ryan & Deci, 2000; Ryan & Martela, Chap. 7, this volume).

It would be hard to argue, in principle, against the idea that we should check whether the things called 'well-being' are actually well-being, i.e. that they are prudentially good for the people whose being is under consideration. People can be mistaken about their well-being, or about other people's well-being, and they can and do deliberately offer false promises and false self-presentations in this regard. An important function of the study and promotion of well-being should be to rectify mistakes and fakery, and to provide more people with the kinds of cautionary lens that can help us avoid and prevent them. Few would disagree with moderate arguments in favour of self-reflective introspection. This proposal becomes morally and diplomatically problematic, however, when those who have the luxury to spend a large chunk of their lives deliberating then start disparaging people who for various reasons aren't so philosophical. It is pure snobbery to insist that philosophy is the main pathway to virtue. It is also naïve to claim that more introspection is better, or that contemplation necessarily takes us towards truth and goodness.

No-one has yet come up for a sound reason for believing that life must have a 'purpose'. And everyone has a bewildering and ultimately unknowable variety of potential achievements and identities, so Polonius's idea of a 'true self' is obviously absurd. So you can seriously mislead people if you try to persuade them that they ought to crave a sense of existential purpose, or that there is a single 'true' self and a 'true' potential or destiny that they should spend their lives 'fulfilling'. In a post-Enlightenment world, social planners have no more right to peddle 'true self' or 'meaning in life' fantasies than they have to promote belief in witches or deities.

Either from force of circumstances or from active choice, some people just get on with their lives and try to live well without endlessly asking whether their pleasures are adequately sophisticated or whether their identities and roles are 'authentic'. Indeed, there is a basic contradiction that runs through eudaimonism, between an anti-subjectivist ideology of objective verification, on the one hand, and a very different ideology that privileges subjectivism, individualism, and that idea that hidden 'inside' ourselves we will find some elusive entity that we may eventually recognize as our 'true self' and which is bound to offer us better moral guidance that we will get from anyone else. Arguably, there is a moral case for bringing in some degree of 'negative utilitarianism' back into well-being policies: a good society should teach people how to avoid inauthentic forms of selfhood and enable them to pursue their own visions of what it means to live well. But if you recognize that 'true selfhood' is a mirage, then you wouldn't want parents, teachers, or counsellors sending people off in pursuit of authenticity, would you?

37.3.2 Active Virtue: Functional Well-being

The idea of making an inseparable link between practical virtue and happiness is one of the more appealing features of Aristotle's ethics, and one that has obvious merits for social planners. However, Aristotle also saw virtue as inseparable from human nature, which is problematic for two reasons: first, lots of natural dispositions and capabilities are nasty – bad for us and/bad for society; second, some of Aristotle's beliefs about human nature now seem very antiquated and culture-bound.

Few would disagree with Aristotle's basic idea that in order to think about human flourishing we should think about what kinds of 'ergon', or functionings, are distinctively human. For him, as for Plato, the concept of 'arete,' which is often translated as 'virtue,' effectively equates goodness with an entity's proper function. Beyond this descriptive approach to virtue, any effort to use descriptive information about human genetic traits to guide moral conduct is highly suspect. Scholars disagree on whether Aristotle thought that you could 'get an ought from an is', but neo-Aristotelians have a hard job explaining any kind of principle by which we should select some natural dispositions (wisdom, kindness, etc) as indicative of 'flourishing' and worth cultivating, while rejecting others (proneness to pleasure addiction, social anxiety, aggression, etc) as worth inhibiting.

Aristotle's version of this argument is idiosyncratic and perplexing, deriving from his obsession with the idea of distinguishing humans from animals. There is certainly merit in considering distinctively human evolved genetic dispositions, including of course our dispositions for social cooperation and cultural learning (Grinde, 2003). Contra Aristotle, however, we need to recognize humans as animals. We should embrace rather than denying or downplaying the importance of basic animalistic pleasures. Few scholars or planners today would agree that there is a single version of human nature that serves as a good model for virtue, still less with Aristotle's particular version of whatever that 'nature' might be.

37.3.3 Excellence: Personal Growth and the Pursuit of Exceptional Well-being

If Aristotle's functionalist argument from nature is morally problematic and in need of modernising, it does at least make the valid point that we would consider evolved human traits and dispositions when planning for well-being. Complementary to his reference to the human *ergon* is Aristotle's recommendation that we should also consider *kalon*, which is variously translated as the human ideals of nobility, excellence, beauty, or perfection. The 'perfectionism' associated with this line of thinking is considerably more problematic than the relatively down-to-earth functionality of ergonomic well-being. This is because aspiring and struggling to become ideal specimens of nobility is considerably more challenging than simply trying to be true to human nature. Particularly problematic for modern rationalists is Aristotle's idea that humans should suppress their animality and enhance their approximation to deities.

A useful general idea is that insofar as the pursuit of lifelong self-improvement is a good human trait, well-being assessors should explore whether people's lives entail substantial progress towards fulfilment of well-chosen and reasonably ambitious goals. Many psychologists have argued that the desire for interest, complexity, or novelty is satisfied by different kinds of psychological reward than the desire for competence, and have consequently argued for distinction between the emotions of 'interest' versus 'pleasure' or 'happiness' (Silvia, 2006, ch1). Interest has been plausibly described as a 'eudaimonic' emotion, in contrast to the 'hedonic' satisfactions of more comfortable, less challenging stimuli (Vittersø, Søholt, Hetland, Thorsen, & Røysamb, 2010). While it is helpful to recognize that interest and the pursuit of cognitive challenges are important functions, it is less clear that our appreciation or understanding of interest is enhanced by the claim that this isn't 'pleasurable'.

As with the pursuit of truth and virtue, the pursuit of excellence can be taken too far, and may be more suitable for some socio-economic and cultural contexts than others. The idea that the good life involves lifelong challenges in pursuit of self-improvement is relatively uncontroversial in cultures where adults are expected to keep trying to self-improve through the life course. It would make less sense in a culture in which maturation is expected to finish soon after the completion of childhood. But even in cultures that are generally keen on the idea of lifelong self-development, many people choose to reject the ideology of self-improvement, along with the idea that a good life needs a coherent narrative (Strawson, 2004). Personal growth ideology becomes more problematic still when it is coupled with the belief that individuals have some kind of hidden 'true self' or personal 'destiny' to which they should aspire.

Beliefs about destiny-fulfilment no doubt derive from complex interactions between two important features of human nature: *genetic diversity*, and *versatility of genetic expression*. Genetic diversity means that as a species, we are highly diverse in our aptitudes, and hence it makes sense to encourage people to consider their personal aptitudes when choosing self-improvement goals. If you want to flourish in sport, for example, it helps to appreciate whether your genetic make-up would pre-dispose you towards excellence as a long distance runner or a wrestler. However, we are also a uniquely versatile species. As individuals, we face a seemingly infinite variety of capabilities that we could choose to develop. We can also choose whether to pursue one form of excellence, or to be an all-rounder doing moderately well at lots of things, or not to bother pursuing any form of excellence. Baffled by choice, we may find it privately and collectively convenient to restrict choice by invoking beliefs about destiny. The modern phrase 'follow your bliss' shows contemporary ambiguity about this existential problem: we could interpret this as 'find the one true path that is written for you in the stars', or as 'just do whatever takes your fancy'.

Whether we choose to believe that our optimal growth pathways are fixed or arbitrary, we also need to address the question of how vigorously we should pursue personal growth. It is instructive to note the ambiguity of the concept of 'perfectionism': for philosophers and some eudaimonic psychologists, it seems mainly to mean that Aristotelian idea of striving for excellence, whereas for many psychologists perfectionism is a harmful psychological trait that leads to unrealistic goals, obsessions, narcissism, disappointment and a lack of balance in one's activities. Aristotle is often associated with perfectionism, despite his repeated contradictory insistence on the virtue of moderation. However it is easy to understand why he should have that reputation. Even the generally astute neo-Aristotelian interpreter Martha Nussbaum approvingly describes Aristotelian eudaimonia as 'a kind of living that is active, inclusive of all that has intrinsic value, and complete, meaning lacking in nothing that would make it richer or better' (2012: 342). Reminiscent of the World Heath Organization's utopian ideal of health as 'complete' well-being, this is obviously an absurd way to describe human flourishing. Even if a human could achieve a state of utter perfection, it hardly sounds like an interesting or enviable condition to be in for very long.

37.3.4 Intrinsic Value: Purposeful Well-being

For Aristotle, a major reason for engaging in eudaimonic discourse was to work out a hierarchy of goals such that ultimately one of them would be so good that it required no further justification. And it was clear that he meant this in the sense of prudential for the agent in question. If you examine your hierarchy of motives and find out you are pursuing something for some other end, then that must be an instrumental good and you need to keep thinking until you arrive at ultimate happiness, which is self-sufficient. Unfortunately, in places Aristotle overstates his case, saying that you never can pursue happiness for the sake of something else. We can, of course, harness short-term happiness for instrumental reasons – for example cheering ourselves up in order to boost our immune system to fight a common cold, or promoting happiness in a class for the sake of creative learning.

Some have extended Aristotle's 'telic' line of thinking to the assumption that to live well, our enjoyments must be coherently linked with some overarching sense of purpose or meaning. A problem with this line of thinking is that some proponents seem to believe that there 'is' some final, overarching purpose or meaning that people will find. A reasonable counter-argument would be that while it may be good to think about how our goals are hierarchically related, this doesn't entail any assumption about our lives having any single purpose or meaning at all. Existentialists are free to enjoy eudaimonically excellent lives while rationally recognizing that there is no single purpose or meaning to any human life, or to humanity in general. Also, since meaning and purpose are both subjective mental constructs, it should be obvious that to declare a respect for 'meaning in life' or for the 'purposeful life' is not consistent with 'objectivist' denigration of people's own views about the quality of their mental experience. This doesn't stop eudaimonists from claiming that we can objectively distinguish some kinds of meaning-in-life as better than others.

37.4 Objections to Hedonism in Policy and Planning: The 'Bread and Circuses' Problem

One important way of talking about both value and subjectivity in the planning process is to talk about desires, and how these are influenced – deliberately or otherwise – by policies and leaders. The first-century Roman poet Juvenal is best remembered for his tenth 'Satire' poem, 'On the vanity of human wishes', in which he berates the Roman masses for having been distracted from the pursuit of freedom and dignity by their leaders' ploy of pampering them with 'bread and circuses'. The phrase has become synonymous with cynical happiness policies that rob people of agency, and the poem has inspired many famous writers to ponder the difficulty of discerning 'true goodness from a host of opposites' as Juvenal puts it in his opening line.

If it is possible for individuals to lazily adopt a life of shallow hedonism, it is also possible for governments and organizations to exploit populations by encouraging this. Juvenal also popularised the phrase 'sound mind in a sound body', so it is easy to discern in his philosophical outlook a eudaimonic objection to non-nutritious comfort food and to the mental blunting that might result from excessive indulgence in simple entertainment. To live well, we need to challenge our bodies and minds, and to achieve this we must learn to resist any attempts to control us into passivity by offering us shallow, undignified comforts.

Going beyond comforts at the individual level means pursuing a more challenging but also more meaningful and ultimately rewarding life. But public interest in well-being is about social progress and societal-level planning and learning, not just about individual morality. Debates about the importance of 'eudaimonic well-being' and 'eudaimonist' approaches aren't just about the relationship between pleasure and value, they're about the complex intertwining of individual and social interests. We all hope to flourish as individuals, but most of us also want to be part of good societies, and more generally we value self-transcendent goods and hence we value and require self-transcendence in order to live well. Social goods, social quality, and social well-being are crucial aspects of living well (Keyes, 1998).

So if you recommend that the core purpose of social planning should simply be to maximise good feelings, you are asking for trouble. The British unofficial leader of well-being policy, the economist Richard Layard, did just this in his *Happiness* book, one of the most influential and popular texts on nationally planned well-being: 'happiness is feeling good, and misery is feeling bad' (2005: 4). In doing so he offered a gift – or perhaps an intentional wind-up – to neo-Aristotelian ethicists. As noted above, he could mount a defence of hedonism by arguing that there are lots of different ways – including highly challenging and sophisticated ways – of 'feeling good'. But why risk confusion, why not just accept right away that planners should enable and encourage citizens to choose a sensible composition of diverse life pursuits that includes challenging and prosocial activities rather than just selfish or short-termist pleasures?

Conversely, if you insist on complaining, with philosopher Raymond Belliotti, that *Happiness Is Overrated* (2003), you had better find a defensible definition of the entity you believe people are over-valuing. This is going to be hard, because in normal speech 'happiness' has so many meanings that it's hard to imagine anyone over-valuing all of them. Happiness doesn't point to specific entities, but serves, like 'well-being,' and 'flourishing', and eudaimonia, as a starting-point for conversations about how to live well. There is no single 'thing' to be overrated or underrated. Normal understandings of happiness include both hasty quantitative judgements about feelings as well as much more complex narratives about the quality and meaning of lives.

Whether you're a quantitative hedonist like Layard or a conscientious objector like Belliotti, you invite unnecessary arguments if you don't recognize that well-being is too diverse and complex to be promoted or 'rated' in any simplistic way. Whether we call our ultimate value 'pleasure', or 'happiness' or 'well-being', it is futile to try reducing policy purposes to the promotion of any single kind of goodness. Nor does it make much sense to 'maximise' something that we learn about through potentially unreliable reports of pleasurable experiences that may not have been reliable indications of well-being in the first place. These kinds of objections aren't at all the same kind of thing as denying the value of subjective well-being (SWB) research. Whereas many prominent well-being scholars have quite reasonably defended the use of 'hedonic' measures of SWB, few have gone as far as to defend the idea of equating happiness itself with a single measure of pleasures minus pains. Unsurprisingly, Layard's avowed 'good friend' Amartya soon weighed in by criticising Layard's 'imperialistic' promotion of pleasure as the sole measure of value (Sen, 2009: 273–276).

37.5 A 'Well-being Lens' in Social Planning

Another thing well-being promoters should try to transcend is the ego-centred individual. Humans value *social goods* that transcend their own individual well-being. Indeed, our well-being depends heavily on various qualities of the social environment we live in. Humans are an evolutionary anomaly: we are a highly social species that nonetheless values and respects individuality. Anomalies and moral debates seem likely to increase as global cultural trends increasingly valorise and facilitate individualistic and idiosyncratic pathways to well-being, while at the same the scope of the social web and the circle of empathy expands. Eudaimonists seem unavoidably enmeshed in the awkward synergies and trade-offs involved in these two sources of well-being – personal freedom and self-determination on the one hand, and sociocultural approval and belonging on the other. Shout too loudly in favour of the freedom of individuals to choose their own forms of happiness and to subjectively rate their own well-being, and the prudish disapproval of eudaimonists will remind you that individuals aren't really so free after all. Insist on culturally approved and prosocial pathways to well-being, and eudaimonists will remind you of the values and virtues of individual 'authenticity' and self-determination.

When 'happiness' or 'well-being' are proposed as social policy themes, the two most common kinds of objection are, first, that some undignified or false varieties of well-being might be promoted, and second, that an emphasis on the well-being of individuals might promote egocentrism and detract from need to nurture social quality. These two categories of objection sometimes combine in complaints about forms or pursuits of well-being that are deemed undignified or false precisely because they are antisocial or meet with sociocultural disapproval. Conversations about well-being in policy and governance are hence about conventional standards of value, and about the ways in which subjective experiences are mediated through sociocultural and political contexts.

Perhaps because of the threats often posed to personal dignity by various forms of sociocultural exploitation, the positive roles of social quality tend to get short shrift in eudaimonic discourse. The loose set of traditions called 'eudaimonism' has generally focused on approving or disapproving varieties of well-being, and has only tangentially addressed Aristotle's interest in social quality and relational goods (Bruni, 2008). The odd choice of 'self-determination theory' as a rubric for one of the most prominent versions of contemporary psychological eudaimonism is paradoxical, given the proponents' frequent protestations that they don't want to promote individualism or portray social influences as antagonistic to personal autonomy (Ryan, Huta, & Deci, 2008; Huta, Chap. 15, this volume; Ryan & Martela, Chap. 7, this volume). Although Seligman's PERMA formula for flourishing includes positive relationships as a key dimension of human flourishing (Seligman, 2011), his earlier work on 'authentic happiness' paid minimal attention to social life and was explicitly pessimistic about the prospects for enhancing happiness by changing the social environment (2003: 50). Keyes, a leading social theorist in the positive psychology movement, proposed a useful model for 'social well-being' (1998), but by this he didn't mean social quality, he meant the individual's engagements with other people. Most eudaimonic psychology, if it addresses social aspects at all, looks at relationships egocentrically rather than looking at the overall social environment.

To appreciate whether discussions about pleasurable versus worthy lives might be useful in policy discourse, we first need to consider what kinds of difference it makes to consider 'well-being' in social planning. When we insert a 'well-being' or 'happiness' lens into the discourse of social planning, we ought to notice at least three main kinds of significant impact. The whole policy process (thinking, decision-making, and cumulative learning) ought to become more:

- *Value-based* – aspirational, and appreciative, paying more explicit and systematic attention to life enhancement – to what we ultimately value and why (axiological questions), and what we can and should do to promote this (pragmatic and normative questions)
- *Introspective*, i.e. mental (since the mind is our most valued feature) – considering more carefully the ways in which human subjectivity (goals, motivations, experiences, evaluations, and deliberations) influences the processes through which external conditions promote or inhibit well-being
- *Integrative*, paying systematic attention to interactions between life domains, to the narrative development of the quality of people's lives through the life course, and to the interactions between minds, bodies, and sociocultural and well as physical environments

Linking this value-introspection-integration policy triad with the above question about the basic pleasure/value distinction, evidently we do need to consider pleasure in relation to other values. We need to consider how social planning interacts with people's minds. And we need to think integratively about how people's whole lives are composed, rather than just relying on fragmentary thinking about heaps of momentary pleasures. In principle, then, eudaimonist questioning can help promote intelligent well-being policy discourse, and if it makes us pause before committing silly hedonistic or welfarist or subjectivist mistakes of the 'bread and circuses' variety it may serve some useful functions. In principle, it is easy to see why social researchers and social planners need to engage with psychologists and moral philosophers in order to optimise the potential of the well-being lens to transform social planning in these ways. It is much less obvious that the multifarious jumble of considerations and ideologies that have been promoted under the header of *eudaimonia* represent a coherent set of principle our outlooks, let alone that the more specific use of 'Aristotelian' discourse – a diverse set of intriguing and inspiring but often baffling thoughts based on papyrus lecture notes from 23 centuries ago – is likely to enhance contemporary policy discourse.

37.6 Beyond the 'Greatest Happiness Principle': Prioritising and Quantifying Well-being

Utilitarianism in policy makes two main ideological claims: that well-being should have the *highest priority* in policy and planning, and that *more of it is better*. Commentators on utilitarianism rarely question the supremacy of well-being in the hierarchy of axiological 'what matters' questions, but many have doubts about what happens when you try to quantify and maximise well-being.

Both the prioritising and the quantifying aspect of utilitarianism are implicit in the 'Greatest Happiness Principle' (GHP), one of the most profoundly influential cultural innovations of the Enlightenment. This was first articulated by Francis Hutcheson, a neo-Aristotelian or 'eudaimonist', in 1725. Hutcheson, who later served as teacher of Adam Smith, also coined other formidably influential political sound-bites such as 'all men are created equal' and 'inalienable rights'. The single most important source of utilitarian philosophy, Hutcheson was also an arch-opponent of David Hume's hedonism, and was pretty close to Aristotle in seeing virtue as the cause of happiness: 'That action is best, which procures the greatest happiness of the greatest numbers' (1725/2008: 2.3.7). Happiness matters in that it is the outcome of virtue. Happiness and virtue are inextricably linked – they are valued together. So to those who see eudaimonism as the opposite of hedonism, it must seem ironic that the GHP is today mainly associated with the 'hedonist' Jeremy Bentham, who popularised it towards the end of the eighteenth century.

In its day, Hutcheson's GHP was strikingly humanistic and humanitarian, a *rhetoric of prioritisation* (axiological and normative) that put citizen well-being ahead of any other drivers of policy such as order or productivity or divine rules. He followed Aristotle in arguing that there is a single category of ultimate goodness which we can use to steer, motivate, evaluate, rank, and justify our actions and institutions. Both Aristotle and Hutcheson took folk terms associated with good fortune and nonhuman agency, and tried to invest them with new meanings associated with careful deliberation and purposeful human agency in pursuit of ultimate value.

But Hutcheson's phrase also implies a different *rhetoric of quantification*, based on the metaphor of happiness as a heap of goodness that could be measured and compared. If we are persuaded that happiness is what counts, we still need to consider what it is that should be counted, because evidently happiness is too mysterious and various for us to count it directly. Later in the eighteenth century, another Scot, the aristocrat-administrator John Sinclair of Thurso coined the term 'statistics' to promote a new science of national accounting. He argued that the purpose of national surveys would be to assess the 'quantum of happiness' of a population. But to judge from the surveys, what he seems to have meant was that state agencies should assess the conditions and resources for living well, using these as proxies for happiness. There was nothing very hedonic, or eudaimonic, about the basic living conditions covered in his surveys: statistics was about the conditions and resources for meeting minimal standards of decency. Although Bentham and Edgeworth later toyed with the ideas of 'felicific calculus' (1776) and 'hedonimetry' (1881) respectively, it has really only been in the twenty-first century that governments and other organizations worldwide have begun vigorously pursuing the possibility of measuring and promoting national happiness, as in positive psychological experience. Before then, the GHP had only served loosely as a kind of moral signpost until the twentieth century, when the quantification of happiness and domain satisfactions gradually transformed from a minority academic sport into national systems.

So it is crucial to bear in mind that prioritisation, which is about value and importance, is not at all the same thing as quantification. The trajectory of 'Gross National Happiness' rhetoric in Bhutan is an iconic example of the kinds of slippage that occur between prioritisation and quantification. When the new teenage King used this phrase in the early 1970s, it was just a rhetorical quip about the hierarchy of values – a reminder that 'the economy' only matters insofar as it contributes to well-being. It was 40 years before substantial efforts were made to turn GNH rhetoric into national policies and learning tools. In this recent internationalised and heavily aid-funded phase of institutionalising GNH, the rhetoric of quantification seems to have taken over with the development of a major new industry of GNH 'statistical' indicator development (Ura, Alkire, Zangmo, & Wangdi, 2012).

Hutcheson's contemporaries would have interpreted and used the term 'happiness' in many ways. This matters because you can only give something priority, in thoughts or in deeds, if you know what it is, and what it isn't. Generally, pre-twentieth-century happiness concepts would have been more holistic and hence more closely synonymous with 'well-being' than is the case today. Since today the default meanings of happiness tend to be both psychological and hedonic, 'well-being' is the more favoured if somewhat blander term in policy discourse. In Hutcheson's day, most people would also have included the anticipation of heavenly rewards in their understanding of happiness, and this is still true in many countries today. So anyone who argues in favour of GHP or 'maximising' well-being begs a lot of questions and isn't being very practical.

One way of clarifying matters is to distinguish *axiological* questions (what matters?) from *normative* questions (what goods should we pursue and promote?). There are also *epistemological* arguments concerning how embed well-being in our learning strategies. Often, the epistemological arguments take the much more specific form of 'measuring what matters', most familiarly represented in the currently fashionable 'beyond GDP' slogan. Both Aristotle and Bentham are invoked in support of the 'beyond GDP' movement – Aristotle reminding us that GDP is mainly about the means not the ends of our activities, and Bentham reminding us that what matters are the pleasures and the pains, not the economy. Epistemology and norms combine in claims that we should 'measure' and 'maximise' happiness – an idea which can obviously only be rhetorical because even Benthamites must admit that you can't literally measure something as vague as happiness, nor can you literally maximise anything unless you force yourself into the belief that only one thing matters (which, perplexingly, much of Aristotle's writing seems to be attempting).

Beyond agreeing on well-being as the overarching policy priority, planners and citizens need to address further (axiological and normative) questions concerning such factors as components (what kinds of well-being should we prioritise?); interactions (what kinds of balance, or mix, or harmony between these various components should people aspire to?); and sequencing (in what ways does the sequencing of well-being, through the day and over the life course, matter? Does it matter how well-being is distributed across the life-course? Do anticipated post-life enjoyments count?). To establish the priorities needed for policies and actions we also have to ask *epistemological* questions about how we can and should try to learn about these various goods:

- **Subjectivity**: How much priority should we accord to people's own subjective assessments of their well-being, versus external assessments based on objective criteria?
- **Reliability**: Under what conditions, and with what kinds of questioning, should we judge someone's well-being according to their own present subjective views? Should private and momentary self-assessments have higher priority over other kinds of self-assessments that are prone to social desirability and memory biases?
- **Extractive versus dialectical**: do we understand well-being as an essential condition that we could in theory find a true expression of, or as a dialectical process, i.e. as an emergent product of interactions between minds and environments?

These kinds of important questions can be further subdivided with greater sophistication, and the point of asking them isn't hard to grasp. So Hutcheson must surely have been aware that despite the Aristotelian naivety of his 'maximum happiness' phrase, there was no single good that could be maximised. What he presumably meant was that people should think and converse as intelligently as they could about how our actions affect the various desirable qualities of people's lives. None of these qualities can be maximised, because obviously you can't maximise multiple goods. But in a loose sense an insistence on happiness in our moral discourse stands a reasonable chance of steering us towards benign decisions, because it helps us distinguish instrumental from ultimate values, and to cultivate aspirational goals rather than merely thinking about the avoidance of harms.

Having thought about what well-being is, how valuable the various components are, and how we should learn about them, individuals and social planners may be in a stronger position to consider normative and practical matters – what aspects of well-being ought we to pursue and promote, and how? We may, for example, believe that some aspects of well-being are so elusive or idiosyncratically personal that they are beyond the scope and responsibility of social planners.

37.7 Is Pleasure More Quantifiable Than Eudaimonia?

One of the most important remarks in Aristotle's *Nichomachean Ethics* is this:

> It is the mark of the man experienced in the world and interested in studying it to look for no more precision than the subject matter allows.

Politicians and planners need a rough outline of the kinds of goodness worth promoting, not mathematical guidance. We should not, in other words, allow the rhetoric of quantification to run on towards pseudo-science. Nor should we give undue attention to phenomena just because they happen to be quantifiable. In their critique of sloppy hedonia-eudaimonia distinctions, Kashdan et al., have argued that the dichotomy is unhelpful, and that 'eudaimonia is not well-defined and lacks consistent measurement' (2008: 221). Eudaimonists have not, however, been shy of developing measures for an immense variety of ways of talking about the good life. Perhaps the problem lies not with shortage of measures but with inadequate consideration of the severe limits of measurability.

There seem to be two problems here. The first is the unwieldy variety of eudaimonic concepts, and consequently the lack of any single adequate overall measure of eudaimonia. So even if you approve of the proliferation of new eudaimonic measures, you would have to be concerned about how useful all of this diversity is likely to be for planners. The second problem is more fundamental: perhaps the usefulness of measurement diminishes as our interest shifts from relatively simple pleasures and impromptu life satisfaction assessments to more complex eudaimonic considerations. If the full experience of living well is ultimately ineffable – unavoidably vague and uncertain – then quantification may be an unsuitable way of learning about it. Yet since it matters more than anything else, well-being promoters need to find ways of expressing and interpreting at least some important aspects of what it means to live well. Insofar as happiness is a social or 'conversational' phenomenon – something that occurs through relationships between people rather than just in the privacy of individual minds – it is not only 'effable' but it actually comes into existence through expression. It is those life narratives and dialogues we need to listen to if we want to gain deeper wisdom into how well people's lives are going.

Could it be that the opposition between 'hedonia' and 'eudaimonia' is not so much about different values, but about different modes of expression? Are 'hedonists' better understood as intuitive underthinkers who rely more on quantitative metaphors to understand well-being, and 'eudaimonists' more ponderous overthinkers who rely more on complex reflective narratives? Are the debates really about preferences for pseudo-certainty versus vagueness? A lot of the debate about hedonic versus eudaimonic well-being does seem to be about epistemological matters rather than about values or norms. Much of it is really about indicators and measurement, and the most telling eudaimonist objection is against scientistic reductionism and the numerical pretence of certainty. The trouble with measuring pleasures and satisfactions and calling these 'happiness' is rather like the trouble with measuring economic transactions and calling GDP 'the economy'. You are measuring proxies, not the real thing, so the measures can sometimes give you perverse readings.

If quantification is the problem, there are two different strategies worth adopting to make planning more 'eudaimonic'. You can de-emphasise quantification, so that social planners use a more balanced set of methods and indicators and explore well-being in qualitative and narrative ways that better capture the rich variety of ways in which people experience well-being. Or you can try to quantify as many aspects of well-being as you can, including not just pleasures and satisfactions, but people's sense of meaning or purpose, or authentic selfhood, or whatever. But these may be harder to assess quantitatively. Pleasures and pains seem to be kinds of experience that we more readily quantify. Indeed the default mode of hedonic thinking seems to be a simplificatory mode. It tells us roughly how good or bad any experience is, in defiance of the ultimate incommensurability of pleasures. Sometimes, in order to prioritise and to take decisions, we have no option but to pretend that very different kinds of value are comparable. It is hardly surprising, therefore, that national statisticians and policy makers find hedonic indicators appealing despite their evident shortcomings.

In short, exploring pleasures and satisfactions using quantitative methods is a moderately useful and relatively cheap proxy for learning about happiness, but exploration of the full range of well-being themes, i.e. eudaimonia, is a much more complex, time-consuming, and expensive task. The 'eudaimonic turn' in positive psychology has produced some helpful debates on the relationship between positive and humanistic psychology, and consequently on the kinds of important values and experiences that are likely to be missed if we overemphasise the kinds of pleasures and satisfactions that are readily susceptible to quantification. There may be some value in trying to develop methods for quantifying people's sense of 'meaning', 'personal authenticity', and so on, but it should be evident that the resulting numerical results give us much more unclear information than numerical reports about pleasure.

This doesn't mean we can only waffle about the more complex aspects of well-being and never hope to investigate them scientifically. Nor does it mean that we need to resort (as has become increasingly fashionable) to the ancient mystical concepts like 'soul' and 'spirituality' to refer helplessly to the tantalizing elusiveness of happiness. It does mean that reductionist approaches to happiness are unscientific unless they take great care not to lead people to confuse specific indicators (such as numerical self-reports or electrical activity in the brain) with happiness. Happiness science must avoid the kinds of statistical or biological reductionism and unscientific pseudo-precision that are sometimes indulged in by happiness scholars, and considerably more often in popular misrepresentations of their work in popular media. Measuring self-reported happiness may be interesting and instructive, and some ways of doing this are more scientifically credible than others, but we should not expect to develop 'reliable' and 'valid' measures of something that is itself permanently volatile and endlessly open to debate and doubt.

37.8 Conclusions

Perhaps the main contribution of eudaimonism has been to remind us to think and talk about well-being in sophisticated ways. And if that's all the fuss is about, if it's really just a reminder that complicated things sometimes need to be discussed in complicated ways, it seems a little unnecessary and patronising. Even if cheeky Benthamites do occasionally stick their hedonistic heads above the parapets from time to time, do most of us really need to be reminded that pleasures and satisfactions can sometimes be unreal, unsustainable, undignified, unkind, meaningless, harmful, antisocial, selfish, deluded, inauthentic, or complacent?

The interdisciplinary science of well-being is still in its formative years but it has rapidly been thrust onto a global media stage, raising high expectations of its roles in shaping public discourse and planning. We have wonderful opportunities to influence the pursuit and planning of well-being, but we also have fragile reputations that can quickly be lost. When we share our key concepts with the rest of the world, we had better be sure to share terms and concepts that are clear and memorable. When we publicise our arguments, we had better be confident that our disagreements are real, important, and potentially generative, i.e. that they stand a good chance of changing people's understanding and life choices for the better.

I hope the above review has shown that while many of the debates invoked by the concept of 'eudaimonia' have been fruitful and important, there is no coherent 'eudaimonia' concept. Even if there were, we would still need to know more than eudaimonists typically tell us about what it is supposed to influence – our values, our norms, our personal or collective life goals, our learning strategies, or what? There are 'serious problems in the translation of eudaimonia from philosophy to psychology' (Biswas-Diener, Kashdan, & King, 2009: 209), but there have always been equally serious sources of potential misunderstanding between Aristotle's different lectures, let alone among his modern neo-Aristotelian interpreters. Even if there were a clear 'ism' that can be usefully contrasted with other 'isms', its proponents would still have a lot of work to do to clarify whether their arguments are about what kind of life is ultimately worthwhile, what kind of goals people ought to pursue for themselves, what kinds of good people ought to promote for society in general, or what kinds of indicator and means of assessment should be used to learn about well-being.

More specifically, I hope that I have thrown useful doubt on several of the concepts commonly associated with eudaimonism. While it may well sometimes be useful to consider vague concepts such as 'authenticity', 'meaning', and 'fulfilment,' the meanings and values of these are far too vague and ambiguous to serve as moral guidance. More worryingly, they have in many instances seemed to provide an excuse for cultural dogma that ought to have no place in serious scholarship or policy discourse. The three main sources of 'eudaimonist' theory are Aristotle, neo-Aristotelian moral philosophy, and psychology. None of these three, let alone eudaimonism in general, offers a single coherent approach. It is not clear what proponents seek to be contrasted with, nor is it clear what they promote.

So whatever benefits might ensue from resorting to the term eudaimonia, they would have to be pretty substantial to offset the many rather obvious disadvantages and dangers, as outlined in the box below.

Box: Nine Problems with Eudaimonism

1. *Gratuitous jargon*: we shouldn't use potentially confusing foreign terms where we have perfectly good alternatives in plain English. Doing so is impolite, inefficient, and pretentious.
2. *Residualist vagueness*: vagueness is a characteristic of terms like happiness, well-being, and flourishing. Vagueness gives them the flexibility to serve well as general invitations for conversations and enquiries about better living, but they can't plausibly serve as labels for any particular kinds of entity or experience. Eudaimonia is similarly vague, but compounds this with the problem of residualism: it often stands for all those aspects of well-being that aren't captured by the concept of pleasure.
3. *False opposition to hedonism*: pitting eudaimonia *against* hedonia doesn't make sense to anyone who (like most ancient Greek philosophers including Aristotle) believes a well-lived life tends to be accompanied by a lot of diverse pleasures, or – more specifi-

(continued)

cally – recognizes that the ability to enjoy diverse goods is an important and active human capability of paramount moral importance.

4. *False opposition to subjectivism*: nor does it help to propose 'eudaimonic' objectivism against subjective self-reports of well-being, or against the view that people should be free to choose their own well-being criteria. Even so-called 'objective' goods need to be subjectively experienced and evaluated. Value is an unavoidably subjective concept: there is no non-subjective position from which humans can judge the value of anything. Well-being research requires subjective self-reports of both pleasures and active functionality.
5. *Snobbery*: insofar as eudaimonism is associated with suspicious or disparaging attitudes towards simple pleasures, it runs the risk of encouraging snobbery, as exemplified most famously by Aristotle's elitist and egocentric confidence that the philosophical life is the best, and J.S. Mill's disparagement of the 'happiness of swine'. It is fine to offer the view that challenging and sophisticated activities are worth pursuing, but quite wrong to assert dogmatically that they are simply better for everyone.
6. *Perfectionism*: although for most people the association of eudaimonia with striving and thriving is commendable ('perfectionism' in the sense that philosophers use it), its more inflationary association with perfectionism in the psychological sense is problematic. When psychological eudaimonists promote aspirations such as achieving 'the best within us' (Waterman 2013) this is likely to alienate anyone who favours a 'good-enough' rather than a perfect life.
7. *Getting-an-ought-from-an-is*: although conversations about the good life certainly require some consideration of human evolution and human nature, but this is no excuse for pretending that evolution has a purpose or that humans have some divinely-inspired ergonomic destiny. After Darwin, we should know better. Aristotle and his followers come uncomfortably close to the dogmatic but naïve ideology of a 'natural' model for human flourishing. Yet anyone can see that there are many aspects of human nature (violence, laziness, greed, jealousy, social anxiety, etc) that don't offer good inspiration for moral conduct.
8. *Culture-bound spirit beliefs*: the 'good spirit' etymology may not always have been salient in the minds of ancient Greek users, but as with the contemporary global fashion for talking about 'spiritual well-being', beliefs in occult 'spiritual' beings are unavoidably implicated in the term eudaimonia, rendering it suspect to atheists and rationalists.
9. *'Authenticity' dogma*: several self-declared eudaimonists have also advocated ideological commitments to highly uncertain and questionable goods such as 'authentic happiness', 'self-actualisation', and 'meaning in life'. Moderate versions of these ideas seem harmless enough: it probably is good for people to pursue a modest variety of intrinsically valuable self-chosen goals, and to try to establish some sense of self-awareness, coherence or personal purpose. But existential and identity issues are endlessly uncertain and it is dangerous to pretend otherwise.

Regarding the pursuit and promotion of well-being, it certainly makes sense to consider the important differences between valuing something, making it a salient goal, and measuring or 'maximising' it. At both personal and collective levels, the pursuit of pleasure soon leads to perverse outcomes if easy-access but short-lived and unhealthy or undignified pleasures are targeted. Nonetheless, most people would agree that good lives and good societies are pleasurable, and that pleasure is a key part of what we value about them. But even if personal and social values coincide, we should also think carefully about the different normative implications of well-being at personal and social levels. It has, for example, been persuasively argued that utilitarianism is a good normative guide for social policy but not at all suitable for individual decision-making (Goodin, 1995). This is because as individuals we are bound to prioritise the good of people with whom we are most intimately related, whereas governments and organizations are obliged to consider the benefits and harms of a much larger number of people.

Despite all of the above warnings about the shortcomings of eudaimonist discourse and the lack of justification for eudaimonia as a jargon term in public policy debate, it does seem likely that eudaimonistic objections and questioning have been constructively provocative. Pursuers and planners of well-being who engage in these debates seem likely to adopt better thinking habits that will help them avoid naive short-termist, passive, or lazy hedonism, and to take account of the many kinds of capability and value that people have reason to pursue and to foster.

References

Bates, W. (2013). Should we choose eudaimonia over hedonia? http://wintonbates.blogspot.co.uk/2013/10/should-we-choose-eudaimonia-over-hedonia.html

Belliotti, R. A. (2003). *Happiness is overrated*. Lanham, MD: Rowman & Littlefield.

Bentham, J. (1776/1907). *Introduction to the principles of morals and legislation*. Oxford, UK: Clarendon.

Biswas-Diener, R., Kashdan, T., & King, L. (2009). Two traditions of happiness research, not two distinct types of happiness. *Journal of Positive Psychology, 4*, 208–211.

Bruni, L. (2008). Back to Aristotle? Happiness, eudaimonia, and relational goods. In L. Bruni, F. Comim, & M. Pugno (Eds.), *Capabilities and happiness* (pp. 114–139). New Delhi, India: Oxford University Press.

Coyne, J. C. (2013). Highly correlated hedonic and eudaimonic well-being thwart genomic analysis. *Proceedings of the National Academy of Science USA, 110*(45), E4183.

Crespo, R. F., & Mesurado, B. (2015). Happiness economics, eudaimonia and positive psychology: From happiness economics to flourishing economics. *Journal of Happiness Studies, 16*, 931–946.

Deci, E. L., & Ryan, R. M. (2008). Hedonia, eudaimonia, and well-being: An introduction. *Journal of Happiness Studies, 9*(1), 1–11.

Diener, E., & Seligman, M. (2004). Beyond money: Toward an economy of well-being. *Psychological Science in the Public Interest, 5*(1), 1–31.

Disabato, D. J., Goodman, F. R., Kashdan, T. B., Short, J. L., & Jarden, A. (2015). Different types of well-being? A cross-cultural examination of hedonic and eudaimonic well-being. *Psychological Assessment* [advance online].

Edgeworth, F. Y. (1881). *Mathematical psychics*. London: Kegan Paul.

Fleurbaey, M., & Blanchet, D. (2013). *Beyond GDP: Measuring welfare and assessing sustainability*. Oxford, UK: Oxford University Press.

Goodin, R. E. (1995). *Utilitarianism as a public philosophy*. Cambridge, MA: Cambridge University Press.

Grinde, B. (2003). *Darwinian happiness: Evolution as a guide for understanding human behavior*. Princeton, NJ: Darwin Press.

Henderson, L. W., & Knight, T. (2012). Integrating the hedonic and eudaimonic perspectives to more comprehensively understand well-being and pathways to well-being. *International Journal of Well-being, 2*(3), 196–221.

Huta, V., & Waterman, A. S. (2014). Eudaimonia and its distinction from hedonia: Developing a classification and terminology for understanding conceptual and operational definitions. *Journal of Happiness Studies, 15*(6), 1425–1456.

Hutcheson, F. (1725/2008). *Inquiry into the original of our ideas of beauty and virtue*. Indianapolis, IN: Liberty Fund.

Joshanloo, M. (2016). Revisiting the empirical distinction between hedonic and eudaimonic aspects of well-being using exploratory structural equation modelling. *Journal of Happiness Studies* [advance online].

Kashdan, T. B., Biswas-Diener, R., & King, L. A. (2008). Reconsidering happiness: The costs of distinguishing between hedonics and eudaimonia. *Journal of Positive Psychology, 3*(4), 219–233.

Keyes, C. (1998). Social well-being. *Social Psychology Quarterly, 61*(2), 121–140.

Keyes, C. L. M., & Haidt, J. (2002). Introduction: human flourishing – The study of that which makes life worthwhile. In C. L. M. Keyes & J. Haidt (Eds.), *Flourishing: Positive psychology and the life well-lived* (pp. 3–12). Washington, DC: American Psychological Association.

Layard, R. (2005). *Happiness: Lessons from a new science*. Harmondsworth, UK: Penguin.

Maslow, A. H. (1943). A theory of human motivation. *Psychological Review, 50*(4), 370–396.

Nozick, R. (1989). *The examined life: Philosophical meditations*. New York: Simon and Schuster.

Nussbaum, M. C. (2008/2012). Who is the happy warrior? Philosophy, happiness research, and public policy. *International Review of Economics, 59*(4), 335–361.

Ryan, R. M., & Deci, E. L. (2000). Self-determination theory and the facilitation of intrinsic motivation, social development, and well-being. *American Psychologist, 55*, 68–78.

Ryan, R. M., Huta, V., & Deci, E. L. (2008). Living well: A self-determination theory perspective on eudaimonia. *Journal of Happiness Studies, 9*(1), 139–170.

Ryff, C. D. (1989). Happiness is everything, or is it? Explorations on the meaning of psychological well-being. *Journal of Personality and Social Psychology, 57*, 1069–1081.

Schlegel, R. J., Hirsch, K. A., & Smith, C. M. (2013). The importance of who you really are: The role of the true self in eudaimonia. In A. S. Waterman (Ed.), *The best within us: Positive psychology perspectives on eudaimonia* (pp. 207–225). Washington, DC: American Psychological Association.

Seligman, M. E. P. (2003). *Authentic happiness: Using the new positive psychology to realize your potential for lasting fulfillment*. London: Nicholas Brealey.

Seligman, M. E. P. (2011). *Flourish: A visionary new understanding of happiness and well-being*. New York: Free Press.

Sen, A. (2009). *The idea of justice*. Cambridge, MA: Harvard University Press.

Silvia, P. J. (2006). *Exploring the psychology of interest*. Oxford: Oxford University Press.

Strawson, G. (2004). Against narrativity. *Ratio, 17*, 428–452.

Ura, K., Alkire, S., Zangmo, T., & Wangdi, K. (2012). *A short guide to gross national happiness index*. Thimphu, Bhutan: Centre for Bhutan Studies. www.grossnationalhappiness.com/

Vittersø, J. (2013). Functional well-being: Happiness as feelings, evaluations, and functioning. In S. David, I. Boniwell, & A. C. Ayers (Eds.), *Oxford handbook of happiness* (pp. 227–244). Oxford, UK: Oxford University Press.

Vittersø, J., Søholt, Y., Hetland, A., Thorsen, I. A., & Røysamb, E. (2010). Was Hercules happy? Some answers from a functional model of human well-being. *Social Indicators Research, 95*, 1–18.

Waterman, A. S. (Ed.). (2013). *The best within us: Positive psychology perspectives on eudaimonia*. Washington, DC: American Psychological Association.

York, P. (2015). *Authenticity is a Con*. London: Biteback.

Part VI

Epilogue

The Future of Eudaimonic Well-Being: Subjectivism, Objectivism and the Lump Under the Carpet

38

Valerie Tiberius

This volume brings together leading researchers in the social sciences and philosophy, who are all concerned with what it is to live a good human life. What could possibly be more important? And what could be a more deep and difficult question? It shouldn't be terribly surprising that there is controversy in the field; philosophical controversy about the nature of the good life has persisted for millennia! Social science research on the topic has introduced new controversies, some of which are internal to the particular field and some of which arise from the fact that the same topic is being considered by very different fields. Given this situation, one might fear that the appropriate adage for the occasion is the one that says "too many cooks spoil the broth". I incline more toward the thought that "two heads are better than one". Indeed, I believe that one of the great contributions this volume makes is that it brings together competing voices from different disciplines so that we can face the controversies squarely and learn what we can from each other.

What are the areas of controversy? The following is not an exhaustive list of the questions covered in this book, but all of the authors cover at least one of these questions:

- What is eudaimonia and how is eudaimonia different (if it is) from other constructs or concepts (like well-being, happiness, subjective well-being, flourishing, fulfillment, perfection)?
- Granted a particular definition and/or a theory of eudaimonia, what is its value? Is it the highest good or a component of the human good, or something else?
- Granted a particular definition and/or a theory of eudaimonia and a theory of its value, how should it be measured (if at all)?
- What are the causes and consequences of eudaimonia (as theorized and as measured)? Relatedly, how is it connected to other constructs and concepts such as virtue and subjective well-being?
- How should eudaimonia (as theorized and as measured) figure into social policy and planning?

The first question – about the very concept of Eudaimonia – is probably the most contentious. According to the editor, "The most fundamental dispute in the handbook, and it is a big one in the general happiness literature as well, concerns the question of whether the concept of eudaimonic well-being is warranted at all". The arguments that the concept is not warranted do not assume that eudaimonistic elements (such as meaning, achievement and so on) are unimportant to human life. Rather, the point is that these elements

V. Tiberius (✉)
University of Minnesota, Minneapolis, MN, USA
e-mail: tiberius@umn.edu

J. Vittersø (ed.), *Handbook of Eudaimonic Well-Being*, International Handbooks of Quality-of-Life,
DOI 10.1007/978-3-319-42445-3_38

should be studied separately as important elements of human life that are related in various ways to (but not the same as) well-being.

This might lead us to think that there is no fundamental dispute, but a mere terminological disagreement. If this appearance is correct, one way forward would be to regulate our terminology. We could go with Happiness 1 and Happiness 2, eudaimonia and subjective well-being, flourishing and happiness, or some other pairing. There are a number of ways people have labeled a distinction between happiness as a psychological state and happiness as something more or other than a psychological state. It might be helpful for particular communities of researchers to agree on some technical terms so that they can share data in meaningful ways. Legislating technical vocabulary for a large community of researchers is not easy, but it probably could be done. The prospects for regulating the vocabulary of a multidisciplinary group of researchers, however, are dim. Bemoaning these dim prospects would make for a very short (and dull) epilogue, and in any case I think it is worth considering whether there might be something deeper at issue in this apparent battle over words.

Persistent and heated terminological disputes often hide something more fundamental and, when this is the case, agreeing on terms just moves the battle somewhere else: the lump under the carpet is pushed to a different quadrant, but it doesn't go away. I want to explore one possible interpretation of the real lump under the carpet, namely, a very deep disagreement about the nature of a good human life. Some of you reading this epilogue might think that I'm changing the subject – from happiness and eudaimonic well-being to the lofty notion of *a good human life* – but I hope you will bear with me. To make my point I need a term that isn't the direct subject of terminological disagreements, and (as I hope to make clear) I do think that ideas about this lofty notion are fueling the debate.

The lump under the carpet, I suggest, is a persistent difference of opinion about the fundamental explanation of value or goodness. On one side of this debate we have those who think that the essence of a good human life is found in our psychological attitudes toward our lives, or the subjective quality of our experiences. Let's call this the subjectivist camp. Life satisfaction theories of well-being are squarely in this camp (Sumner, 1996). On the other side we have the view that the essence of a good human life is found in the quality of our activities and achievements themselves (as distinct from how we experience them); a good human life is one spent in pursuit of *worthwhile* goals, in which we attain things that are themselves good. Let us call this the objectivist camp. Aristotle (though not all who claim to follow him) is squarely in this camp, as are so-called "objective list theories" (Finnis, 1980; Fletcher, 2013).

I suspect many social scientists will find this an odd or even an incoherent distinction. Social scientists are often skeptical about the idea that there are objective goods: facts are objective, values are subjective, and never the twain shall meet. This way of thinking is tremendously controversial in philosophy, and (as you would expect in a case of controversy), there are strong arguments on both sides. For my purposes, it isn't important to decide which side is right: what matters is seeing that there are two sides, that there is a coherent view according to which the good is objective (in the sense that what is good is not simply defined by what "subjects" value or take to be good). To show this, I think it will help to say a bit more about the philosophical question that gives rise to the disagreement. Moral philosophy or ethics is a normative practice where one object of inquiry is the nature of "the good", and in particular, the good life, the ultimate "end" of our existence. The question "what is the good?", when asked by philosophers, is not a psychological question. It is not in the first instance a question about what people find to be good, or what goods people pursue. Rather, it is a question about what, if anything, we *should* pursue. We philosophers are not writing *about* an ethical practice, looking at it from the outside and describing it. Rather, we are engaged in it, trying to follow its norms and see where they lead. What are the norms of philosophical thinking about the good? They are the norms of good thinking in any domain (consistency, attending to evidence, and so on). Further, answers to questions in ethics have also been judged by how well they provide a *justification* for valuing whatever it is that's supposed to have value. Importantly, justification is different from causal explanation. What is sought is an account of why we *should* take some putative good to have value. The subjective and objective camps differ in the kind of justification they provide.

Now let's return to the two ways of thinking about a good human life. The two different ways of thinking about a good human life offer different explanations (again, justifying explanations, not causal explanations) of why something is good for a person, or not. The subjectivist camp explains why something is good for a person by reference to that person's experience of it. The objectivist camp explains why something is good for a person by reference to the external (that is, independent of our experiences) value of that thing. For example, subjectivists will say that physical health is good for us because we enjoy or want health (or perhaps because health is necessary for pursuing other things we enjoy or want). Objectivists will say that health is good for human beings because of the kind of organism a human being is, or because health is objectively good. According to the second camp (but not the first), someone who didn't want health would still be someone for whom health is good.

The concern about the coherence of this distinction can now be put more precisely. Ultimately, to many social scientists, the objective view about "the good" looks at best mysterious and at worst incoherent, because it makes no sense to say that some things are good independently of our experience of them. The underlying thought here is that there is nothing other than our subjective reactions to things that could justify our valuing them. This is not the place to rehearse the centuries of arguments for the idea behind the objective view, but it is worth saying a few things. First, we should distinguish between ideas that make no sense and ideas that are incorrect. There is a long tradition of arguments in philosophy for what is sometimes called "value realism", which is full of sophisticated arguments for the objective reality of values or the good. This by itself is compelling evidence that the possibility of such values isn't just incoherent. To illustrate with a rather simple example, someone defending value realism might argue that values are determined by a Divine being; God creates value just as He creates everything else. You may not agree with this proposal (I don't), but it isn't incoherent. There are also many secular defense of value realism (for one of the best contemporary versions see Shafer-Landau, 2003). The Aristotelian version relies on the idea that the good for something is dependent on its function or telos (Kraut, 2009). That is, what is good for a person is to be an exemplary member of the human kind as defined by human nature, where "our nature" includes many facts about us in addition to how we experience our lives. Second, from my experience of teaching ethics, I think it is fair to say that many people think about goodness in this "realist" way. They think that there are good things in the world that they should try to achieve, teach their children to care about, choose political candidates for, and so on. For people who see the world in this way, it is deeply important that there is some explanation for why it is better to be a family doctor than a Ponzi schemer, better to be a loyal friend than a fink, better to raise your kids to be kind than greedy, that doesn't just boil down to "you'll feel better". Social scientists may be inclined to dismiss the realist views of my students (and some of their fellow citizens) as naïve or misguided. But on what basis would they do this? Dismissing this way of thinking about values would require engaging in the philosophical argument about what the justification for valuing this or that really is.[1]

Notice that when you attend to the question "what explains why something is good for a person?", there is actually substantial agreement about the concept of eudaimonia. What is distinctive about eudaimonia is that it offers an explanation of the second, objectivist type: it is the kind of thing you are – your nature – that makes something good for you. It isn't what you want (though your desires may be *part* of your nature) or what you find satisfying or pleasant. It is what you are, physically, psychologically, spiritually, and maybe even biologically. Of course, this understanding of

[1] Thanks to Blaine Fowers for drawing my attention to this issue.

eudaimonia, which is very broad, does not tell us what our nature is or how we might fulfill it. It's not a definition of eudaimonia that is ready to go for psychological research. But it does represent a distinct view about what it is that makes certain kinds of lives good for us. This explanation is clear in Besser's (this volume) definition of eudaimonia as well-functioning and Haybron's (this volume) definition of eudaimonia as nature fulfillment: whether or not you are functioning well or fulfilling your nature is not simply a matter of how you feel.

Does this disagreement about the basic explanation of what makes something good for a person make any difference? I think it does. First, the two different theories create different challenges. Theories in the first (subjectivist) camp – that explain what's good for us by reference to our experiences and psychological states – face the challenge that our reactions to the world can be "off" in various ways that intuitively seem bad for us. For example, if people are satisfied with very little in life because of adaptation to oppressive environments, their life satisfaction seems a bad indicator of something very important about their lives. Subjective theories have to find a way to explain how our subjective responses could count as misguided or mistaken. The second camp's eudaimonist explanation does not have this problem because it leads us to think about human beings as aiming at an ideal that is beyond individual experience. The challenge for the eudaimonist is to establish a compelling basis for this ideal.

Second, the two different explanations do tend to have different implications for how we think about practical questions and what problems we thereby encounter. At least on first sight, the two camps have different implications for how we ought to think about, for example, the well-being of children and people with disabilities. Because eudaimonist theories posit an external ideal, they seem committed to holding everyone to the same standard. This is intuitive in the case of children, because we tend to think that children should be raised to develop the capacities to be exemplary adults. It is less intuitive when it comes to people with disabilities; here, eudaimonist theories are at risk of having to say that people with disabilities are defective as human beings and that they would be better off if they were not defective in this way. Subjective theories do not imply that people with disabilities cannot live lives that are just as good as the lives of anyone else; if what matters is whether people with disabilities are satisfied with their lives, then their well-being depends on this and not on whether they are able to function in typically human ways. But subjective theories need to do some maneuvering to explain why we ought to raise our children in the ways we intuitively think we ought. That is, to be agents who are capable of working, playing, loving, and so on (even if what they like to do is watch violent movies and eat marshmallows).

These differences are interesting, but for my purposes in this epilogue, what's more important than the practical upshot of the difference between these two ways of thinking about well-being is the fact that there really are two different ways of thinking about the good. Some people think that what explains the goodness of something must have to do with our experience of or reaction to it, while others think that what explains the goodness of something must have to do with value that is inherent in the thing itself. We can trace this difference back to Plato's dialogue, "The Euthyphro", in which Socrates asked whether piety was good because the Gods love it, or if the Gods love piety because it is good. The reason I think this is important in the context of this book is that I believe that this deep disagreement fuels the fire over what counts as "well-being".

I've been calling the general, overarching notion "the good life". This highlights the evaluative dimension of the debate. Of course, "well-being" has the word "well" in it, which is also an evaluative notion and I've suggested that the fact that it is an evaluative notion is the reason there are such tenacious disputes about the term. In other words, I'm suggesting that people see "well-being" as aligned with "the good" and this is why those in the objectivist camp do not want to accept a subjective definition of "well-being" without a fight. Fowers (this volume) observes, in his chapter for this volume, that you cannot think about eudaimonia in value neutral terms. I am suggesting, in agreement with Hirata's contribution to this volume, that it is also pretty hard to think in value neutral terms about well-being.

If I'm right about this, what is to be done? We could hope to fight it out, to the death, about the question of what kind of life has value and why. I think it's unlikely that this fight would result in a victory for anyone. A philosophical disagreement that has spanned thousands of years is not likely to be resolved in our lifetimes. A second possibility is that we could move to hybrid theories of well-being that accommodate both sides of the divide. According to such theories, what makes a human life a good one is the combination of objectively valuable things experienced in the right way (Woodard, 2015). This isn't a bad option, though it does depend on establishing that there are objective values that it is good for us to want, enjoy or appreciate. It seems to me that this is less likely to be a path that psychologists are eager to follow.

The most promising path, I think, is to recognize that the ethical work of exploring what we mean by a good human life does not settle on a univocal answer. In other words, people think differently about what makes human life good – not just about what activities, resources or experiences contribute to a good life, but about the explanation for why anything makes a life go better or worse. How could this path change philosophy and psychology? Philosophers who tend toward universal theories with single, overarching principles might benefit from the thought that different ways of thinking about value are useful for different kinds of problems in different contexts. Psychologists who sometimes seem to assume that everything that matters can be measured, might benefit from the realization that there are people whose conceptions of a good human life are built on assumptions about what they take to be objective goods, and that SWB is not the be-all-and-end-all for such folks. Insofar as *well-being* has become the term that stands in for "good human life" in psychology, thinking of us all as in the subjective camp leaves some people out.

I am now suggesting that we embrace what amounts to a sort of pluralism about good human lives, and hence about well-being (insofar as I'm right that those two notions are inevitably intertwined). Perhaps this is disappointing for those who hoped we might settle once and for all whether well-being is hedonistic or eudaimonistic, subjective or objective, a matter of our attitudes or a matter of what we actually achieve. As I've suggested, I don't think settling things once and for all is the right goal for a topic like this. Of course, this doesn't mean that we shouldn't try to be very clear about our technical definitions and how we are using them in our research. Certainly we should. But the topic of well-being is important and complex, and – more importantly – it is a subject of deep reflection that is itself a valuable and quintessentially human activity. Like it or not, social scientists who use the concepts that structure this activity are engaged in this deep reflection too. In this way, the subject of well-being is different from other research topics. If we were to find a cure for cancer that eliminates it from our lives, we would not have to think about cancer anymore. If we find the right kind evidence for the existence of a new planet in our solar system, we can stop deliberating about whether it is there or not. But I think we will always reflect on what it is to live a good human life. This collection of papers contributes to that ongoing reflection and that should make us happy.[2]

References

Finnis, J. (1980). *Natural law and human rights*. Oxford, UK: Clarendon Press.

Fletcher, G. (2013). *A fresh start for the objective-list theory of well-being*. *Utilitas* 25(02) (2013): 206–220. http://philpapers.org/rec/FLEAFS

Kraut, R. (2009). *What is good and why: The ethics of well-being*. Harvard University Press. http://books.google.com/books?hl=en&lr=&id=jq_u6DWjMFcC&oi=fnd&pg=PR7&dq=Kraut,+Richard&ots=OPVOoZa-bo&sig=t3jW5Yn1KZgnYvN5Xxyaub4EX38

Shafer-Landau, R. (2003). *Moral realism: A defence*. Oxford, UK: Oxford University Press.

Sumner, L. (1996). *Welfare, happiness, and ethics*. Oxford, UK: Clarendon.

Woodard, C. (2015). Hybrid theories. In G. Flectcher (Ed.), *The Routledge handbook of the philosophy of well-being*. London: Routledge.

[2]I would like to thank Blaine Fowers and Joar Vitterso for helpful comments on a draft of this epilogue.

GPSR Compliance
The European Union's (EU) General Product Safety Regulation (GPSR) is a set of rules that requires consumer products to be safe and our obligations to ensure this.

If you have any concerns about our products, you can contact us on

ProductSafety@springernature.com

In case Publisher is established outside the EU, the EU authorized representative is:

Springer Nature Customer Service Center GmbH
Europaplatz 3
69115 Heidelberg, Germany

www.ingramcontent.com/pod-product-compliance
Ingram Content Group UK Ltd.
Pitfield, Milton Keynes, MK11 3LW, UK
UKHW051028041026
15470UKWH00015B/1733
* 9 7 8 3 3 1 9 4 2 4 4 3 9 *